RADIOLOGICAL ATLAS
OF COMMON DISEASES OF
THE SMALL BOWEL

RADIOLOGICAL ATLAS
OF COMMON DISEASES OF
THE SMALL BOWEL

J. L. SELLINK M.D.

Department of Radiology, Leiden University Hospital

H. E. STENFERT KROESE B.V. / LEIDEN 1976

ISBN 978-90-207-0476-1

ISBN 978-90-207-0476-1   ISBN 978-94-011-8088-7 (eBook)
DOI 10.1007/978-94-011-8088-7

Photography: C. T. Ruygrok and M. Popkes, Leiden.
Translation: G. P. Bieger-Smith, Wassenaar.

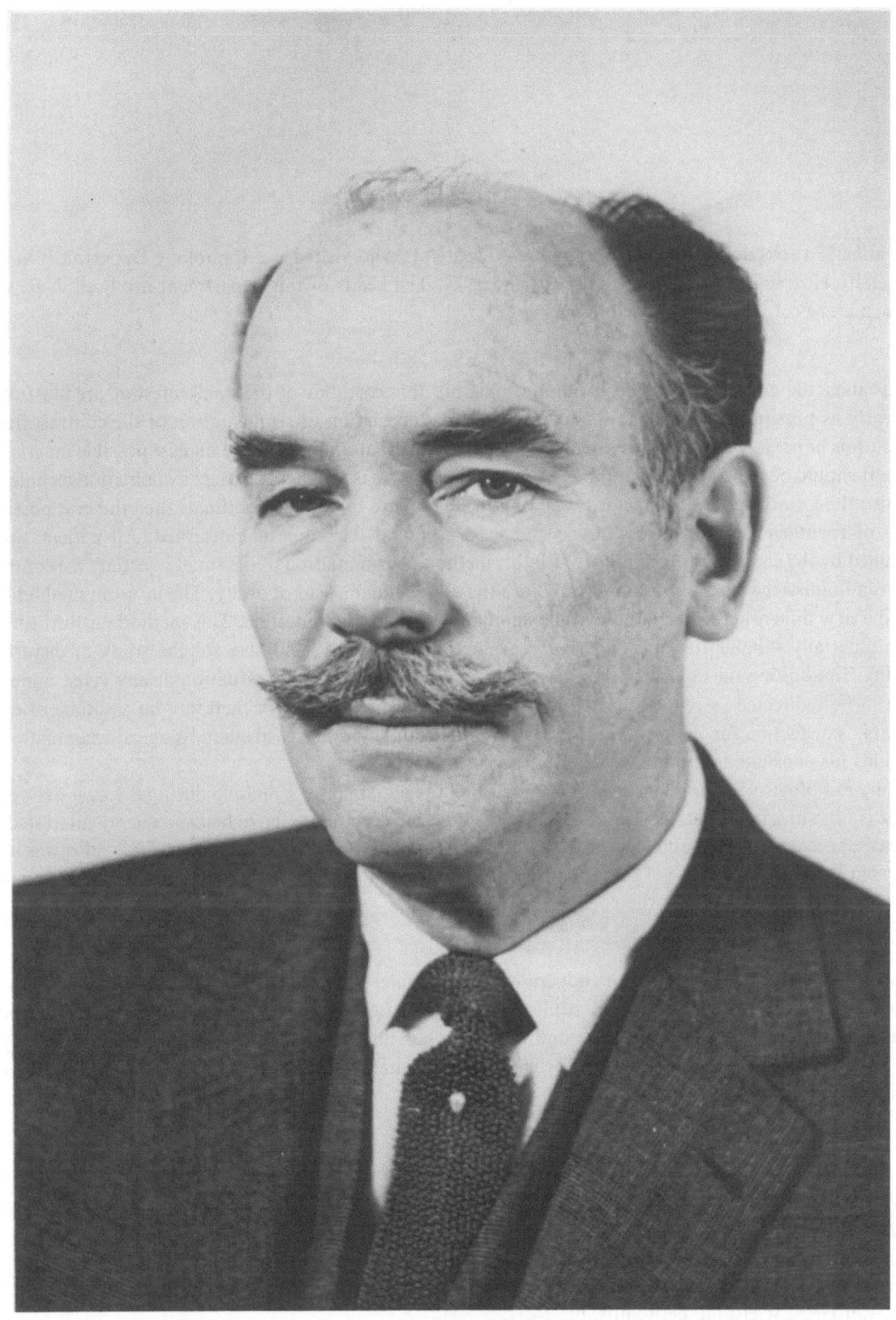

J. R. VON RONNEN

PREFACE

This atlas is a selection of the roentgenograms of patients who visited the Radiology Department at the University Hospital in Leiden between 1970 and 1974. The heads of this department are Prof. J. R. von Ronnen and Prof. A. E. van Voorthuisen.

In this atlas, the most frequently occurring radiological abnormalities of the small intestine are illustrated as clearly as possible – without the shadows caused by flocculation or segmentation of the contrast fluid. The author hopes it will be a positive contribution towards the attainment of the highest possible diagnostic score. It should be remembered that the key to good diagnostics is not only a perfect examination technique, but also the knowledge and character of the physician. If these factors are optimal, then the best possible series of roentgenograms will be obtained, at least as far as technique is concerned. All patients were examined by the enteroclysis technique. With this method of examination of the small intestine, the contrast fluid is administered via an infusion directly into the duodenum instead of orally. The infusion method has added a new dimension to the radiological examination of the small intestine. This method has turned out to be especially suitable for the comparative evaluation of motility, and also for the study of disturbed motility. In addition the course of the examination can be adapted to the situation at any given moment and can be redirected as required. Each new enteroclysis examination can therefore be a source of considerable satisfaction for the physician since it – more than any other gastro-enterological examination – demands his constant attention and all of his skills.

Many radiologists in our department have mastered the enteroclysis technique during the past five years and it is not surprising that, as a result of their great enthusiasm, many have become deeply interested in a particular aspect of the pathology of the small intestine. The author and compiler of this atlas was able to benefit from the experience of these associates and was given permission to use their data which in most cases have been published elsewhere.

I wish to thank the following for their cooperation: J. R. Achterberg (staff) – drug-induced atony; C. A. van Hees – Meckel's diverticulum; W. F. Müller – celiac disease (awarded with the Boris Rajewski medal at the A.E.R. congress in Edinburgh in June 1975); J. Th. Schlangen – radiation enteritis; W. H. B. Tuynman – melanoma metastases; P. J. van Wiechen – yersinia enterocolitica infections and C. J. L. R. Vellenga – a-specific ulcerations.

The following former members and consultant radiologists of the Department of Radiology at the Leiden University Hospital sent me interesting photographic material and we hereby thank them for their efforts:
Dr. A. S. J. Botenga; mesenterial cyst, fig. 10.3
G. Coerhamp; amebic abscess, fig. 9.68
J. G. van Dorssen; adenocarcinoma of the jejunum, figs. 8.40N and 10.24
C. A. van Hees; sclerosing peritonitis, fig. 14.12
J. O. op den Orth; mesenterial thrombosis, fig. 11.13
Dr. G. R. Prager; carcinoid lesion, figs. 8.40L and 10.17

F. Rodenboog; jejunal intussusception, fig. 14.18, lipoma, fig. 10.12.

J. Th. Schlangen; lymphoid hyperplasia, fig. 9.76

Dr. H. E. Schütte; appendicular abscess, figs. 9.65 and 9.67 PQ, cong. lymphedema, fig. 8.8ABC

H. Verhoef; lymphosarcoma of the jejunum, fig. 10.26

We are also grateful to the following colleagues for the use of their exceptionally fine roentgenograms:

D. M. A. Agenant and Dr. G. N. Tijtgat (gastroenterologist of the Wilhelmina Gasthuis, Amsterdam University) Whipple's disease, figs. 8.23 and 9.54FG, eosinophilic gastroenteritis, fig. 9.46; Naish syndrome, figs. 12.4 and 12.5 amyloid disease, figs. 12.35–1,3 and 12.36; ascaris, figs. 8.29–1,2.

Dr. G. Rosenbusch and Dr. J. M. H. van Tongeren (gastroenterologist of the St. Radboud Hospital, Nijmegen University) reticulum cell sarcoma, figs. 8.8E and 10.27K; ascaris, figs. 8.29–5; Whipple's disease, figs. 9.55, 9.56–2; Zollinger-Ellisons disease, fig. 9.71.

Dr. R. W. Radder; a-specific jejunal ulcer, fig. 8.36

W. P. L. van Ouwerkerk; primary amyloidosis, figs. 12.33 and 12.35–4

Dr. G. P. Gooris-Namur; Peutz-Jegher syndrome, fig. 10.11B.

It can be regarded as a special coincidence that the publication of this atlas coincides more or less with the retirement of Professor von Ronnen and the transfer of his position as head of the Department of Radiology at the Leiden University Hospital to his successor Prof. Dr. A. E. van Voorthuisen.

During Prof. von Ronnen's 20 years as head of the above-mentioned department, he succeeded in raising its status to a level in accordance with the glorious history of the 400-year-old Leiden University. In addition he improved, at least on a national level, the position of radiology as an independent specialty as well as that of the radiologist to such an extent that colleagues of most other European countries are justifiably envious.

Many years ago Prof. von Ronnen realized that radiology is much too broad a field for one professor and several residents to be able to work within the university on further developments and that for this purpose the formation of a permanent staff of enthusiastic associates was indispensible. The magnetism of the considerably higher fees in peripheral hospitals however made this task impossible. Prof. von Ronnen then made the decision – unique at that time – to form an association with his close co-workers and to divide the revenues of the collective practise with them equally. That he not only regarded this move as inevitable but also was on friendly terms with his younger associates and wholeheartedly approved of their increased income is characterized by the fact that in later years he even went so far as to limit his own share. It was many years before this vision and his approach were understood and even longer before they were adopted on a broader scale. Only recently in the last few years have the means been found in most other university clinics to form a scientific staff in a more or less similar manner. The early introduction of these concepts by Professor von Ronnen was however certainly one of the reasons that his department assumed a leading position in the Netherlands. Under his guidance, post-graduate courses were organized and annual reunions were held for radiologists who had studied in Leiden. Although the social function of the latter was certainly not unimportant and was greatly appreciated, they were in fact mainly scientific in character. Only recently in the past few years has the Dutch Association of Radiologists organized periodic post-graduate courses and courses for the training of residents on a national level.

It is not surprising that a leader with the stature of Prof. von Ronnen, a man who during his career could be considered the undisputed Master of Radiology in the Netherlands, fulfilled numerous prominent administrative functions, not only within the Netherlands but also internationally. Quite recently, at the Third A.E.R. Congress in Edinburgh, he turned the presidency of the Association Européenne de Radiologie over to a man of similar capabilities, the Swede Olle Ollson.

One basic requirement for good leadership, and certainly not the least important, is the ability to delegate responsibility adequately. It is even questionable whether one can fulfill an executive position satisfactorily without this characteristic, which is highly developed in Prof. von Ronnen. Prof. von Ronnen was a master of the art of delegation and was able to let others do the work even when he knew that he could do it better himself. In his criticism, which was always very constructive and stimulating, he avoided at all costs offending the individual involved, although this must have required considerable effort now and then. His 22 Ph.D. students in particular acquired the deepest respect for this attitude and will remember with gratitude and esteem the dignity of this personality – a dignity which is seldom encountered today.

In addition to his daily practice which he always pursued with the greatest satisfaction and dedication and in spite of the time-consuming chores arising from his many functions and the management of the department, Prof. von Ronnen was able to prepare countless lectures and more than 60 publications, some in collaboration with one or more of his colleagues or colleagues of other disciplines; this certainly can be attributed, at least partly, to his ability to delegate.

During the first 15 years of his career as a radiologist, 10 in diverse functions in the former Dutch East Indies and 5 in Bronovo Hospital in the Hague, his interests were diversified as required by the demands made of a radiologist with a general practice. Although his publications covered numerous subjects in diagnostics, his major concerns in this period were the urogenital tract, the digestive tract, aortography and arteriography and later also mammography; the latter was the subject of his Ph.D. thesis in 1956.

During the next 20 years as professor in Leiden, he was still interested in the diagnostics of the gastro-intestinal tract. However in the course of time he turned his attention to an ever increasing degree to the diagnostics of the skeleton, in particular of bone tumors. Fifteen years as secretary of the Dutch Commission for Bone Tumors gave him considerable experience in this field. His impressive contribution to the book compiled by this group 'Radiological Atlas of Bone Tumours', which can be considered an unparalleled standard text on this subject, must be regarded as his most extensive scientific work.

The assignment to determine whether it would be possible to improve the disappointing results of the transit examination of the small bowel was given in the fall of 1969; as far as the outcome was concerned, expectations were probably not very high. The conclusion of this study, which was carried out partly under the stimulating influence of the head of the Department of Gastroenterology, Prof. Dr. A. J. Ch. Haex, was not just that the quality of the contrast fluid required improvement but in the first place that the examination technique had to be adapted to the conditions existing in the gastrointestinal tract. Once convinced that enteroclysis of the small bowel signified a not unimportant improvement over all other procedures used at that time, Prof. von Ronnen became in this respect the author's most loyal supporter. Furthermore it was a source of considerable satisfaction that during these past years he, more than any other, could become enthousiastic about the continual new surprises which we still encounter regularly. It was moreover a great privilege during this initial period, when an adequate opponent is in fact of the greatest importance, to be able to talk with a man of such stature. Last but not least the author is grateful to his chief, supervisor and associate for his frequent, friendly and often paternal advice as well as his wise, usually mitigating influence in situations which threatened to boil over. Thus an esteem for his personality and gratitude for his role in the developments which led to this atlas, to which so many of his associates and former students have contributed, have led the author to dedicate this work to Professor von Ronnen.

In addition to the members of the photography section of our department who handled a gigantic amount of work, I am finally and especially also very grateful to and have the deepest admiration for my wife, Mia. In spite of the many chores resulting from our large family, she has in the past 5 years still managed to do all of my typing – not only for this Atlas but also for the book which preceded it (Examination of the small intestine by means of duodenal intubation, 1971) and a book published in 1973 (Dutch antique domestic clocks).

Leiden, August 1975. J. L. Sellink

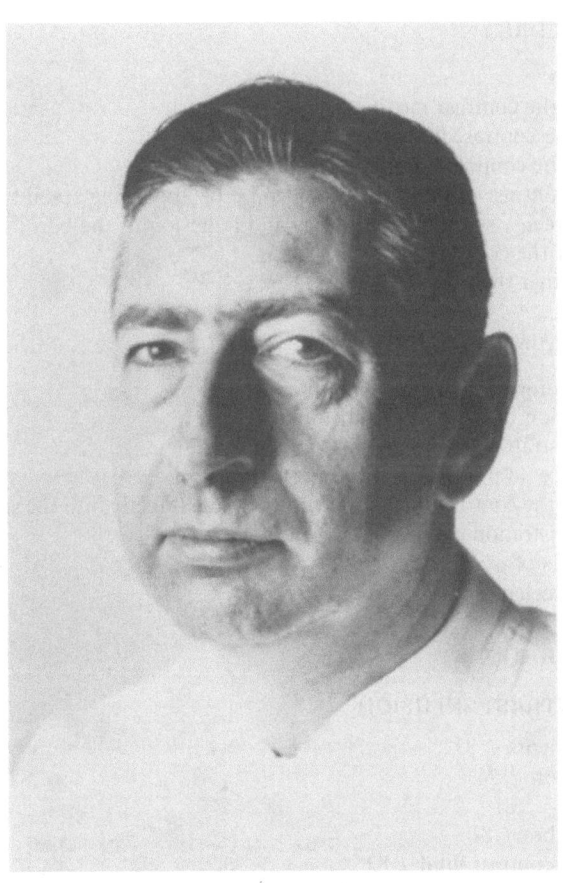

J. L. SELLINK

CONTENTS

I

INTRODUCTION

Although there has been some improvement over the past few years, the radiological examination of the small intestine must still be regarded as a stepchild of radiology and even of the examination of the digestive tract. The net gain of a transit examination of the small intestine was so disappointing for so many years that the negative attitude on the part of many radiodiagnosticians is certainly understandable. Gradually, however, steady improvement has changed this somber situation and nowadays an adequately executed roentgenological examination of the small intestine is definitely worthwhile and its contribution to diagnostics can be considerable.

Early in the fifties, Golden showed that even if the examination techniques are not at an optimum and the contrast fluids are not the best, good results can be achieved if the radiologist himself at least approaches the examination enthusiastically.

Somewhat later in the same decade, Marshak pointed out that better results are obtained if larger amounts of contrast fluid are used. Then not only is there better filling of the intestinal loops so that abnormalities are not as easily overlooked, but in addition an examination carried out in this manner is more efficient since more intestinal loops are visualized per exposure and the examination as a whole is shorter. Moreover, an even shorter examination as well as an improvement in the mucosal patterns was achieved by using drugs to accelerate passage.

Quite often in the past ten years, Bodart has demonstrated very effectively that smaller abnormalities of the mucosa need not escape the attention of the physician if he studies the intestinal loops carefully by using fluoroscopy and the compression technique in combination with detail spot films.

More recently as a result of the introduction of the enteroclysis technique the many meters of small intestine have become much more accessible for radiodiagnosis. With this method, optimum filling of the intestinal loops is obtained and the fear of malabsorption, the major testimonium paupertatis for the conventional transit examination of the digestive tract, has disappeared from the scene forever.

To a certain extent the enteroclysis technique demands more of the radiologist since this examination must be executed properly in every respect. Neglecting one or more of the factors, which will be discussed in detail, leads without fail to disappointment and perhaps even to reinstatement of less adequate procedures. Because of the rather high degree of filling achieved with enteroclysis, careful compression of the superimposed intestinal loops has become essential since otherwise, as before, numerous abnormalities will be overlooked.

Unfortunately it has also been established that the diagnostic output of the radiological examination of the small intestine, even more than that of other examinations, can vary greatly depending upon the technique used and the care and skill with which the examination is carried out.

Although the radiological examination of the small intestine has always been referred to the radiologist with a general practice – and this should continue to be true because of the high frequency of abdominal complaints – it may be to the advantage of these patients if the examination is carried out by those radiologists especially interested or specialized in this aspect of radiodiagnostics.

The scala of radiologically demonstrable abnormalities has by now become quite extensive; furthermore diseases of the small intestine appear to occur much more frequently than previously assumed.

In addition to complaints such as abdominal pain, unexplained high fever, blood loss in the digestive tract, diarrhea and diseases accompanied by malabsorption, all of which clearly require radiological evaluation of the small intestine, this type of examination must also be carried out in the event of unexplained hypoalbuminemia, whether accompanied by edema in the lower extremities or not. Since without a doubt a well-executed enteroclysis examination must be considered the best possible method of examination, every conceivable aspect and pitfall of this procedure has received special attention in this atlas.

ANATOMY

1. Normal mucosa in the small intestine

More important for a correct interpretation of the pictures obtained than for the technical execution of the examination is a thorough knowledge of the anatomical structure of the wall of the small intestine. It is, however, difficult to differentiate between examination and interpretation, at least when the radiologist is actively involved in both as is the case for gastric and colon examinations.

The wall of the small intestine, shown schematically in fig. 2.1, consists of the following layers, starting from the outside:

1. the serosa;
2. the tunica muscularis, which consists of an outer longitudinal layer and an inner circular layer;
3. the submucosa, which contains many blood and lymphatic vessels in a loose connective tissue so that the tunica muscularis can move freely with respect to:
4. the mucosa; this layer is made up of three parts:
   a. the muscularis mucosae which, like the tunica muscularis, consists of an outer longitudinal layer and an inner circular layer. The muscular strands of this inner circular layer extend into the folds of Kerkring and some even extend through the tunica propria into the villi which cover the surface of the mucosa. The villi vary in number from 10 to 40 per mm^2; they are 0.2–1 mm high and contain a centrally located, blindended lymphatic vessel. Between the villi are the crypts of Lieberkühn.
   b. the tunica propria, like the submucosa, consists of a loose connective tissue containing blood and lymphatic vessels as well as nerve

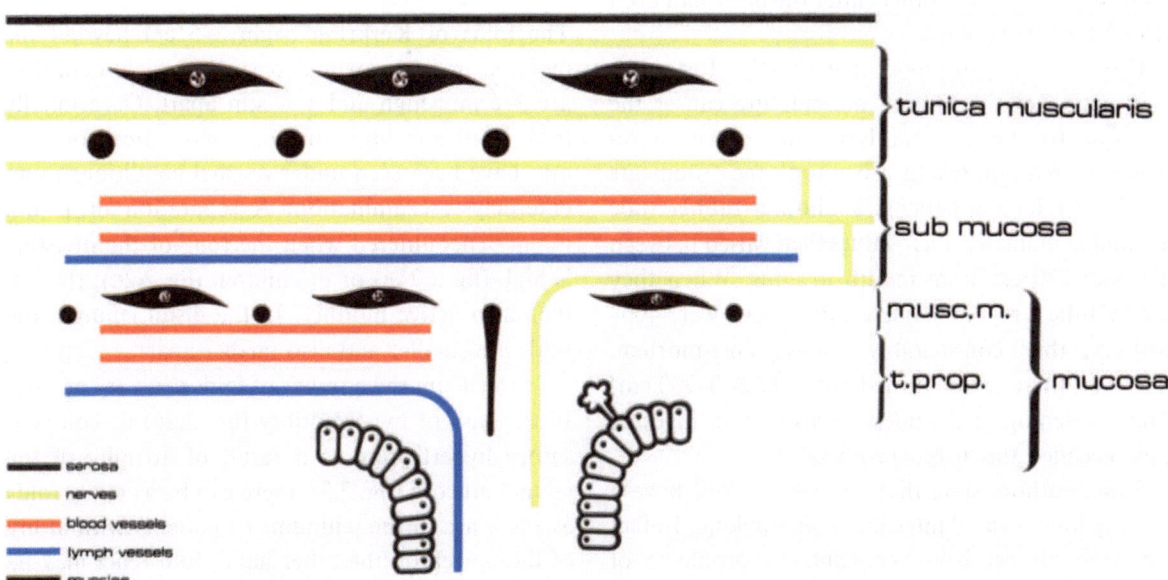

tunica muscularis

sub mucosa

musc.m.

t.prop. } mucosa

serosa
nerves
blood vessels
lymph vessels
muscles

Fig. 2.1
Schematic drawing of a cross-section of the intestinal wall.

fibres. Occasionally conglomerates of lympho-cytes are found in this layer.

c. a layer of simple columnar epithelial cells which can move freely with respect to the tunica propria. The surface of each epithelial cell is covered with hundreds of microvilli, which are 0.2–1 mm high and together form the so-called 'brush border'.

Although several studies have been published concerning the length of the small intestine, the definitive answer has yet to be found. Most handbooks list values varying between 5 and 7 metres and the small intestine is assumed to be 3/5 of the total length of the digestive tract. The distance from nose or mouth to the duodenojejunal flexure varies only slightly; a length of 90 cm is assumed here. It is known that the length as well as the diameter of the small intestine is highly dependent upon the tone, so that the results of measurements taken post-mortem or under anesthesia will be too high. A length of 12 m need not be unusual for American negroes and in India. X-ray films of the small intestine occasionally show that individual variations can be enormous. However, when several measurements are taken of the same patient, the results appear to differ by only 10 per cent at the most (87). Underhill (225) obtained post-mortem values of 4.7–9.7 m with an average length of 6.9 m. Unfortunately she took some measurements several hours after death and others after the body had been stored for several days.

Hirsch et al. (90) report that shortly after death contraction of the smooth musculature causes the intestine to shorten; autolysis later causes a renewed increase in length. They took measurements in vivo by having patients swallow a rubber tube 3.5 mm in diameter; their values then varied between 220 and 270 cm from mouth to anus. When they used a tube 2 mm in diameter, the results were 400–540 cm, thus considerably longer. Post-mortem, however, these values turned out to be 800–900 cm! The shortening of the intestine around an ingested tube is called the 'telescope effect'.

Some authors state that an asthenic will have a slightly longer small intestine than a pyknic. In fact we have almost never encountered problems of superposition of a convolution of ileal loops in the small pelvis in our pyknic patients.

For the jejunum, the diameter is normally assumed to be 2.5–3 cm and for the ileum 2–2.5 cm. Values have also been reported of 1 and 0.5 inch respectively, which are probably a closer approximation of the diameter in vivo and during a conventional transit examination. During an enteroclysis examination, the diameter of the loops of the small intestine is generally greater and more variable, as a result of the more active peristalsis, than during a conventional examination. With a dosage of 600–900 ml and a rate of flow of 80–100 cc per minute, as used in our department, the maximum diameter of the proximal jejunal loops will be 4 cm in normal cases. Generally the diameter of the distal ileal loops depends to a large extent on the counterpressure caused by a contaminated cecum. A diameter of 3 cm for those segments which are in the rest phase can be considered normal in this region. During a conventional transit examination the diameter of the contrast column in the distal ileum depends partly on the degree of thickening of the contrast fluid which in turn is determined by the length of the examination. At the transition between the jejunum and the ileum the diameter of the intestinal lumen differs only slightly from the standard values for a conventional transit examination. Of course in the event of a greater rate of flow, an increased dosage of contrast medium or transit retarding factors, the diameter of the intestinal lumen will increase.

The folds of Kerkring begin 3–5 cm beyond the pylorus; in the proximal part of the jejunum, they are 3–6 mm high and 1–6 mm apart. Occasionally folds 7–10 mm high and local separations of 7–12 mm have been seen under normal conditions in an enteroclysis examination. A separation of 1 mm is only encountered when the tone of the intestine is high (fig. 2.2AB) or in children (fig. 2.2c); there is then also active motility. In the distal jejunum the folds are smaller and also farther apart.

In the ileum the number of folds can vary greatly. In the case of hypermotility (fig. 2.2B) or compensatory hypertrophy as a result of atrophy of the jejunal mucosa (fig. 2.3), there can be as many folds as there are in the jejunum. In patients with atony of the bowel, on the other hand, fold relief may be completely lacking in the ileum; even in normal cases, it can be barely visible (fig. 2.4). In comparison

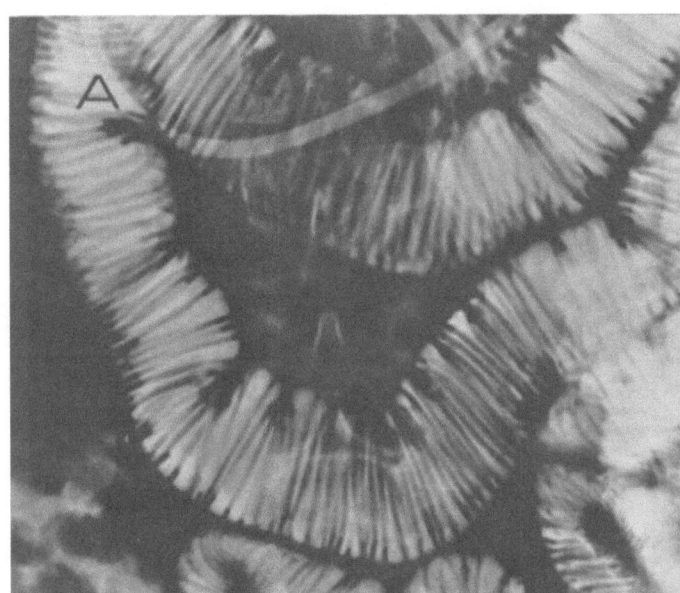

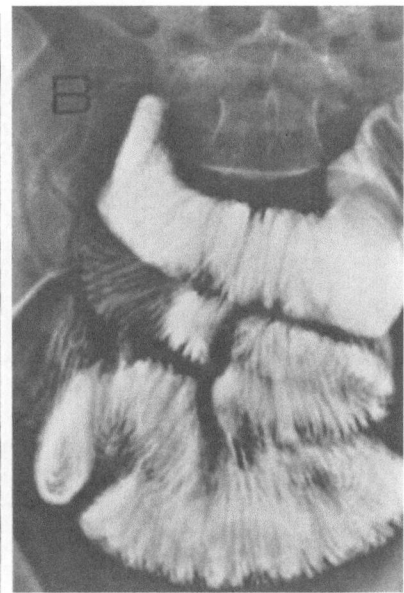

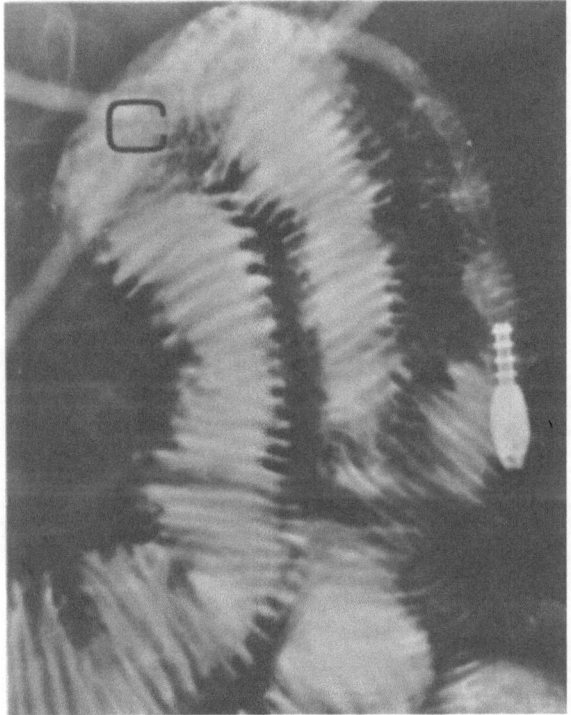

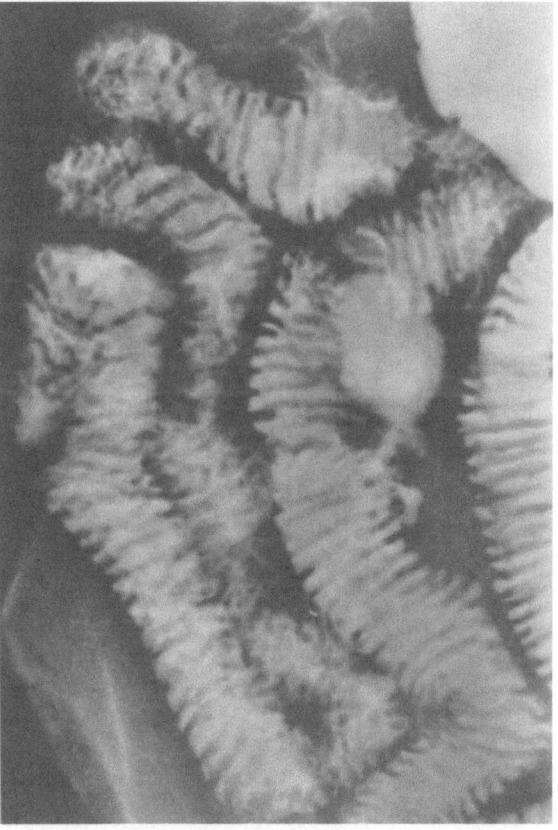

Fig. 2.2
The folds in the jejunum and the ileum are more numerous as a result of the high muscular tone of the intestinal wall (A-jejunum, B-ileum, C-child, 12 years old).

Fig. 2.3
Increased number of folds in the ileum ('jejunization') in a patient with atrophy of the jejunal mucosa as a result of celiac disease.

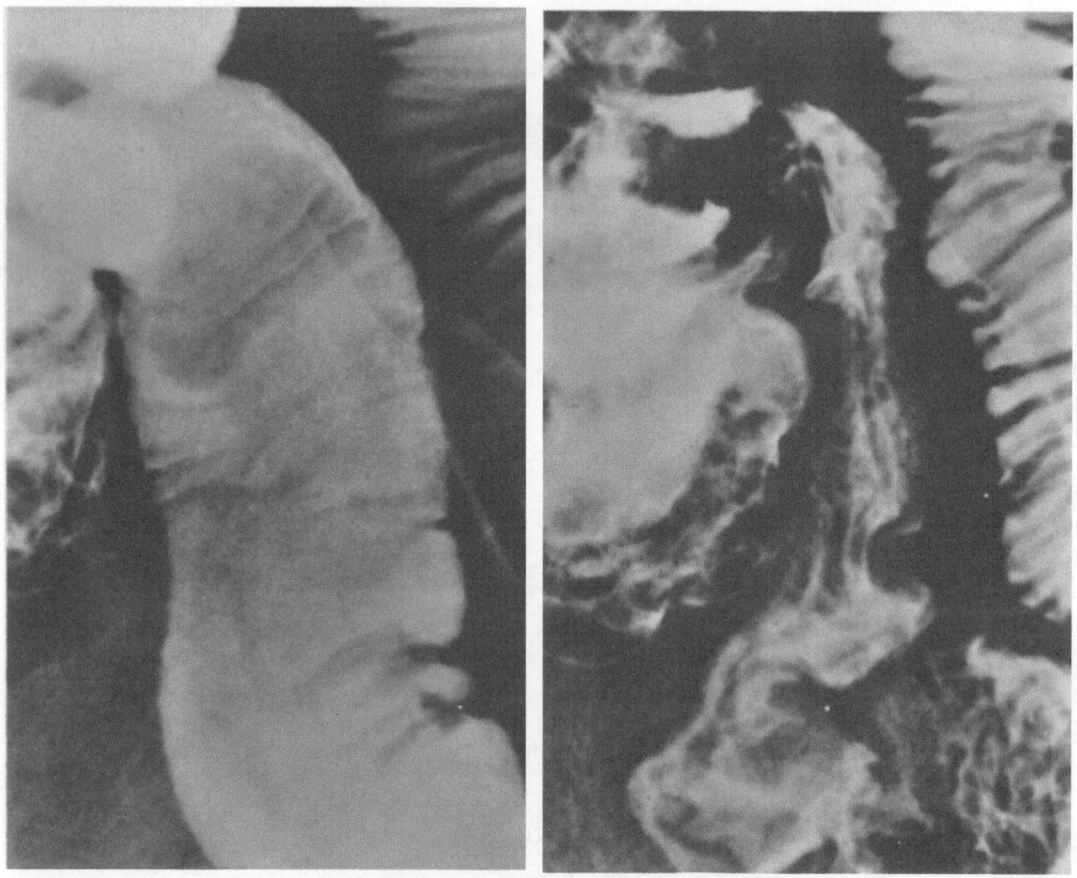

Fig. 2.4 When the ileum is stretched, the fold relief is barely visible.

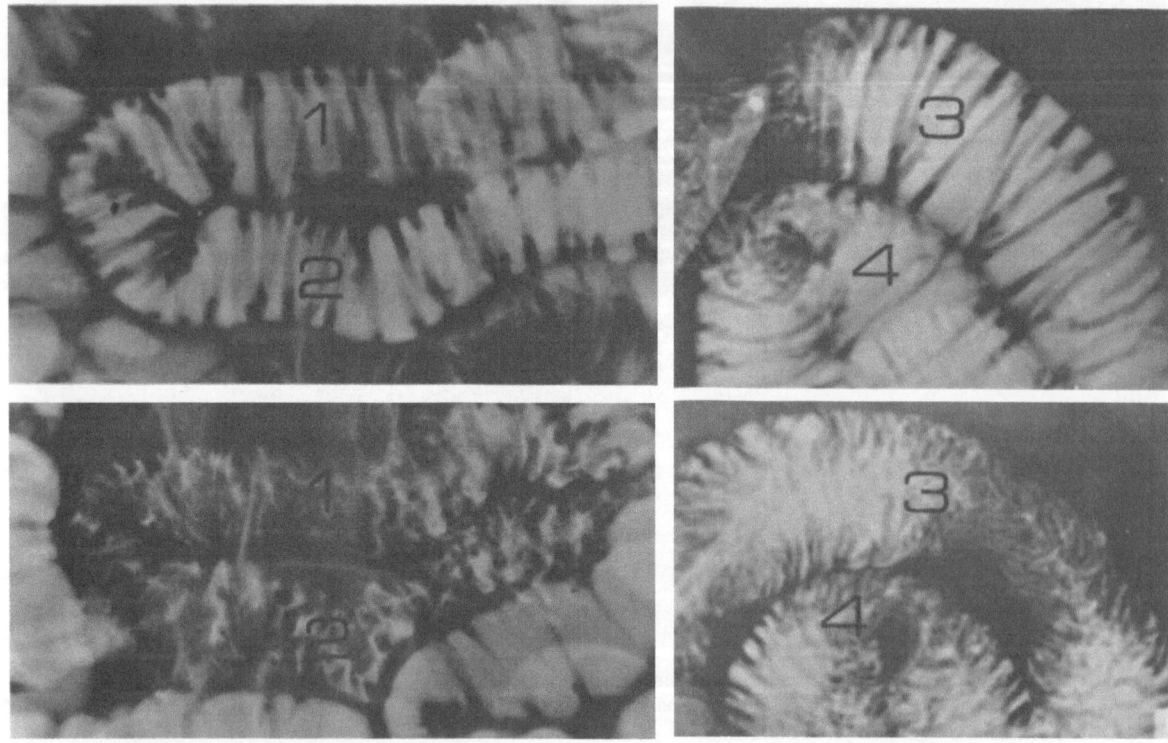

with a conventional examination of the small
intestine therefore the height of a fold may possibly
be somewhat less on an enteroclysis film but the
thickness will barely change. Evaluation of the
height of a fold is much easier with enteroclysis
because the more active peristalsis induces stronger
contractions as well as more pronounced dilatations
during the rest phases (fig. 2.5). When the intestine
is in a state of dilatation, the folds are stretched and
quite orderly with respect to one another so that
they are easy to measure; in addition minor anatomical abnormalities are less likely to be overlooked
(fig. 2.6).

The margins of a normal fold of Kerkring extend
in parallel into the intestinal lumen; the transition
from fold to intestinal wall can best be described
as a rounded corner (fig. 2.7). On the roentgenogram the space between two intestinal loops is
2–3 mm depending upon the phase of contraction;

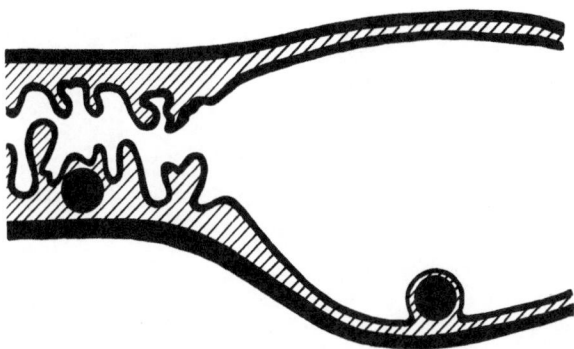

Fig. 2.6
An abnormality of the mucosa is more clearly visible when
the intestine is in a state of dilatation than in a state of
contraction.

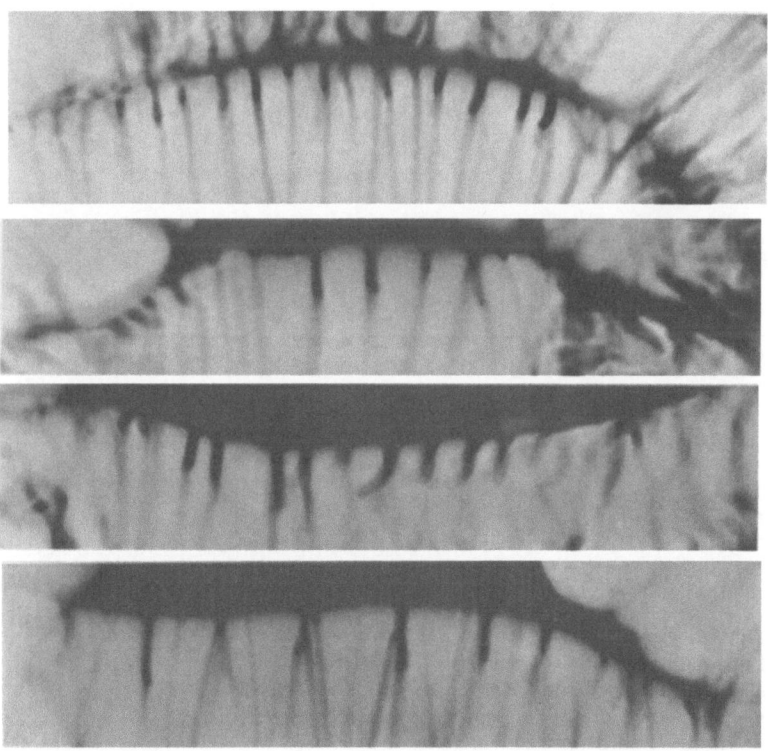

Fig. 2.7
The margins of a fold of Kerkring
extend approximately in parallel; the
transition from fold to intestinal wall
has the shape of a rounded corner.

Fig. 2.5
Circular course of the mucosal folds in the proximal part of the jejunum. Evaluation is much easier when the intestine is
stretched than during the rest phase (below).

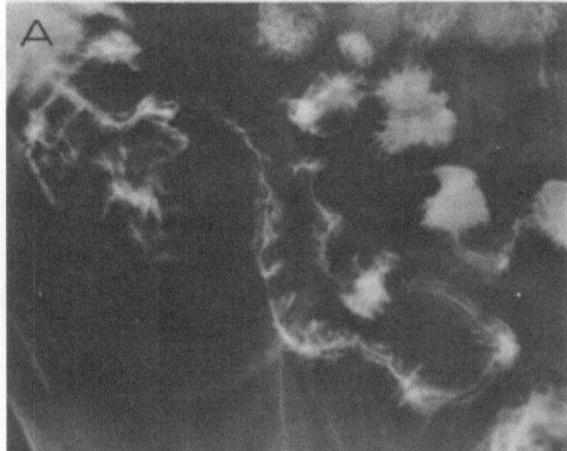

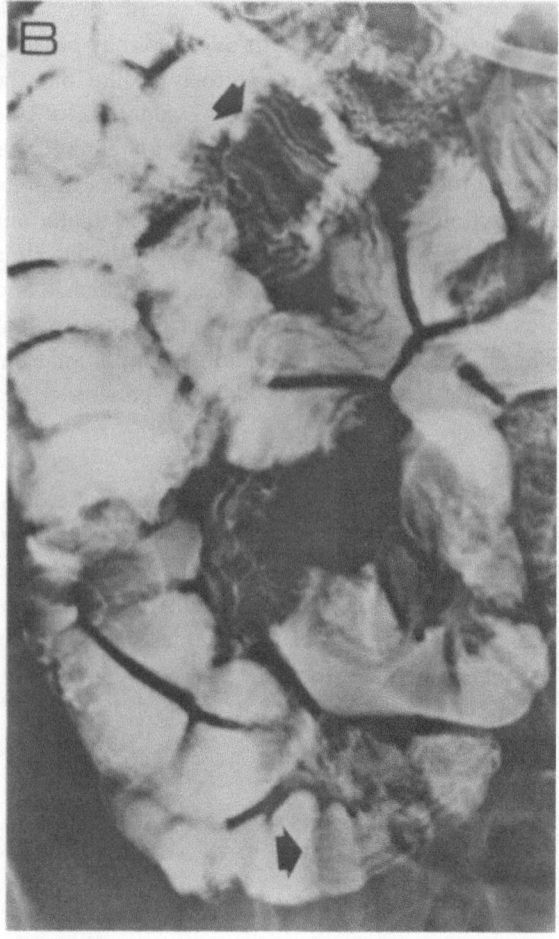

Fig. 2.9

Longitudinal folds in the ileum.

A. in a contracted intestinal loop.
B. due to collapse of an atonic loop in which the circular folds have disappeared (cured Crohn's disease).

the thickness of the intestinal wall is therefore only
1–1¼ mm.

In the proximal half of the jejunum, the folds lie
in a more or less circular configuration (fig. 2.8),
but in the distal half of the jejunum and the proximal
half of the ileum, the course becomes spiral-shaped.
In this region it can be seen that the folds follow a
true spiral course in some segments of the intestine
while in other segments they resemble more or less a
chain of tridents along each wall which mesh
together in the center of the lumen (→). We have
the impression that the latter configuration is more
common in the distal jejunum and that the spiral
course occurs predominantly in the proximal ileum.

In the literature it is generally stated that the
folds in the distal ileum often follow a longitudinal
course. In our opinion, however, this is not true;
the configuration of the folds is just as circular as
in all other parts of the small intestine. The ileal
folds are in fact smaller, thin and farther apart and
do not contribute significantly to the fold relief –
irrespective of the state of contraction of the intestine. The longitudinal folds frequently seen on
x-rays of the ileum are obviously wider and higher
than the circular ones. Like those on the evacuation
films of a colon with few haustra, they must be
explained as puckering caused by collapse of the
intestinal wall, possibly enhanced by contractions
of the circular muscle fibers (fig. 2.9). Circular folds
of Kerkring which extend in a longitudinal direction
do not exist.

Occasionally in the most distal part of the ileum,
an abnormal mucosal pattern is seen: the folds
have a longitudinal course on the mesenterial side
and a circular course on the other side of the loop
(fig. 2.10).

The mucosal pattern can, depending upon the state
of contraction or dilatation, show very pronounced
changes. During a contraction, the folds in the
jejunum can extend in a more longitudinal direction,
like they do in the ileum.

In the rest phase, the folds lie in a very disorderly
fashion if the intestine is empty and especially if the
muscular tone of the intestinal wall is high. Com-

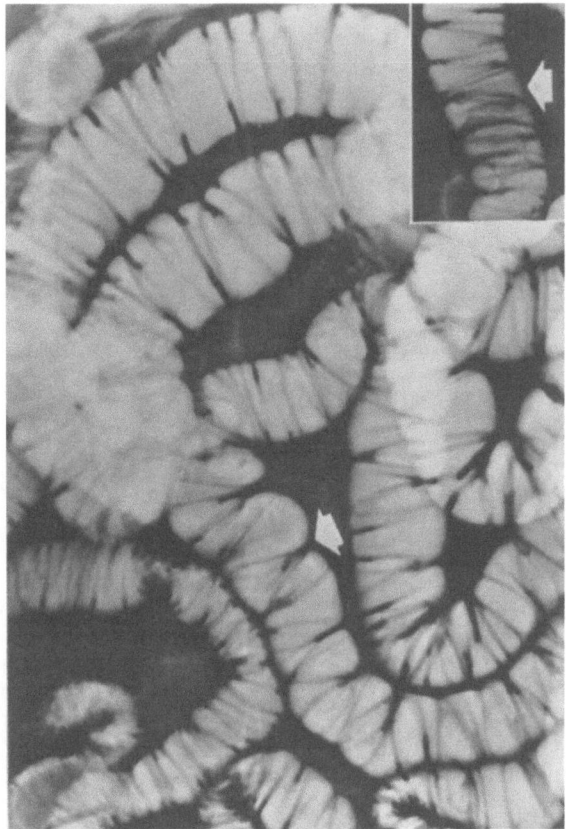

Fig. 2.8
Trident-shaped mucosal folds which mesh together in the
region of the jejunoileal transition.

parison of the mucosal patterns of one intestinal
segment in the various stages of contraction (fig.
2.11) illustrates this quite clearly. In this figure it is
also obvious that the thickness of the folds is fairly
constant and is therefore not influenced by the different phases of contraction.

Whatever the degree of stretching of the intestine,
they are about 2 mm thick in the jejunum and about
1 mm in the ileum. In the first decimeters of the
jejunum, however, the folds can sometimes be
2½–3 mm thick – although no visible reason can be
found. If these folds are normal in shape, they
probably have no pathological significance.

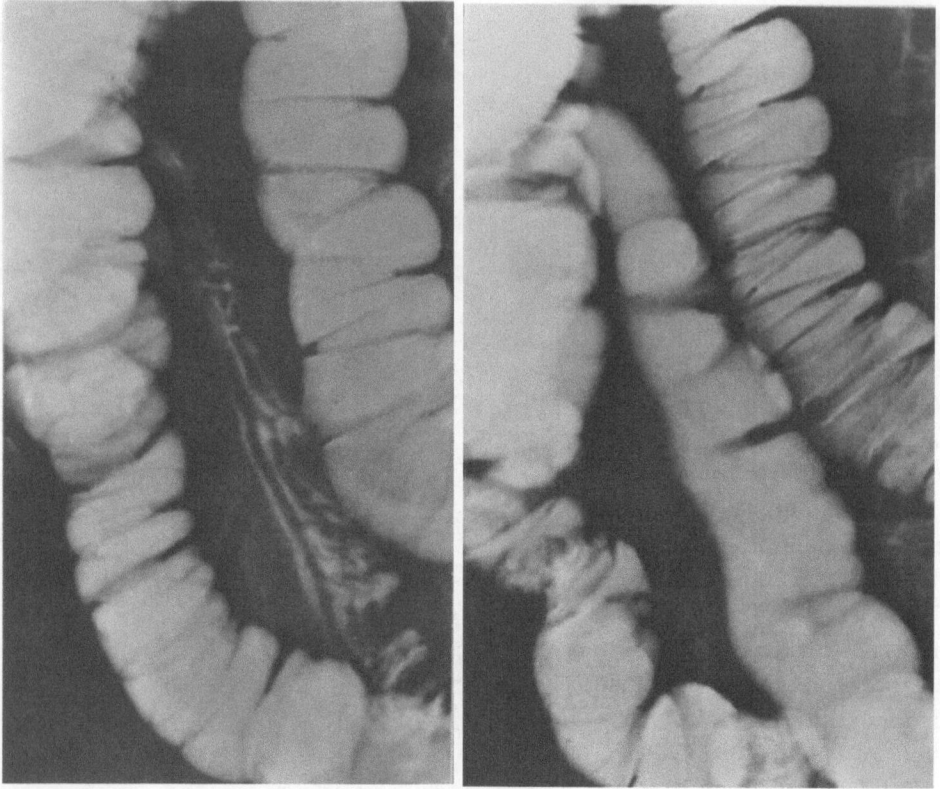

Fig. 2.10
Fold relief occasionally seen in the distal ileum. Longitudinal folds on the mesenterial side of the intestine and a circular course on the opposite side.

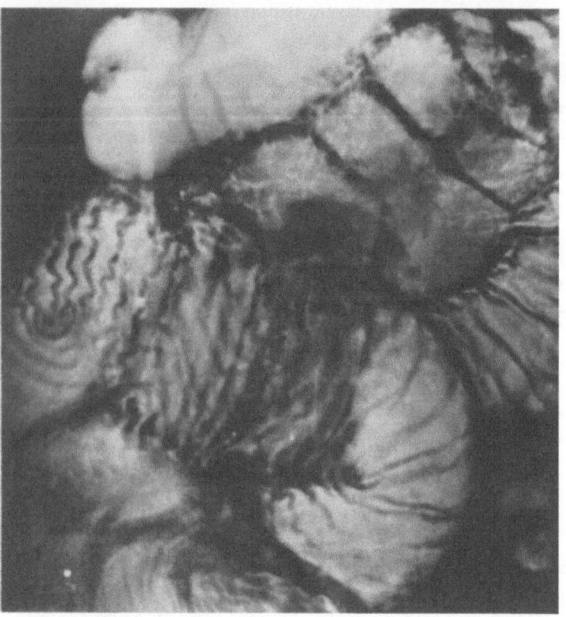

Figure 2.12 shows that even if there is marked stretching of the intestinal wall, as in the case of total mechanical obstruction, the folds of Kerkring retain their thickness fairly well. The folds do become somewhat shorter and are smoothed out, which implies that the shorter and thinner ileal

Fig. 2.12
Pronounced stretching of the intestinal wall causes the mucosal folds in the jejunum and ileum to become shorter but barely thinner than normal.

Fig. 2.11
Various phases of contraction of the same intestinal loop. Disorderly arrangement of the folds in the rest or contracted phase, orderly in the dilatation phase or when well-filled.

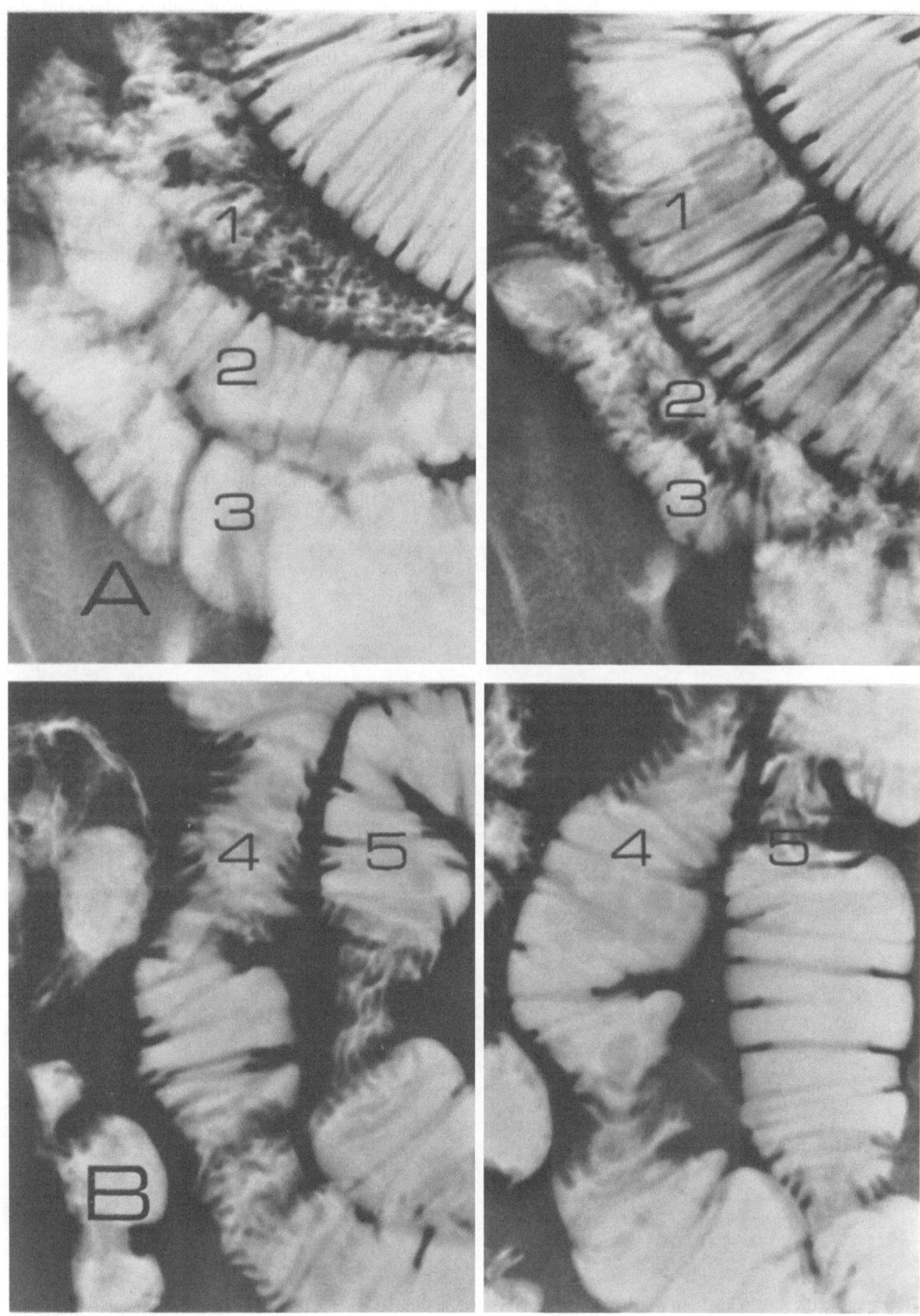

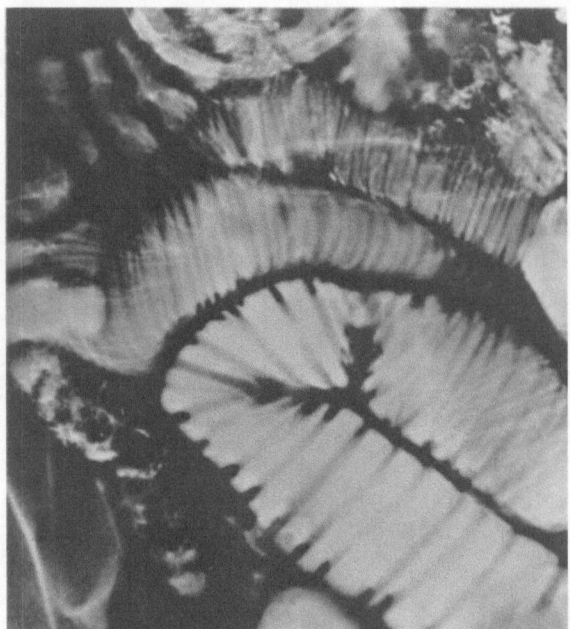

folds may only be visible as minute ridges (fig. 2.4).

It can be seen on the x-ray in fig. 2.13 that the thickness of the folds as well as the space between adjacent intestinal loops and the ileal loop dilated as a result of the obstruction has clearly increased. This is due in this case to Crohn's disease accompanied by lymphedema (see page 112). Only in the proximal part of the jejunum could this fold relief be attributed to dilatation alone; then, however, the intestinal wall would have to be thinner and the distance between the folds less.

Fig. 2.13
Crohn's disease with obstruction in the ileum. Mucosal folds as well as intestinal wall are thickened.

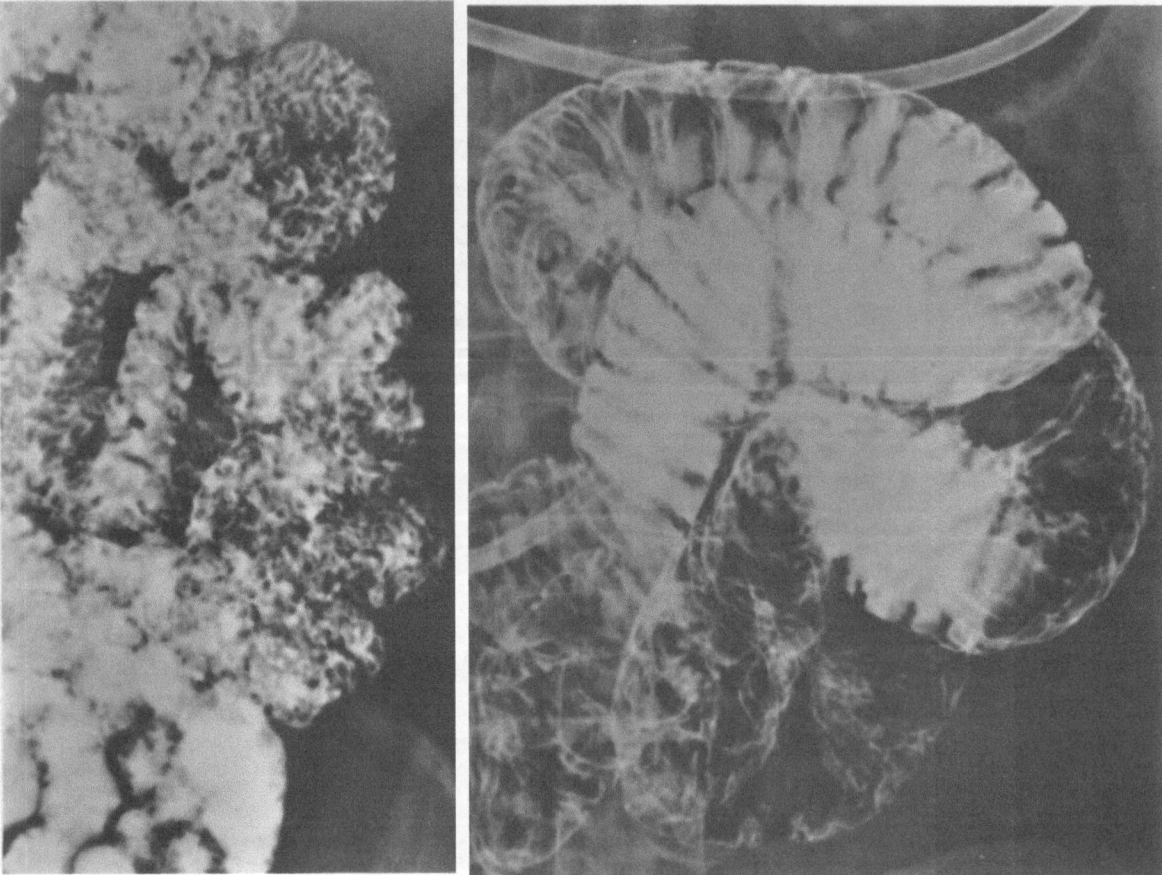

Fig. 2.14
Clear spots in the mucosal pattern which resemble enlarged lymph follicles are due to the fact that contractile intestinal loops intersect many times. After administration of a hypotonic agent, the illusory pattern disappears completely.

If the jejunum is in the rest phase and there is moderate filling with contrast medium, then evaluation is difficult as we know from the conventional examination. Because the folds intersect one another frequently, particularly in a highly contractile intestine, multiple small round bright spots appear in the mucosal patterns which are highly suggestive of lymph follicles. Since dilatation and a high degree of filling are often impossible to achieve in a contractile intestine, it may be necessary to induce hypotonicity for the purpose of evaluation (fig. 2.14). Because there are fewer folds in the distal ileum, the presence of true lymph follicles is easily demonstrated there. These follicles are frequently encountered in small children under normal circumstances; they disappear when the children are 10–14 years of age. The much larger Peyer's patches can also be seen in the distal ileum in older patients. They are recognized by the cushion-like configurations which occur mainly on the mesenterial side of the intestine (fig. 2.15).

A fine circular sawtooth pattern, like that often seen in the mucosa of a colon irritated by laxatives, may also be found in the distal ileum; this presumably is a result of contractions of the muscularis mucosae (fig. 2.16).

Until the second world war, it was assumed that the intestinal mucosa and the intramural nervous system of infants were still markedly underdeveloped, because for the first 3–6 months mucosal patterns were never seen on the x-ray films, not even in the duodenum. The appearance of a baby's small intestine on the x-ray films at that time was strikingly similar to that of an adult with a severe malabsorption or 'deficiency state' (less stable contrast medium and therefore flocculation caused by mucin and lactic acid). It was assumed that this deficiency state must be ascribed to damaged nerve cells since the pathologist found vacuolar degeneration in these cells. The x-ray films often showed flattening or even disappearance of the relief of the mucosal folds (Golden 75).

Bouslog (21, 22) and Weltz (230) were also not able to observe mucosal patterns on the x-ray films of infants but their studies had shown that the mucosal folds are more highly developed both absolutely and relatively than those in an adult and are even present in the third fetal month. The folds are, however, thinner and not as high. Vascularization and cellularity are pronounced in the mucosa. The submucosa is thinner than that in an adult so that the muscularis, the mucosa and the submucosa

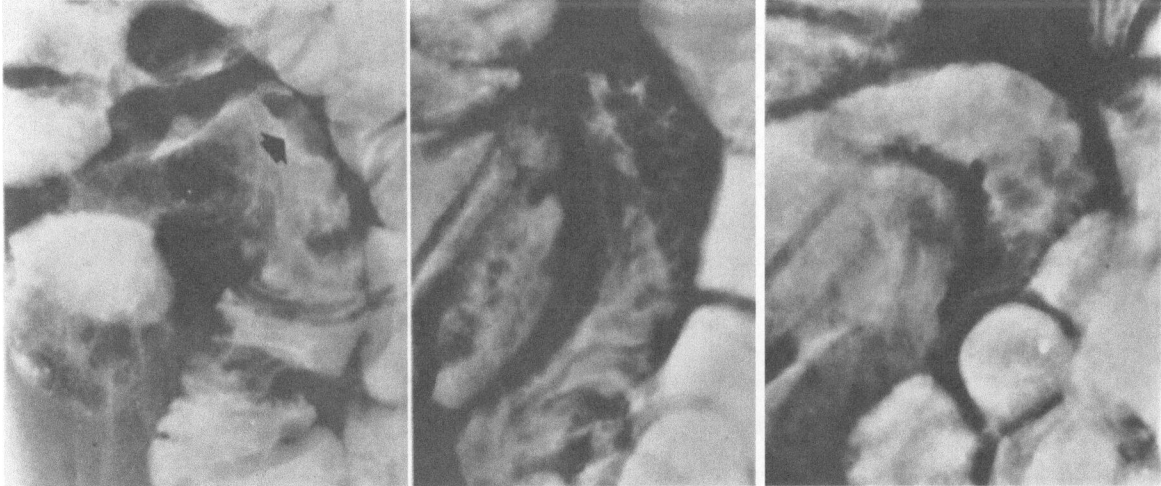

Fig. 2.15
Cushion-like configurations in the mucosal pattern in the distal ileum caused by Peyer's patches.

of an infant are all of approximately equal thickness. The relative underdevelopment of the muscularis, also in the mucosa, could cause the mucosal folds to be flattened completely by the barium column. All x-ray films published before the second world war show only a pronounced segmentation of the barium column, even in the duodenum. In general therefore one suspects that these examinations were in vain and that the conclusions were probably more often incorrect than correct.

Although the composition of many contrast media has been greatly improved, articles still appear today reporting that mucosal patterns cannot be observed until the infant is several months old. It is also stated, however, that no conclusions may be drawn from this fact.

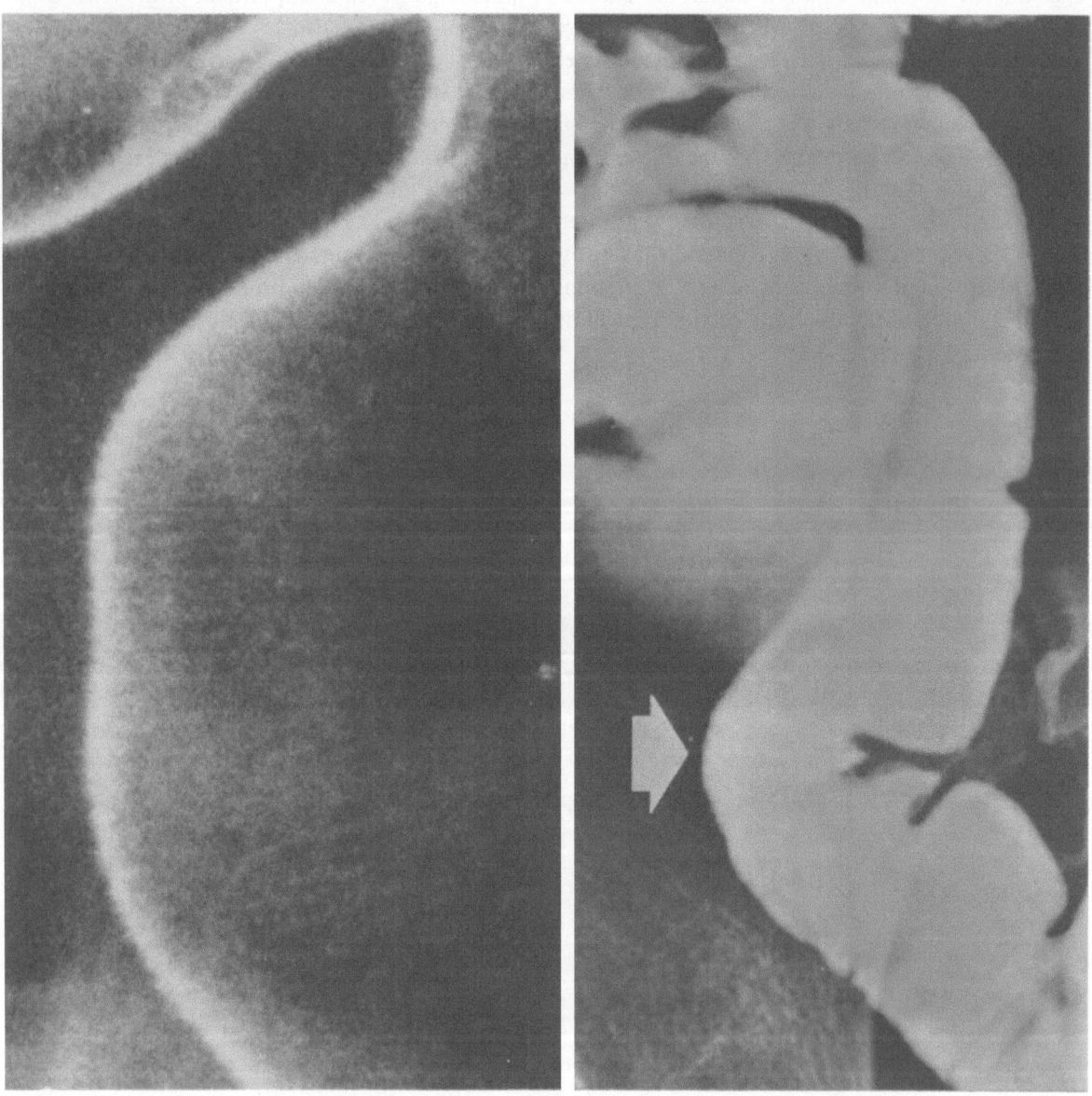

2. Normal position of the intestine

To be able to understand why a specific configuration of the small intestine is abnormal, as well as how it developed, knowledge of the development under normal conditions is required. An important phase in this respect is the rotation phase which occurs between the fourth and tenth weeks of fetal development. In the early stages of embryonal development the digestive tract is a tube-like organ called the archenteron. The superior mesenteric artery already exists; the liver is large and there is little space in the abdominal cavity.

The intestine increases rapidly in length but the mesentery which attaches it to the abdominal wall does not grow at the same rate so that loops are formed. This elongation is the greatest in the region supplied by the superior mesenteric artery, thus the small intestine and the colon, and is much less in the area of the rectosigmoid and especially the esophagus and stomach.

Since the initial enlargement of the fetal abdominal cavity is not sufficient to contain the rapidly lengthening intestine, part of the intestine with the omphalomesenteric duct as midpoint herniates physiologically into the umbilical cord (fig. 2.17A). The steadily growing intestine then rotates 90° with the omphalomesenteric duct and the superior mesenteric artery as axis such that the distal ileum and proximal colon lie on the left side and the jejunum and the proximal ileum on the right (fig. 2.17B). Further growth of the liver is slow so that the space in the abdominal cavity now increases faster than the total volume of the intestinal loops and the latter can again return into the abdominal cavity. During this so-called reduction of the umbilical herniation the jejunal loops pass behind the superior mesenteric artery to occupy the left posterior abdominal cavity (fig. 2.17C). The left anterior region contains the distal

ileum and the ascending colon and the right half of the abdomen, the still relatively large liver. After the return of the physiological herniation, there is again a rotation around the omphalomesenteric duct and the superior mesenteric artery. As a result of the pressure of the jejunal loops which occupy the left posterior part of the abdominal cavity, the ileocoecal section rotates another 180° in the same anticlockwise direction as the first time. The cecum is now to be found to the right in the upper abdomen with the ileum, at least the distal half, below it (fig. 2.17D). The loops of the small intestine continue to fold and as a result of the elongation of the colon, the cecum descends into the lower right abdomen and finally becomes fixed.

When the rotation process is completed, the loops of the small intestine are grouped in the abdominal cavity as seen in fig. 2.17E; the jejunum then lies to the left in the upper abdomen and the ileum to the right and in the middle of the lower abdomen.

According to recent studies the position of fully developed intestine is not achieved by rotation; the word 'malrotation' therefore should not be used to indicate an abnormal position of the bowel. Normally, the embryonic intestine is embedded in a mesenchymal mass, which is by no means compatible with the later mesentery, without a coelomic cavity between the intestine and the mesenchyme. As a result of extension of the coelom, segmental growth of the intestine takes place inside the mass, in the area surrounded by the coelomic activity and situated between two parts of the intestine which are still fixed in position within the mass. As the development of the intestine reaches completion, the mesentery develops as a very thin duplicature at the same time.

Welvaart, K., Etude du développement de l'intestin envisagée parallèllement à la genèse du mésentère. *Bulletin de l'Association des Anatomistes*, March 1965, 921: 926.

Fig. 2.16
←
Saw-toothed margins of the wall of the distal ileum due to contractions of the muscularis mucosae (→). Similar configurations are also seen in the colon, especially if a laxative is added to the contrast fluid (left).

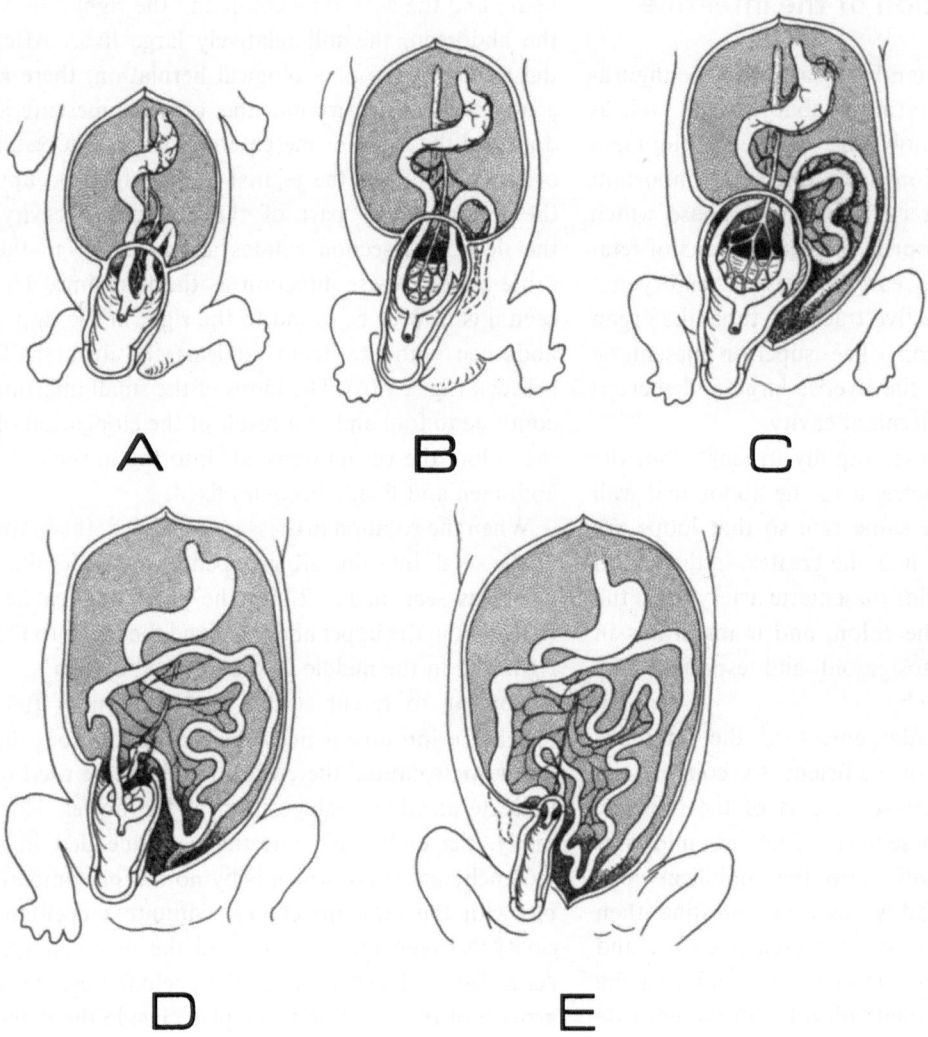

Fig. 2.17
A–E. Stages of development and rotation of the convolution of intestinal loops in the abdominal cavity.

3. Normal impressions on the intestine

Impressions can be caused by other intestinal loops, adjacent organs, vessels, inflammatory infiltrates, tumor tissue and fat. In enteroclysis the degree of filling of the intestinal loops is greater than in a conventional follow-through examination so that mutual compression of these loops occurs much more frequently.

a. BY OTHER INTESTINAL LOOPS

In the jejunum indentations in the contrast column may be seen, which in later films is shown to be caused by other jejunal loops (fig. 2.18). In general these impressions are most clearly visible on the largest loops, which usually have the lowest tone or are at that moment in the rest phase. We see fewer impressions on an intestine with active peristalsis, which therefore must have good tone, than on an atonic intestine. Since atony usually affects the proximal intestinal loops sooner than the distal ones, the most distal loops are more likely to push against the most proximal. An impression of the ileal loops on those in the jejunum is therefore likely; we have never seen the opposite (fig. 2.19). It is not always possible to explain an

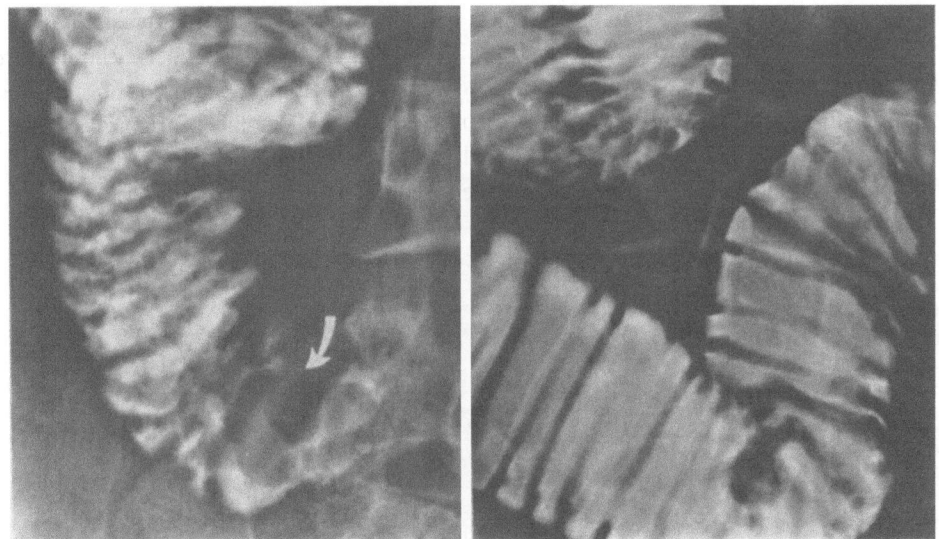

Fig. 2.18
Impression of a jejunal loop on a jejunal loop caused in this case by a sharp curve in the loop.

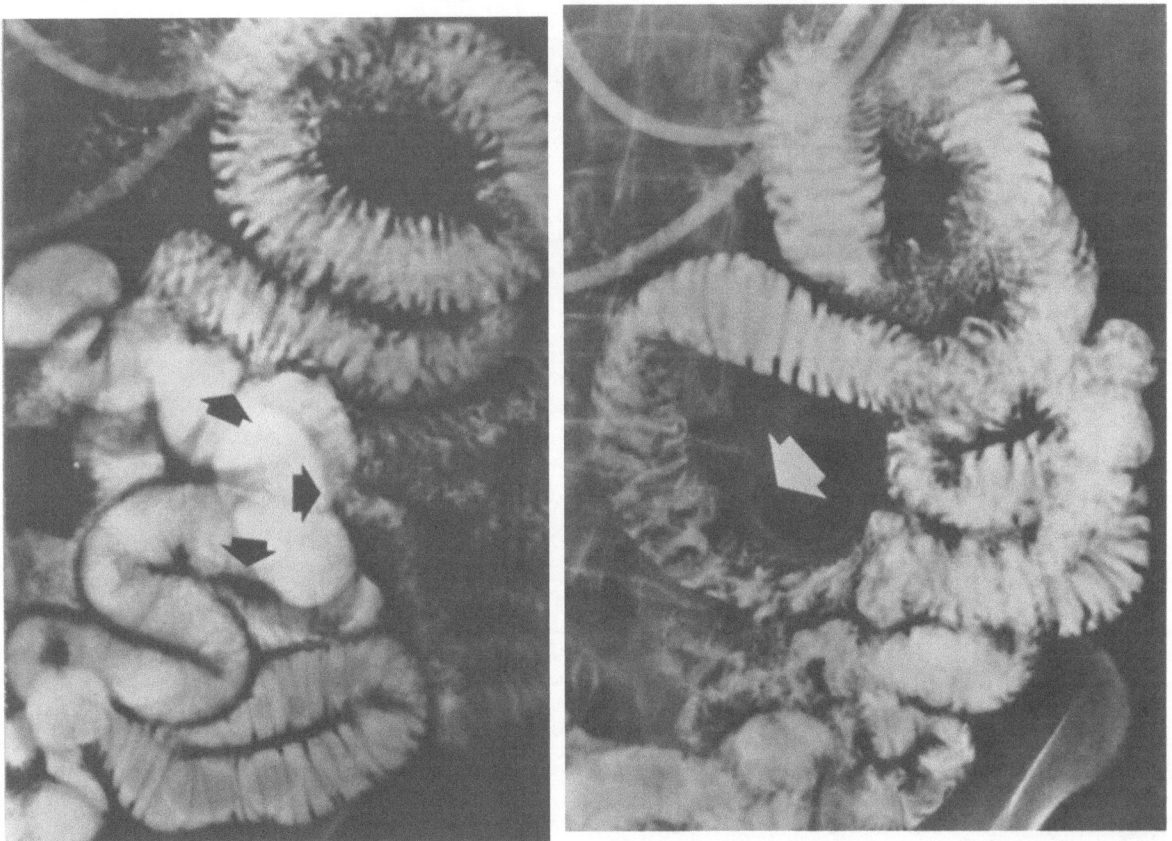

Fig. 2.19
Impressions on the jejunum caused by ileal loops which were not yet filled with contrast fluid when the x-ray was taken.

impression even though later films prove without a doubt that they were temporary (fig. 2.20AB). The most frequently encountered impression of one intestinal loop on another is that of the colon on the small intestine. The most likely explanation for this is the considerable difference in the viscos-

ity of the contents of these two sections of the intestine. The most common are impressions of the cecum or sigmoid on the ileum; occasionally we may see an impression of the descending colon on the jejunum (fig. 2.21A — D).

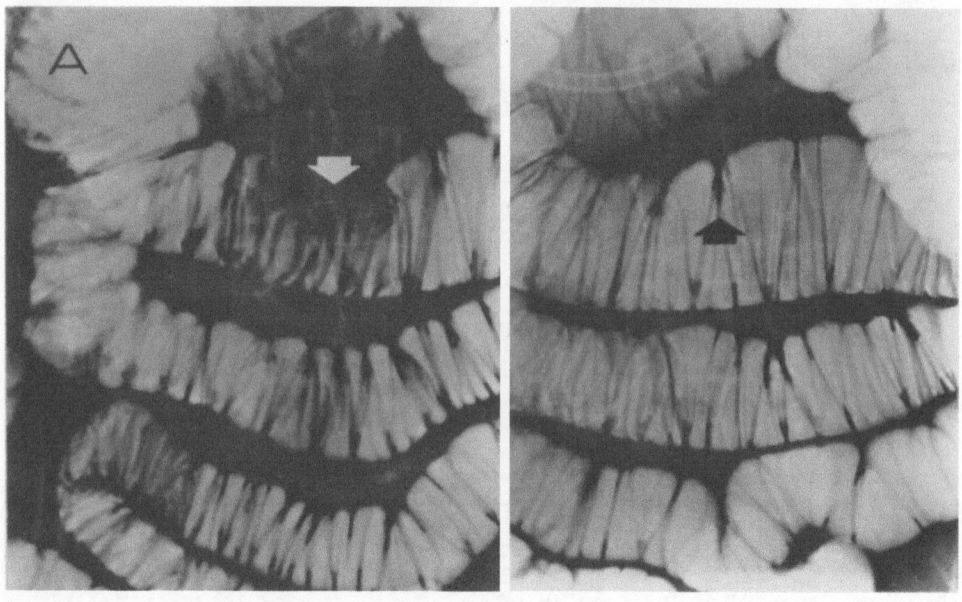

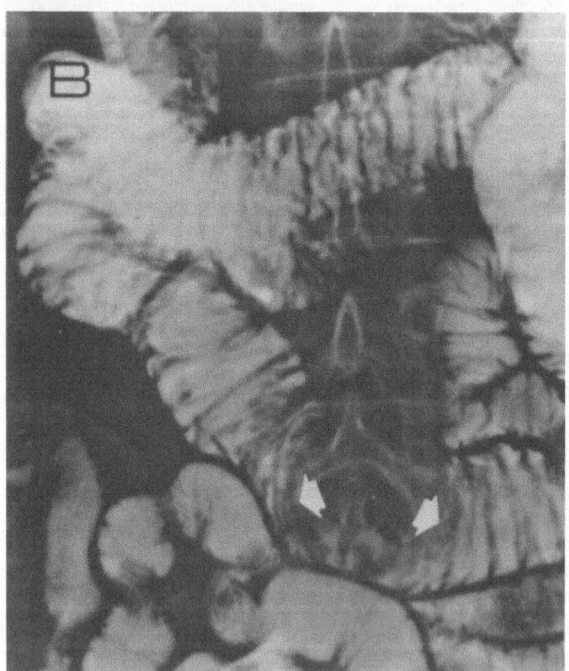

Fig. 2.20
Temporary impression of unknown origin (abdominal aorta?) on the jejunum.

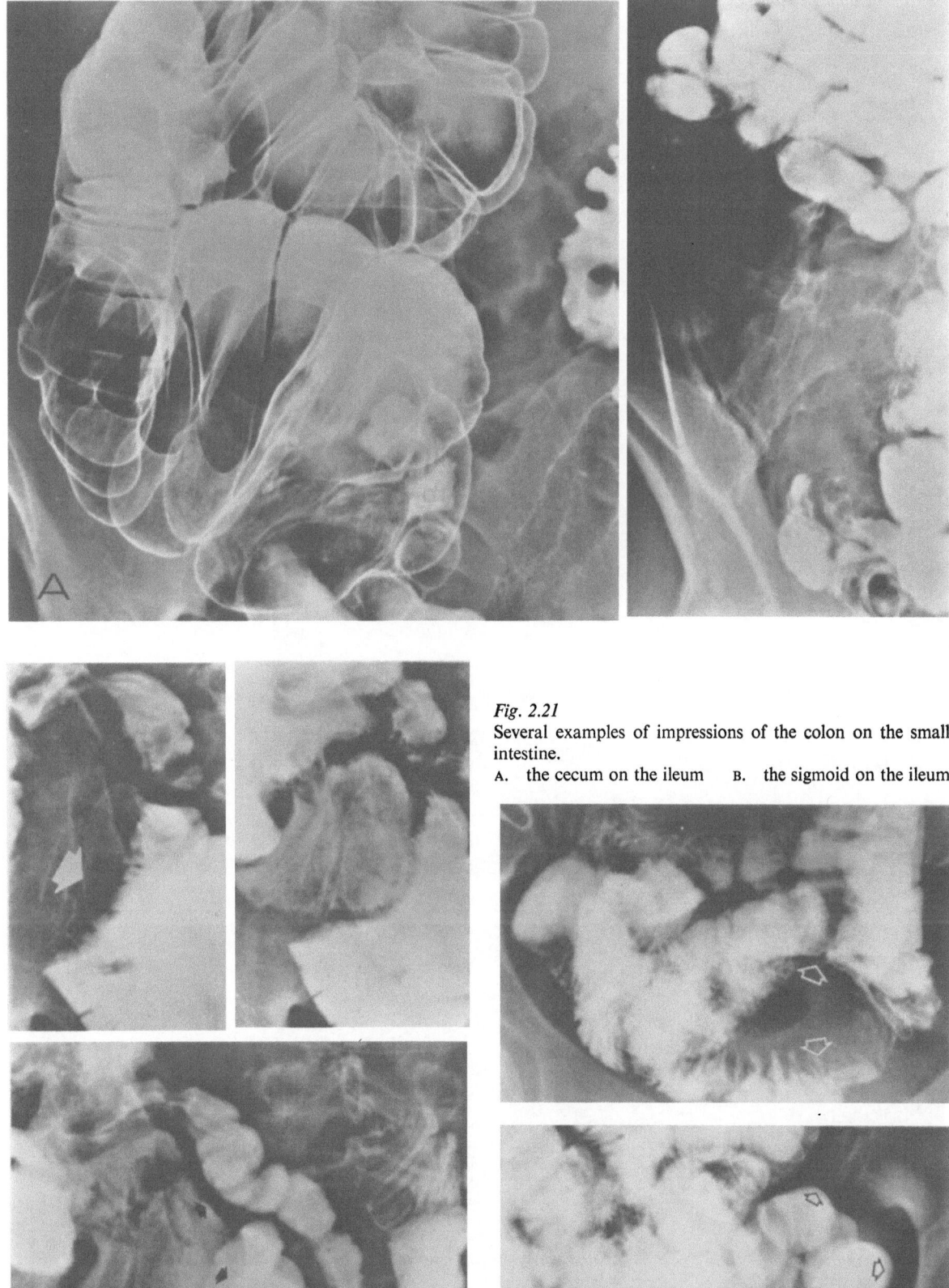

Fig. 2.21
Several examples of impressions of the colon on the small intestine.
A. the cecum on the ileum   B. the sigmoid on the ileum

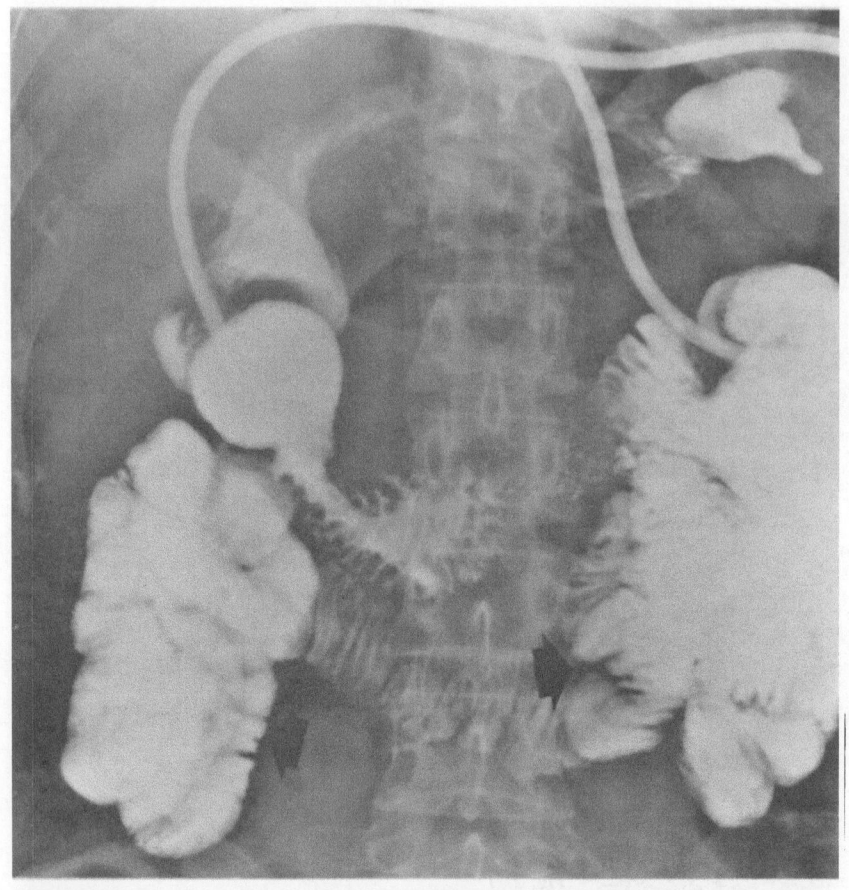

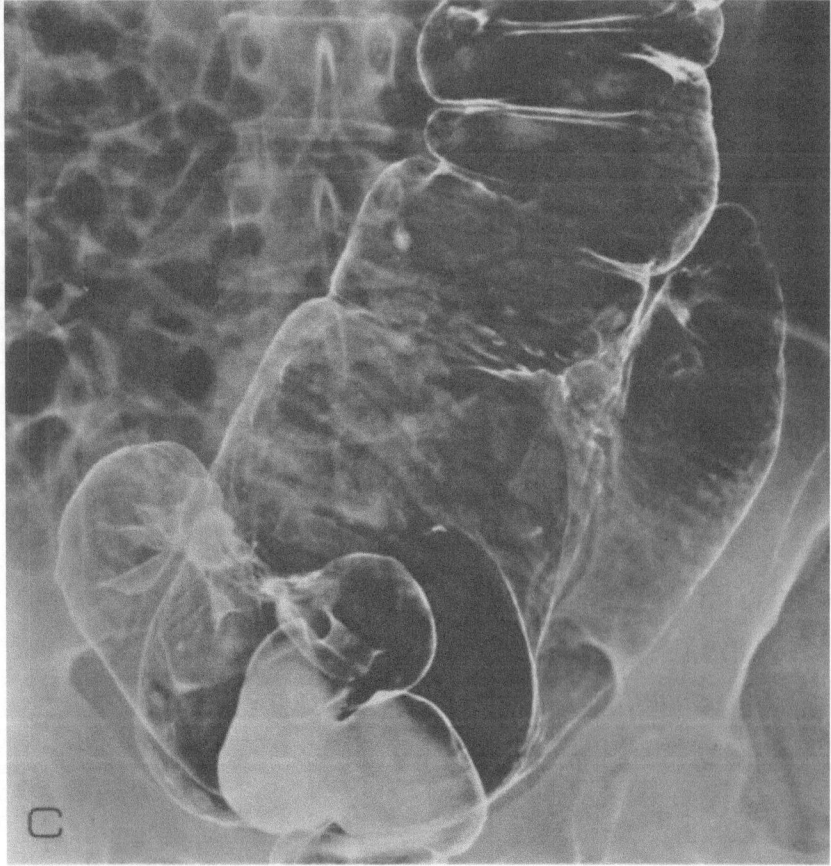

Fig. 2.21
c.   megasigmoid on the jejunum

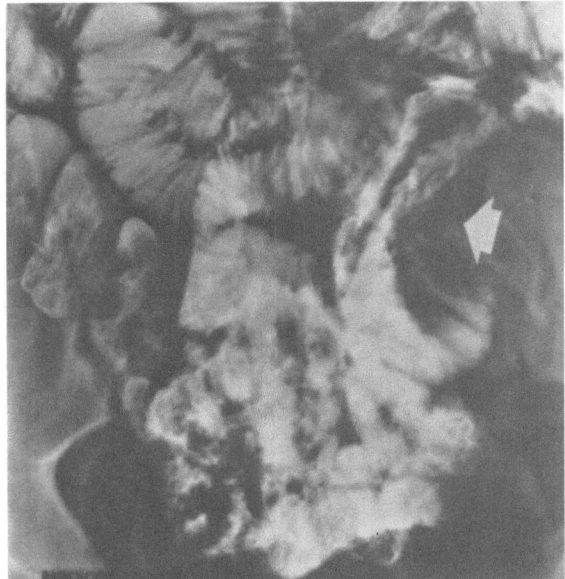

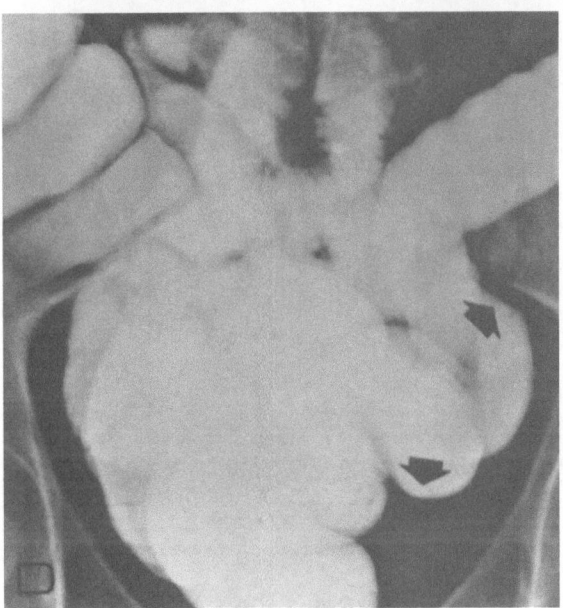

Fig. 2.21
D. the descending colon on the jejunum and ileum.

b. BY VESSELS

The pressure in the veins is so low that indentation by a vene in an intestinal loop is not conceivable. On the other hand the large arteries frequently cause an impression on the small intestine. Usually we see an indentation in the duodenum due to the aorta where the former passes between the aorta and the superior mesenteric artery (fig. 2.22). An impression of the superior mesenteric artery on the duodenum is rarely visible; it is probably completely 'overshadowed' by the much larger impression of the aorta.

Another common indentation in an intestinal loop by a large vessel is that of the iliac artery in the ileum at the somewhat narrower pelvic outlet (fig. 2.23). Here too as in the duodenum and the jejunum, it is striking that such cases involve fairly wide and highly filled intestinal loops, usually as a result of an iatrogenic atony (see chapter XII).

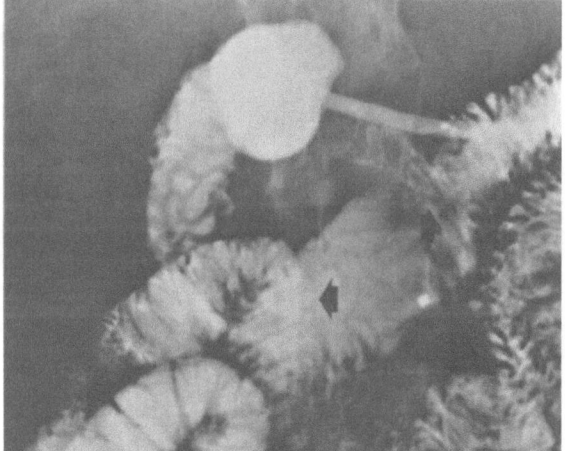

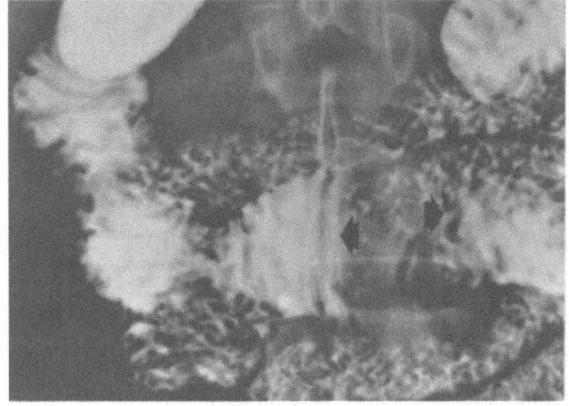

Fig. 2.22
Impression of the abdominal aorta on the duodenum.

4. Filling defects between the intestinal loops

a. CAUSED BY OTHER ORGANS

Exactly in the middle of the abdomen we sometimes observe an abnormality in the convolution of intestinal loops which is seen only when the patient is in the prone position; it is due to the fact that a sagging loop of the transverse colon is filled with feces (fig. 2.24). A fairly recent phenomenon is the appearance of a large abnormality in the convolution of intestinal loops in the lower left or lower right abdomen due to the presence of a hetero-

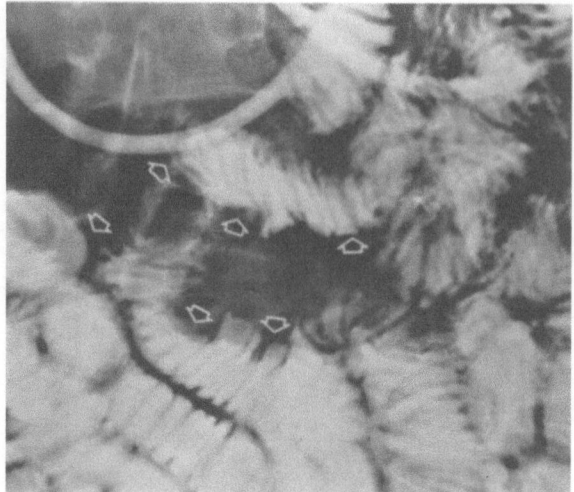

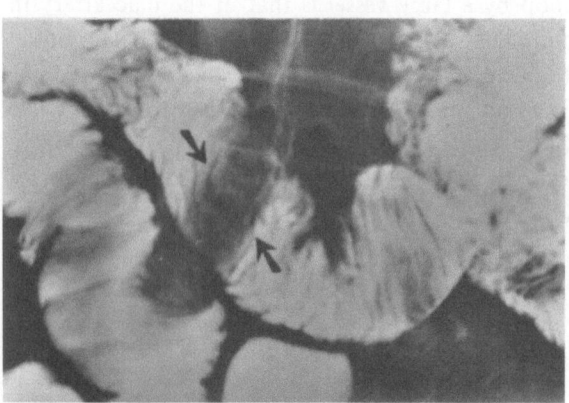

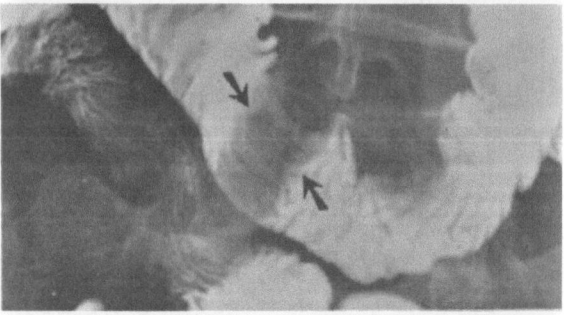

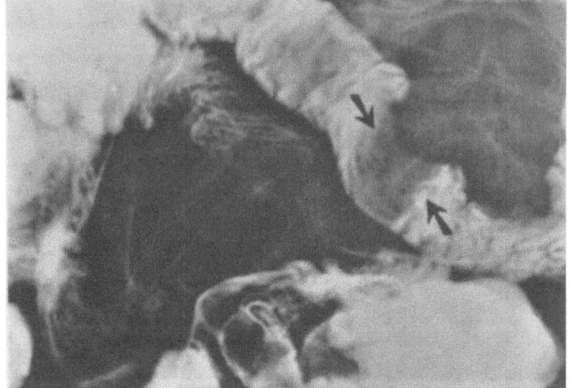

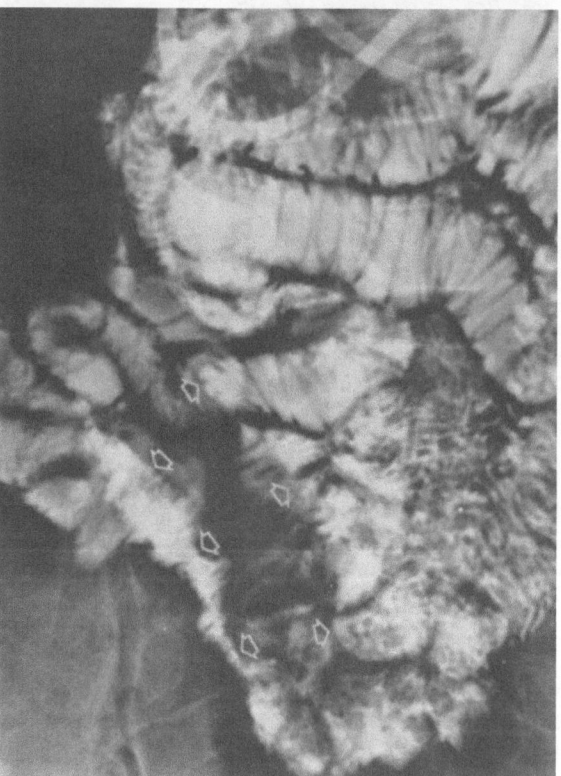

Fig. 2.24
Empty space between the intestinal loops in the mid- and right lower abdomen, caused by the transverse colon.

Fig. 2.23
Impression of the iliac artery on the ileum.

topically transplanted kidney (fig. 2.25). Recognition of this abnormality is, however, exceedingly important since the use of compression in this region could cause heavy damage to the transplanted kidney.

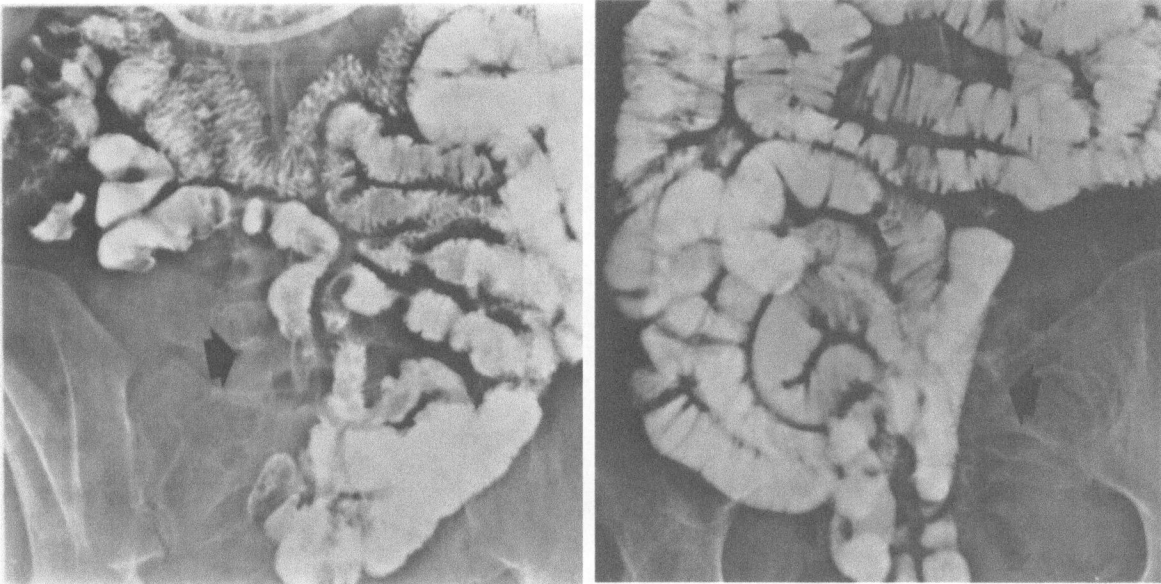

Fig. 2.25
Empty space in the right or left lower abdomen, caused by a heterotopically transplanted kidney.

b. CAUSED BY OTHER TISSUE STRUCTURES

This is not considered a normally occurring phenomenon. A voluminous greater omentum or fatty degeneration or shriveling of the mesentery can result in empty spaces in the middle of the abdomen or scattered among the intestinal loops; these defects are even larger than those visualized in pyknics (fig. 2.26). In pyknics, there is almost never a convolution of intestinal loops in the pelvis minor (fig. 2.27). An empty space within the convolution is, however, usually caused by an inflammatory infiltrate, for instance in Crohn's disease (fig. 2.28), or an inflamed appendix (fig. 2.29). The intestinal loops adjacent to the infiltrate often show deformation and adhesions as well as edematous or irregularly altered mucosal folds. Approximately the same pattern is seen when the infiltrate is not caused by inflammation but by tumor growth in the intestinal wall or the mesentery (fig. 2.30). A tumor causes more pronounced destruction and stenosis than an inflammation.

Tumors or cysts in the wall of the abdomen can sometimes only be visualized when the patient is in the prone position or when compression is used. The opposite may be true of tumors, nodular masses or cysts located in the mesentery (fig. 2.31).

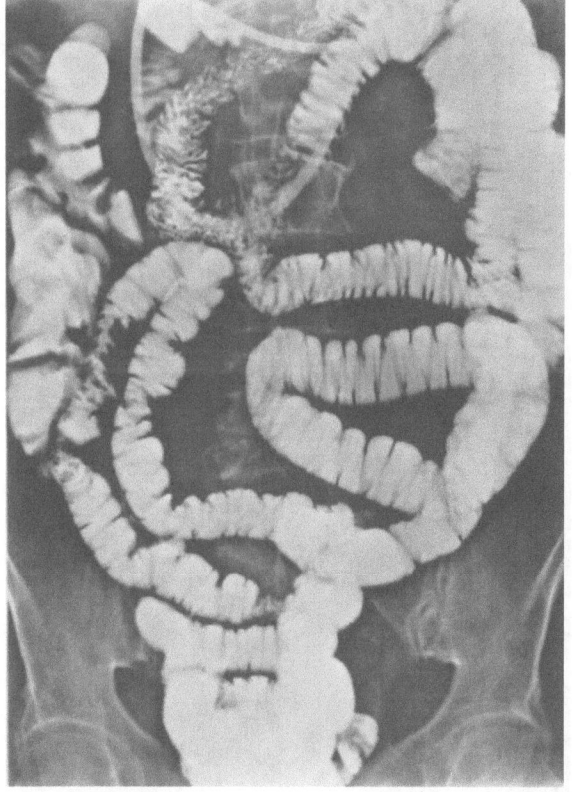

Fig. 2.26
Unusually large spaces between the intestinal loops in the center of the abdomen, possibly due to mesenterial fat or a copious greater omentum.

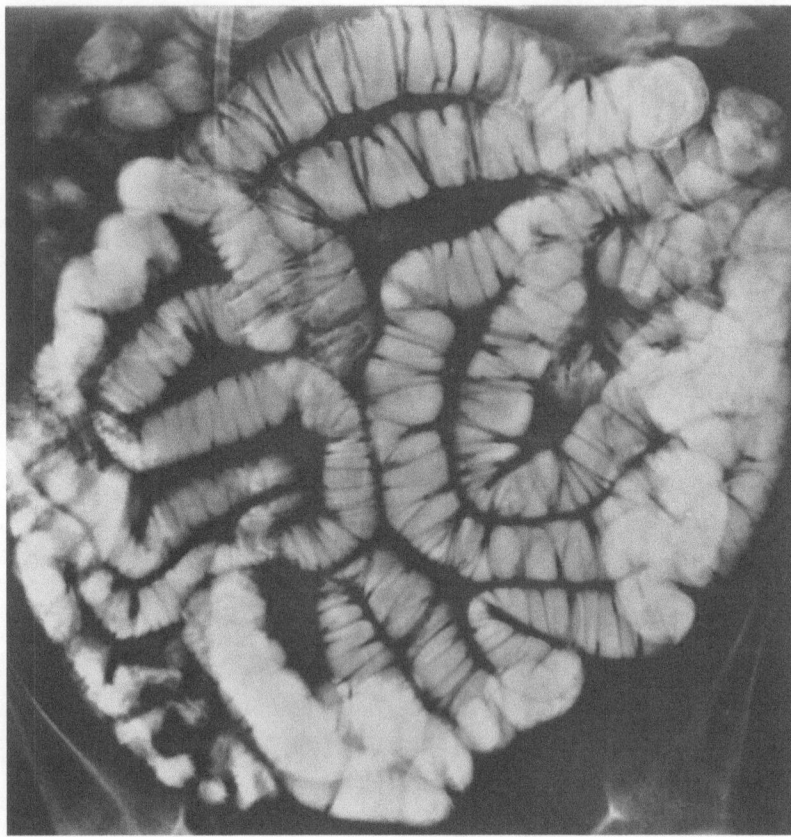

Fig. 2.27
Small intestine of a pyknic, filled with 1200 ml contrast fluid and 600 ml water. No hindrance of superposition.

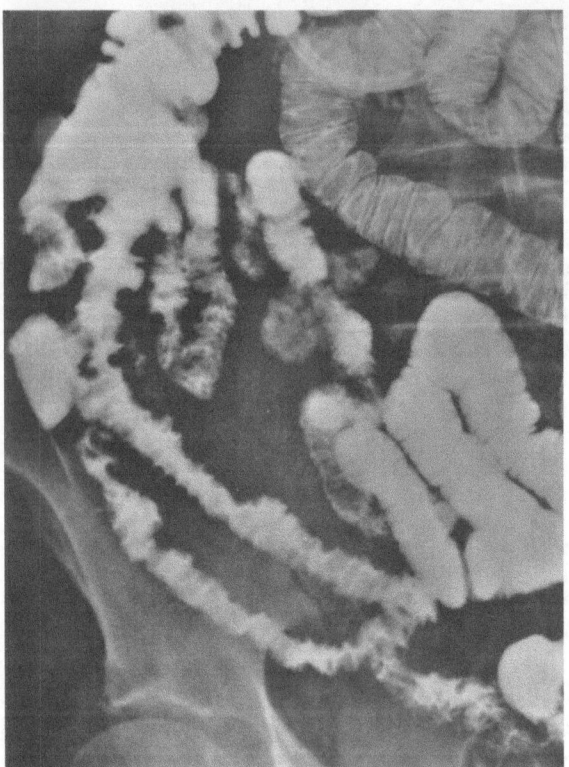

Fig. 2.28
Greater spaces between intestinal loops as a result of an inflammatory infiltrate or a layer of fat encircling the intestine in Crohn's disease.

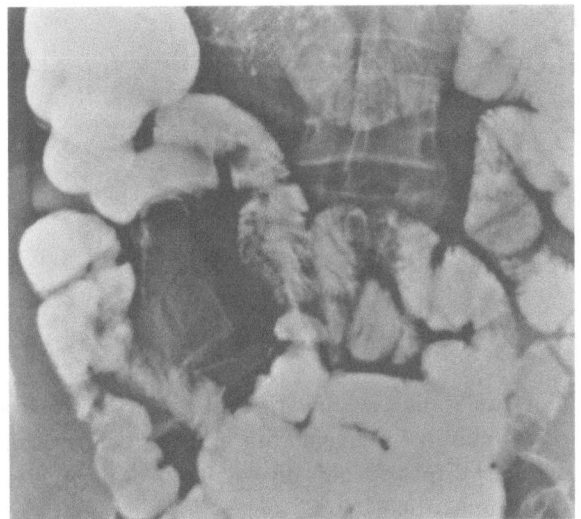

Fig. 2.29
Empty space between the intestinal loops in the right lower abdomen as a result of an appendicular infiltrate.

Fig. 2.30
Increased space between intestinal loops caused by tumor growth which has involved the mesentery.

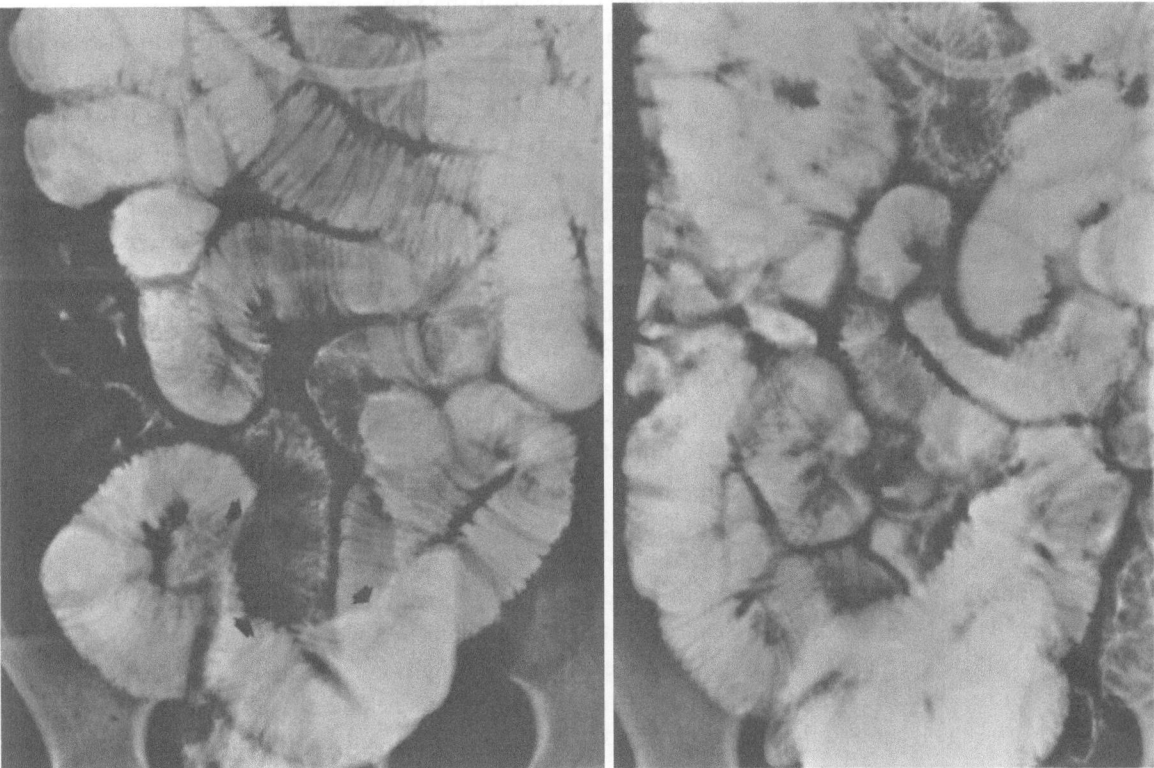

Fig. 2.31
AB. Mesenterial cyst, visible when the patient is in the supine position (left) and hardly visible in the prone position (right).

III

PHYSIOLOGY

1. Innervation and motility

The parasympathetic innervation of the small intestine occurs via the celiac ganglia by fibers of the right vagus nerve. Cutting the vagus causes a decrease in the motility of the small intestine and therefore a reduced rate of transit. The sympathetic innervation occurs via the splanchnic nerves. The fibers of both systems lie in the mesentery and belong to the central nervous system.

The intramural autonomic nervous system is exceedingly important for the small intestine. It consists of the plexus of Auerbach in the tunica muscularis and the plexus of Meissner in the submucosa (see fig. 2.1).

Loewi (1921) and Dale (1929) showed that when the parasympathetic nerves are stimulated, acetylcholine is produced; in 1933 Cannon demonstrated that stimulation of the sympathetic nerves produces adrenin which has the same effect as adrenalin. Acetylcholine plays an important role in the transmission of nervous impulses; it is not soluble in fat and cannot pass through the lipoidal membranes of the nerve fibers. Acetylcholine causes contraction of the muscle fibers. Termination of this contraction is caused by the repeated inactivation of acetylcholine by the enzyme acetylcholinesterase. This enzyme can be inactivated by neostigmine; when this occurs, the breakdown of acetylcholine is retarded and the state of contraction or the tone lasts longer. This heightened tone causes an enhancement of the peristalsis, especially in the jejunum.

In 1923, Forssell (54) showed that the movements of the muscularis mucosae are independent and not, as was generally assumed, dependent upon contractions of the tunica muscularis. Using x-ray films and autopsy material, he observed that a given intestinal segment with a lumen of a specific diameter displays highly divergent mucosal patterns. He assumed that the movements of the muscularis mucosae might fulfill an important role in the digestion of food.

In 1922, the physiologists King and Arnold (109) made similar observations but it is not clear whether Forssell was aware of this. They noted that mechanical stimulation of the ends of the villi only caused contractions of the stimulated villi, usually once but occasionally several times in succession. Stimulation at the base of the villi caused contractions of the villi as a group. The mucosa appeared to be stimulated not only locally but also via the splanchnic nerves. The plexus of Meissner probably regulates only the tone. Stimulation of the muscularis mucosae is not possible via the plexus of Auerbach; however, stimulation of the mucosa does cause a relaxation of the tone of the tunica muscularis, followed by a recovery. The rate of this recovery increases as the stimulation is intensified. Physiologically, mechanical stimulation by the food mass is the most important factor causing contractions of the tunica muscularis. The reflex mechanism for these peristaltic waves is regulated via the plexus of Auerbach and it will only respond to stimulation of this plexus (109). Peristaltic waves of the tunica muscularis are characterized by relaxation before and contraction behind the area stimulated. Although similar in motion to milking, the mechanism involved is not known precisely since it is highly complicated (124). The longitudinal fibers shorten behind the advancing circular contractions. The frequency of the peristaltic waves is approximately 1 per sec. In the case of hypermotility, this frequency increases only slightly, but the contractions clearly become more pronounced. There are fewer peristaltic contractions in the ileum than in the jejunum and the latent period between stimulation and contraction is the longest in the distal part of the small intestine. In addition, the movements of the villi decrease in the distal direction. This gradual decrease in diverse vital functions from proximal to distal is called the 'metabolic gradient'.

Normally peristaltic contractions should not occur in the ileum; they are seen, however, when there is an increased irritability of the intestine or a lowered stimulus threshold. The ileum is characterized by segmentation moving in the aboral direction; the intestinal contents are constricted at regular intervals and divided up into the so-called 'segments of Cannon' (125).

Nicotine and stimulation of the vagus influence the tunica muscularis but not the muscularis mucosae (109). The development of the mucosa appears to be highly dependent upon the blood supply (109, 76). Abbott and Pendergrass (1) found that when morphine is administered directly into the duodenum, there is a pronounced increase in the tone which decreases in the distal direction. 15 to 20 minutes later, the tone decreases; it is once again the greatest in the duodenum and decreases in the distal direction. Using a double balloon to register the change in the pressure in the small intestine, they observed that the motility is highly dependent upon the differences in tone and that the intensity of the peristaltic waves increases with an increase in the tone of the intestinal wall. Lenz and Kreppel (126) studied the influence of prostigmin, pilocarpine and arecoline on the motility of the small intestine of a cat, which is structured similar to that of man. The movements of the contrast column were filmed. After prostigmin was injected, the tone increased and the Cannon constrictions become more pronounced and more frequent; the number of peristaltic contractions also increased. The prostigmin was ineffective 9 minutes later and hypotonia occurred.

The intensification of peristalsis produced by neostigmine or prostigmin is used in intravenous pyelography to remove troublesome small gas bubbles from the small intestine. It is well-known that air in the small intestine moves so fast in the distal direction that it takes only several minutes to travel from the stomach to the cecum. Large gas bubbles generally remove themselves from the digestive tract since they cause sufficient stretching of the intestinal wall to induce peristaltic contractions (133).

The effect of prostigmin is cancelled by atropine. Neostigmine has no effect on patients with sprue; it is tentatively assumed that this is due to a disturbed functioning of the nerve cells. In this respect the role of vitamine B deficiencies is still unknown.

The results with pilocarpine and arecoline were similar but more pronounced. In particular pilocarpine enhanced secretion so that dilution of the contrast medium was greater than with prostigmin. The mucosal folds were clearly broadened; autopsy showed that this was due to edema. Overdosage of prostigmin and arecoline caused spasms and dyskinesia; peristaltic waves no longer occurred. An overdosage of pilocarpine did not cause dyskinesia, but there was such heavy secretion and edematous swelling of the mucous membrane that peristaltic waves were no longer possible mechanically.

In 1931, Pansdorf had already observed swelling of the folds of Kerkring caused by pilocarpine in 18 healthy persons. The effect of these 3 substances, called the muscarine effect, is similar to that of postganglionic sympathetic stimulation and can be neutralized by atropine. Pilocarpine and arecoline act directly on the smooth musculature; prostigmin acts on cholinesterase.

2. Gastric emptying and transit time

a. PERISTALSIS

The rate of transit of a contrast fluid through the small intestine depends almost entirely on the rate and intensity of the peristaltic movements in the intestine. This motility is in turn dependent on diverse factors which can be utilized by the physician at will, such as caloric value, temperature and osmosity of the contrast fluid. However, the most important factor, as far as the stimulation of peristalsis is concerned, is the gastric emptying time since this determines the degree of stretching of the duodenum and the proximal jejunum. The latter is essential for the stimulation of good peristaltic movements. If there are no factors inhibiting peristalsis (these are described in detail in chapter XII) and if mechanical passage through the pylorus is unimpeded, then the gastric emptying time depends to a large extent on the degree of filling. These considerations shall now be discussed in more detail.

b. QUANTITY

Henderson (87) studied the gastric emptying time for 110 infants using specific amounts of contrast medium; he found values of 8–24 hours for a newborn child, 4–5 hours for a baby 2 weeks old and 2–3 hours for babies 3–4 months old. He therefore advised that the fasting period before examination of the baby should be longer than the usual 4 hours. He observed that 2/3 of the contrast medium leaves the stomach rather quickly but the remaining 1/3 takes considerably longer. He also saw that the stomach empties faster when the babies are in the prone or right lateral position and that good mucosal patterns sometimes even of the proximal ileum, can be obtained only under these conditions. He was not able to find an explanation for this observation.

Even the size of the meal influences the gastric emptying time. Van Liere et al. reported emptying times for 200 ml, 400 ml, and 600 ml in normal individuals. They found that 400 ml of a watery barium suspension took only 16.83 per cent instead of 100 per cent longer to leave the stomach than 200 ml; 600 ml took 38.33 per cent longer. The use of two decimal places suggests an accuracy in conflict with the small number of persons tested. It is also improbable that the second supplementary dosage of 200 ml took $38.33 - 2 \times 16.83 = 4.67$ per cent longer to leave the stomach than the first supplementary dosage of 200 ml. However, the inaccuracies caused by these small numbers does not change the importance of their observations (129). This phenomenon can only be explained by the greater supply which, especially in the beginning, is comparable to a continuous supply in the right lateral position. Henderson observed that the gastric emptying time for a child decreases gradually; this follows in the same line of thought (87).

c. TEMPERATURE

Gershon-Cohen, Shay and Fels (66) found that barium test meals cooled to 35–40° F left the stomach sooner and (therefore) passed through the small intestine more quickly than contrast meals heated up to 140–145° F. The mechanism of this accelerated gastric emptying and rapid transit after cold meals is not known. The assumption that it is due to insufficient digestion and absorption resulting from decreased secretion is speculative. Gastric secretion decreases markedly when the gastric contents are cold; however, when the gastric contents are warm, secretion increases to only slightly above the norm. For cold gastric contents, secretion returns to normal more rapidly than the increase in the temperature of the gastric contents suggests.

d. NUTRIENTS

The influence of nutrients on gastric emptying and transit time through the small intestine can best be studied using carbohydrates. Glucose was chosen because it mixes easily with the contrast fluid and with it, the contrast fluid can easily be made hypertonic. Hypertonic gastric contents first become isotonic; during this process, the volume can increase considerably. For example 215 ml of a 50 per cent glucose solution increases to more than 500 ml after 1 hour in the stomach (129); 100 ml of a 10 per cent glucose solution increases to 128 ml and 12 min later, it is still 122 ml. When a 3.5 per cent glucose solution is administered orally, then 1 hour later the glucose concentration in the small intestine is 2.6 mg per 100 ml. If a 50 per cent glucose solution is used, this concentration is only 5.3 mg per 100 ml, a relatively small difference.

Reynolds et al. (189) compared the gastric emptying time for 33 children using 5 different mixtures of the contrast medium. They examined each child five times; their values are given below:

Contrast medium:	Gastric emptying time:
1. 60 g Ba + 120 g water	1.9 hours
2. 60 g Ba + 120 g milk (2.33 per cent fat)	3.1 hours
3. 60 g Ba + 120 g cream (13.33 per cent fat)	4.8 hours
4. 60 g Ba + 90 g water + 30 g syrup	3.3 hours
5. 40 g Ba + 200 g water + 100 g protein (3.5 per cent fat, 7 per cent protein)	5.0 hours

If we consider the fact that the high value of the 5th test is due to the greater amount administered, then we can conclude from the above that fat is the slowest to leave the stomach. This conclusion is in agreement with that of Menville and Ané (151) who carried out similar tests with adults and found that proteins and carbohydrates retard gastric emptying to the same extent, but fats considerably more. Fat was also the most important factor causing retarded transit through the small intestine. Although the gastric emptying time is shorter after a partial gastrectomy, here too the addition of nutrients to the contrast medium has a delaying effect. Because of the presence of glucose in the proximal part of the small intestine, entero-gastrone is produced, a hormone which inhibits the peristalsis of the stomach. Similar mechanisms also exist for fat and possibly protein.

Van Liere et al. (129) introduced 50 ml of an indifferent mixture into the stomach of dogs who had first received an intravenous glucose injection. Autopsy showed that a half hour later this mixture had moved an average of 141 cm in the small intestine in contrast to 183 cm for the control group. The blood sugar was then 183 mg per cent versus 99 mg per cent for the control group. According to their report, the inhibitory influence of a high blood sugar concentration on the peristalsis of stomach and intestine has been known since 1924. A low blood sugar concentration on the other hand causes contractions of the stomach and a feeling of hunger.

e. OSMOSITY

In 1907 it was reported that isotonic solutions leave the stomach faster than hypotonic or hypertonic solutions (129). Gershon-Cohen et al. (67) showed that a hypotonic solution leaves the stomach almost as fast as an isotonic solution. However, when these solutions are introduced directly into the duodenum, then the hypotonic solution causes the pylorus to remain closed until isotonicity is achieved. A solution becomes isotonic much faster in the duodenum than in the stomach although the stomach also attempts to make a hypertonic solution isotonic by fluid secretion.

Using HCl and Na_2CO_3, Shay and Gershon-Cohen demonstrated that the responses of the stomach and the pylorus are the same, whether the hypertonic solution is administered into the stomach or directly into the duodenum by intubation (202). Johnston and Ravdin (101) administered glucose-barium to dogs after a partial gastrectomy to demonstrate that severe contractions of the small intestine compensate to some extent for the absence of the pylorus. They also observed this in patients. This peristalsis can vary greatly for the same tone. For a rapid increase in pressure in the intestinal lumen, the stimulus threshold for the development of peristaltic waves is lower than for a slow increase in pressure. The stimulus threshold is also lower for an increased tone than for a decreased tone (39). If there is a marked increase in pressure or pronounced stretching of the intestinal wall, which physiologically probably do not occur, motility is inhibited after a latent period of 2–3 seconds. This entero-intestinal 'inhibitory reflex' (235) develops more rapidly as the stretching or pressure as well as the length of the intestinal segment involved increases.

f. pH

In addition to the caloric value of gastric and duodenal contents and osmosity, the pH also plays an important role (202). The contents of the duodenum are usually slightly acidic, depending upon the composition of the ingested food. It appears that prolonged closing of the pylorus is not caused by highly acidic contents alone; this also occurs when sodium bicarbonate is introduced via a tube causing the duodenal contents to become alkaline (36). This mechanism of duodenal neutralization is the most highly developed in hyperchlorhydria and the least in achlorhydria. The most sensitive reactions to tone and acidity occur in the proximal part of the duodenum and decrease in the distal direction (202).

In an empty stomach, the pyloric ring is relaxed which explains why the bulb is so often well-filled immediately after administration of the first few mouthfuls of barium in a gastric examination. Shortly afterwards the pylorus closes; the latent period for this reaction is several seconds. The tone of the gastric musculature depends upon the conditions in the duodenum and is the stimulus for the development of peristaltic waves. These peristaltic waves are, however, not necessary for gastric emptying; the stomach can also empty if there is sufficient tone and an open pyloric ring. The pylorus is more relaxed in achlorhydria than when there is free acid in the stomach. If the other conditions remain the same, then the stomach empties faster in achlorhydria.

g. EMOTIONS

Another well-known fact is that fear and emotions influence the small intestine by causing an increase in tone and an enhancement of the peristalsis. Because there is not enough time for the absorption of fluids, diarrhea develops. The opening and closing of the pylorus is a very complicated mechanism which is only partially understood. Almost everyone who has studied this mechanism has found that a peristaltic wave in the stomach is not necessarily followed by relaxation of the pyloric ring.

IV

THE CONTRAST MEDIUM

General considerations

During the second world war barium was the generally accepted contrast medium for examination of the small intestine. The 40-year-old custom of mixing nutrients with the contrast medium was abandoned since this appeared to be the main reason that good mucosal patterns could not be obtained. The importance of good reproduction of anatomical detail had become considerable since the morphological examination of the small intestine had replaced the functional examination. The omission of nutrients, however, did not improve the characteristics of the contrast medium such that it could now be regarded as ideal and was considered satisfactory by everyone. It had been recognized that a good contrast medium suited for examination of the digestive tract must satisfy many requirements, namely (240):

1. sedimentation may not occur after prolonged standing,
2. must mix easily with all secretion and digestive products found in the stomach and the small intestine without the development of flocculation and segmentation. The contrast medium must therefore also be insensitive to pH changes,
3. must adhere readily,
4. the viscosity may vary between that of water and that of cream but no more. In order to prevent the formation of stones due to fluid absorption in the colon and the distal ileum, a specific maximum viscosity may not be exceeded,
5. barium content must be high enough for good contrast,
6. must have a homogeneous structure,
7. must have a pleasant taste,
8. must be non-toxic,
9. must be inexpensive and easy to prepare without clumping or formation of foam. Later these characteristics were expanded to include:
10. must stimulate peristalsis.

Obviously it is not easy, if at all possible, to find a contrast medium which satisfies all of these requirements. Several of these factors will be discussed separately in more detail.

1. Sedimentation of the contrast medium

A well-known characteristic of barium powder is that it precipitates quickly in aqueous solutions, as does bismuth. In 1931 Holzknecht wrote in his handbook (94) that the colon mixture must be stirred until just before use. In the same book, Jozef Paluguay wrote that colloidal barium suspensions were on the market which gave a better reproduction of relief and which settled less quickly. He did not see the usefulness of these new media, however, because the same could be achieved by first boiling and then cooling the barium suspension.

The problem of sedimentation had already been studied extensively in 1947 by the pharmacologist Braeckman (23). He suggested that the formation of clumps of barium particles can be separated into an orthokinetic and a perikinetic coagulation. The former pertains to the larger particles and is caused by gravitation, the latter applies to the smaller particles and is caused by Brownian movement. Although an increase in the viscosity of the solution will cause a decrease in both types of clumping, perikinetic coagulation is more effectively combatted by adding an electrolyte or peptizing agent to the contrast suspension. In addition, there is of course less coagulation when the particles are smaller; it is also important that the particles be of equal size, otherwise the larger will act as nidus (Brown, 25).

Barium sulfate particles in water have a slight negative charge due to the OH groups on their surface. The agglomeration of these particles is decreased by increasing their negative charge. Brown achieved this by adding a small amount of an electrolyte with many hydroxyl groups, such as sodium carboxymethylcellulose. Braeckman obtained the best results in his experiments with a mixture of 7.5 per cent arabic gum and 0.01 N. sodium citrate. On a graph, he showed the differences between the rate of sedimentation of a mixture of $BaSO_4$ and 0.01 N. sodium citrate and the rate of sedimentation, of the same mixture with 7.5 per cent arabic gum (fig. 4.1). If too much hydrophilic colloid is added, then the negative charge will become too high and clumping will again occur as a result of the strong mutual repul-

sion. During this phenomenon, called 'super settling', a barium mass develops which is so hard and compact that it can no longer be dissolved. A suspension with such a high negative charge has the advantage of being almost insensitive to pH changes in the digestive tract. Therefore mucus and other substances found in the digestive tract will not cause flocculation. Since in any event 'super settling' must be avoided, some tendency toward flocculation is unfortunately necessary. The rate of sedimentation of many barium sulfate preparations now on the market is so low that this factor no longer plays a role in the examination of patients. The stomach and the intestine are in sufficient continuous motion to prevent pure sedimentation. Letters and Gaul (128) had already reached this conclusion in 1951.

2. Flocculation of the contrast fluid

A phenomenon which perhaps appears quite similar to sedimentation but must definitely be differentiated from it is the flocculation of barium particles in the contrast suspension when it comes into contact with specific substances found in the digestive tract, such as hydrochloric acid, gall and mucin. Mucin is coated with colloidal protein polymers which are usually amphoteric: it is therefore positive in acidic and negative in basic surroundings. Under normal circumstances therefore a massive clumping with the negatively charged barium particles will occur in the stomach. We observe this phenomenon as flocculation. It had already been reported in 1931 by Berg and in 1932 by Frik (62). Knoefel et al. (112) demonstrated that a 10 per cent solution of barium sulfate flocculates 10 times as fast in gastric juice as in water. An increase in the amount of gastric juice causes a further increase in the rate of flocculation until a specific limiting value has been reached, apparently when all the mucoprotein has combined. Sedimentation appears to be mainly a physical process, flocculation a chemical process. A contrast medium prepared from barium powder with very tiny particles of approximately the same size, which in addition has a cream-like viscosity and contains a peptizing agent, will produce practically no sedimentation. Experience with patients has, however, shown that

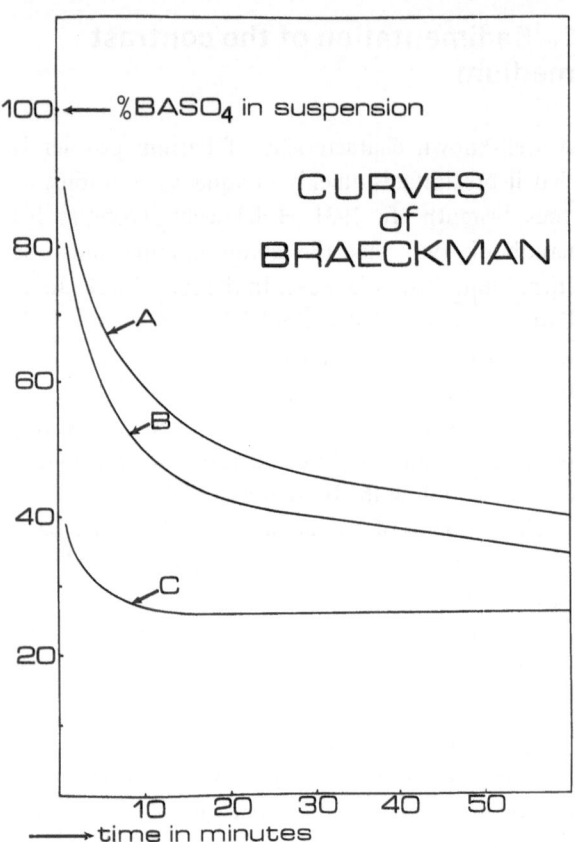

Fig. 4.1
Difference in rate of sedimentation of following mixtures:
A. $BaSO_4$ + 0.01 citr. Na + 7.5% gum. arab.
B. $BaSO_4$ + 7.5% gum. arab.
C. $BaSO_4$ + 0.01 N. citr. Na

this same medium can, in spite of continuous movement, still produce pronounced flocculation when gastric acid or other juices found in the digestive tract are added. The precipitation caused by sedimentation in vitro has a homogeneous structure. Flocculation on the other hand produces a precipitation with a coarse, splotchy structure; a complete change in the viscosity of the contrast medium is even possible (fig. 4B). Also in vivo, flocculation can be recognized by the coarse, splotchy structure of the contrast medium in the intestinal lumen; this is called the 'snowflake pattern'. The finely spotted pattern usually left behind after the contrast medium has passed through the jejunum is also caused by flocculation of the barium residual. In general it can be stated that these floccules will be smaller when the contrast fluid adheres less readily to the mucosa so that less barium is left behind.

Deucher (42) introduced barium into isolated intestinal loops in surgical patients during the operation and induced peristalsis with an injection of prostigmin. He then made roentgenograms which showed a finely spotted distribution of the contrast medium in the intestinal loops. In addition he noted that the outline of the intestinal lumen could not be distinguished clearly (fig. 4.2). Deucher was not able to give a convincing explanation for these phenomena. The retention of contrast fluid between swollen folds which were not able to contract seemed to him the most likely explanation. He assumed that the mucosal swelling was caused by a disturbance in the blood circulation since there were no indications of an infectious process in the intestinal wall. It is clear that in fact we are confronted here with such a complete flocculation of the contrast fluid that there is no barium left in the suspension at all. The difference between the specific gravity of the suspension fluid and that of the tissue of the intestinal wall has therefore become so small that the outline of the intestinal lumen can no longer be seen.

Deucher showed quite clearly with this experiment that no further morphological information can be obtained once flocculation has occurred. Many radiologists have found that a small dose of contrast medium causes more flocculation than a large dose. It has long been known that flocculation

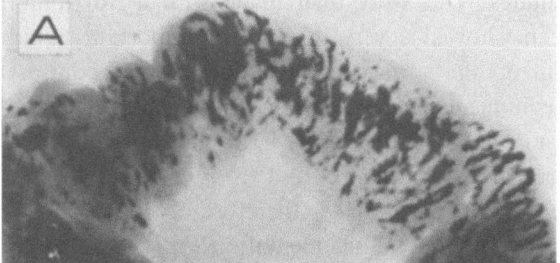
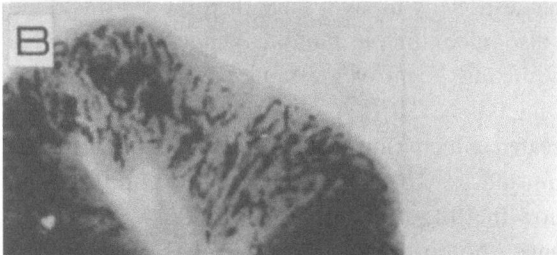
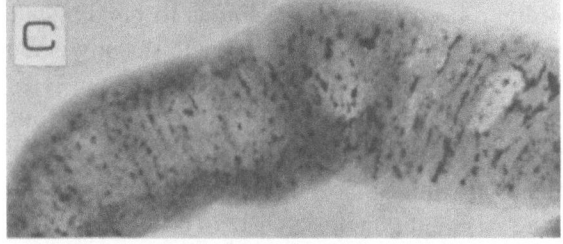
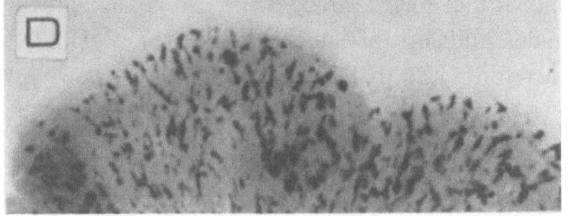

Fig. 4.2
Contrast fluid in isolated intestinal loop during surgery. There is practically no barium left in suspension. Peristalsis induced by injection of Prostigmin.
A, B. beginning of clump formation.
C, D. flocculation (snowflake pattern) (Deucher 1949).

occurs in the foremost part of the contrast column, which disappears as soon as more contrast medium is administered (175). Patterson even saw flocculation develop with the exceedingly stable Raybar which he introduced directly into the duodenum. For the patients he examined in this way, however, he only used 40 ml of this contrast medium (170).

In a series of in vitro experiments we studied the occurrence of sedimentation and flocculation. Five barium suspensions of various brands were placed in test tubes, agitated and then set aside for 30 minutes. The x-ray then made with a horizontal beam showed a very thin and unimportant liquid film on the surface of several brands of contrast medium and some sediment at the bottom of the test tube for others (fig. 4.3A). In particular the structure of brands (2) and (3) appears to remain very homogeneous. It is therefore obvious that the annoying effect of sedimentation no longer plays a role, especially in vivo, since then the contrast fluid is also in continuous motion. The test was repeated by mixing 15 ml of the same contrast media with 5 ml 0.1 N. HCl. A contrast-acid ratio is then created which can occur under physiological circumstances. The films made after 30 min (fig. 4.3B) show that the structure of brand (2) is definitely no longer homogeneous (flocculation). The contrast medium has acquired a gelatinous to pudding-like consistency and only after energetic shaking could it be removed from the test tube. Brand (3) appeared to be insensitive to the addition of the acid while brand (4) flocculated completely. Although most brands of contrast medium on the market can withstand basic substances better than acidic, tests have shown that their characteristics can change greatly under influence of intestinal juice (57, 241). It is therefore clear that barium suspensions can lose

their most valuable characteristics completely in vivo.

It was exceedingly difficult for the chemical industry to produce a contrast medium which retains its stability in both acidic and basic surroundings. Fig. 4.3AB shows that not every manufacturer has been successful in this respect.

The fact that the factors responsible for flocculation of the contrast medium were not recognized is certainly the most important reason for the slow development of the radiological differential diagnosis of diseases of the small intestine. Golden assumed that the flocculation and subsequent disintegration into segment clumps of the contrast column resulted from a disturbed motor function of the small intestine, which is a dominant symptom of sprue and is caused by abnormalities in the intramural nervous system of the intestinal wall (75). Bouslog (22) agreed with Golden's interpretation because the nervous system in the intestinal wall of babies only a few months old is still underdeveloped and during the examination of the small intestine of these babies, he observed only that the contrast fluid flocculates and finally disintegrates into segment clumps. Caffey supported the assumption of a disordered motor function by reporting

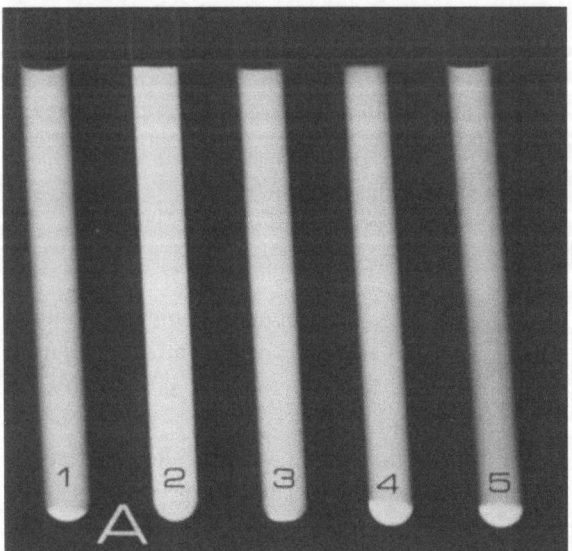 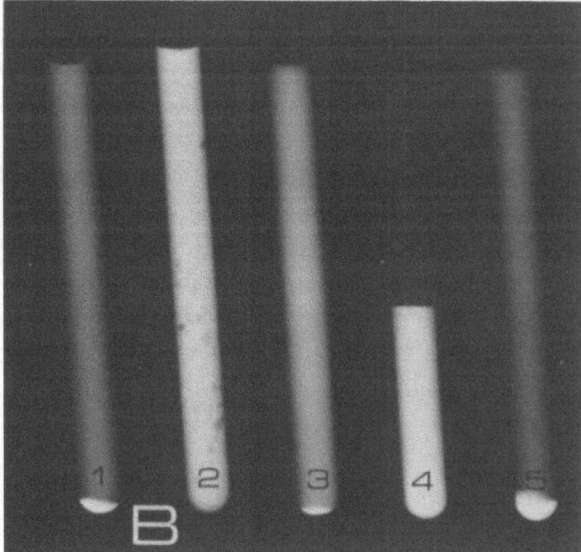

Fig. 4.3
In vitro tests with 5 current brands of contrast medium, numbered 1–5.
A. After standing for 30 min, only slight sedimentation of barium particles.
B. 15 ml of the same contrast fluids used in (A) mixed with 5 ml 1/10 N. HCl. x-ray after 30 min brand (2) shows flocculation; for brand (4), there is practically no barium left in suspension.

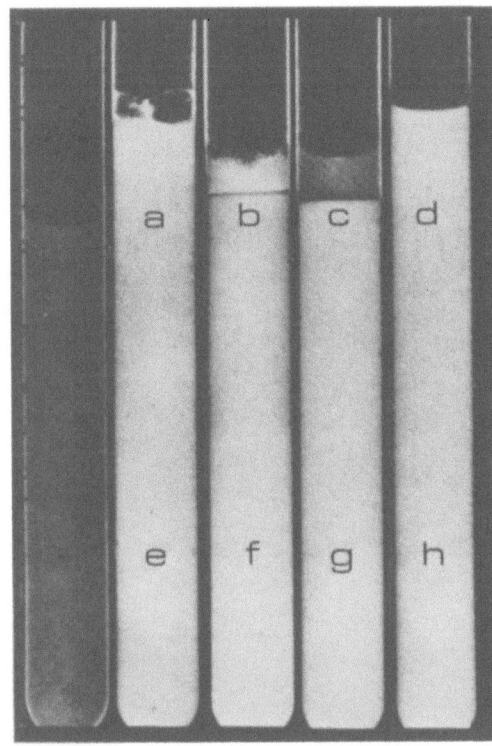
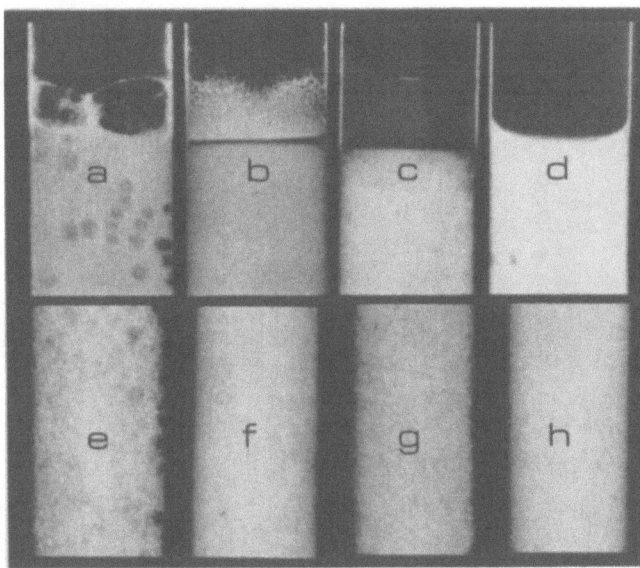

Fig. 4.4

A. X-ray of 4 barium sulfate suspensions to which artificial gastric juice (pH 1.8–2) is added.

a, e pure barium sulfate; b, f high quality brand; c, g low quality brand; d, h Alubar 'Wander'.

Suspensions a, e and c, g show flocculation.

a, b, c, d: detail exposures of fluid surface; e, f, g, h: detail exposures below fluid surface.

that passage through the small intestine lasted 5 to 6 hours for new-born children. In addition some radiologists, including Golden, Friedman (60) and Goin (72), had found that fear and emotions could cause sudden flocculation of the barium suspension, a phenomenon which is said to have also been observed in animals.

Many other radiologists, even including Reynolds et al. (189) in 1940, proved convincingly that flocculation of the contrast fluid can at least be caused by factors other than the above-mentioned, such as gastric acid, hypertonic solutions, proteins and fats. The authority of Golden was, however, so great that his neurogenic theory was still generally accepted.

Not until 1949 were many converted by the publication of Frazer, French and Thompson (57), who used an extensive series of tests to show that flocculation of the barium suspension in the small intestine of completely normal individuals can be caused by many factors. To avoid the influence of gastric acid, the contrast medium as well as the substances to be tested were administered through a tube directly into the duodenum. They observed flocculation followed by segmentation after adding: hypertonic solutions, acetic acid, lactic acid, fatty acids, olive oil, unsaturated fatty acids (sprue patients) and gastric mucus. Gall only caused flocculation in acidic surroundings, not for a pH greater than 6.4. To rebut Golden's theory in a spectacular manner, they demonstrated that the barium suspension also flocculated in the intestines of a deceased person where a disordered motor function such as Golden supposed cannot possibly exist. Furthermore it appeared that flocculation followed by segmentation developed in persons who had consumed a meal rich in fats the evening before the examination.

In the same year, Zimmer (240) compared the characteristics of Alubar, which he considered to be a superior contrast medium, with those of an ordinary barium sulfate suspension and two com-

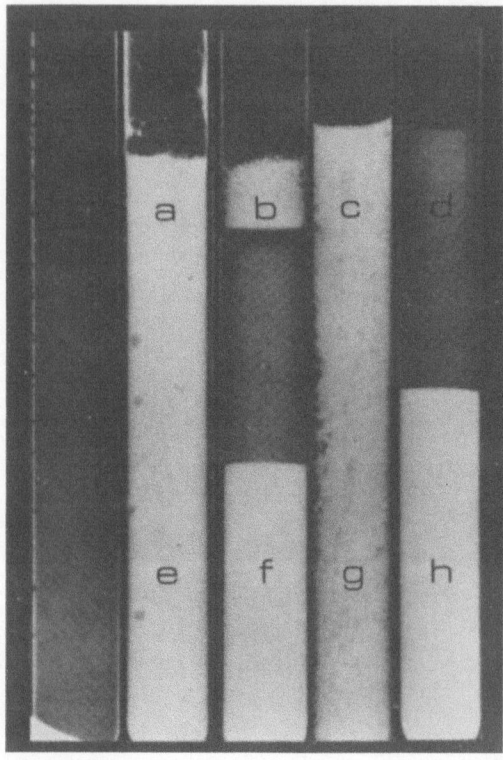
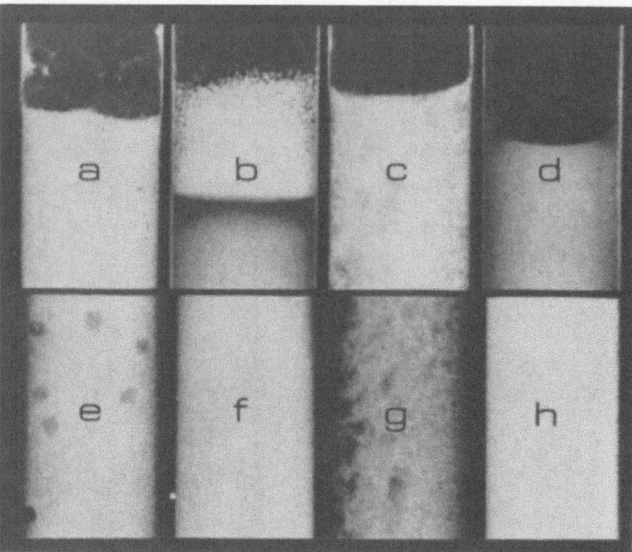

Fig. 4.4
B. Same test as A, but with artificial intestinal juice (pH 8.2–8.4).

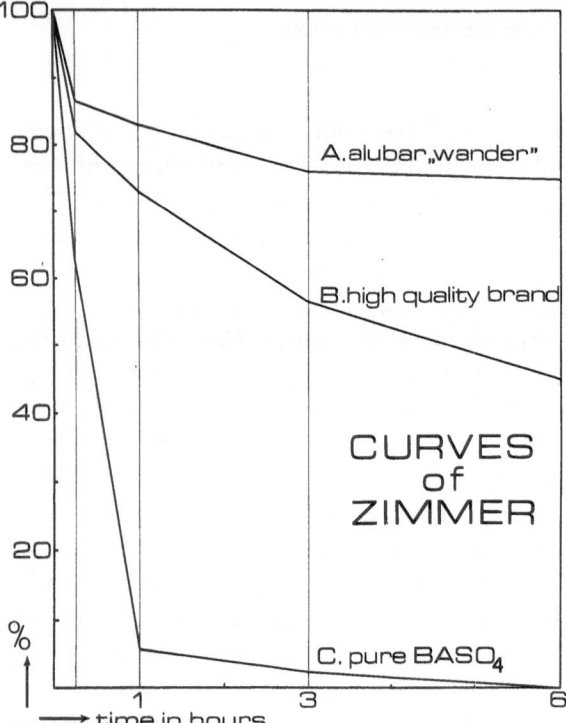

Fig. 4.5
Sedimentation curves of ZIMMER (1949). Difference between Alubar 'Wander', a high quality brand and a barium suspension without additives.

mercial products by adding artificial gastric juice with a pH of 1.8–2 and artificial intestinal juice with a pH of 8.2–8.4. The roentgenograms made show varying degrees of structural change for at least 2 of the 4 contrast fluids which are highly similar to the changes noted for brand (2) during our experiments (fig. 4.4AB). The rate of flocculation under the influence of gastric and intestinal juices was also measured for these 4 contrast fluids; the resulting values were plotted on a graph (fig. 4.5). He then studied the homogeneity and the adhesion for these suspensions. Alubar appeared to be better than the ordinary $BaSO_4$ in all respects. In his conclusion he writes that the use of a pure $BaSO_4$ suspension will often lead to the unjustified diagnosis of sprue.

One year later, Ardran, French and Mucklow (9) also proved that a colloidal barium suspension does not flocculate in children with celiac disease, but that a normal barium suspension does. After these publications many others of similar intent followed, but there are still radiologists who have remained more or less loyal to Golden's theory of disordered motor function. In 1959, Golden himself seemed to have similar difficulties in abandoning his original line of thought when he wrote:

'Flocculation is undoubtedly caused by the contents of the intestine and has been attributed to mucus. In as much as mucus is always present the question arises as to whether this effect is related to the quantity or to some unknown quality of the mucus. Flocculation may occur as a result of emotional disturbances. It may appear and disappear in an individual during a period of an hour or two for no obvious reason '(74). Meanwhile, he prefers barium suspensions which do not flocculate but does not see any advantage in all kinds of special examination techniques.

He still administers 240 ml contrast medium orally and if necessary, takes spot films. Since Gianturco's article in 1953, he uses the 'high voltage' technique because with a low voltage only marginal information is obtained (fig. 4.6).

At a congress in 1960, in reference to a demonstration of the radiologic examination of the small intestine where a tumor was not localized, Golden clearly indicated that his opinions had changed in the meantime by stating: 'It would seem that a tumor such as this should easily be detected by a small intestine study (barium follow-through). The segmentation was so great and the distribution so uneven that the tumor could not be demonstrated. It seems possible that this might have been demonstrated by a small bowel enema'.

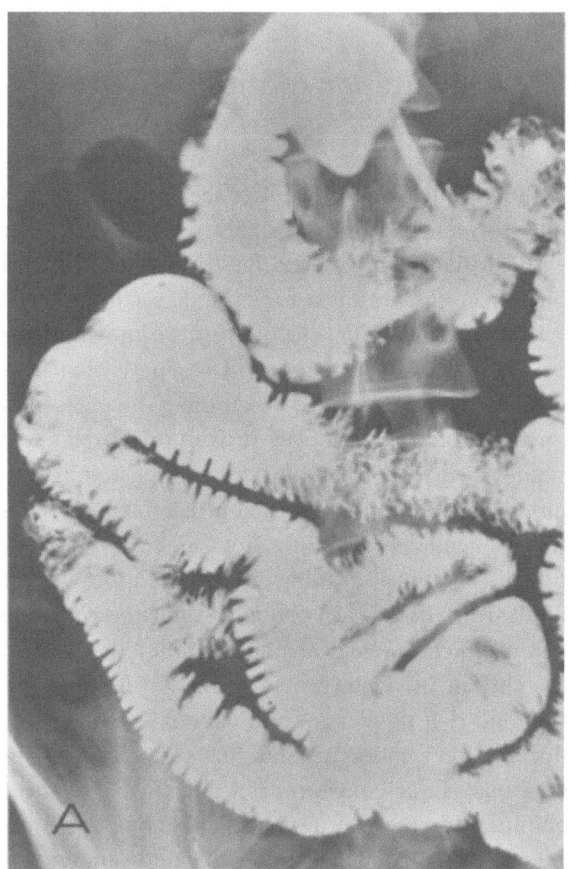

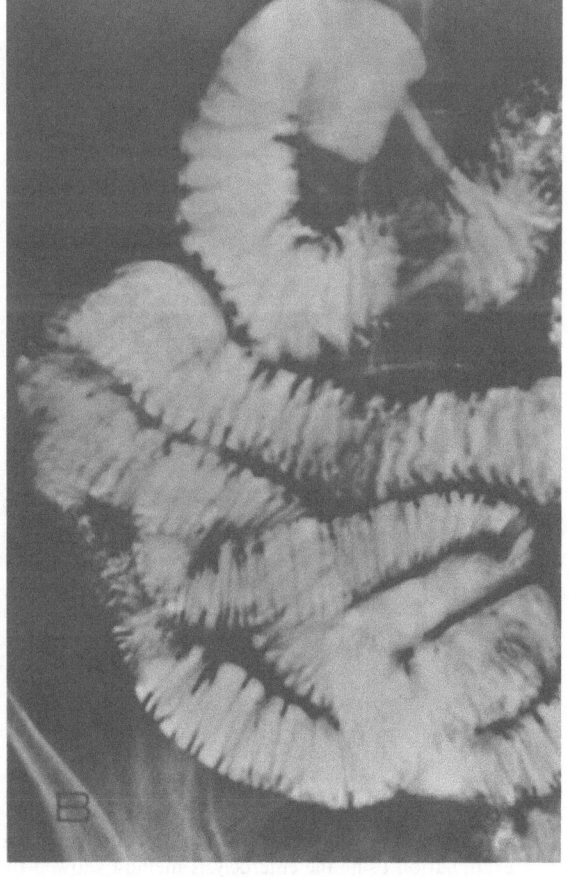

Fig. 4.6
Decrease in contrast and increase in information when a higher voltage is used (A: 80 kV, B: 120 kV). Film density equal for both exposures.

3. Segmentation of the contrast column

Although the disintegration of the contrast column into segment clumps is usually observed together with flocculation, a separate discussion of this phenomenon is justified for several reasons.

The segmentation picture was known long before that of flocculation. The reason is that flocculation is only obtained when the patient receives a reasonably homogeneous suspension of relatively small particles. When it was still customary to mix nutrients through the contrast medium, this requirement was certainly not satisfied. As mentioned previously, owing to the withdrawal of fluids from the contrast column, segmentation in the colon is a physiological phenomenon: this is also the case in the ileum when transit is very slow. In the fluid-rich duodenum and jejunum such massive flocculation can occur that this can result in increasingly large conglomerates and finally segment clumps. In the thirties, this phenomenon was frequently seen in the duodenum and jejunum of infants; a reasonable explanation was unknown

(22). Autopsy material had shown that mucosal folds were definitely present; the fact that Henderson had indeed observed these folds on roentgenological films when the stomach emptied rapidly also could not be explained (87).

In 1934, Snell and Camp described the segmentation of the contrast column in sprue. They saw clumping of the barium and disappearance of the fold relief. They are to be respected for the fact that even then they believed that this was not a specific symptom but that the same could be observed for other 'diffuse infections'. In 1939 Kantor (105) described the 'moulage sign' which can be seen in the duodenum or jejunum, where the rigid barium column resembles a wax mold without fold relief (fig. 4.7AB). He only saw this picture in highly advanced cases of sprue and therefore he thought that in these cases the fold relief was greatly flattened or absent altogether. In fact there will probably always be a heavy and early occurrence of clumping of the barium suspension in such cases. When the

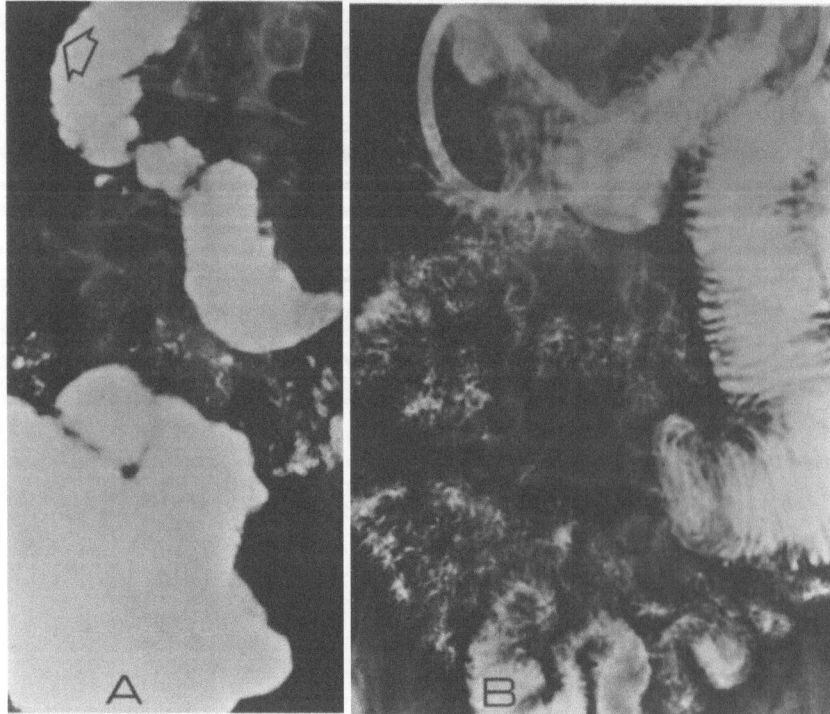

Fig. 4.7

AB. 'Moulage' sign in the duodenum of a patient with celiac disease is caused by total disintegration of the contrast fluid and a pronounced increase in viscosity so that reproduction of the mucosal folds has become impossible (A). A repeat examination using the enteroclysis method showed that the mucosal folds do in fact exist (B).

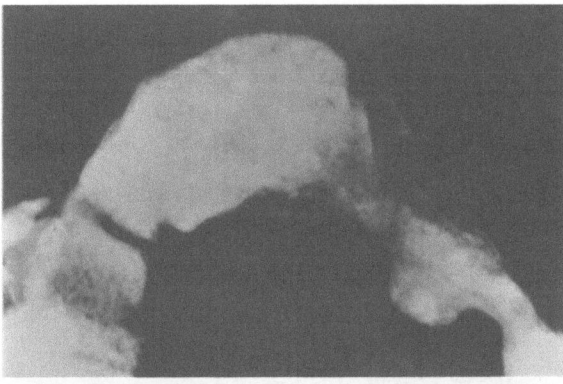

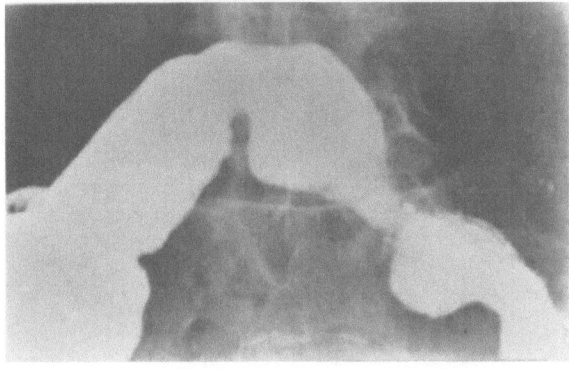

Fig. 4.8
Only when the radiation dose is high enough can it be seen that the structure of a disintegrating barium suspension has become granular; in other words underexposure completely masks the fact that a contrast fluid can no longer be used.

roentgenograms are overexposed, then the barium-column has a grainy structure (fig. 4.8). In a case of pure mucosal atrophy, without signs of malabsorption, this structure must be homogeneous. Kantor's conclusion that the moulage sign could be considered an indication of the severity of the sprue often might still be correct, in spite of the opinion of Snell and Camp; however, this picture has absolutely nothing to do with the condition of the mucous membrane.

In 1961 Marshak (139) was of the opinion that the moulage sign could be the result of hypersecretion and segmentation but in the same article he does mention his surprise that he also saw string sign-like configurations and coarse mucosal folds, which do not seem to agree with the normal autopsy findings. The quality of the published roentgenograms is, however, poor and they are so distorted by flocculation and segmentation that this incongruity between radiological and autopsy findings is not strange. Fig. 4.9 shows that flocculation and segment

formation of the barium suspension led to an apparent flattening and coarsening of the mucosal folds. Patterns are even possible which do not resemble the actual situation in the least.

From the above it must be concluded that a radiological examination of the small intestine should be terminated when the contrast fluid shows clear signs of disintegration and is apparently no longer able to provide real images of the intestinal mucosa. It would be ideal if a contrast medium was available which is highly stable, moderately viscous and adheres readily. In order to prevent the annoying effect of dehydration and thickening of the barium column in the distal ileum during slow transit, it is also desirable that the contrast medium be protected against unlimited fluid withdrawal. Of the numerous attempts undertaken to improve the characteristics of the contrast media, only the most important shall be discussed.

4. Additives to the contrast medium for the purpose of improving stability and adhesion

Many radiologists have tried this method to increase the adhesion of the contrast medium to the mucous membrane of the digestive tract. An improvement in adhesion is usually also accompanied by a decrease in the sedimentation and flocculation tendencies of the contrast medium; therefore an attempt aimed specifically at the latter cannot easily be distinguished from the former. Due to the importance of double-contrast exposures for the colon examination, good adhesion is even more important for this examination than for an examination of the small intestine, while the reverse holds for sedimentation and flocculation. Adhesion of the barium meal to the intestinal mucosa could be increased by adding tannin since this substance causes precipitation of proteins on the cellular surfaces and decreases the mucin secretion.

For a long time, tannin was used for the colon examination in concentrations of 0.3 to 3 per cent in the cleansing enema and in the contrast medium. Since it has become known that tannin is absorbed by the mucous membrane (113) and 8 fatal cases resulting from necrosis of the liver have been described, use of this substance has been forbidden in

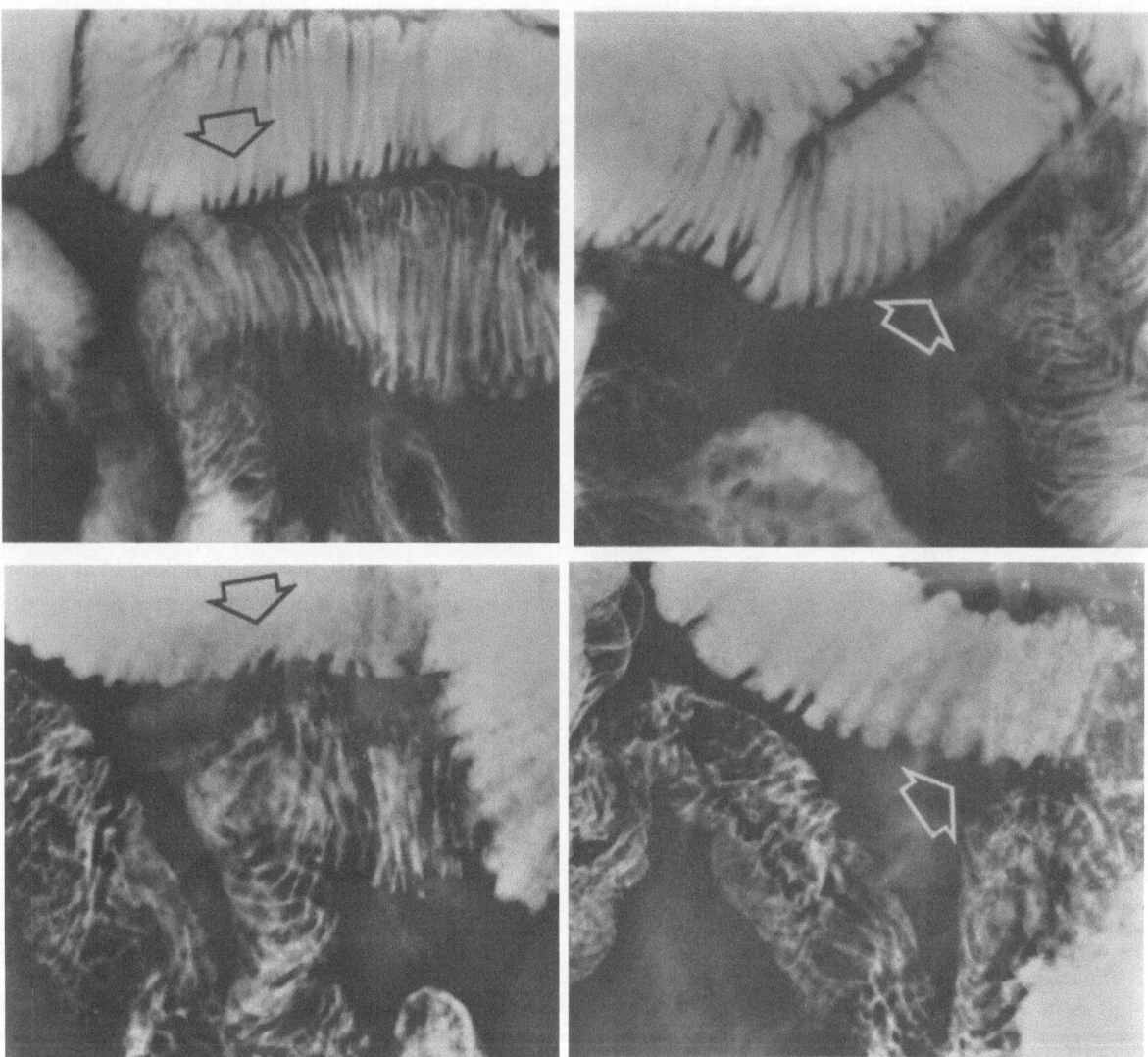

Fig. 4.9
On the 2 uppermost exposures the mucosal folds appear normal; disintegration of the contrast fluid then developed rapidly with flattening and apparent coarsening of the mucosal folds (2 lowermost exposures). The structure of the contrast fluid has become granular.

America (6). Some do not agree with this decision since they believe that in these cases, the possibility of overdosage exists (96). Tannin is found in tea and, it is said, in red wine. It is not only hepatotoxic but is also believed to be carcinogenic. When perforations occur and the barium mixture containing tannin enters the abdominal cavity, a serious chemical peritonitis develops. To avoid lethal termination acute surgical intervention and cleaning of the abdominal cavity is absolutely necessary.

As far as we know, tannin has never played a role of any importance in the examination of the small intestine although the influence of a cup of strong tea consumed the evening before the examination has never been studied.

In 1938 Wooldman (232) reported that the addition of colloidal aluminum hydroxyde to the contrast medium produced good results. This substance is slightly astringent, does not irritate and is amphoteric. He had noticed during operations and in autopsy material that a contrast medium containing this substance adheres quite readily to the mucosa.

In 1953, Schufflebarger et al. (206) tried to improve adhesion to the mucous membrane by decreasing the secretion from the intestinal wall in animals and later also patients. They injected histamine and atropine but were not successful. They did note that the best results were obtained in patients with hypotonic, ptotic stomachs.

Alexander (5) believed that adhesion would be improved if the barium suspension mixed easily with the mucus; he therefore added 1 per cent mucin. He reported improvement for the examination of the small intestine and the colon, but not for the esophageal and gastric examinations.

Embring and Mattsson (46) added a wetting agent (tweens, sodium lauryl sulfate and saponins) to enhance the mixing of 2 different water phases, but they were not very enthusiastic about their results.

Many radiologists (25, 46, 111, 174 and others) added carboxymethyl cellulose or its sodium salt to the barium suspension and in general reported good results with this combination. The sodium CMC does cause an increase in viscosity but does not dissolve in gastric juice and does not appear to adhere as readily as the CMC in a 0.5 per cent concentration. Both substances are highly hydrophilic and therefore accelerate transit.

Both the binding of water and the acceleration of transit protect the barium suspension against excessive fluid withdrawal in the ileum. A slight disadvantage of the contrast media containing hydrophilic colloids to restrict dehydration in the ileum is that they cannot be used to diagnose a disacchari-dase deficiency (118). Micropaque therefore does not contain these colloids; however, for prolonged transit times there is the disadvantage of pronounced dehydration in the distal ileum as a result of fluid withdrawal. Other substances which have occasionally been used to improve the adhesion of the contrast medium are tragacanth and arabic gum (2, 87). The results described vary widely; this may be a result of the various dosages used. Henderson did not see any improvements when 10 ml 2 per cent arabic gum was added, an observation which we can confirm. We have found that the addition of 10 volume per cent of the total amount of the contrast medium, thus a considerably higher dosage, does produce satisfactory results. This suspension, however, is rather viscous and only becomes thinner and more liquid in patients with sufficient

gastric acid. This decrease in viscosity is not accompanied by flocculation at all; in this case the gastric acid is apparently bound chemically. This chemical combining of the gastric acid must be regarded as specifically preventing flocculation; substances which bind mucin have the same effect. In addition to the above-mentioned substances, many others have been tested; as a result it has been demonstrated clearly that no single additive has been found which is ideal. Some of these substances are: buttermilk, olive oil, sodium oleate, fecal fat from sprue patients, diverse carbohydrates, lactic acid, citric acid, gelatin, agar and pectin.

5. Relationship between viscosity, particle size and adhesion of the barium suspension

Although the adhesive capacity of a suspension can be increased by adding several substances, a minimum viscosity is also a necessary requirement. An increase in the viscosity, however, has the disadvantage of retarding the rate of transit through the pylorus and small intestine. An additional difficulty is that when the viscosity of the contrast medium is too high, the adhesive layer left behind can become annoyingly thick (fig. 4.10). The correct (creamy) viscosity for the suspension, however, does not guarantee that adhesion will be good.

Some radiologists have tried to obtain a clearly visible adhesive layer by preparing solutions with a high specific gravity and a very low viscosity. One example is Brown's mixture (25). He used sodium carboxymethyl cellulose, heparin and sodium dextran sulfate or sodium cellulose acetate to obtain a thin, liquid suspension containing 75 weight per cent barium. Embring and Mattsson (45) also obtained a thin, liquid, as well as stable barium suspension with a specific gravity of approximately 3 as follows: they added 1 g sodium citrate and 9 g Sorbitol to a paste-like mixture of 100 g $BaSO_4$ and 40 ml water; a pronounced decrease in viscosity resulted. However, for filling exposures of even the relatively thin ileum a barium suspension with a specific gravity of 3 is much too high and therefore not desirable; only marginal diagnoses can be made with this medium.

For double-contrast exposures, it is in principle

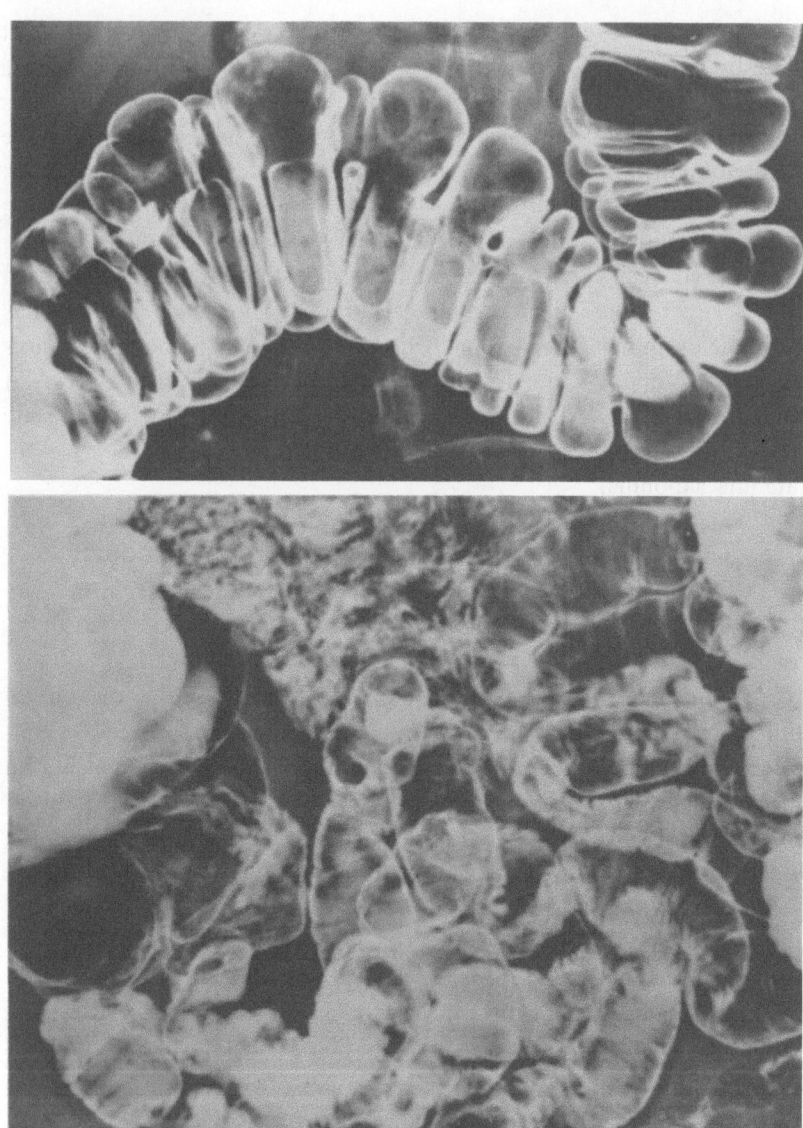

Fig. 4.10
Layer of barium suspension on the intestinal wall is too thick because the viscosity of
the contrast fluid is too high. Double contrast exposure of the colon at the end of the
small intestine examination.

a question of personal preference whether a thin
liquid suspension with a high specific gravity or a
thicker liquid suspension with a lower specific
gravity is used; a clearly visible layer can be obtained
with both.

Various radiologists, even including Adam (2) in
1932, have shown that for a good adhesive layer in
double-contrast exposures, the colloidal chemical
relationships are more important than the particle
size. For suspensions with a low viscosity a particle
size of less than 0.4 microns can even be a disadvantage instead of an advantage. Both the
specific gravity and the thickness of the adhesive
layer are then insufficient for the double-contrast
examination and thus all the factors for a barely
visible adhesive layer are present.

Brown pointed out that for the same weight of
barium, the viscosity of a suspension increases as
the size of the particles decreases and that the adhesion decreases as soon as the barium content in a

suspension becomes greater than 45 weight per cent. Many who have prepared barium suspensions themselves for an examination of the esophageal varices will have experienced the truth of this observation.

When requested, the manufacturers of contrast media usually do not supply adequate information about the chemical composition of their product. It was found that often the data supplied were not even correct; this was also true for the particle size given.

Microscopic studies have proven that the grains were usually much larger than indicated, sometimes even significantly larger than prescribed by the American pharmacopeia (154). In addition the relative differences in the grain size of the diverse products on the market appeared to be a factor of 4 (45). Schufflebarger et al. (206) made diagrams of the grain size distribution of 6 different brands of barium sulfate and showed that most of the powders also displayed a marked lack of homogeneity. Moreton and Yates (156) compared 4 commercial preparations and obtained similar results.

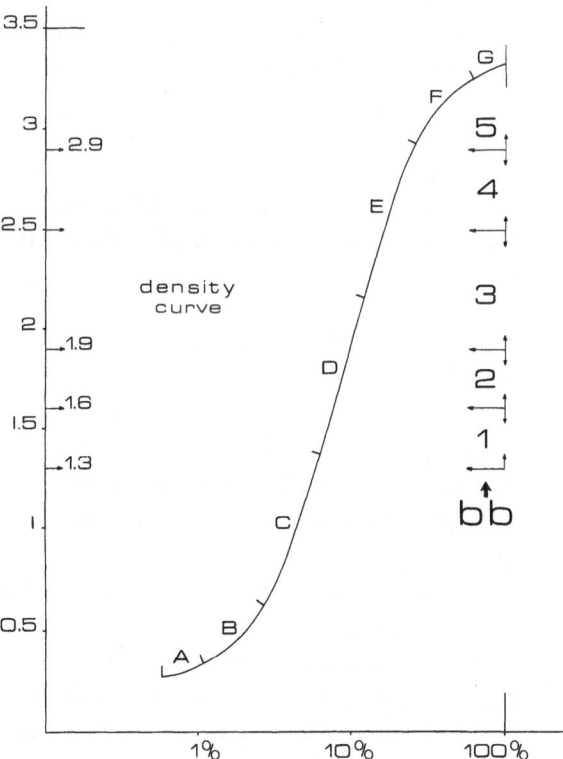

Fig. 4.11
Schematical representation of a film density curve. Background blackenings 1, 2, 3, 4 and 5 (figs. 4.12/4.18) are indicated on the curve.

6. Specific gravity of the contrast fluid

We have found that generally this exceedingly important factor has not received sufficient attention and often barium suspensions are used with a specific gravity which is much too high. The choice of the barium content for a suspension is apparently influenced by the spectacular sight of snowwhite intestinal loops, preferably against the background blackening of a normally exposed abdominal survey film. As long as there are no annoying effects of superposition, only small abnormalities on the contours of the intestinal loops can be seen clearly on these photographs. In addition the other organs in the abdomen will also be seen since their blackening falls in the midportion of the density curve (fig. 4.11, section D). Masses in the lumen of the intestine, however, will be easily missed since there is insufficient contrast difference with the intense white parts of the intestinal loops which lie in the lowermost part of the density curve (fig. 4.11, section A). It will be obvious that with this exposure technique, only 2 very small segments of the contours of these snow-white intestinal loops are visible. The specific gravity of the human body differs only slightly from that of water and can be set at approximately 1. The specific gravity of a concentrated barium suspension, such as undiluted liquid Micropaque, is approximately 1.75. The difference in specific gravity between this contrast fluid and the human body is approximately 0.75, thus even less than the difference in specific gravity between the human body and air which is slightly less than 1.

From this it could be concluded that air could perhaps be an ideal as well as very inexpensive contrast medium for the examination of the digestive tract. However, a disadvantage of air is that its specific gravity cannot be regulated by means of dilution like the positive contrast media. In addition air is not capable of adhering to the mucosa and therefore cannot leave traces of its presence. Air is also not able to mix with mucus secretion and therefore cannot penetrate the narrow spaces which are filled with fluids. The greatest disadvantage of air, however, is that disturbing contrast differences caused by solitary gas bubbles are located in approximately the same section of the density curve as contrast differences of the intestinal loops filled with gas. The result is that an isolated gas bubble for instance could not be differentiated from a diverticulum of either the anterior or the posterior intestinal wall. Unhindered evaluation of the intestinal loops and the contrast fluctuations caused by diverticula and polypoid tumors can best be made when:

1. the density of these loops differs markedly from that of the (irrelevant) background and its fluctuations,
2. the contrast fluctuations caused by pathological processes of the intestinal wall fall in the steep part of the density curve and can therefore be seen as clearly as possible,
3. the background fluctuations fall in the highest possible section of the density curve, and therefore cause the least possible disturbance.

From the above, it can be seen that theoretically the density of the intestinal loops can best fall in section C and the density for the rest of the abdomen in section G of this curve. The specific gravity of the contrast fluid should then be chosen such that small bulges of the intestinal lumen and narrow fistulous tracts can be seen clearly on the one hand, while on the other hand, mucosal folds and small masses, even in the lumen of wide loops, do not escape our attention. It is known that a high voltage exposure technique levels out the contrasts; this has a favourable effect on the density of both the background and the intestinal loops filled with contrast fluid (fig. 5.6). A film blackening such that the background falls in section G of the curve would, however, mean a very high radiation dose for the patient.

Therefore we thought it would be useful to experiment with a phantom to determine how much the background blackening with its fluctuations can be decreased without interfering with the evaluation of the contrast differences in the intestinal loops. It also seemed worthwhile during these experiments to test contrast fluids of different specific gravity in order to determine which specific gravity (s.g.) gives maximum information.

In a 15 cm thick phantom filled with water which acted as scattering medium, we placed plastic pipes with diameters of 22 and 34 mm. The plastic pipes were filled with barium suspensions with s.g. of 1.65, 1.32 and 1.2. In each plastic pipe was a nylon thread holding wooden beads with diameters of 5, 7, 9, and 12 mm. Roentgenograms were made with a voltage of 125 kV and increasing degrees of density of the background (henceforth designated as: d.b.), numbered from 1 to 5. These 5 levels were chosen such that they adequately represented the upper half of the density curve (fig. 4.11). The walls of the plastic pipes could still be seen with d.b. 3; with d.b. 4 they were no longer clearly visible.

The results were as follows:

I.   For the contrast medium with a s.g. of 1.65 in the 22 mm pipe, the largest bead could be seen vaguely with d.b. 2; not until d.b. 4 were 4 beads visible in this pipe. They could be observed most clearly with d.b. 5 in the 34 mm pipe, the 3 largest beads were just visible with d.b. 5 (fig. 4.12).

II. For the contrast fluid with a s.g. of 1.32 in the 22 mm pipe, visibility of all 4 beads increased as the d.b. increased from 2 to 4.

Although clearer with d.b. 4, all 4 beads in the 34 mm pipe were already visible with d.b. 3; the smallest was very vague. With d.b. 2 no beads were visible in the large pipe (fig. 4.13).

III. For the contrast fluid with a s.g. of 1.2, the visibility of all 4 beads in both pipes increased as the d.b. increased from 1 to 3 (fig. 4.14).

IV. In the small pipe, the beads in the contrast fluid with a s.g. of 1.32 and a certain d.b. were as clearly visible as the beads in the contrast fluid with a s.g. of 1.2 and one d.b. lower.

V.   When the film density is even higher, the same applies for the large pipe.

The contrast fluid with a s.g. of 1.2 revealed the beads in the large pipe somewhat more clearly with d.b. 2 than the fluid with a s.g. of 1.32 with d.b. 3. This difference in visibility of the beads in the large pipe increases as the d.b. decreases to the advantage of the contrast fluid with the lowest specific gravity.

The experiment was repeated but this time the wooden beads were not located in the middle of the plastic pipes but along the wall. Fig. 4.15 shows the results, which are similar to those of the previous experiment. Once again it was apparent that the wooden beads are most clearly visible when the film density is high; in all cases, however, with the same d.b. they are more clearly visible than in the previous experiment. There is again no difference in clearness in the small pipe between a s.g. of 1.32 with a certain d.b. and a s.g. of 1.2 with one d.b. less. In the large pipe, however, as the d.b. decreases the beads were significantly clearer in the contrast fluid with the lowest specific gravity.

The results with a s.g. of 1.65 were again very disappointing, although somewhat less than in the previous experiment.

For the actual examination of the digestive tract, the results of these experiments offer the following:

1. A s.g. of 1.65 is always much too high for the contrast fluid and a d.b. in the lower half of the density curve is always too low. A combination of these 2 factors is particularly unfavourable, especially for a colon examination.
2. The combination of a relatively high d.b. (approx. 3) and a contrast fluid with a low s.g. yields the most information. When the s.g. of the contrast fluid is decreased, the d.b. can also be decreased without a loss of information. This means a lower radiation dose for the patient.
3. For the colon examination, the specific gravity of the contrast fluid must be lower than for a transit examination and the density of the background must be higher.
4. The loss in information due to underexposure of the x-ray films is less when a contrast fluid with a low specific gravity is used. The loss in information due to a contrast fluid with a high specific gravity can be compensated by overexposure of the x-ray film.

In order to evaluate the disturbance caused by fluctuations in the density of the background, a new experiment was carried out. A transverse, air-filled plastic pipe 22 mm in diameter was introduced into the water phantom. This pipe crossed the 2 pipes filled with contrast fluid. This time we used barium suspensions with specific gravities of 1.32 and 1.16, and once again exposures with varying d.b. were made.

The results were as follows (fig. 4.16):

1. The disturbing influence of the differences in contrast of the lumen and the wall of the air pipe is the least for the background when the density is high (sections F and G) and for the pipes filled with contrast fluid, when the density is low (sections A and B).
2. The disturbing positive and negative influences of the air pipe are greater for the background as the density decreases and for the contrast column as the specific gravity of the barium suspension decreases.

In spite of the fact that disturbance by background fluctuations is greater for a contrast fluid with a s.g. of 1.16 and a d.b. 3 than for the 1.32–4 combination, a s.g. of 1.16 is still to be preferred since in the larger pipe the wooden beads are then seen more clearly even with one d.b. less. In practice, the combination of a contrast fluid with a s.g. of 1.32 or higher and a d.b. 1 (normal exposure) is generally used. Fig. 4.16 shows that in this way no information on the presence of filling defects is obtained in the large pipe and in the thin pipe only a little. It can also be seen that a s.g. of 1.16 obviously gives us more information for the same film density.

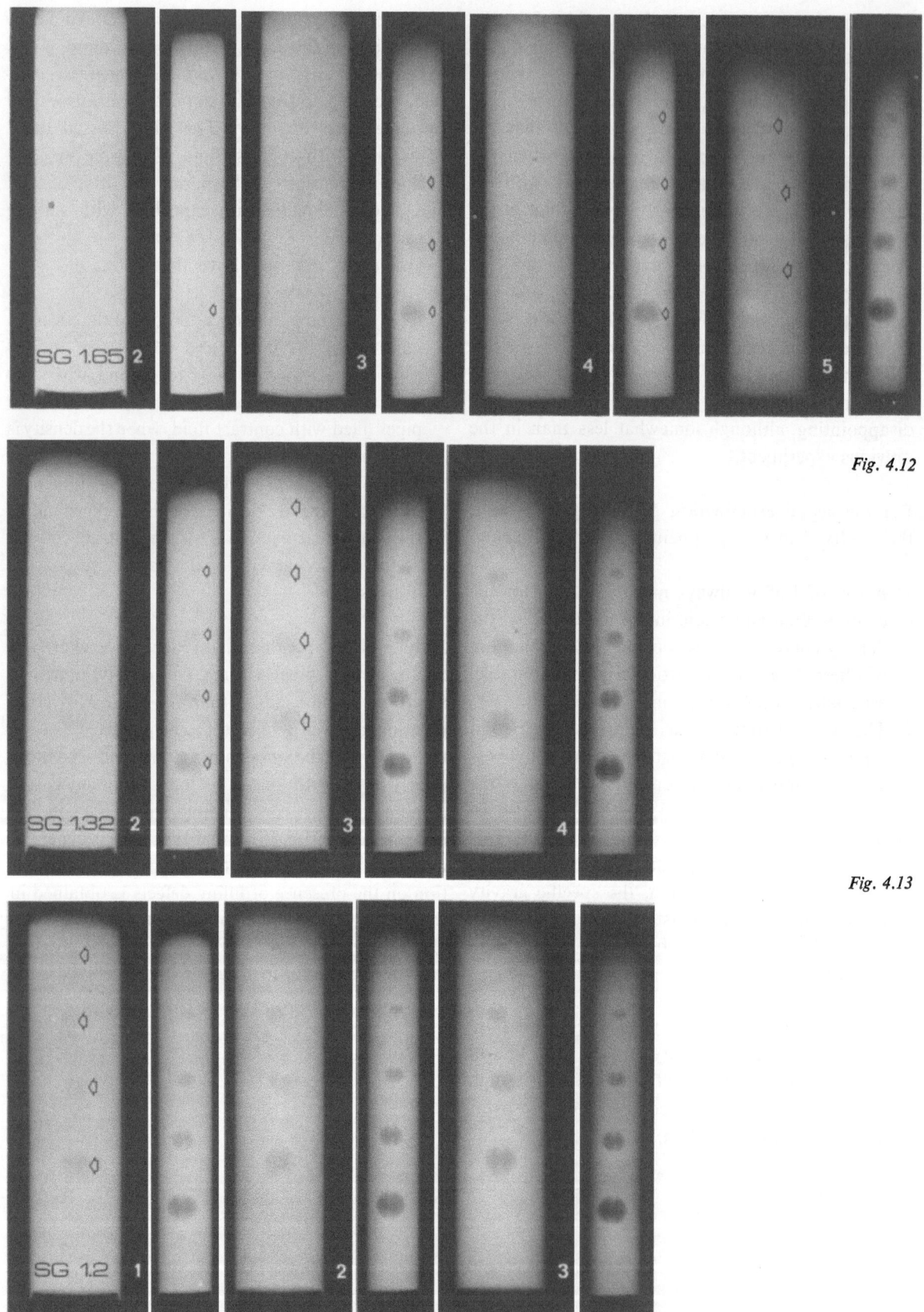

Fig. 4.12

Fig. 4.13

Fig. 4.14

Fig. 4.12/4.17

Tests on the s.g. of the contrast fluid. The diameters of the plastic pipes are 14, 22 and 34 mm and of the wooden beads, 5, 7, 8 and 12 mm.

The density of the background (d.b.) is shown in white numbers; the values 1 through 5 correspond to the following values on the density curve (fig. 4.11):

1→1.3—1.6   2→1.6—1.9   3→1.9—2.5   4→2.5—2.9

5→>2.9.

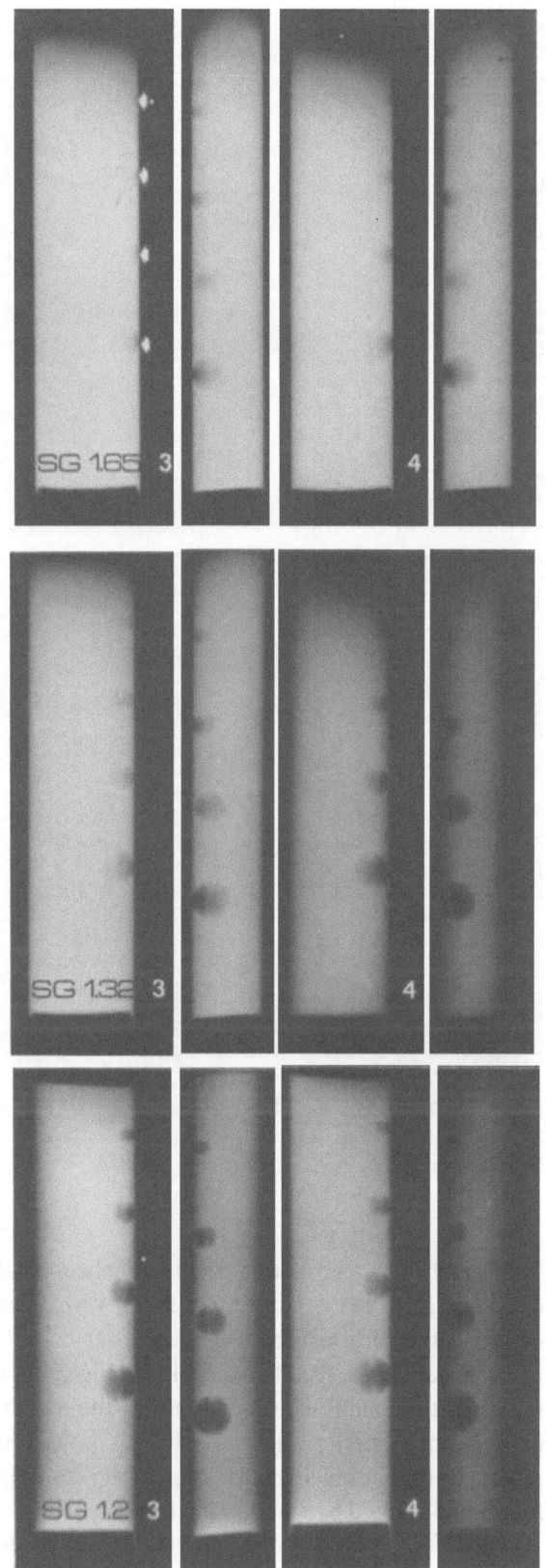

Fig. 4.15

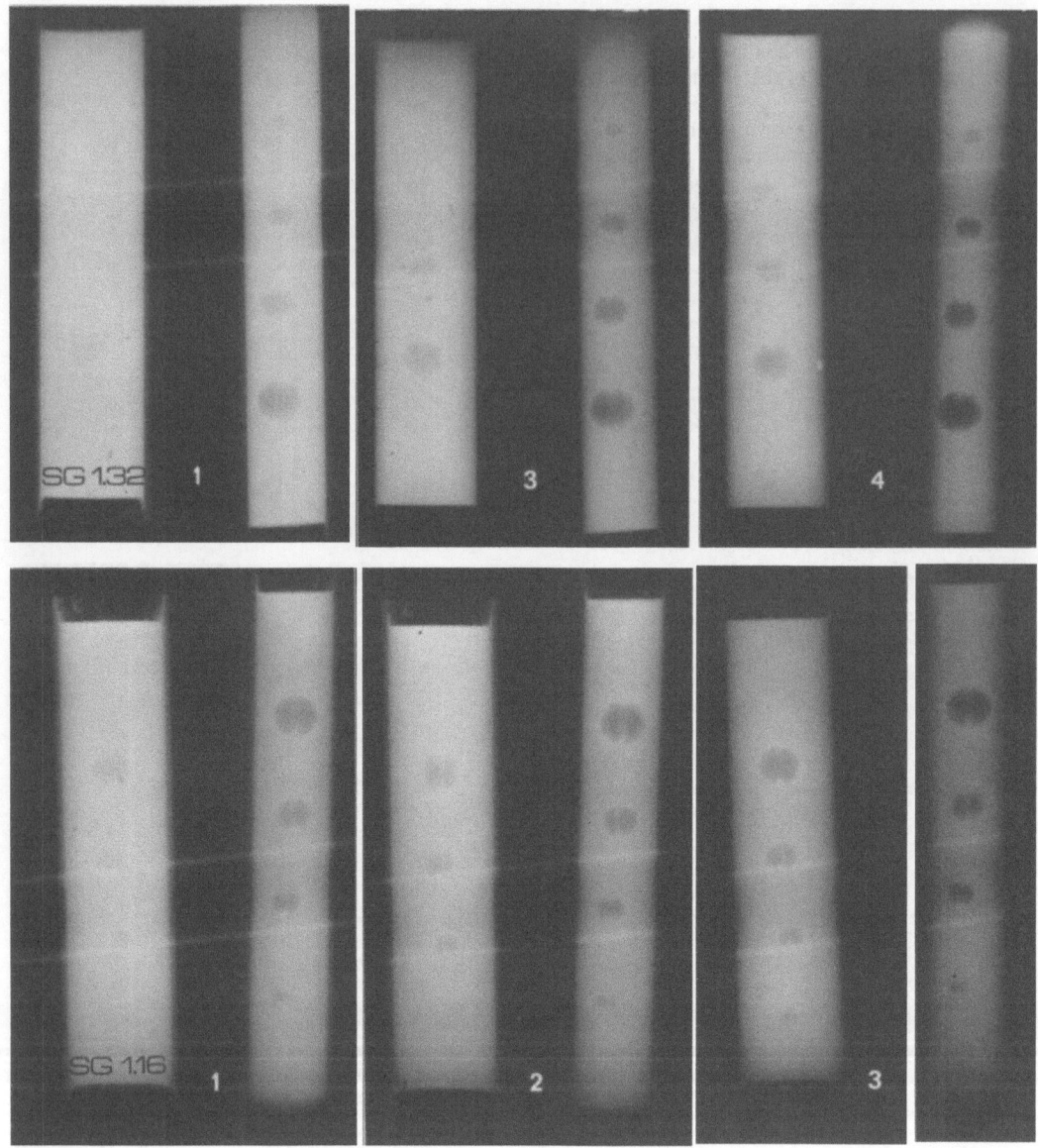

Fig. 4.16

The practical confirmation of these theoretical considerations was demonstrated nicely with films of the rectum of a patient who visited our department because of rectal blood loss. Fig. 4.18A shows that the filling exposures made of the rectum in anterior-posterior, $\frac{3}{4}$ and lateral projection revealed no abnormalities. The s.g. of the contrast fluid is 1.32; the d.b. is approximately 2.

The difference in contrast between air and tissue is greater than between the contrast fluid and tissue so that we need not be surprised that the double-contrast films made with the same d.b. revealed a large polypoid tumor in the right posterior wall of the rectum (fig. 4.18D).

New films of the rectum were again made using the same contrast fluid, this time, however, with a d.b. of approximately 4 and 5. On these films, the polypoid tumor can be seen (fig. 4.18B).

Finally after thorough evacuation, a third series of filling exposures was made. The s.g. of the contrast fluid was 1.16 and the d.b. was approximately 2 and 3. These last films show the filling defect in the rectum very clearly. In addition, the contours of the sigmoid loops which cross each

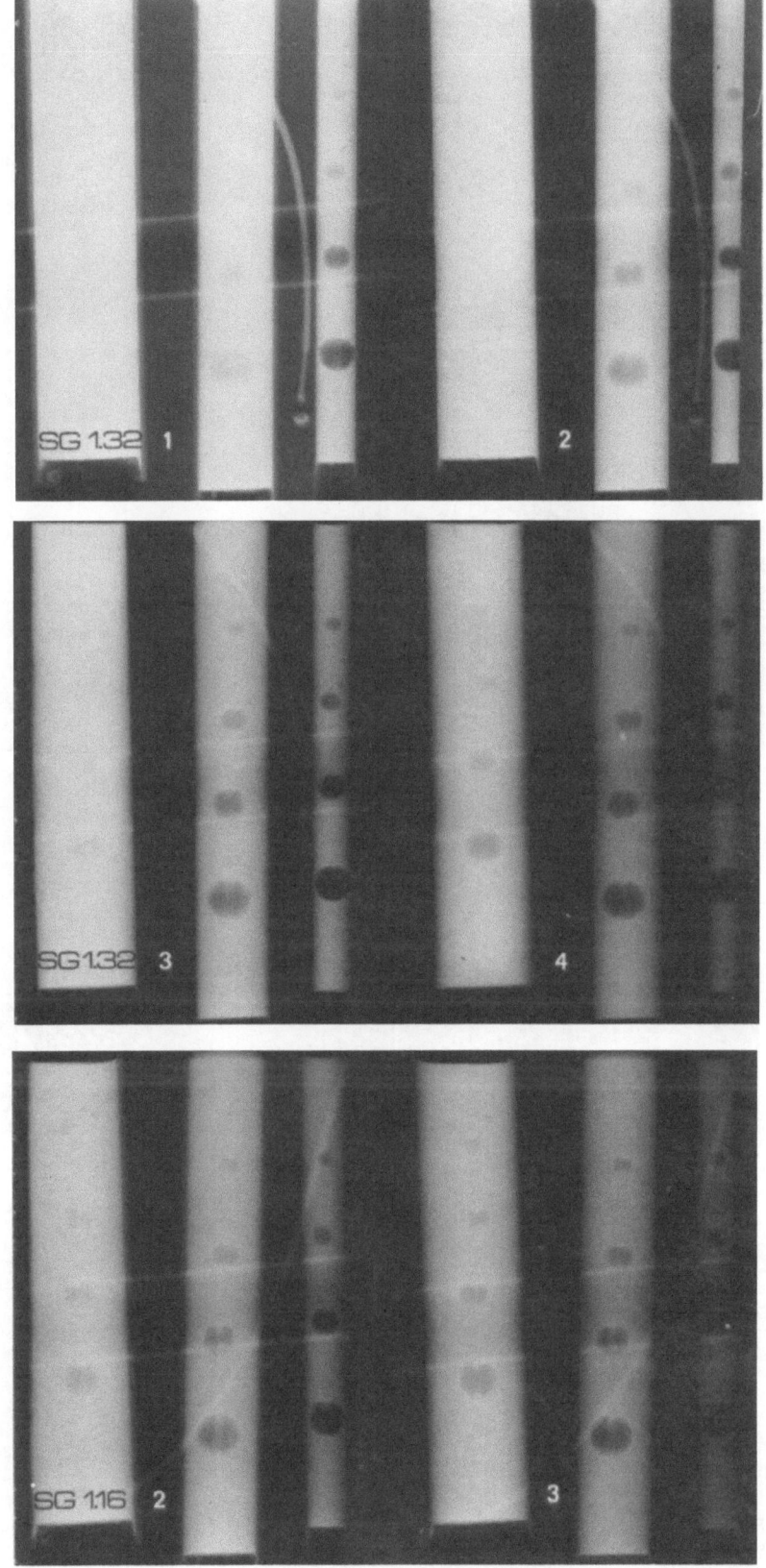

Fig. 4.17

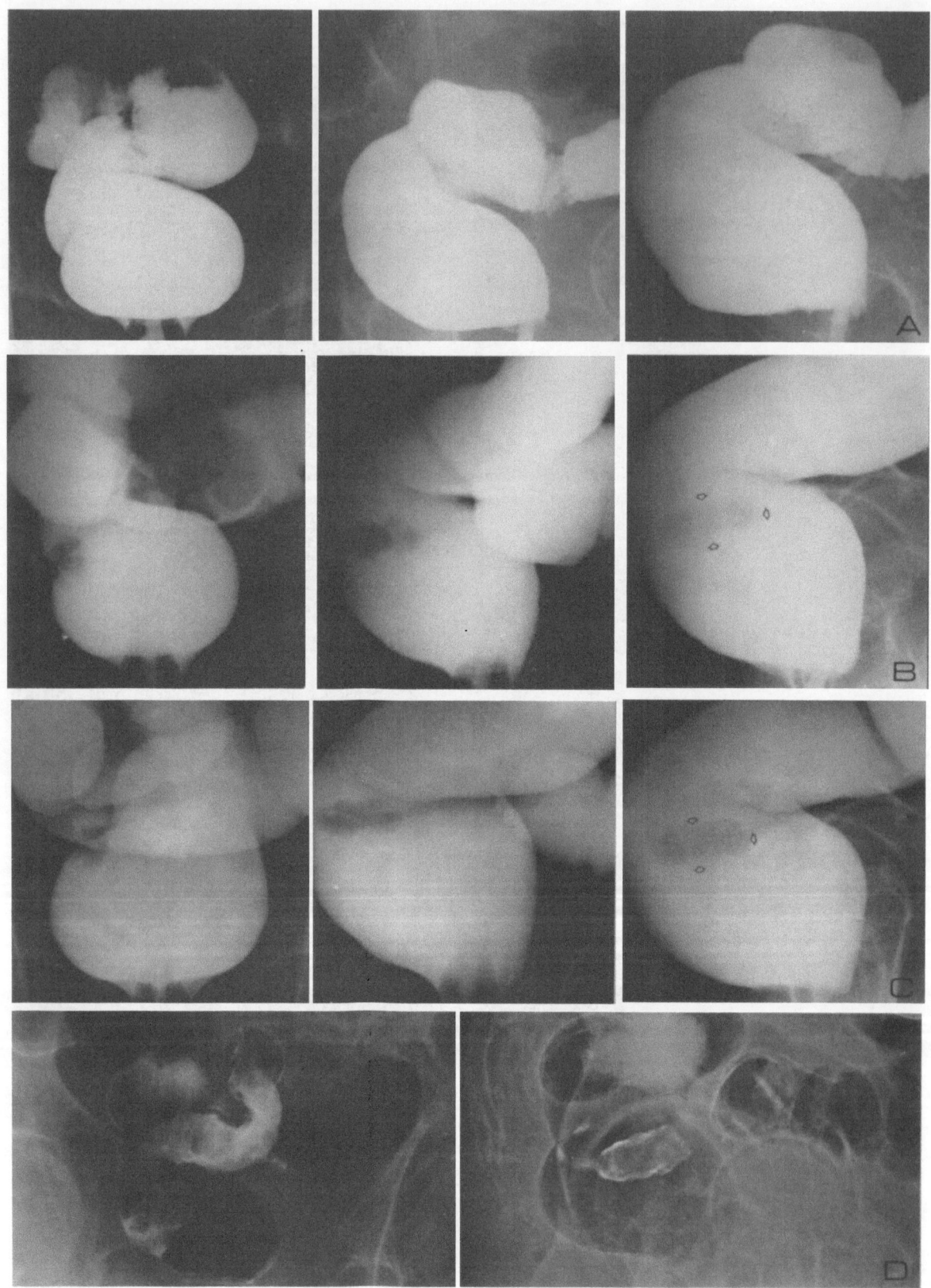

Fig. 4.18
Visibility of polypoid mass in rectum under various exposure conditions.
A. s.g. contrast fluid 1.32   d.b. 2
B. s.g. contrast fluid 1.32   d.b. 4—5
C. s.g. contrast fluid 1.16   d.b. 2—3
D. double contrast exposures d.b. 2

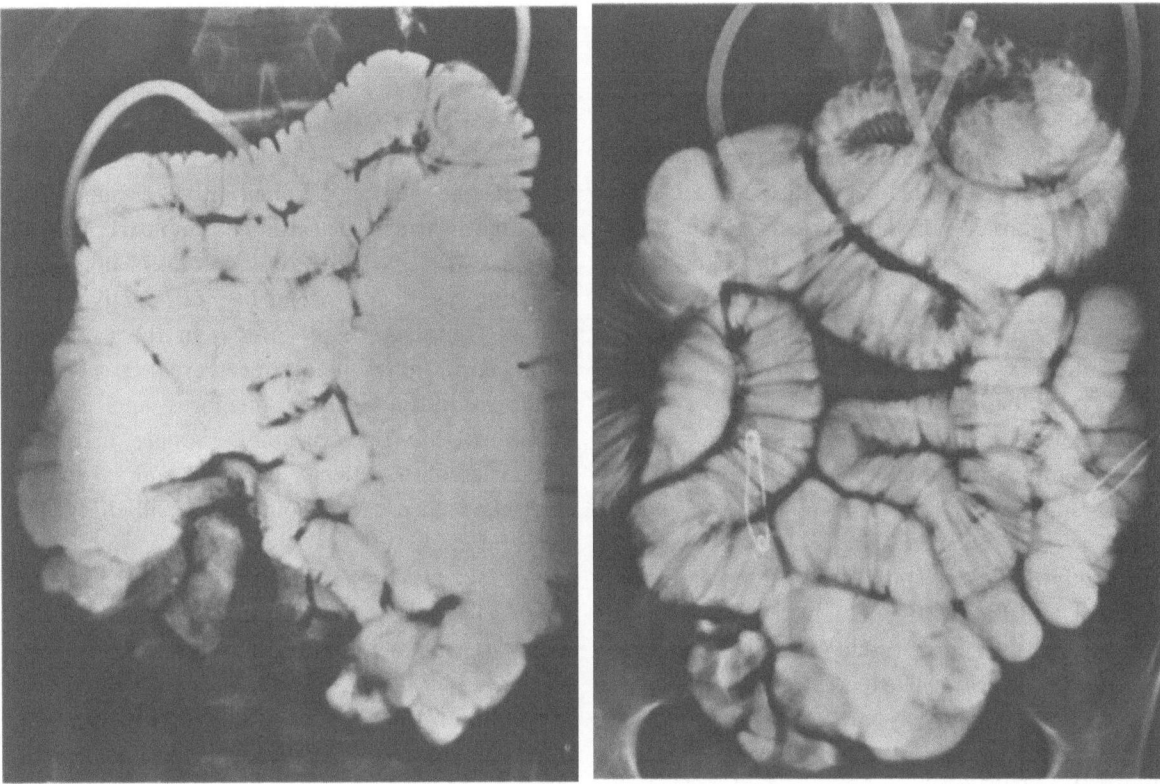

Fig. 4.19
Survey film of an enteroclysis examination executed elsewhere (left). Although the background density is rather high, the information obtained is only marginal. Therefore it must be concluded that the s.g. of the contrast fluid was much too high. There are no indications that the kilovoltage was low (see fig. 4.6).
When the examination was repeated in our department, the results (right) were better because a barium suspension with a lower s.g. was used so that the density of the background could be lower and therefore the x-ray dosage used was much lower.

other can be followed more easily with the contrast medium of lower specific gravity than on the first two series of exposures (fig. 4.18c).

If the importance of the s.g. with respect to the examination of the small intestine is neglected, the survey films obtained will inevitably be useless, especially with the enteroclysis technique (fig. 4.19).

The two pipes with the contrast fluid can only be considered representative of a colon which is not too wide and for filling of the duodenum and the jejunum in the manner described in this study (duodenal intubation). The ileum, however, is less wide and mucosal folds only 2 mm thick must also be visible over their entire length without overexposure of the margins.

Furthermore small ulcers, diverticula and fistulous tracts may not escape our attention. The test

procedure was therefore expanded to include a 14 mm plastic pipe containing the 4 wooden beads described previously. This pipe can be considered representative of a loop of the ileum. Finally, a thin plastic tube with a 2 mm lumen was introduced into the phantom such that it crossed several barium columns.

The 3 pipes and the tube were successively filled with contrast fluids with specific gravities of 1.16 and 1.32. For s.g. 1.16, films were made with d.b. 2 and 3 and for s.g. 1.32, with d.b. 1, 2, 3, and 4 (fig. 4.17).

It is striking that for this series of experiments the greatest amount of information is again obtained with s.g. 1.32 and d.b. 4 or with s.g. 1.16 and d.b. 3. Here the preference for the 1.16–3 combination is greater than in the other experiments because for the 1.32–4 combination overexposure almost occurs for the 2 mm tube and the density of the largest bead in the 14 mm pipe is so high that the central hole is no longer clearly visible.

With a contrast fluid with a s.g. of 1.32, the information in the 'ileum pipe' is greater with a d.b. 3 than with a d.b. 4, the tube is also more clearly visible with d.b. 3. For the 'colon pipe' the lower specific gravity was usually to be preferred; it is therefore sensible to be guided by this factor so that for less wide loops, the density can be decreased from 3 to 2 without loss of information, which means a reduction in dosage for the patient. Although the tube is most clearly visible with the 1.32-2 combination, the opacification caused by the two smaller beads in the 'jejunum pipe' is too vague.

Probably the best results for the examination of the small intestine will be obtained with a d.b. 2 and a s.g. for the contrast fluid somewhere between 1.16 and 1.32. Practical experience has confirmed this hypothesis completely.

The results of this series of experiments can best be summarized as follows:

For a colon examination, a contrast fluid can best be used with a specific gravity of 1.15 for a thin and at the most 1.2 for an obese patient. The density of the background must lie in the upper fourth of the steep part of the density curve.

For the examination of the small intestine, a contrast medium can best be used with a specific gravity of 1.2 for a thin, 1.25 for a normal and 1.3 for an obese patient. The density of the background must lie in the third quarter of the steep part of the density curve.

The density for an examination of the digestive tract may therefore never lie in the lower half of the density curve.

If the conditions described here are satisfied, then the density of the intestinal loops filled with contrast fluid will fall in the lower fourth of the steep part of the density curve.

7. Contrast media other than barium sulfate

a. BARIUM CARBONATE

In 1959 the gastric examination of a number of patients was carried out using barium carbonate. In 8 patients there were severe symptoms of poisoning, including cyanosis, irregular heart activity, intestinal complaints and paresis. In the 6 patients who died as a result, autopsy revealed a hemorrhagic infiltration of the meninges and cerebral edema. Before the barium carbonate had been administered to patients, extensive animal experiments had been carried out and no ill-effects had been found (135).

b. DISADVANTAGES OF BARIUM SUSPENSIONS

In addition to the great difficulties still encountered in producing a sufficiently stable barium suspension which is at the same time protected against fluid withdrawal, several other disadvantages of this contrast medium are mentioned in literature.

1. owing to the higher viscosity of a barium suspension in the ileum, it cannot deeply penetrate narrow fistulous tracts in this area.
2. as a result of leakage from perforations or fistulas, the formation of barium granulomas can occur.
3. as a result of aspiration, a necrotizing bronchopneumonia can develop.

Some radiologists have therefore tried to find a contrast medium which does not have these disadvantages. They considered organic iodine compounds since the thin liquid aqueous iodine solutions are just as unsatisfactory; this will be discussed in more detail in this chapter.

c. SUSPENSIONS OF AN ORGANIC IODINE COMPOUND

Jones et al. (103) studied tetraiodophtalimidoethanol; they were able to produce a very homogeneous suspension with a particle size of 1–2 microns. This fluid contains 73 per cent iodine, barely precipitates and adheres more readily to the mucosa than barium suspensions. By adding gelatin, the characteristics of the suspension were further improved. From animal experiments it appeared that the toxicity of this contrast medium is as low as that of barium sulfate; for the latter it has been shown that particles varying from 0.04 to 0.1 microns in size can be absorbed by the intestinal mucous membrane. These particles, which do not end up in the blood stream but in the lymphatic channels, form less than one ten-thousandth of the normal barium suspension (4). The organic iodine compounds were tested in several experiments with dogs; it appeared that much smaller mucosal lesions could be localized with this contrast medium than with barium.

In 18 patients and a number of students, a total of 56 follow-through studies and 4 colon examinations were carried out. The resulting roentgenograms were very clear. One objection was that fluid absorption in the distal ileum and the colon caused even greater dehydration of the contrast fluid than barium. Unfortunately the preparation of this contrast medium was so time-consuming and expensive that the experiments had to be terminated.

d. AQUEOUS IODINE SOLUTIONS

In 1958, the first publications appeared on the use of Urokon, Hypaque and Renographin as contrast media for examination of the digestive tract. Shortly thereafter, similar articles were also published in England and Germany. A true avalanche of reports from enthusiastic users broke loose after the introduction of Gastrografine about 1960. After Gastrografine, which consists of 76 per cent Urografine mixed with a wetting agent, a sweetener and a flavoring, several other brands were introduced but they have never been generally accepted. Most radiologists believed that Gastrografine was ideal for use when barium fails due to flocculation or when barium is contra-indicated. The following examples of the latter are mentioned:

1. atresia or fistulas in the tracheo-esophageal area (danger of aspiration).
2. special cases of pre- and post-operative diagnosis of the digestive tract, such as bleeding ulcers, suture leakage or perforations.

3. partial obstructions which cannot be passed by barium or where dehydration and thickening of the barium suspension might occur.

There were, however, also publications reporting the use of Gastrografine for all patients, for the colon examination as well as the examinations of the stomach and the small intestine. Shehadi even reports a series of 1500 patients (203). Robinson and Levene (193) prefer Renografin over barium for the gastro-intestinal examination. In 1959, Lessman and Lilienfeld (127) had already studied and compared the experiences of various radiologists. It appeared that the amount of Gastrografine used per examination varied widely. Some used only 25–50 ml of a 76 per cent concentration and others used 10 times as much. There was general satisfaction with the reproduction of the gastric mucosal relief and the greater ease with which a pyloric stenosis could be diagnosed or a fistulous tract filled. However, they all discovered that dilution of the contrast medium in the small intestine was so great that morphological evaluation of this area was absolutely impossible. In addition, no-one succeeded in making acceptable double-contrast exposures; and some authors report that more than 50 ml can cause abdominal cramps, vomiting and diarrhea. Reasonably satisfactory colon films can be made because absorption of fluid causes an increasing contrast in this area (203). In this way it was often possible to obtain good filling of the colon on the proximal side of a stenosis which could not be passed by the barium from the distal side. It remained impossible to localize tumors in the small intestine, although the diagnosis 'obstruction' could often be made on the basis of the presence of wide loops.

Some radiologists believe that when the Gastrografine has not yet reached the colon 4 hours after oral administration, a post-operative ileus is due to an obstruction and not a paralysis (226).

Rubin et al. (195) were not able to confirm this opinion. Berger of Philadelphia agrees with Rubin and at a conference he showed slides of 4 patients. In these cases the Gastrografine was visible in the colon within 15 minutes although a definite obstruction did exist in the small intestine which apparently could easily be passed by the thin liquid Gastrografine. In approximately 2 per cent of the patients, some of the iodine contrast medium is excreted into the urine (89). This is believed by some to indicate an obstruction, perforation or other pathological condition in the digestive tract (157). Although surgical confirmation has often supported this line of thought and Tosch has shown with radioactive Gastrografine that this can indeed occur (223), disappointments (236) and false positive results have also been reported in this respect (194). In 1959, Lessman and Lilienfeld already pointed out the strong hyperosmotic characteristics of Gastrografine and the dangers this can cause for intestinal obstructions (127). Since the osmotic value of 50 ml 70 per cent Urokon is equal to that of 15 g magnesium sulfate, a dose of 6 ml per kg body weight can cause such excessive fluid withdrawal that the circulating plasma volume can decrease 15–30 per cent. Harris et al. have described lethal complications in children due to the hypovolemia. They also showed that the osmotic force of Gastrografine in isolated intestinal loops can be so great that blood circulation in the intestinal wall can be seriously disturbed (84). In addition the vomiting and diarrhea caused by Gastrografine can further disturb an already critical electrolyte balance (165). It has therefore become clear that for cases of suspected obstruction in the small intestine it is far from certain that Gastrografine is the most suitable contrast medium. If considered desirable, then it must in any event be handled with extreme caution and used only when the clinical condition of the patient permits it. Furthermore when Gastrografine is used, it must be realized that this contrast medium does not adhere easily and therefore reliable morphological information can only be obtained when filling is complete. In addition Gastrografine is such a thin liquid that fistulous tracts or perforations may not be discovered because the contrast medium passes so rapidly that there is not enough time for penetration.

Shehadi wrote in 1960 that the introduction of the aqueous iodine contrast medium could be considered a milestone in the diagnosis of the digestive tract (204). Fortunately since then application of Gastrografine has lost some of the ground it had taken by storm; however, a new land-mark in the diagnosis of the digestive tract will be reached when use of this medium is only a rare exception.

e. GASTROGRAFINE-BARIUM MIXTURES

A number of radiologists did not simply stop using Gastrografine but have attempted to obtain better results by mixing it with barium (71, 217). They expected the mixture to have the better adhesive characteristics of a barium suspension on the one hand, and the transit acceleration and the ability to mix with gastric and intestinal juices without flocculation of Gastrografine on the other. The combination of these two entirely different contrast fluids was tested in every possible ratio, especially in Japan where it is still used extensively for gastric and duodenal examinations. During these tests it appeared that the tendency of barium to flocculate does not decrease; it even increases as the amount of barium in the mixture decreases. The transit acceleration of the Gastrografine-barium mixture does not depend particularly on the ratio but is almost directly dependent upon the absolute quantity of Gastrografine.

Both Shehadi (203) and Stecken et al. (217) report the strange phenomenon of separation of barium and Gastrografine already occurring in the jejunum. The Gastrografine produces less contrast as a result of the absorption of fluid and it travels rapidly to the cecum while the barium remains in the jejunum. Furthermore Stecken et al. observed that not only stenosis and hypotonia but also meteorism clearly delay the rate of transit. Various radiologists believe that 150 ml barium suspension and approximately 30 ml Gastrografine is still the most satisfactory ratio. This is probably because there is so little Gastrografine in this mixture that it barely affects the barium suspension; furthermore it is not impossible that the 30 ml Gastrografine does not visibly separate from the barium in the duodenum and the jejunum and absorbs sufficient fluid to cause transit acceleration. Due to the faster transit a larger portion of the intestine can be photographed with the still usable barium suspension than would otherwise have been the case.

V

METHODS OF EXAMINATION

1. 'Physiological' examination of the small intestine

In Chapter III it was noted that addition of nutrients to the contrast medium was abandoned during the second world war. The problems involved in the functional examination were found to be considerably greater than those for the morphological examination. Furthermore it was recognized that a functional examination must also be evaluated morphologically. It is therefore necessary that the morphological examination of the small intestine first attain a much higher degree of perfection. In the sixties, only Mattsson et al. (46, 149) advocated a return to this method; however, their published photographs of the ileum were very poor. The nutritional composition of the 300 ml contrast meal administered by Mattsson et al. is approximately the same as Borgström's and is as follows:

153 g BaSO$_4$
12½ g protein
15 g fat
12½ g lactose
25 g dextrose
200 ml water.

In one of their articles they report that their examination technique gave very constant transit time, in contrast to the highly variable data from literature. The authors hereby show that they have no insight into the reasons for these variations.

It is customary for many radiologists to give their patients something to eat or drink whenever a standstill of the contrast column has occurred in the ileum; this has of course nothing to do with a physiological examination. This additional food is usually given to renew stimulation of the peristalsis, sometimes, however, only to remove the patient's feeling of hunger.

Some radiologists have set rules; Pirk and Vulterinová (177) for instance give a small meal after 3 hours if the stomach is empty and the cecum has not yet been reached. Patients who have undergone gastrectomy even receive this food after 2 hours.

If this is done, it must be realized that a large, liquid meal will induce more active peristalsis and faster transit than a small, more viscous meal. In the first case, therefore, the additional food is more likely to disturb the roentgenograms of the ileum, insofar as this has not already occurred as a result of the long transit time.

2. Single administration of the contrast medium

a. NORMAL AMOUNT

For examination of the small intestine, most radiologists including Golden have the patient drink approximately 250 ml of the contrast fluid. Usually this is preceded by a gastric examination whereby the mucosa is studied using approximately 50 ml contrast fluid. The number of exposures subsequently made of the small intestine is highly dependent upon the rate of transit but possibly even more upon the attitude of the radiologist. Many are in the habit of making films at equal time intervals even when the rate of transit continues to decrease. This of course is not correct, in this case the patient receives an unnecessarily high radiation dosage and in addition, it means a waste of film material.

There is no waste of film material for those who believe that an examination of the many meters of small intestine can be carried out with only 3 (237) or even 2 (159) exposures. It is not necessary to demonstrate that this method is very dangerous and therefore should be rejected, even when each of these exposures clearly shows practically the entire small intestine.

b. SMALL AMOUNTS

Some radiologists use small quantities of contrast fluid, such as Laws et al. who administer only 100 ml undiluted Micropaque even for sprue patients (120). This is probably done to avoid the annoying effect of superposition, but this exaggerated fear must be paid for with flocculation and segmentation. Morton, who only used 70 g Micropaque powder mixed with 200 ml of an ice-cold physiological salt solution (159), also obtained poor results. He made only 2 exposures, but probably the information would not be increased by an increase in this number.

c. LARGE AMOUNTS

For many years, an increasing number of radiologists have switched over to the use of large quantities of the contrast medium for examination of the small intestine.

Although there was no response, Weltz in 1937 had already pointed out that the quality of the x-ray films of the small intestine is highly dependent upon the degree of filling (230). He also reported that this requires rapid gastric emptying and that stretching of the small intestine is the main stimulus for the induction of good peristaltic waves. Furthermore he believed that a large amount of contrast medium offers the best buffer action against the detrimental effects of secretion and absorption in the intestinal canal. He had noted that the contrast intensity in the ileum is greater than in the jejunum but that this phenomenon is less pronounced for a rapid transit because there is apparently not enough time for fluid absorption.

In view of the time in which he worked, his insights can be regarded as brilliant. If he had had a better 'sales technique', the development of the radiological examination of the small intestine would certainly have advanced much further.

According to the articles published, Marshak had similar views but did not reason them as well as Weltz. In any event, Marshak's great contribution was that these improvements in the examination technique were widely publicized in his numerous articles after 1954 (139–145). He routinely used 480 ml contrast fluid and when the small intestine was dilated, sometimes 600 ml or more (144).

In 1963, Caldwell and Floch examined 32 patients twice and thereby showed that the transit time is significantly shorter when the amount of contrast medium is chosen according to Marshak (480 ml) rather than Golden (240 ml). For the former, the average transit time was 2.25 hours and for the latter, 3.25 hours (32).

Many authors believe that it is desirable to make compression exposures of the ileum, whereby the loops which cover one another are forced aside (139, 216).

Numerous radiologists also find that diagnosis is considerably improved when several exposures are made, one immediately after the other; the same intestinal loops are then seen more often in approximately the same stage of filling (233, 237). Caldwell et al. (33) pointed out that delayed gastric emptying can still cause flocculation and segmentation even when 500 ml stable barium is administered.

It is striking that none of the radiologists who use large quantities of the contrast medium feel that either the use of ice water or drugs to accelerate passage is necessary.

3. Fractional administration of the contrast medium

a. METHOD OF PANSDORF

In 1927 Pansdorf (169) had already introduced this method based on the entirely reasonable assumption that the best technique for administering the contrast medium must be·extreme fractionation. He gave his patients one tablespoon to drink every 5 min and thought that only in this way distribution of the contrast medium throughout the small intestinal loops could be guaranteed; furthermore the annoying effect of superposition would be very slight, at the most. He reasoned that each roentgenogram would then show as many loops as possible. ·

Pansdorf was probably not sufficiently aware of the numerous factors which can completely disturb this theoretically uniform supply. Ideal fractionation only exists when administration of the contrast medium is matched by gastric emptying through the pyloric canal (fig. 5.1). In addition the stability of the contrast medium is too low to be able to withstand such an unfavourable ratio with respect to the intestinal fluids. It is, however, possible that at the time of Pansdorf, this technique of fractional administration of the contrast medium was not as unfavourable as it is now. After all, the contrast medium then used was highly unstable even without the addition of food and disintegration occurred anyway in the proximal part of the intestine. Possibly a distribution of the flocculation or segmentation was still to be preferred over large segment clumps. Should there ever be completely stable contrast media in the future, then it is conceivable that the principle of fractional administration will regain a place of honor.

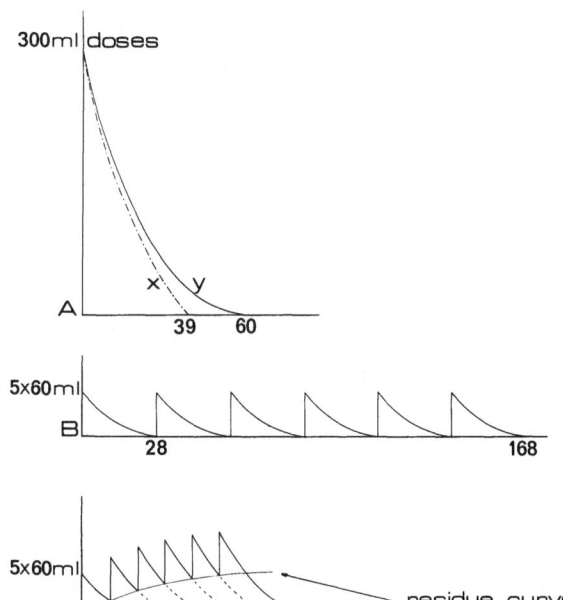

Fig. 5.1
A. Gastric emptying curve
    Y. sitting or standing position ———
    X. right lateral position —·—·—
B. Ideal fractionation: rate of supply equals rate of emptying.
C, D. Fractionation: rate of supply is greater than rate of emptying so that an increasing residual is found in the stomach.

b. MODIFICATION OF WELTZ

In 1937, Weltz (230) introduced important changes in the method of Pansdorf by first giving a single dose of 200 ml contrast medium for the gastric examination. For the subsequent follow-through study, the patient drank approximately 30 ml every 5 minutes. As mentioned previously, Weltz believed in a large dosage of contrast medium. Although his method appears to resemble fractionation, this is in fact not true. The stomach is continuously filled to a large extent and fractionation is probably only meant to keep the patient from feeling that his stomach is much too full.

c. MODIFICATION OF NAUMANN

Naumann (163) administered two doses of 200 ml a half hour apart. Again this method cannot be regarded as true fractionation; it is used to administer a slightly larger amount of contrast medium without discomfort to the patient.

d. FRACTIONATION BY THE PYLORIC MUSCLE

It is probably useful to realize that every quantity of contrast medium administered orally is passed on to the small intestine in fractions by the pylorus. The size of these fractions differs for every patient and is partly dependent upon:

pylorus function   right lateral position

peptic ulcer or tumor   drugs to enhance peri-
                                stalsis

gastric acid concentration   temperature, osmosity
                                and caloric value of the
                                contrast fluid.

4. Administration of cold fluids with the contrast medium

a. METHOD OF WEINTRAUB AND WILLIAMS

In 1941 Weintraub (229) noted that drinking ice water after a meal enhanced peristalsis and caused diarrhea. Using this observation he gave ice water after a barium meal and found that in about 50 per cent of the cases, the cecum was reached within a half hour. The quality of the pictures, however, was not very good although it improved when he replaced the ice water with cold physiological salt. It was remarkable that passage of the contrast medium through the small intestine proceeded even more rapidly. After some experimentation, he finally settled on the following technique:

1. gastro-duodenal examination with a mixture of 120 g barium and 120 g isotonic salt solution at room temperature.
2. after this examination, 240 g ice-cold physiological salt is administered and after 5 minutes, a new roentgenogram is made.
3. immediately after this x-ray film, another 240 g ice-cold physiological salt is administered and again a new roentgenogram is made after 10 minutes.
4. 15 minutes later, still another film is made and if necessary, every 30 minutes afterwards.

As a result of the large amount of fluid given in total (700 ml) transit is rapid and the barium does not thicken in the ileum. He even reports that when the transit time is short, the quality of the films is good and it is poor when the transit time is longer. It is understandable that this method of examination is not very pleasant for the patients.

b. SIMPLIFIED VARIATIONS

Golden found the method of Weintraub too arduous and believed in addition that the great haste involved was not opportune since precise following and evaluation of the transit films already cost so much time. Many other authors also found this method of examination too laborious but they did want to profit from the passage acceleration caused by a cold liquid. The simplifications introduced are so similar that they will not be discussed as separate modifications.

Ettinger (48) gave a glass of ice water after first examining the stomach with a mixture of 120 g barium and 120 ml water. Hudak (96) gave a glass of ice-cold physiological salt solution 10 minutes after a small barium meal and 10 minutes later, 1 mg prostigmin.

Bendick (15) gave 200 ml ice-cold soda water after the contrast meal. He had noted that the gas formation which is then caused induces peristalsis. This gas travels to the cecum rapidly and completely independently and therefore certainly does not accelerate passage of the contrast medium. Apparently Brown's experiences were similar (24). In spite of the fact that he even gave 3 glasses of ice-cold soda water, in only 60 per cent of his patients had the cecum been reached within 2 hours. He tried to prevent the pronounced flocculation and segmentation of the contrast fluid which then occur by using Raybar, the most stable contrast medium known. Morton (159) gave the patient a mixture of 200 ml ice-cold salt solution and only 70 g Micropaque powder. Like those of Hudak, his photographs show only flocculation and segmentation of the contrast fluid and therefore demonstrate quite clearly how unsuitable this technique is.

All the authors in this group report a transit time to the cecum of 1.5 to 2 hours, thus considerably longer than with the method of Weintraub. No-one apparently recognized the importance of the large quantities; they all used 200 ml instead of 700 ml like Weintraub. In this connection it is very interesting to note the technique of Brown who did give approximately 600 ml fluid. The passage acceleration which this large dosage should have produced was completely neutralized by the retardation caused by the development of gas.

5. Administration of the contrast medium through a tube directly into the small intestine (enteroclysis)

Publications between 1920 and 1925 by Einhorn, who introduced the contrast fluid into the duodenum through a tube and obtained outstanding films, gave Pesquera the idea in 1929 of using this method for filling the entire small intestine (175). He administered a mixture of barium and water, which also contained a small amount of gum acacia. Although no quantities are reported, the article indicates that he let the infusion run slowly and as long as necessary to reach the cecum, usually no longer than half an hour. He reports that he was able to diagnose a lymphosarcoma in the distal ileum in this manner; this can certainly be regarded as a success in radiological diagnosis at that time.

Ten years later, Gershon-Cohen and Shay (65) did some experiments on the function of the pylorus and noted that the closing mechanism was very good. After the duodenum had been filled using a tube, the entire contents quickly disappeared into the jejunum; reflux into the stomach occurred only when the pressure of the infusion was too high. They used this method to administer 800–1200 ml contrast fluid and they were surprised by the rapid rate of transit through the small intestine. The cecum was reached in 8–15 minutes. This interval would probably have been even shorter if the pressure of the infusion had been higher; their level difference was only 25 cm.

In 1943, a publication by Schatzki (197) appeared reporting on 75 patients examined in this manner. He intubated a supple Rehfuss tube with an olive-shaped metal end into the duodenum and let 500–1000 ml barium suspension with a lower specific gravity than he normally used for a gastric examination run through this tube. In half of his patients the cecum was reached in 15 min. For 4 patients, reflux into the stomach occurred; in these cases the average transit time was more than 40 minutes, thus considerably longer. The rather low percentage of reflux and the relatively long transit time for such an examination with large amounts of contrast fluid probably indicate that his infusion was given under low pressure.

Once reflux into the stomach had occurred, Schatzki tried to end it by sliding the tube further into the duodenum, decreasing the pressure of the infusion or acidifying the barium mixture. He was not successful with any of these methods, so that he concluded that these factors do not influence the development of reflux. The correctness of this conclusion is, however, very doubtful since it is obvious that once reflux has occurred, the pylorus will continue to open to allow the gastric contents to pass on to the duodenum. While the infusion is flowing, the pressure in the duodenum will probably be higher than in the stomach and opening of the pylorus will therefore have a reverse effect.

Schatzki's great contribution is that he pointed out the importance of administering large quantities of the contrast medium in the right lateral position. He had found that interruption of the contrast column lengthens the transit time considerably, thus allowing more time for dehydration in the ileum.

In 1951 Lura (132) reported on a series of 300 patients; he examined the small intestine of these patients using the infusion technique and found an average transit time of 15 minutes. It had been difficult to pass the tube through the pylorus in 5–10 per cent of the cases.

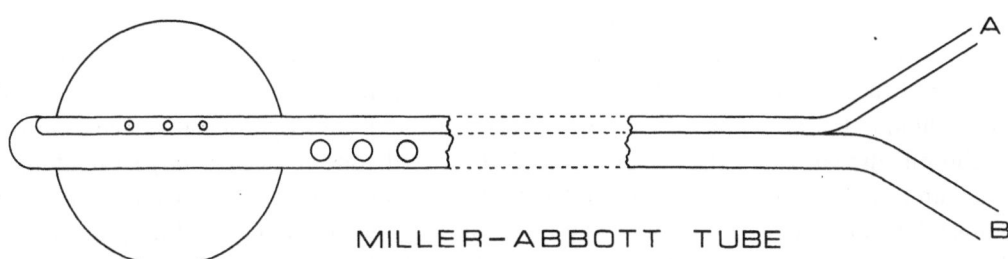

Fig. 5.2
A. air inflow.   B. contrast fluid.

In 1960 Scott Harden et al. (116, 199) and Pygott et al. (184) described an improvement in the technique for duodenal intubation. They passed 2 catheters one inside the other into the pars media of the stomach, which can be felt as well as seen by fluoroscopy since the outer end of both catheters is marked by a metal ring. The outer more rigid catheter has an outer diameter of 5.8 mm and the inner more pliable catheter has a lumen 1.5 mm in diameter. The inner catheter is then slid through the outer into the pyloric canal. It appeared that curling of the catheter could often be prevented by placing the patient in the right lateral position.

In spite of this simplification of the technique, they were still not able to get the catheter into the duodenum in 7 per cent of the patients, which must be considered a high percentage. We have found that beginning this procedure with the more rigid catheter was probably the reason for their failure.

Both catheters remain in place, only the end of the inner catheter with the narrow lumen lies in the duodenum. Pygott et al. then used a syringe to administer 50 ml contrast fluid into the duodenum as often as necessary. It is possible that as a result continuity of the contrast column is occasionally interrupted and probably the outflow through this narrow lumen is too low to cause sufficient stretching of the duodenal wall to induce good peristalsis.

Scott Harden administered only 80 ml of a thin Microtrast solution, directly followed by a $MgSO_4$ solution. It is clear that this method will certainly not lead to good results since both the hyperosmotic $MgSO_4$ solution and the low dosage of contrast medium induce marked flocculation.

In 1965, Patterson et al. (170) reported that they had injected 40 ml Raybar in 15 sprue patients through a duodenal tube. Fifteen minutes later they administered 500 ml ice water as well as a $MgSO_4$ solution. Obviously they obtained flocculation in this manner even with this exceedingly stable contrast medium. Here we are confronted not only with an actual abuse of a good examination technique but also with an entirely misplaced conclusion drawn from their experiments: 'for sprue, an examination technique of duodenal intubation offers no advantages over oral administration of the contrast medium'. It is noteworthy that orally they did not give 40 ml Raybar with ice water and $MgSO_4$, as would be expected, but 120 g undiluted Micropaque solution!

The only techniques which might be regarded as a variation of the preceding are those of Greenspon (79) and Friedman and Rigler (61). In 1960 they reported that they introduced a triple-lumen Miller-Abbott tube (fig. 5.2) into the small intestine just beyond the area they wished to examine.

It can take several days for the end of the tube to reach the desired location. The balloon is filled with 50 to 60 ml air through tube A so that passage beyond this location is not possible. Contrast fluid is then administered through tube B. In this way, according to the authors, one-fourth of the small intestine can be examined without the annoying effect of superposition. Because the intestine is suddenly occluded, the patients cannot easily tolerate more than 600 ml contrast medium. Abdominal cramps can also be caused when the contrast fluid is injected too quickly or its temperature is too low. It is clear that this method of examination is not suitable for routine use and is probably also seldom necessary.

6. Retrograde administration of the contrast fluid

In the twenties and thirties, some authors believed (correctly) that it is better to examine the distal ileum using the colon enema technique rather than the small intestine transit examination.

Although the situation had changed somewhat in 1964, Figiel and Figiel (50) pointed out that retrograde filling of the ileum could still mean a welcome supplement to the transit examination for the diagnosis of strictures, adhesions, ulcerations, fistulas and diverticula. They demonstrated this with the x-rays of a number of patients examined in this manner. They found abnormalities which were confirmed surgically while the normal transit examination had revealed nothing.

Miller (153, 155) found that the appearance of the ileum in particular is determined by peristalsis and tone to such a large extent that constricting lesions in an early stage and smaller mucosal lesions are definitely missed during a transit examination. The functioning of the pylorus causes intermittent, irregular and incomplete filling so that the elasticity of the intestine cannot be determined. Furthermore flocculation and segmentation often completely distort the evaluation.

Miller finds enteroclysis a good method of examination but the duodenal intubation beforehand too troublesome. He propagates retrograde filling of the entire small intestine. Although it is possible to reach the stomach in 9 out of 10 patients, he advises terminating the filling of the small intestine as the duodenum is approached. It is obvious that this filling must occur under fluoroscopic control and that one must be careful that the contrast fluid does not enter the lungs by way of the stomach and esophagus. In many patients it is difficult to pass Bauhin's valve. This can be overcome in most cases by oral administration of 1 mg atropine before the examination; this may also cause a decrease in the secretion of intestinal juices and in forward peristalsis which would greatly facilitate retrograde filling.

The amount of contrast medium needed to fill the colon and small intestine is sometimes less than 2 liters, sometimes considerably more. More than 4.5 liters are never given, even if the duodenum has not yet been reached.

Miller later changed this method slightly by replacing the barium suspension with a physiological salt solution as soon as the ileum begins to fill. When the infusion of the contrast medium is terminated, the colon is emptied by first lowering the plastic infusion bag below the level of the table and then sending the patient to the toilet. Films of the small intestine are subsequently made, if desired of course, films of the colon can be made at the beginning of the infusion period. In our hospital this later modification of Miller's technique is used to our complete satisfaction. The contrast fluid is of course not a colon enema but the same barium suspension used for oral enteroclysis. If it is possible to pass Bauhin's valve and fill the small intestine without giving a drug to induce hypotonicity, the time available for making roentgen films is quite short since the small intestine will empty quickly. The patient must be permitted frequent but short periods for evacuation.

If retrograde filling of the small intestine is not possible without atropine or Buscopan, then the patient must be allowed to evacuate for much longer periods (fig. 5.4). We have found that the small intestine films are best made as soon as peristalsis resumes.

An enormous advantage of this method is that stenotic processes in the small intestine can be approached very quickly from the distal direction (fig. 5.5). Proximal approach in these cases costs more time and moreover an annoying dilution of the contrast medium can occur in the dilated loops.

Figure 5.6 shows a series of films taken when enteroclysis turned out to be impossible because of a stenotic obstruction in the pars antralis due to Crohn's disease. Retrograde filling of the small intestine revealed multiple abnormalities in the region of the duodenum and the jejunum; the ileum, however, was free of abnormalities.

7. Combined methods of examination

Without a doubt, many radiologists use methods which are not described here or which are made up of elements or variations of specific methods of examination.

An example of such a combination is the approach of Bugyi (28), who first examines the gallbladder and stomach according to the method of Gianturco (69), then the small intestine using a variation of the method of Weintraub and finally takes pictures of the orally-filled colon.

The following procedures occur in the given order:

1. On the morning of the examination, gallbladder photographs are taken first. On the afternoon of the previous day the patient swallowed the necessary tablets.
2. After the gallbladder photographs are taken, the colon is cleansed by means of an enema.
3. The next step is the gastric examination. No details are given.
4. After the gastric examination, the patient receives 100–200 g paraffin oil, which is a laxative and also induces contraction of the gallbladder.
5. A half hour later, photographs of the contracted gallbladder are taken.
6. Patient is given a glass of ice-cold salt solution.
7. Films of the small intestine are now made every 10 minutes.
8. 4–6 hours after the beginning of the examination, films are made of the orally-filled colon.

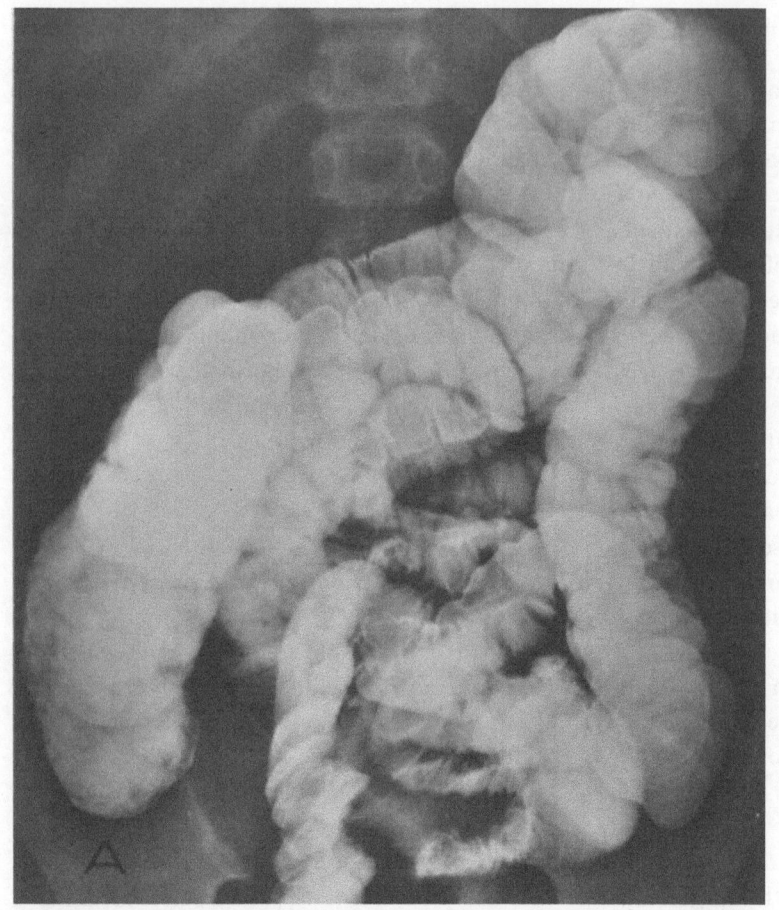

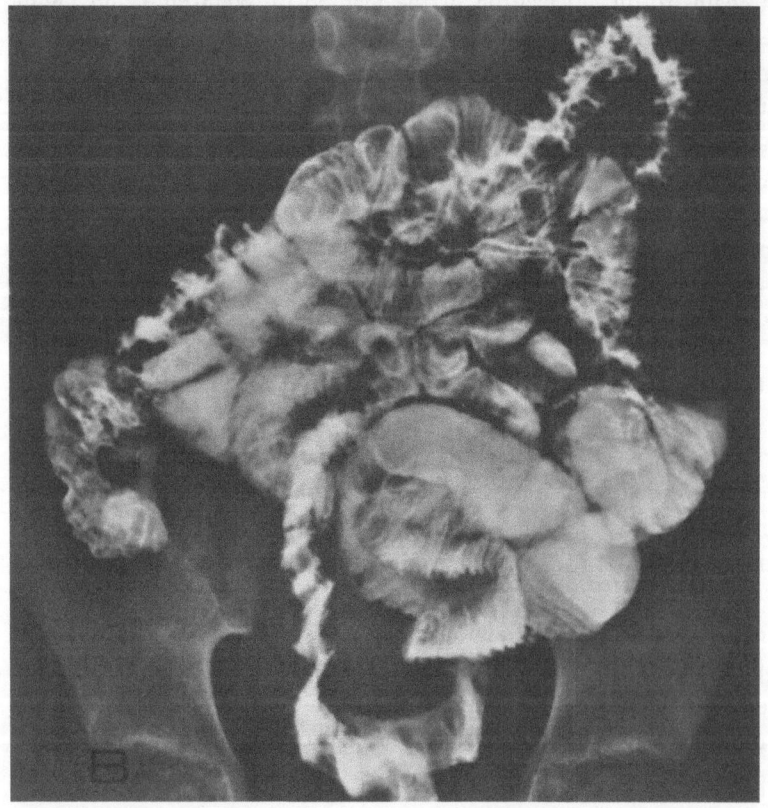

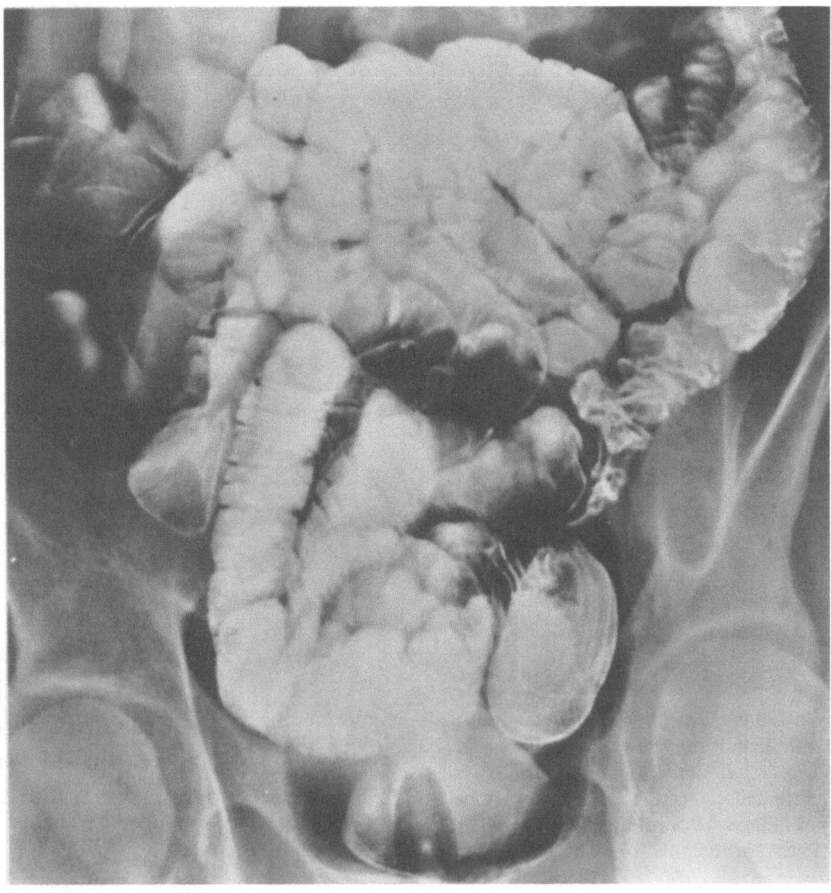

Fig. 5.4
Survey exposure after evacuation; in this case the ileum could only be filled after a hypotonic drug was administered. Evaluation of the colon was of course fairly difficult.

←

Fig. 5.3
Roentgenogram of retrograde filling of the small intestine.
A. Survey exposure after filling of the colon and ileum; hypotonic agent was not administered.
B. Survey film after evacuation; the colon is now empty.

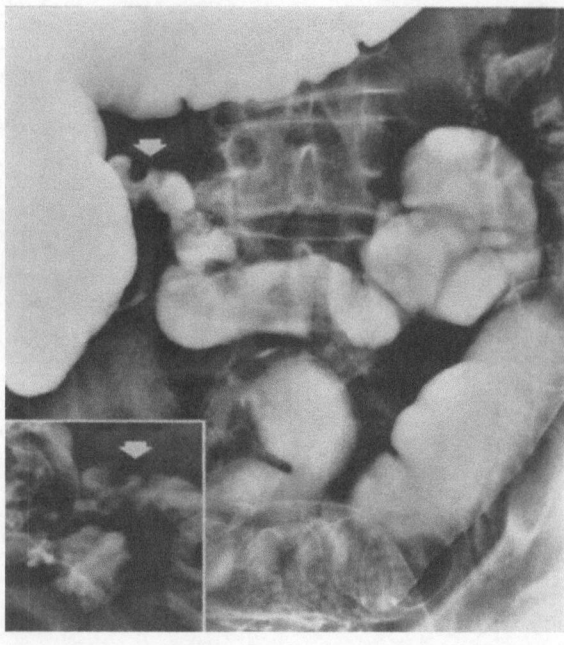

Fig. 5.5
With the enteroclysis technique, this small tumor in the distal ileum was not reached although 2500 ml contrast fluid and water were administered and the examination was continued for one hour. The tumor was quickly visualized via filling of the colon. The patient had been hospitalized 5 times elsewhere because of rectal bleeding.

Unfortunately the article contains no photographs of his results. Bugyi suffices with the statement that he is highly satisfied with this method and that a colon enema examination only occurs upon strict indications.

8. Use of drugs to accelerate transit

The radiologists' growing lack of time and the high demands on the patience and endurance of the patient are the reasons why shortening the length of the examination has been an objective for so many years. This can be accomplished by:

1. drinking very large quantities of contrast fluid.
2. administering the contrast fluid directly into the duodenum by infusion.
3. supplementary administration of cold fluids.
4. mixture of the contrast fluid with Gastrografine. The patient finds methods 1 and 2 more or less unpleasant; method 4 has an unfavourable effect on the quality of the image and method 3 combines both of these unpleasant characteristics.
5. In the past few years, several drugs which are in no way unpleasant for the patient have been used to increase the rate of transit. The effect of these drugs differs greatly; we shall discuss each of them briefly.

a. PROSTIGMIN

A substance long known for its accelerating effect on transit but used only seldom is neostigmine methylsulfate or prostigmin. In Chapter III, we have seen that this substance inhibits acetylcholinesterase so that the acetylcholine is protected against hydrolysis and can be active longer. The effective dosage for adults is 0.75–1.0 mg and for children, 0.25–0.5 mg. It can be administered subcutaneously, intramuscularly or intravenously; with the latter, the effect is the strongest but lasts only a few minutes. The effect of prostigmin can be neutralized by atropine.

Contra-indications for the use of prostigmin are: recent myocardial infarction, volvulus, intussusception and complete obstruction or perforation of the small intestine. Prostigmin has no effect when there is dysfunction of the nerve cells, as in sprue.

An older publication on the use of this substance in a follow-through examination is that of Hudak (96) in 1951. As a result of a combination of factors, however, the photographs published are very poor. Hudak used only a small amount of contrast fluid (not specifically reported) and afterwards he even

Fig. 5.6
AB.   Retrograde filling of the colon and the entire small intestine (A). Because of a highly obstructive abnormality in the pars antralis of the stomach resulting from Crohn's disease, an enteroclysis examination for evaluation of the small intestine appeared to be impossible. After evacuation (B) only the loops of the small intestine are filled. Several skip lesions were found in the duodenum and the jejunum as well as a fistula to the stomach.

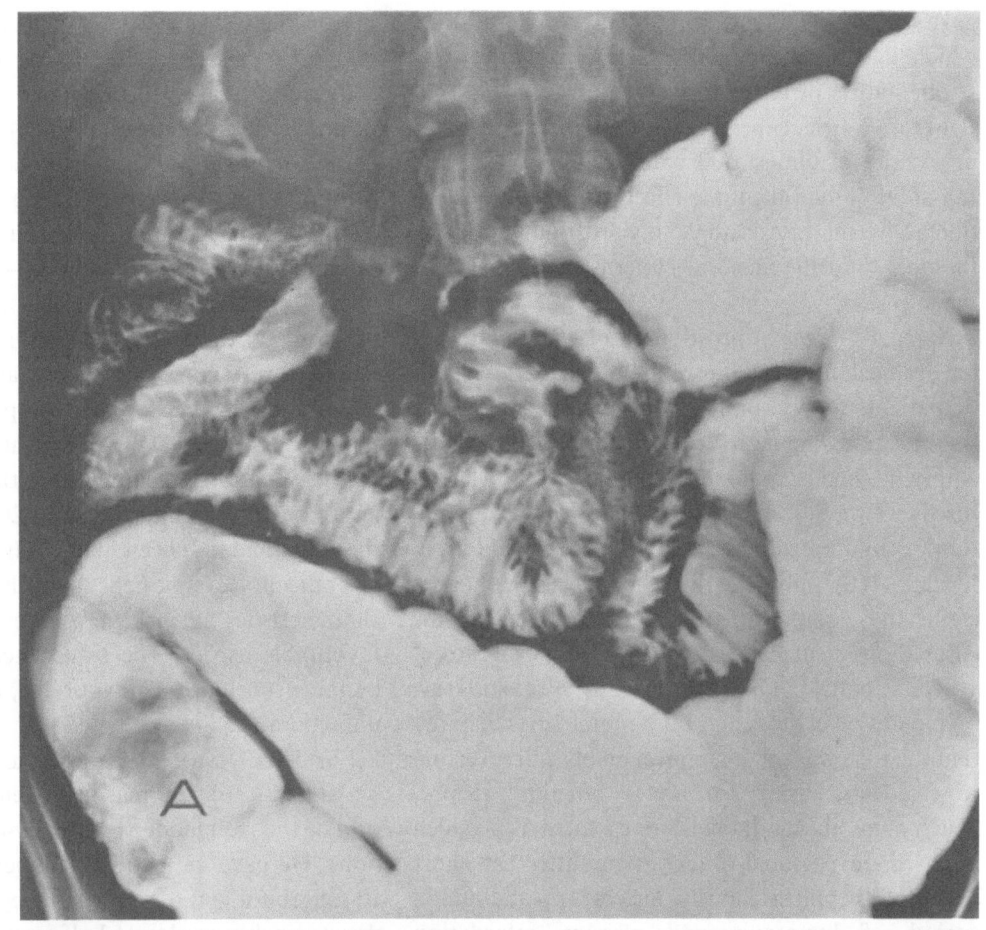

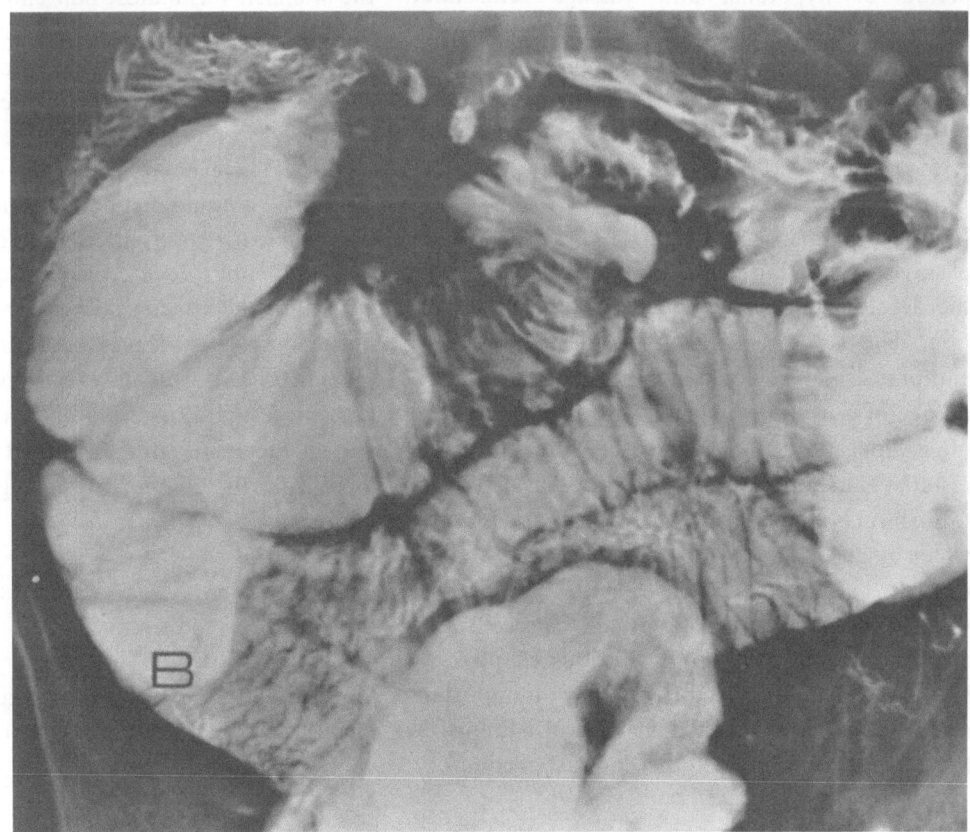

gave a glass of ice-cold physiological salt solution, which had to result in complete flocculation and segmentation of the contrast medium.

In 1962 Friedenberg et al. (59) also found that, in a series of almost 500 patients, 400 ml ice-cold salt solution had the same effect of transit acceleration as 400 ml water with 0.5 mg prostigmin but that the quality of the mucosal patterns was better with the latter.

Margulis has used prostigmin for examination of the stomach and small intestine of many thousands of patients to his complete satisfaction (136, 137). As a result of the more active peristalsis, the gastric emptying time is approximately half as long. Therefore he saw a decrease in the percentage of examination of children with flocculation and segmentation. Müller (160) published his experiences with neoserine in 97 patients; however, 10 per cent of the cases showed side-effects of a respiratory or cardiovascular nature. Like Margulis he also still saw segmentation in the ileum. Both radiologists believed that the tone was too high, presumably still reverting to Golden's 'disordered motor function' theory. Much more likely is the following explanation which is based on personal observations: after the short effect of the intravenously injected prostigmin, a period of hypotonia and passage retardation develops which inevitably results in flocculation and segmentation of the contrast medium.

b. SORBITOL

In 1957 Porcher and Caroli (179) described the passage acceleration caused by 30 g Sorbitol without the development of hypersecretion and segmentation. The latter, however, is contested by many authors although it must be noted that an overdosage of Sorbitol or mixing with other substances often appears to be the reason for their poor results (134, 135).

Sorbitol is a glucose product (hexahydric alcohol) which is absorbed slowly and causes only a slight increase in the blood sugar curve. It has caloric value and is hyperosmotic which can cause indistinct mucosal patterns. In previous chapters we have seen that other factors can play an important role here, such as quantity, method of administration and composition of the contrast medium.

It is likely that the lowest effective dosage will be the best because a higher dosage will cause a linear increase in fluid absorption but a gradual decrease in acceleration of transit. It is therefore probably correct to use 10–20 g as advised by the manufacturer and not to increase to 30 g as some do (214). Manecke and Schmidt (134) found the same; they obtained poor results with 20–30 ml Karion F (variation of Sorbitol) and only 20 ml barium suspension. With 5–10 ml Karion F the mucosal patterns were good, but there was only a slight acceleration of transit. As a compromise they gave their patients 10 ml Karion F at the beginning of the examination. One hour later, the patient received another supplementary dose of 20 ml after films of the ileum had first been made. Furthermore Sorbitol is both cholecystokinetic and cholagogic; these 2 characteristics again have a favourable and an unfavourable aspect. The transit acceleration caused by these substances is favourable, the flocculation is unfavourable.

For Sack (196), the transit acceleration caused by gall was still the reason for enhancing contraction of the gallbladder for follow-through examinations. He gave his patients Diabenol, a mixture of 10 g Sorbitol and 4 g powdered egg, but not before the stomach was almost half empty since Diabenol does accelerate transit but of course also retards gastric emptying. In 20 per cent of the patients, the substance was not successful, usually because of insufficient contraction or absence of the gallbladder. The evening before the examination Sack prescribed a liquid diet and a laxative to cleanse the colon. The mucosal patterns of ileum and colon on the films published are of good quality: it is quite clear that the barium suspension has retained the proper viscosity because of the rapid transit time (30 min!). Unfortunately Sack does not provide any further data; it seems likely that the quantities and characteristics of the contrast medium administered contributed more to his good results than Diabenol.

c. METOCLOPRAMIDE (PRIMPERAN)

Since about 1966, metoclopramide has been used increasingly for transit acceleration. Because of its effect on the brain stem, this substance is supposed to activate and regulate the tone and peristalsis of the small intestine and the stomach without influencing the secretion. This substance can be administered both orally and by injection; the effective dose is 10–20 mg for an adult (1 ampule of 2 ml = 10 mg). Intravenous injection produces of course the quickest effect; within 5 minutes enhancement of peristalsis can already be seen clearly as both the number and intensity of the peristaltic waves increase. We have found that the effect lasts only 15–20 minutes; however, most radiologists report a slightly longer effective period (95, 98).

Diverse authors report that with Primperan (trade name) transit is accelerated to such a degree that the cecum is usually reached in 1 to 2 hours (98). In these publications it is striking that the contrast medium dosage is usually not mentioned although this factor is at least equally important for the transit time (33).

Some authors are justifiably of the opinion that accelerated gastric emptying is an important factor for the transit acceleration caused by metoclo-pramide. Howarth (95) reports that the gastric emptying time is halved by Primperan.

Many also believe that the improvement in the mucosal patterns of the ileum can be ascribed to a decrease in dehydration of the contrast medium as a result of the acceleration of transit. It is strange that the dilatation of duodenum and proximal jejunum frequently seen by accelerated gastric emptying is often believed to be due to a decrease in tone.

The more active peristalsis of the stomach is a time-saving factor for the gastric-duodenal examination and in addition can be useful for duodenal intubation and for cinematographical examination of fixed and immobile sections of the gastric wall.

If it seems necessary to use a transit accelerating drug, metoclopramide (Primperan) appears to be the best choice at present. This preparation is not hydrophilic and, as a result of the accelerated gastric emptying, causes stretching of the duodenum and thus transit acceleration.

VI

GENERAL CONSIDERATIONS

For the examination of the small intestine, it should be realized that this organ is several meters long and lies convoluted in a small space. Owing to tone and peristalsis, the mucosal patterns of each intestinal section vary greatly in different phases.

The objective of the radiological examination is to signalize restrictions in the mobility of the mucosa and anatomical abnormalities of the intestinal wall in an early stage. When the contact between the contrast medium and the mucosa is good, abnormalities can easily be observed. One condition is of course that each intestinal section be shown on at least 2 exposures without superposition. It is often difficult to locate the related intestinal segments on various photographs so that it is wise to make two exposures in succession. In the case of hypertonic, contracted loops, the highly folded mucosa lies even more loosely over the innermost layers of the intestinal wall so that deeper abnormalities in this wall can be concealed completely. In general in a hypotonic or dilated intestine, abnormalities located outside the mucosa are seen more easily since the mucosa then lies against this abnormality smoothly and with few folds (fig. 2.6). We have less difficulty also when an abnormality is seen by chance in the narrow space between 2 loops which are in a more or less hypotonic phase. This combination of favourable factors occurs of course only seldom.

In certain cases, if we should find it desirable, dilatation of the small intestine can be enhanced by an injection of atropine or TEAB (tetraethylammonium bromide). With atropine, the movements of the muscularis mucosa still exist, not with TEAB; the paralyzing effect of this substance is so strong that there is no motion at all (93).

After these preparations are injected, passage comes to a standstill and as a result superposition increases due to dilatation and possibly also lengthening of the loops of the small intestine. Intervention with these drugs is therefore only to be considered in the last phase of the examination after sufficient normal exposures have been made.

Theoretically it would appear sensible to restrict superposition by fractional administration of the contrast medium. The most even distribution of the contrast fluid in the small intestine is obtained by dividing the total amount into as many fractions as possible which are then administered so slowly that the continuity of the contrast column is just maintained. The contrast medium could also be administered until the cecum is reached and then a number of exposures of the entire small intestine are made. In this way, with a restricted number of photographs, the greatest amount of information could be obtained.

Just as sensible theoretically is the method of following a small amount of contrast medium to the cecum without the slightest problem of superposition. With this method, of course, exposures must be made within short time intervals which means prolonged radiation exposure for the patient. With oral administration of the contrast medium, we must realize that we can regulate the supply to the stomach easily but that the passage from stomach to duodenum can only be regulated by influencing the pyloric mechanism.

Orally administered contrast medium does not leave the stomach at a constant rate, but at a gradually decreasing rate. When Henderson's (87) results are plotted on a graph, the resulting curve will resemble curve A in fig. 5.1. It shows clearly that greater gastric filling only slightly lengthens the gastric emptying time while the average rate of gastric emptying increases. It is clear that the

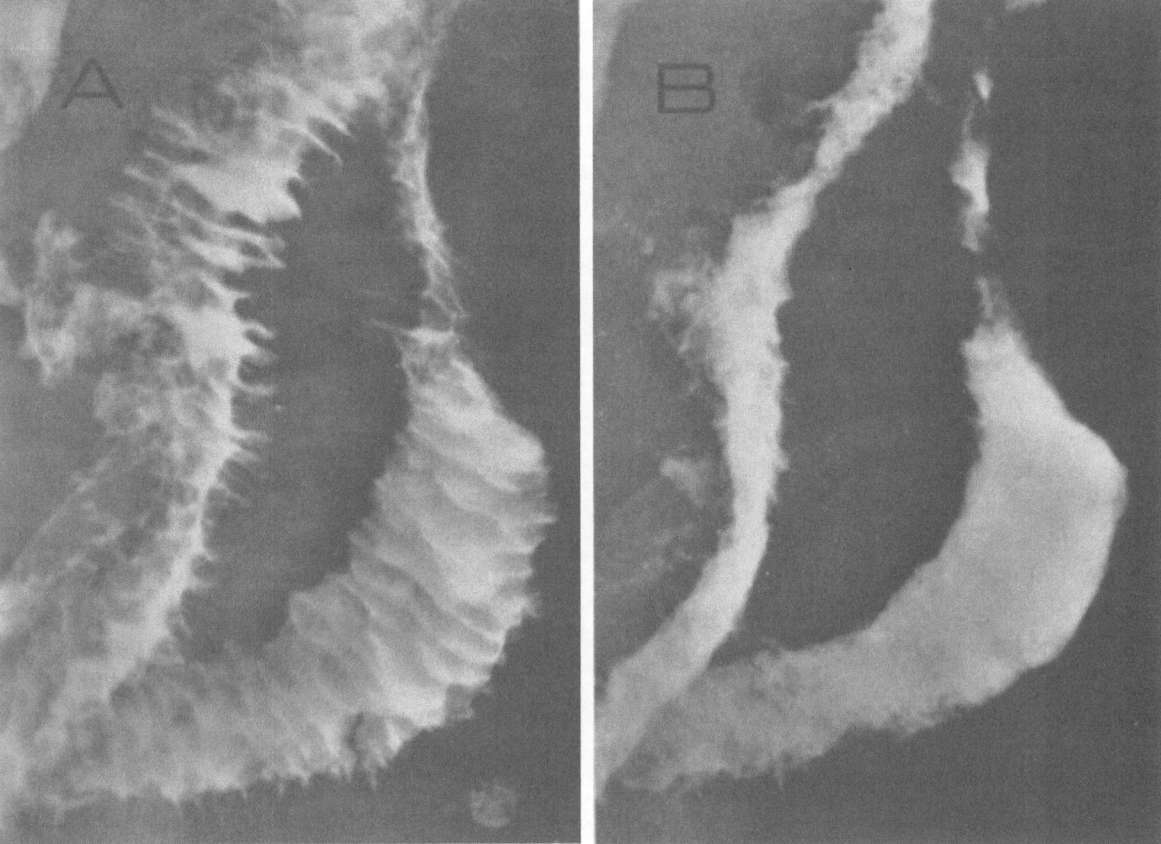

Fig. 6.1
Liposarcoma of the mesentery invading the wall of the jejunum.
A. Coarse irregular mucosal folds.
B. 30 minutes later the contrast fluid has disintegrated (granular structure) and can no longer reproduce the mucosal patterns.

decrease in the tone of the gastric wall and the gradual decrease in the supply of contrast medium to the pylorus cause the curve to become increasingly horizontal as the stomach becomes almost empty. We have seen that the rate of gastric emptying increases in the right lateral position. When the stomach is full, the effect is insignificant; when it is nearly empty, however, there is an obvious gain as a result of the considerably improved supply of contrast medium to the pylorus.

In the left lateral position of course gastric emptying will be the slowest. Some mothers learn to lay a baby on this side after a feeding and to alternate between the right and left sides. It is not impossible that this factor plays an important role in the high average gastric emptying time determined for babies (22).

With fractional administration of the contrast medium, the stomach is only partially filled; in the ideal case, emptying will occur according to curve B of fig. 5.1. For equal fractions administered too rapidly, the stomach will empty approximately as shown on curve C and D of fig. 5.1.

Mixing proteins and carbohydrates through the contrast fluid inhibits peristalsis and keeps the pylorus closed for longer periods. For fats, this effect is even more pronounced; even 8 hours after a meal rich in fats, peristalsis of the stomach is still retarded. In addition it appeared that in healthy individuals flocculation and segmentation of the contrast medium only occurred when they had consumed a meal rich in fats the evening before (57, 189). Experiments with dogs showed that even a high or low blood sugar curve can markedly influence gastric peristalsis and the rate of transit (129). Hunger contractions when the blood sugar is low also occur in humans.

The pylorus remains closed when the contents of the stomach or duodenum are highly acidic or basic. For patients with achlorhydria this closing mechanism does not function as well; the pyloric ring is more relaxed and the stomach therefore empties quickly.

We also saw that isotonic solutions leave the stomach the fastest and that hypotonic solutions do not take much longer. However, when a hypotonic solution is introduced directly into the duodenum the pylorus will remain closed until a condition of isotonicity is achieved (67). Hypertonic solutions retard gastric emptying considerably, even when they are administered directly into the duodenum. In the stomach, a hypertonic solution gradually becomes isotonic as a result of heavy fluid secretion of the gastric wall. This can be accompanied by a considerable increase in volume.

Cold fluids leave the stomach much faster and warm fluids only slightly slower than a solution at body temperature (66). The rapid transit of a cold fluid through the small intestine can certainly be ascribed in part to the accelerated gastric emptying. The reaction of gastric peristalsis and the pylorus to the direct administration of cold or warm fluids into the duodenum has unfortunately not yet been studied; the mechanism for this temperature sensitivity is also unknown. Furthermore it is important to know that the activation of the neutralization mechanism in the duodenum, a reaction to milieu distrubances of all kinds, does not begin until after the bulb and then decreases in the distal direction (1, 12, 67, 108, 124, 188, 202).

The contrast medium has a very difficult time during a gastro-intestinal examination; it must successively endure the influence of gastric acid, intestinal juice and fluid withdrawal without losing its proper characteristics. In some cases, there is also the detrimental effect of fatty acids, gall or lactic acid which practically no contrast medium can tolerate.

Diverse brands can withstand the effect of gastric acid and mucin reasonably well but only a few contrast media can endure dehydration without becoming practically useless. The viscosity then becomes so high that the soft mucosal folds cause few impressions, or none at all. The specific gravity of the contrast mass increases; it retains, however, its homogeneous structure.

We can see that the contrast medium is about to lose the battle when flocculation develops; if in addition segmentation has already developed, then it has definitely lost. The structure of these segment clumps is not homogeneous as in the case of dehydration; the genesis is also different. If it is understandable that a highly thickened contrast medium is no longer able to produce true mucosal patterns, it must then be obvious for a splotchy segment clump (fig. 6.1). In 1942 Bouslog had already seen moulage-like patterns in small children which were not in agreement with the normal mucosal patterns seen at autopsy; the reason for this incongruity was then not understood.

If we study the curves of Braeckman and Zimmer, we learn that disintegration of the contrast medium is a physicochemical process which proceeds gradually and that even in the most unfavourable circumstances we still have to make a number of useful roentgenograms (fig. 6.2AB).

From the preceding it can be seen that it is sensible to give large amounts of contrast medium; the influence of harmful substances on the contrast medium is then less. Furthermore it is obvious that this dosage must pass through the small intestine as rapidly as possible; reaction with the harmful substances is then short-lived and the detrimental effect is as small as possible.

Another important advantage of an extremely rapid passage is the lack of time for dehydration of the contrast medium in the distal ileum and the colon. Because the low viscosity is maintained, mucosal patterns with a maximum reproduction of detail can also be obtained for these sections of the distal intestine. It is not easy to choose among the large number of brands of contrast medium on the market. There are some which are reasonably satisfactory but no single brand can be called ideal.

In 1932, Adam (2) had already reported that the characteristics of the contrast medium suspension are determined predominantly by chemical additives and not the particle size, as is so often suggested by the manufacturers. The requirements for a contrast medium used for a gastro-intestinal examination are much higher than for a colon examination. For the latter good adhesion to the mucosa is of decisive importance; for the former, sufficient stability to prevent flocculation is of even greater importance. Furthermore the viscosity may not be too high and must be maintained insofar as possible under the influence of fluid withdrawal in the ileum.

Supplementary administration of cooled fluids and fluid attracting or secretion enhancing substances is strongly discouraged. Mixture of glucose, Gastrografine or Sorbitol with the contrast fluid has an unfavourable effect in this respect. It is difficult to determine with certainty whether or not prostigmin and metoclopramide are completely free of a secretion enhancing effect.

When Rieder (191) introduced his standard 'meal' at the beginning of the century, this meal was in general use and recording the transit time was probably useful. This harmony, however, did not last very long because the method of examination and the use of contrast media later became highly diversified. It is therefore not surprising that the average transit time reported between 1930 and 1950 by prominent radiologists varied between 2 and 5 hours with extreme values of 1 and 8 hours (130). From the above, it is obvious that including these values on x-ray films and in reports is exceedingly unimportant today. It would probably be better to omit them since they can lead to incorrect conclusions.

Summarizing it must be concluded that a large quantity of contrast medium should be administered by infusion directly into the duodenum. It should be administered so quickly that the stretching of the duodenum induces maximum peristalsis, but not so quickly that peristalsis is inhibited by the enterointestinal reflex mechanism or that the patient will vomit. The amount of contrast medium must be as large as possible but then again not so large that the problem of superposition develops.

The contrast fluid must be hypotonic; hypertonia stimulates fluid attraction and therefore dilution of the contrast fluid; isotonia does not stimulate contraction of the pyloric muscle and in this way enhances the development of reflux into the stomach.

Another advantage of by-passing the stomach is that the detrimental effect of gastric acid on the contrast fluid is eliminated and that the rate of supply to the duodenum is no longer dependent upon the pyloric function.

Since most brands are reasonably stable in alkaline surroundings, we are less restricted now in the choice of contrast medium; the adhesive quality and the viscosity can be the decisive factors. From the above it will be clear that the unrealized ideal of standardization of the contrast medium, desired by so many radiologists, has as a result of this method outlived itself. A continuous supply of contrast fluid without the annoying influence of air bubbles, which possibly also retard transit, is only guaranteed in the right lateral position. The patient may possibly also lie on his back or on his abdomen but in any event, the left lateral position is incorrect.

The question of the most favourable temperature for the contrast medium requires further investigation. It is true that an ice-cold contrast fluid does enhance gastric emptying and intestinal peristalsis but when administered into the duodenum, there is also relaxation of the pylorus so that reflux into the stomach could occur. A warm contrast fluid keeps the pylorus closed longer but could even work as a transit decelerator when administered directly into the duodenum. For our examinations therefore a relatively neutral standpoint is taken; all patients received the contrast medium at room temperature or slightly cooler ($\pm 15°$ C). Also unanswered is the question of the most favourable location for the end of the tube in the duodenum. It is possible that reflux into the stomach is more likely when the end of the tube lies proximal; then when the contrast fluid is administered, maximum stretching of the duodenum occurs quite close to the pylorus which as a result may not close as well.

Another factor is the pyloric ring which is usually relaxed; it takes several seconds before contraction occurs. It is clear that at least some reflux of contrast fluid into the stomach will occur when the end of the tube lies close to the open pyloric canal.

Thirdly a tube located in the proximal part of the duodenum can slip back into the stomach as a result of regurgitation.

On the basis of these somewhat speculative considerations, in our patients the end of the tube is placed in the duodenojejunal area, although it must be assumed that the peristalsis induced by stretching of the intestinal wall is less here than close to the bulb.

It is possible that in achlorhydria reflux of the contrast fluid into the stomach will occur sooner; this question cannot be answered and requires further study. As mentioned previously it is obvious that reflux cannot be terminated once it has occurred. The best thing to do is a supplementary dosage of contrast medium administered at once as well as stimulation of gastric emptying with Primperan. Obviously the patient must lie on the right lateral side between exposures.

In all cases we must concentrate on 'forcing' the contrast medium to the cecum as quickly as possible. Especially in patients with a possible malabsorption syndrome, the disintegration of the contrast medium can occur so quickly that examination of the small intestine must be considered a 'case of great haste'.

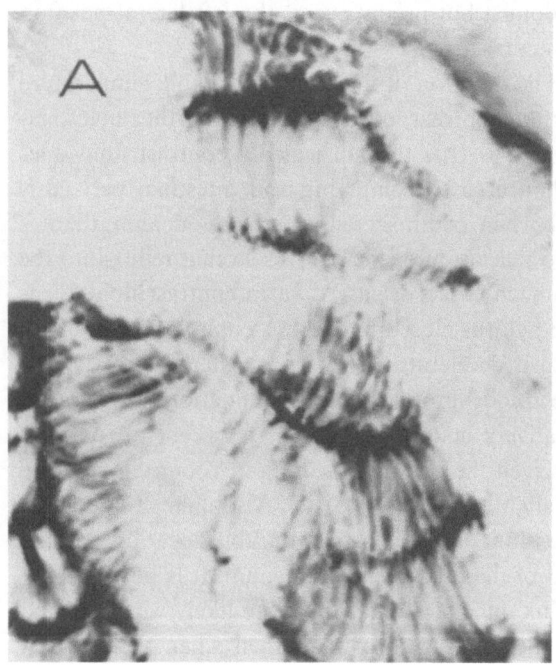

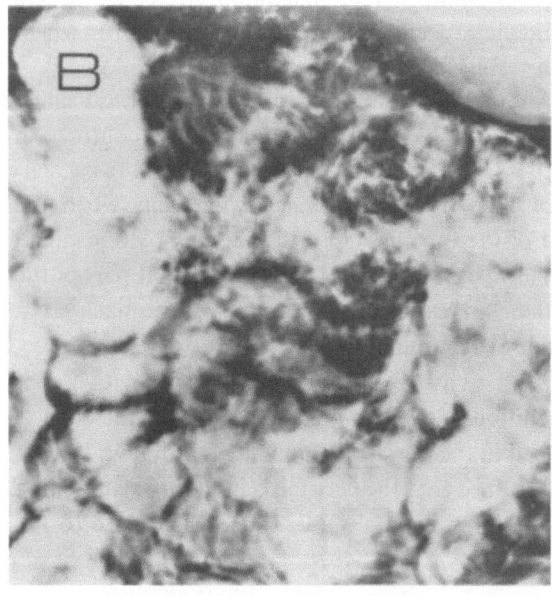

Fig. 6.2 AB
Enteroclysis examination of a 8-month-old baby.
A. Good reproduction of jejunal loops during contrast medium infusion.
B. After the tube is pulled back into the stomach, the rate of flow to the small intestine decreases and within several minutes severe flocculation developed so that the examination had to be terminated.

VII

THE ENTERAL CONTRAST INFUSION

1. Preparation of patients

Even more important than for a conventional follow-through study is the thorough cleansing of the patient; it is even desirable that the stomach be entirely empty and thus contain no fasting gastric residuum. Should there be gastric fluid in the stomach the pyloric ring will not close properly since it is a natural reaction of the stomach to dispel its contents through the pylorus. When an infusion is running, the pressure in the duodenum is probably greater than the pressure in the stomach so that the open pyloric ring will have a reverse effect on gastric emptying and reflux of the contrast fluid into the stomach from the duodenum will occur. Since the presence of feces in the cecum will tend to retard the rate of passage through the ileum, it is obvious that the patient must follow a low-residue diet and that the colon should be thoroughly cleansed. It is therefore preferable that the last meal on the day before the examination be free of fats.

Comparison of the results of examinations when the patients did and did not receive a laxative beforehand has shown that less contrast fluid is required to reach the cecum when it is cleansed than when it is contaminated. Of course it is easier to project the separate ileal loops in the lower abdomen with a low dosage of contrast fluid than with a high dosage which causes greater intestinal filling. An additional advantage of a well-cleansed cecum is that although the x-rays then obtained of this part of the intestine are inferior to the films from a routine colon examination, they are still usable.

It is exceedingly important that castor oil, or any other purgative given for laxation of the colon, be administered orally. It is not advisable to cleanse the colon by means of a rectal cleansing enema. We have found that a cleansing enema can some-times cause extensive reflux of the clyster fluid into the ileum. Some of this clyster fluid is often retained in the ileum and proximal colon and will mix with the contrast fluid flowing in from the proximal direction; as a result the mucosal patterns in this important part of the intestine can only be evaluated with great difficulty or not at all. It is true of course that the disadvantages of a rectal enema can be overcome entirely or to a large extent by waiting 1–2 hours before beginning enteroclysis but then one can no longer speak of a short examination.

Whenever possible preparation of the patient should also include discontinuation of drugs which inhibit peristalsis in the intestine. In general it can be stated that such a drug should be discontinued for a period which depends upon the length of time the patient has been taking the drug (see also chapter XII).

If the patient has received antispasmodics, sedatives or tranquillizers for many months or even years, then discontinuation before the radiological examination will serve little purpose since these drugs must be discontinued for many months before any improvement is noted in the peristaltic movement in the intestine. In addition it should be stated that prior to or during the examination no drugs should be given which enhance the production of bile or contraction of the gallbladder. Bile pigments do in fact stimulate peristaltic action in the intestine but on the other hand also tend to promote disintegration of the contrast fluid. An initial advantage can therefore become a disadvantage if the examination has to be prolonged.

Finally, the patient must be told that large amounts of fluid will be administered during the examination and that as a result he may have to micturate frequently and there may be some diarrhea for several hours afterwards. This should be taken into account when planning the trip home; it might even be wise to remain in the waiting room of the radiology department for 15 minutes or more.

2. Duodenal intubation

Fear of the time-consuming intubation procedure is often the main reason that enteroclysis has not been introduced as a routine procedure in some departments of radiology. If, however, the trouble is taken to practice this technique several times and if the directions described below are followed, then experience will show that this fear is without foundation. After some practice, duodenal intubation of most patients only takes several minutes and fluoroscopy requires 10–30 sec at the most. In only a few patients out of every hundred will intubation prove to be difficult for various reasons; it may then take 10 minutes, sometimes slightly longer. These difficulties are, however, insignificant in comparison to the improved results and the much shorter examination (15–30 minutes). Only in cases of obstruction or drug-induced atony of the small intestine can the examination last 1 or 2 hours depending upon the dose of contrast medium. It is obvious that this is still very short when compared with the conventional follow-through studies which can last all day in such cases, in spite of the administration of large amounts of contrast fluid and drugs to accelerate transit. Furthermore the roentgenograms of a conventional examination will become useless much sooner because of disintegration, pronounced dilution or thickening of the contrast fluid.

Of the tubes on the market today the best choice is the extended Bilbao-Dotter tube (fig. 7.1B) which was designed especially for enteroclysis. The guide wire of this tube has the correct degree of rigidity; those in the catheters used for angiography are too flexible.

In comparison with the original Bilbao tube (fig. 7.1A) designed for duodenography in hypotonic patients, the tube in the new model is not shorter than the guide wire but is instead several centimeters longer. This offers the following advantages:

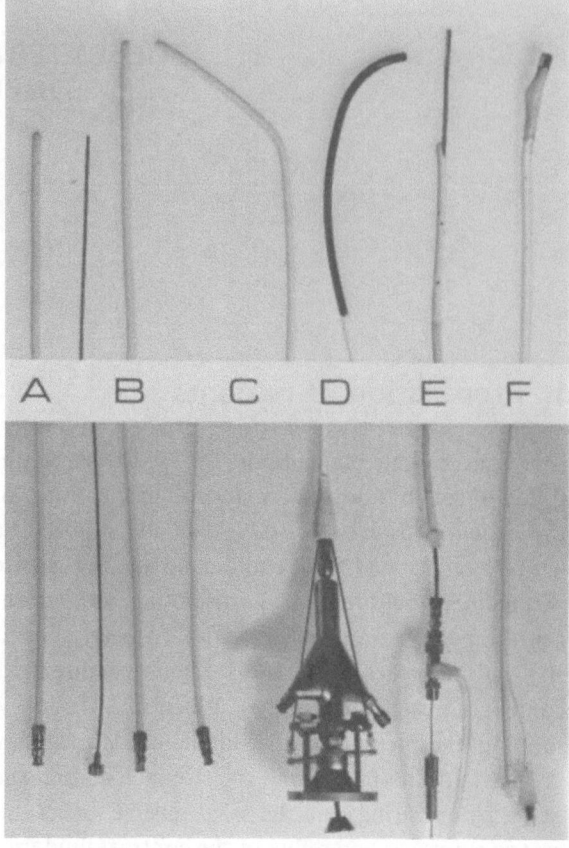

Fig. 7.1
Tubes sold by Cook and Söborg in Denmark.
A. Bilbao-Dotter: guide wire and tube of equal length.
B. so-called Sellink modification: tube 6 cm longer than guide wire.
C. acute angle of 20° in the distal end of the guide wire and the tube.
D. tube which can be guided.
E. tube which is also suited for taking blind biopsies.
F. very long tube with inflatable cuff at the tip, used for selective fillings.

1. Perforation of the wall of the stomach is eliminated since the tip of the guide wire can no longer extend through the side openings in the tube (fig. 7.2).
2. For large atonic stomachs, the old tube was too short and the tip could not reach the distal part of the duodenum.
3. The end of the tube automatically remains flexible which makes it easier to pass through the pylorus.

The tube is best introduced while the patient sits or stands. The stomach is then in a lower part of the abdomen than when the patient is in a supine position; in this way troublesome coiling of the tube in the fundus is often prevented.

Sometimes, however, this is not enough. Then it may help to have the patient breath in or out as deeply as possible as the tube is pushed into the fundus. The gag reflex causes the least trouble if the tube is pushed in as quickly as possible until it is past the glottis. Some radiographers are so proficient in this respect that local anesthesia is completely superfluous. Furthermore we do not advocate anesthetization of the pharyngeal region because we would rather be sure that the patient will not choke after the examination; another undesirable possibility is that the absorbed anesthetic could relax the smooth musculature of the intestinal wall during the examination.

If desired the tube can also be inserted through one of the nostrils instead of the mouth; this port of entry is better in infants since it is easier to secure the tube with tape after it has been positioned. It should, however, be remembered that it can be more difficult to manipulate the guide wire through the fixed curve of the nasopharynx than through the open mouth when the head is tilted backwards. The physician or radiographer quickly slides the tube on until the tip is approximately in the pars antralis of the stomach; this is verified under fluoroscopy. The guide wire is now introduced; it is inserted to within 5 or 6 cm of the tip of the tube, which therefore remains quite flexible. For low atonic stomachs, the flexible part of the tube must be even longer, for instance 10 or 12 cm; it is then easier to pass through the pylorus. The patient himself, now lying on his back or right side, pushes the combination of guide wire and tube further; progress is checked by intermittent fluoroscopy. As soon as the flexible tip of the tube approaches the pylorus, it will begin to flap from side to side. If at that instant it is not possible to pass through the pylorus quickly, we recommend applying light pressure with the tip of the tube and then waiting until the spasm of the pyloric ring subsides. Sometimes it is useful to pull the guide wire back several centimeters. If too much pressure is applied against the pyloric ring, the tube will curl back in the direction of the fundus. If the guide wire is inserted into the outermost tip of the tube, curling of the tube would in fact be prevented but instead of

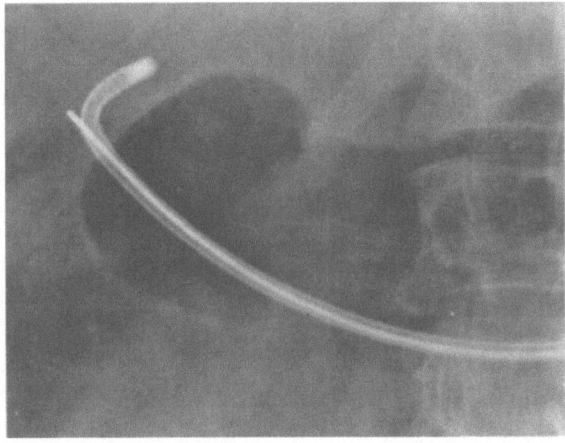

Fig. 7.2
With the original Bilbao-Dotter tube, it was possible that the guide wire would extend through one of the side openings, thus perforating the wall of the stomach or damaging the mucous membrane.

passing through the pylorus more easily, the tube will cause a prepyloric sack-like bulge in the wall of the stomach on the side of greater curvature.

As soon as the tip of the tube has passed the pyloric ring, the guide wire must be pulled back to within 5 or 6 cm of the pyloric ring on the prepyloric side. Take care that the guide wire does not enter the duodenum where it must follow a curved path and is therefore much more difficult to pull back. In cases of doubt the patient must lie on his right side because only in this position can it be determined with absolute certainty under fluoroscopy whether or not the tube has passed the pyloric ring; it will then be seen that the tip of the tube first extends perpendicular to the spinal column and then, in the retroperitoneal region, downwards (fig. 7.3). A rare exception to this rule is seen in fig. 7.4; it is of course also obvious that in the case of a duodenum en guirlande, the descending path of the tube will also be abnormal (fig. 7.5). In the case of seriously ill or highly rheumatic patients as well as accident victims with multiple fractures of the extremities, the patient may have to remain on his back for the introduction of the tube as well as the actual examination. Then it is not possible to have the patient lie on his side in order to check on the position of the tube. When a supine position is mandatory, the following criteria will be helpful (fig. 7.6).

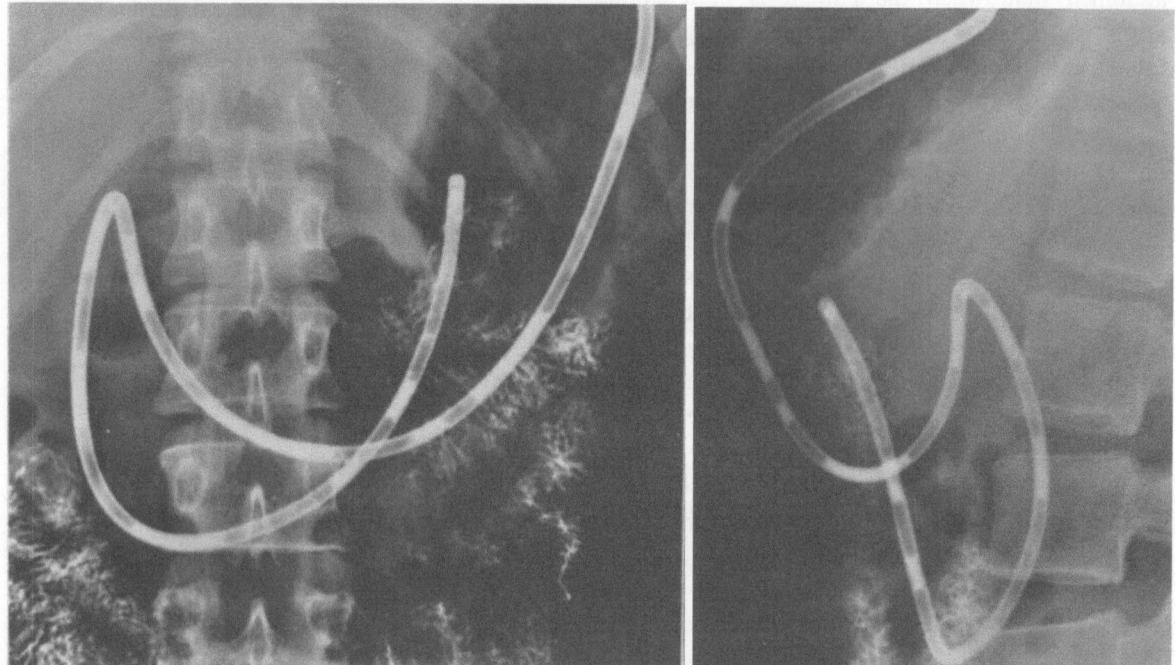

Fig. 7.3
Normal position of the tube after intubation. α-configuration in AP projection, reversed α in right lateral projection.

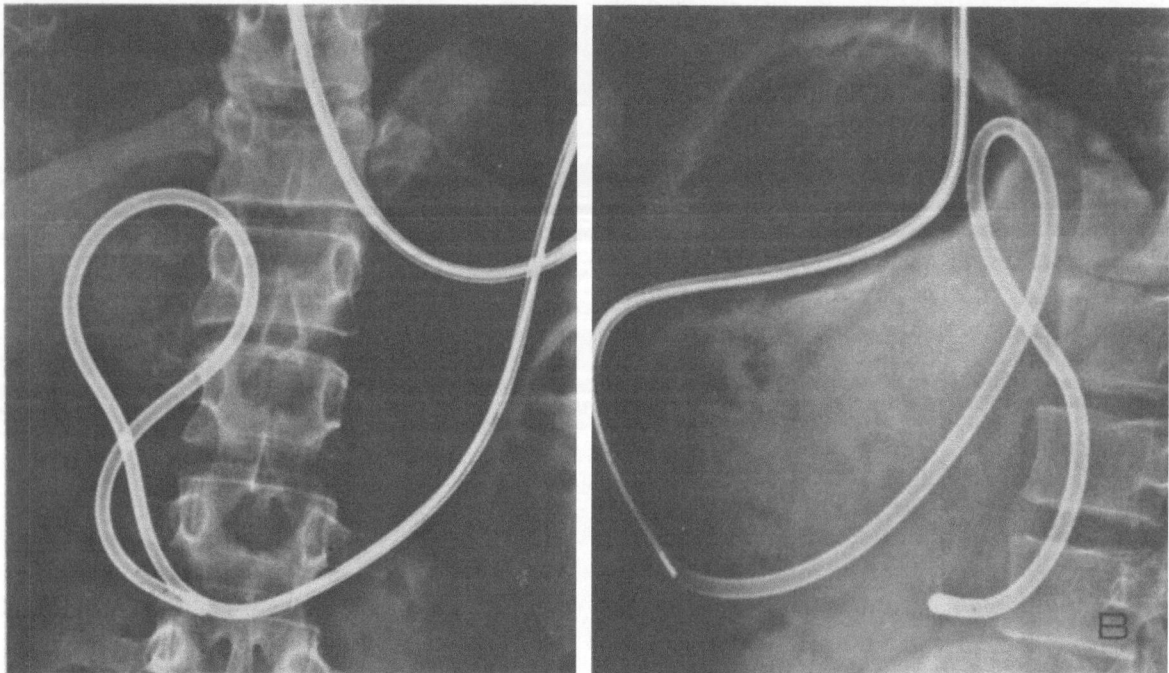

Fig. 7.4
Rare variation of a correct positioning of the tube.
A.   in the AP projection the tube passes through the pylorus in the medial direction and then extends back along the side of
     greater curvature but outside the stomach; it appears, however, as if the tube did not pass through the pylorus but has
     coiled in the stomach.
B.   in the right lateral projection, the tube does not move perpendicular to the spinal column but first extends in the opposite
     direction and then drops down into the retroperitoneal space.

Fig. 7.5
Duodenum en guirlande: after passing through the pylorus the tube first moves downwards slightly and then upwards again.

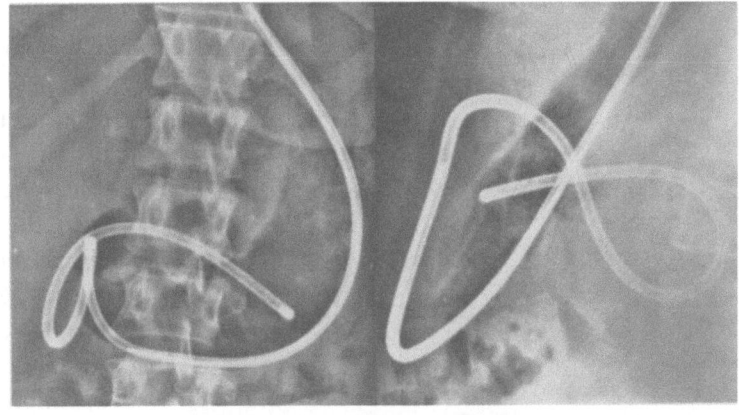

Fig. 7.6
Possible positions of the tube when the patient is in supine position.
1. tube is usually not correct because it passes through the pylorus in the medial direction and turns back along the side of greater curvature in the stomach.
2. the tube is probably correct because it turns back in a plane above the level of the side of greater curvature of the stomach.
3. the tube is almost certainly correctly positioned because it crosses the side of greater curvature and then turns back at a lower level.
4/5. the tube passes through the pylorus in the lateral direction. The tube is then correct even if it turns back at the same level as the side of greater curvature.

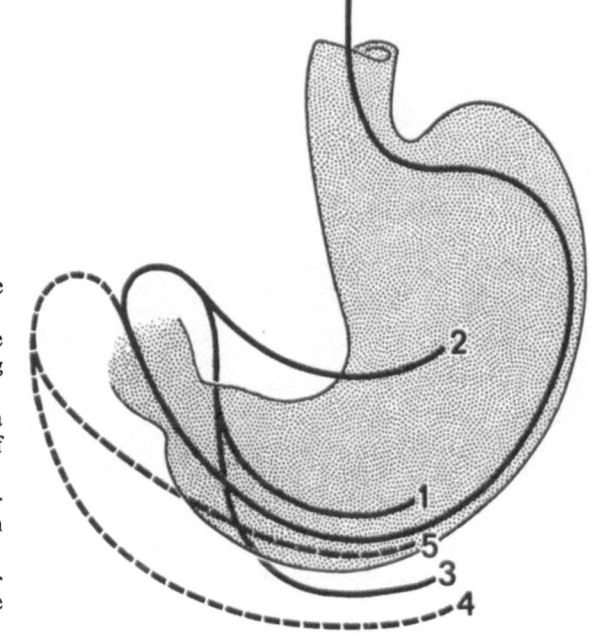

1. The tube with guide wire always lies more or less taut along the greater curvature side of the stomach. If the tip of the tube moves back along this same line in the direction of the pars media, then it is likely that it has coiled in the stomach. It is, however, possible that the tube is in fact located in the duodenum (fig. 7.4); this can be determined by administration of a very small test dosage of 20 cc contrast medium, at the most. As it arrives in the duodenum, the contrast fluid is immediately expelled in the distal direction; if it ends up in the stomach, the mucosal folds typical of this organ will be seen.

2. If the tip of the tube moves back above the level of the greater curvature of the stomach, then it is probably in the duodenum.

3. The tube is almost certainly in the duodenum when it extends towards the median plane below the level of the greater curvature. This is already fairly certain when it is seen under fluoroscopy

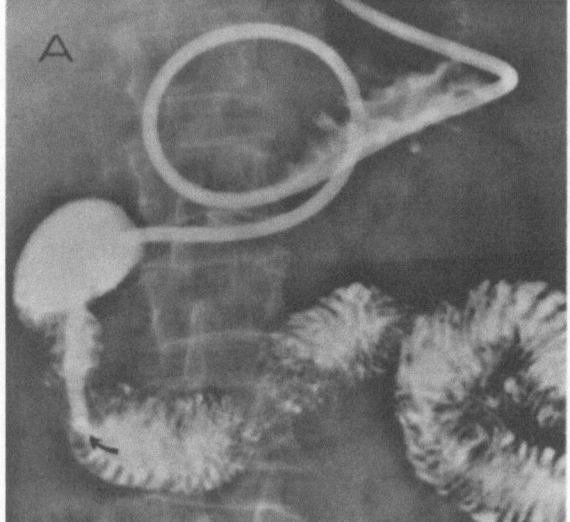
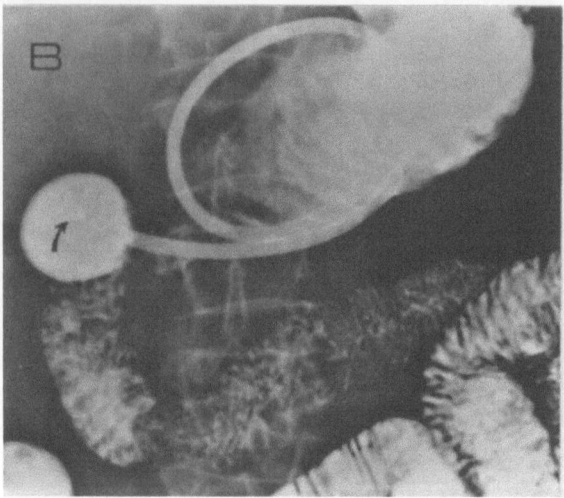

Fig. 7.7
Loop of the tube in the stomach (A). 1 or 2 retroperistaltic movements are enough to jerk the tube out of the duodenum by the loop (B).

that the tip of the tube crosses more or less perpendicular to the part of the tube lying along the greater curvature of the stomach.

4–5. Curling of the tube in the pars antralis of the stomach is almost always directed towards the median plane. Passage through the pylorus can be directed towards either the median or the lateral plane. If the tube curves downwards in the direction of the lateral plane, the pyloric ring has almost certainly been passed even if the tube happens to extend back towards the median plane at the level of the greater curvature side of the stomach.

Once in the duodenum, further positioning of the tube seldom causes problems. This phase can also be executed by the patient himself while the physician checks under intermittent fluoroscopy that the guide wire is pulled back 5–8 cm each time it approaches the pyloric ring. When Treitz's ligament is reached, the guide wire can be removed entirely. In a normal stomach, the tube now appears on the screen to lie in an α-configuration in the AP as well as lateral projection (fig. 7.3); this is of course not true in the event of a steerhorn stomach.

It is important that the tube does not curl in the stomach; otherwise if the patient should become nauseated, one or two pronounced retroperistaltic movements along the loop in the tube will cause the tube to be jerked out of the duodenum (fig. 7.7). When the duodenum is atonic and dilated as a result of the use of certain drugs or in cases of scleroderma (see Chapter XII), a functional stenosis may develop where the duodenum passes between the aorta and the superior mesenteric artery (mesenterial root syndrome). In the prestenotic sacculation the tube tends to curl back in the direction of the pylorus (figs. 7.8AB). In these cases inadequate closing of the pyloric ring enhances the chance of reflux of the contrast fluid into the stomach. Therefore it is better not to push the tube beyond the point where it tends to curl. When the tube has become stiffer due to frequent sterilization, it often slides into the duodenum easily without the help of a guide wire. It is also possible, however, that the tube will become too stiff and can no longer pass along the curve in the duodenum to Treitz's ligament (fig. 7.9). If the tube should remain lodged in the descending limb of the duodenum or is seen to plunge downwards then the tube may have ended up in a diverticulum located in the outer curve of the duodenum (fig. 7.10), or it may have even unexpectedly perforated the wall of the diverticulum; this is, however, a rare phenomenon. When the Bilbao-Dotter tube curls in the fundus of the stomach, as can sometimes occur when the stomach lies high up in the abdominal cavity as in pyknic patients, the following can be attempted:

1. If numerous patients are examined annually then it certainly is worthwhile to buy an extra guide wire with a tip which is bent to form a

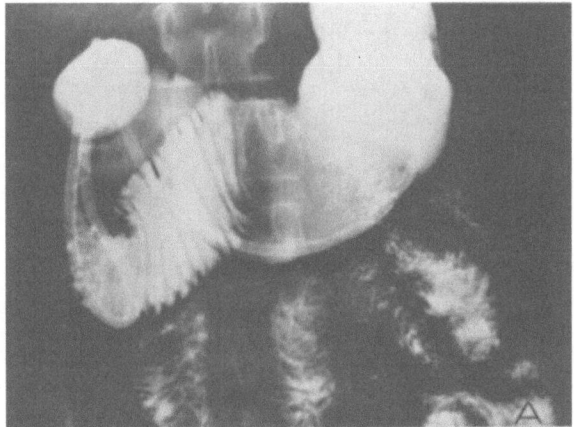

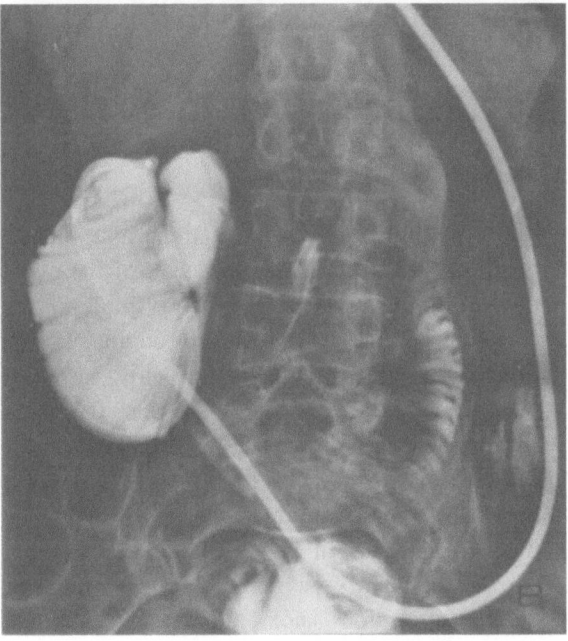

Fig. 7.8

A. The tube turns back in a prestenotic sacculation in the duodenum which has developed as a result of a mesenteric artery syndrome. The tip of the tube is in the duodenal bulb and is therefore close to the pylorus so that a large quantity of contrast fluid flows back into the stomach.

B. The tube coils in the descending limb of the duodenum which is greatly dilated as a result of scleroderma.

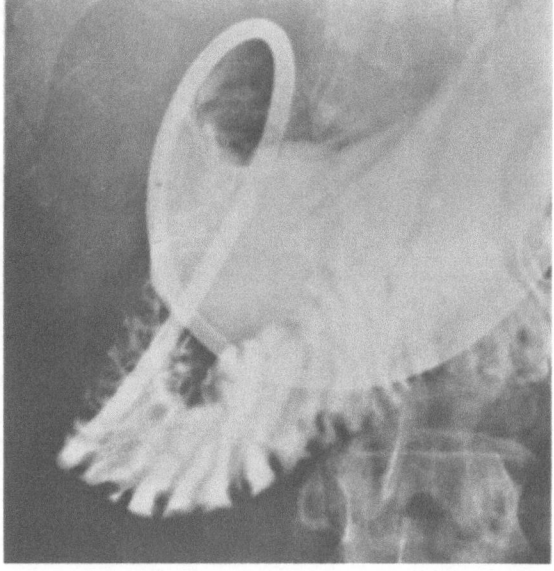

Fig. 7.9
It is no longer possible to pass through the junction between the descending limb and the horizontal portion of the duodenum when the tube has become too stiff as a result of frequent sterilization.

gentle curve of 60–90°. After this guide wire is pushed into the extended Bilbao-Dotter tube as far as possible, whereby the last 6 cm of the tube remain flexible, the unit is introduced until the rounded part of the guide wire is located in the fundus of the stomach and the flexible tip of the tube just touches the wall of the stomach on the side of greater curvature. By rotating the guide wire via a knob, it is now easier to push the unit in the direction of the pars antralis without coiling. As soon as this maneuver has been completed, the curved guide wire is replaced by a straight one. For this procedure, which must be carried out under fluoroscopic control, the physician must stand at the head of the patient who lies in a supine position on the table.

2. If there is only one single loop, one can still try to slide the tube into the required position in the duodenum. The tube should be long enough for this procedure since the stomach is never very long in pyknic patients. As soon as the tube is in position, then it may be possible to uncoil the loop in the fundus; this should be done very carefully, although a sudden tug may sometimes also be successful.

3. Have the patient lie on his stomach and push the tube back and forth quickly several times. To prevent coiling in the esophagus as a result of this maneuver, it is recommended that the guide wire be pulled back so that the last 10 cm of the tube remains flexible. Success is more likely if the same maneuver is carried out with

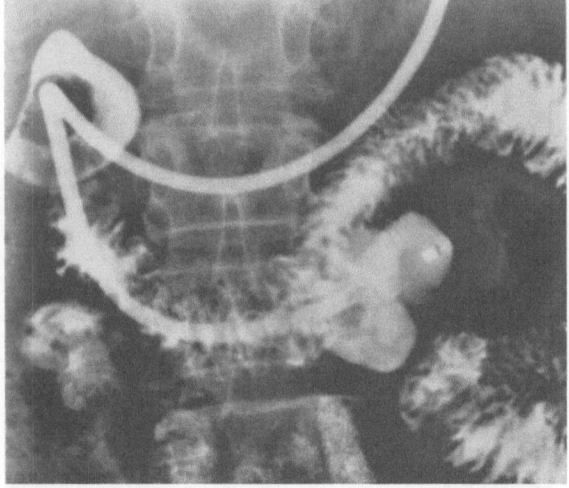

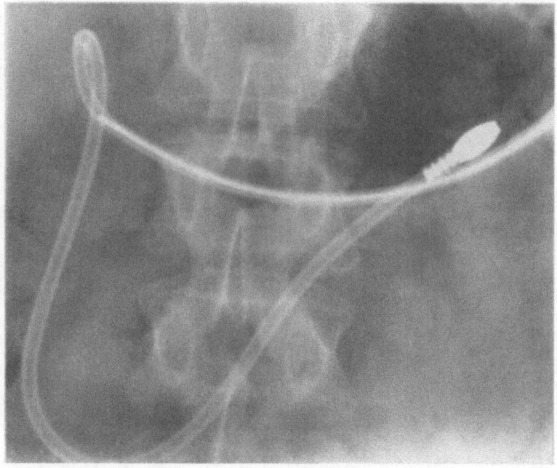

Fig. 7.11
Flexible tube with metal olive on the distal end.

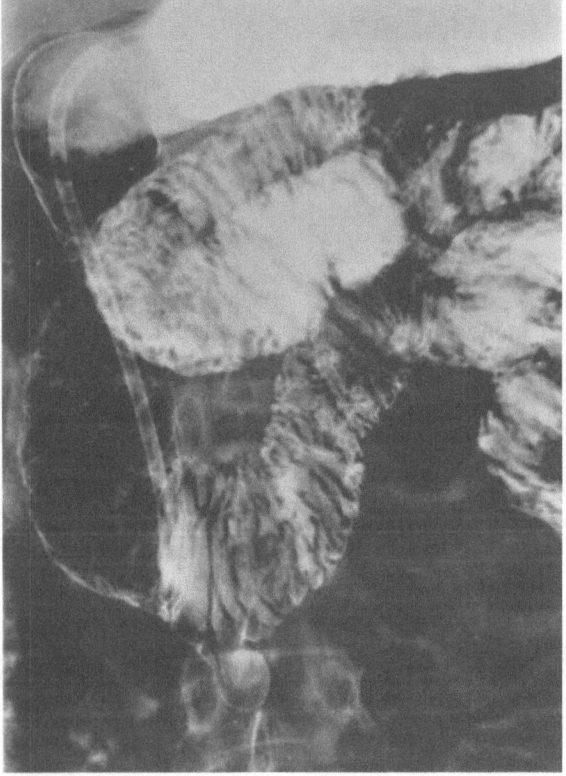

Fig. 7.10
If the tube becomes lodged in the duodenum or if it drops down too far into the descending duodenum, this can be due to diverticula in the outer curve of the duodenum. Beware of perforation!

the patient standing instead of in the prone position.

4. Remove the Bilbao-Dotter tube and use a soft radiopaque tube with a metal olive on the distal end (fig. 7.11). If the patient assumes a prone position and subsequently the right lateral postion, then because of the weight of the metal olive, the tube will almost always fall in the direction of the pylorus without coiling. If it is difficult to introduce the guide wire into this tube, which is often rather thin, then the guide wire should be greased with oil, vaseline or catheter lubricant. Only in very rare cases is it possible to pass the metal olive through the pyloric ring within several minutes. In such cases if the history or a previous follow-through examination does not indicate an organic reason for this failure, we sometimes give a metoclopramide injection and have the patient rest quietly on his right side for several minutes. We have found that this approach is always successful. When metoclopramide is administered intravenously, the rest of the examination must be carried out very efficiently; it should be completed before the peristaltic movements begin to decrease (see page 67). The duration of the examination can be shortened somewhat by slightly increasing the rate of flow of the contrast fluid and by decreasing the dosage. An increased flow is obtained by administering the barium suspension under high pressure using a pneumo-colon apparatus, or by greater dilution of the suspension. If the reduced contrast becomes too troublesome, it can if necessary be compensated for by lowering the kilovoltage.

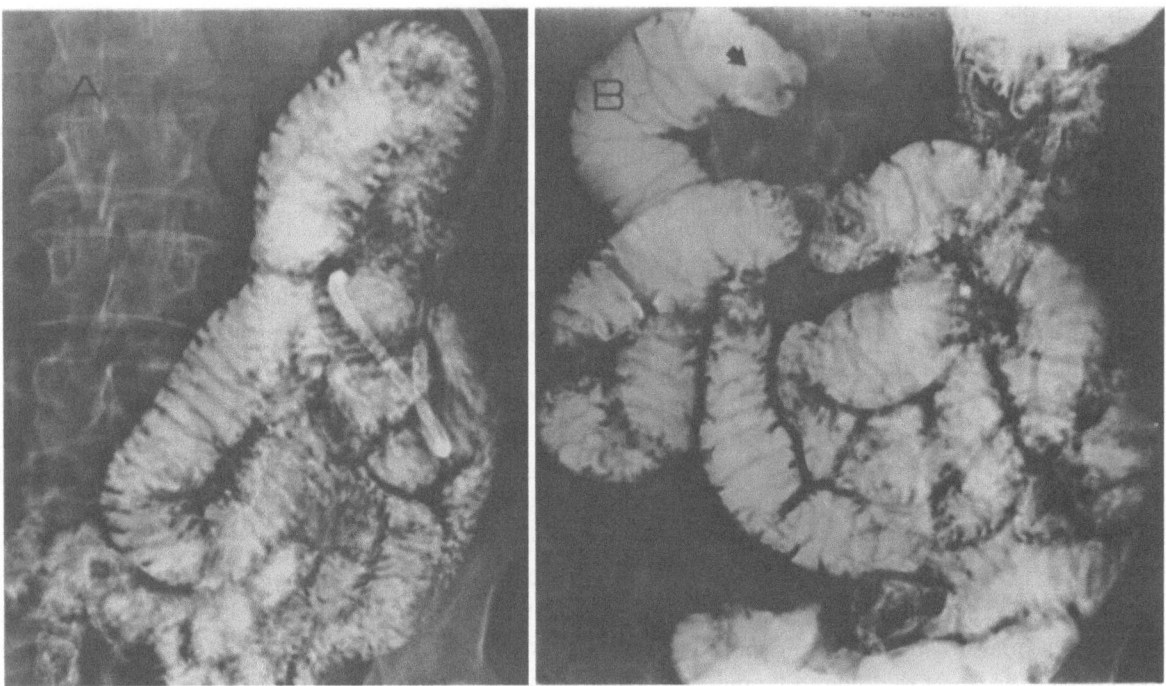

Fig. 7.12
Example of the positioning of the tube after a partial gastrectomy of the B II type. If the tip of the tube extends far enough into the jejunum, there will be no reflux of the contrast fluid into the resected stomach in spite of the absence of a pyloric ring. Many of the loops of the small intestine are in a state of contraction and there is no contrast fluid in the afferent loop (A). It was, however, possible in this particular case to fill the afferent loop after a hypotonic agent had been administered (B). At the end of the duodenal stump is a polypoid lesion resulting from the introverted line of suture (→).

3. Partial gastrectomy

It is a mistake to assume that enteroclysis is not worthwhile in a patient who has undergone a partial gastrectomy. With the exception of the abnormal positioning of the tube (fig. 7.12), these examinations cannot be differentiated from those performed in patients with a normal stomach. Introduction of the tube is never difficult after a BI type operation; after a BII type, the tube may sometimes end up in the afferent loop.

Spontaneous gastric emptying is often markedly reduced after partial gastrectomy of the BI type; on the other hand after a BII type operation, the gastric capacity is exceedingly low. Both groups of patients find it extremely difficult to drink large amounts of contrast fluid whereas one or more liters can be administered without problem via the duodenal tube. Although the absence of pyloric musculature frequently causes reflux of the contrast fluid in a proximal direction, this need not always

occur – not even after a BII type operation. Reflux of course becomes less likely as the length of the tube in the jejunum increases. After a partial gastrectomy of the BII type, whether accompanied by a clinical malabsorption or not, transit through the small intestine can sometimes be so rapid that the rate of flow of the contrast fluid must be increased in order to obtain sufficient filling of the loops of the small intestine. It is therefore not surprising that the afferent loop usually cannot be filled. If visualization of this loop is considered essential, for example because of bleeding, etc., then the administration of a hypotonic agent is indicated (fig. 7.12B).

4. Special types of tubes
(William Cook – Söborg – Denmark)

Because the tube does coil in the fundus of the stomach in some patients, we asked the manufacturer (William Cook-Söborg-Denmark) to design a new unit: the tube and guide wire are almost equal in length and are bent at a 20° angle ± 5 cm from the distal end (fig. 7.1c).

Although we have used this tube successfully many times when the Bilbao tube failed, we have in fact had more favourable results with a guide wire which we bent in the shape of a curve (see page 74); in spite of this, however, we still sometimes have to use the olive tube in order to reach our goal. It is certainly possible that a guide wire with a slightly curved tip will eventually appear to be a more suitable universal guide than the normal straight guide wire of the Bilbao-Dotter tube.

The above-mentioned manufacturer also made another intubation unit which is rather costly because of its limited lifetime; it is the so-called guided unit. In the wall of this tube are four wires which are connected to a revolver-shaped handle; this enables the tip of the tube to be moved in any direction desired (fig. 7.1D). The tube, which is available in any length desired, is not only useful for intubating the efferent loop after a partial gastrectomy of the BII type but can also be valuable when post-operative leakage along the suture line must be bypassed to provide proper nourishment to the patient.

A third modification, also by the same manufacturer, is a tube which can be used to take blind biopsies in the duodenum and proximal jejunum (fig. 7.1E). This last tube, like all the preceding ones, has an outer diameter of only 5 mm.

5. Administration of contrast fluid

By means of a series of tests with a phantom (Chapter 4.6), it was established that the optimum s.g. of the contrast fluid for a normal patient is 1.25, for an obese patient 1.3, for an extremely slender patient or a child ± 1.2 and for a baby 1.15. Moreover the contrast fluid must be hypotonic and fairly cool (± 15°C) (chapter III); however, administration of a fluid which is too cold causes a vomiting reflex.

Addition of Sorbitol and other glucose products to the barium suspension must be avoided since these substances are markedly hyperosmotic and therefore absorb considerable amounts of fluid. As a result, the quality of the mucosal patterns becomes quite inferior (fig. 7.13) and disintegration of the contrast fluid is promoted. Furthermore the barium suspension may not foam; the popular brands Micropaque and Microbar for instance do not satisfy this requirement at all (fig. 7.14).

Tiny gas bubbles can be particularly irritating and are exceedingly difficult to differentiate from multiple lymph follicles or a candidiasis (fig. 7.15).

To obtain high-quality double contrast films, there must be good adhesion of the barium suspension to the mucosa of the small intestine. Moreover, the viscosity must be as high as possible but such that a barium suspension with a s.g. of 1.25 will run through the infusion system at a maximum rate of 100 cc per minute without using a pressure system. Our infusion system is shown in fig. 7.16.

Fig. 7.13   ⟶

A. Dilution of the contrast fluid and vague margins in the jejunum when 40 g glucose was added to the contrast fluid.

B. Enteroclysis was repeated 5 days later using exactly the same procedure but without the glucose. The greater contrast intensity and sharp mucosal patterns are obvious.

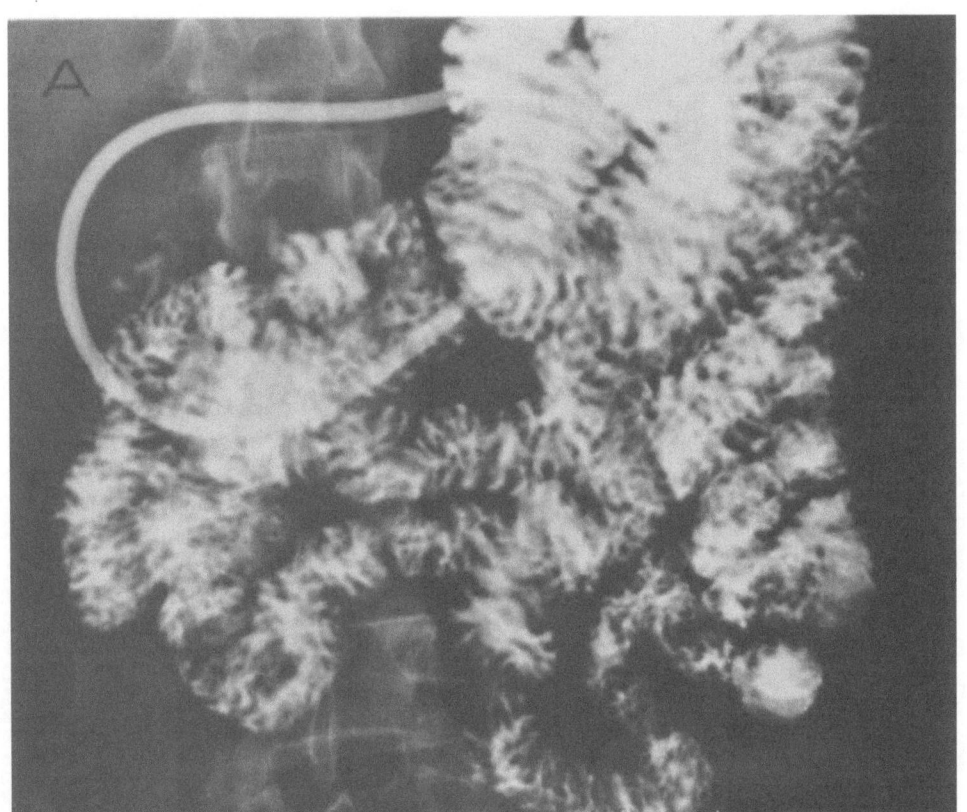

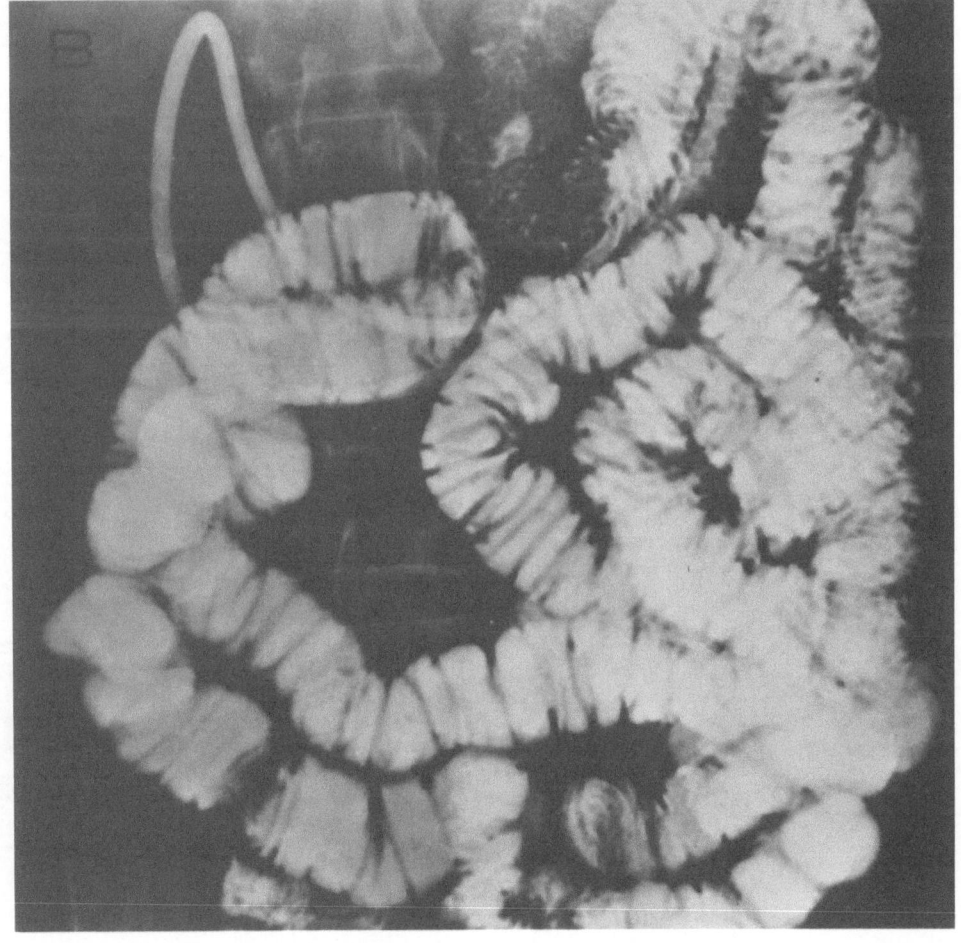

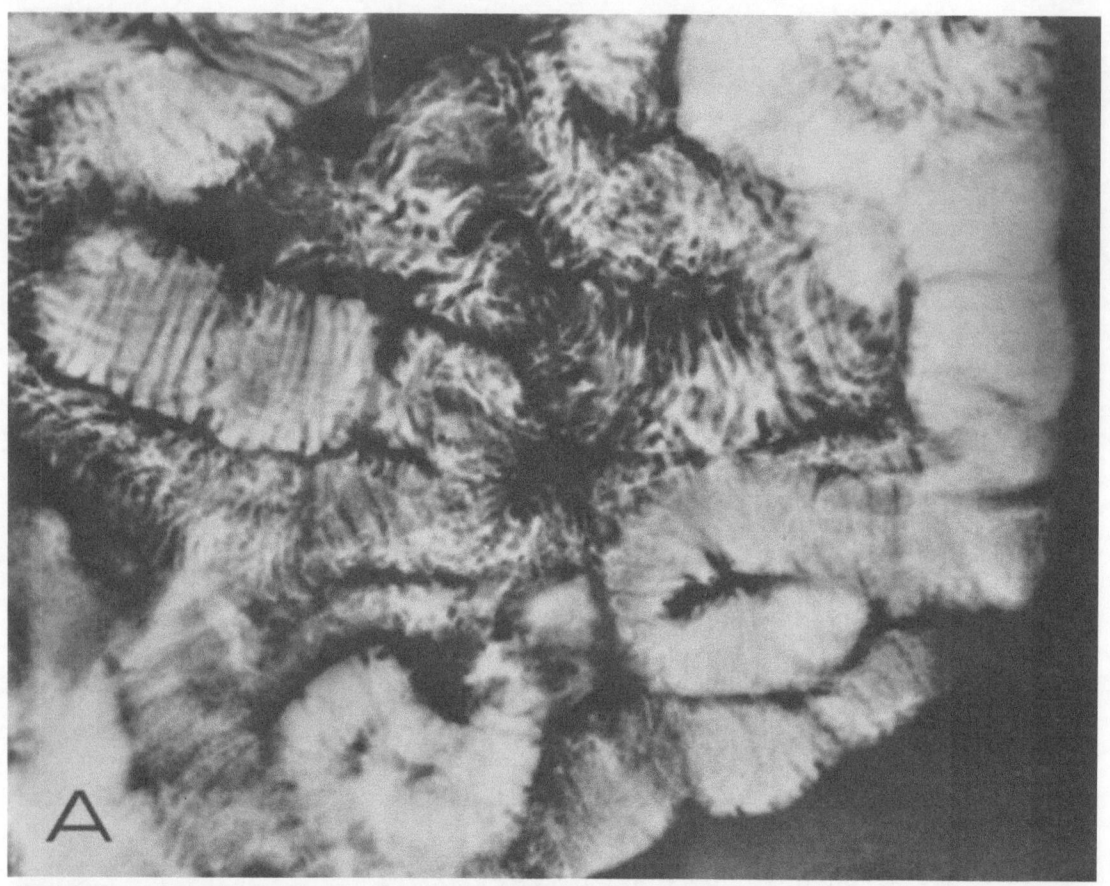

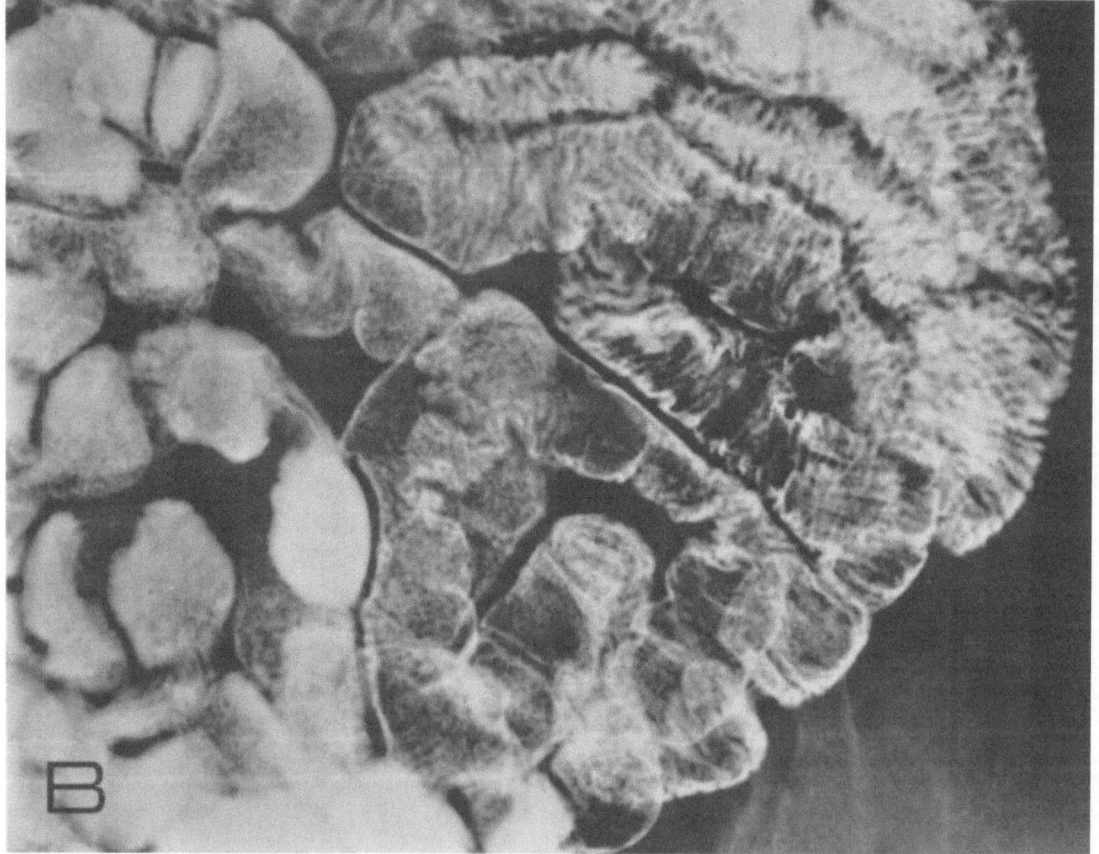

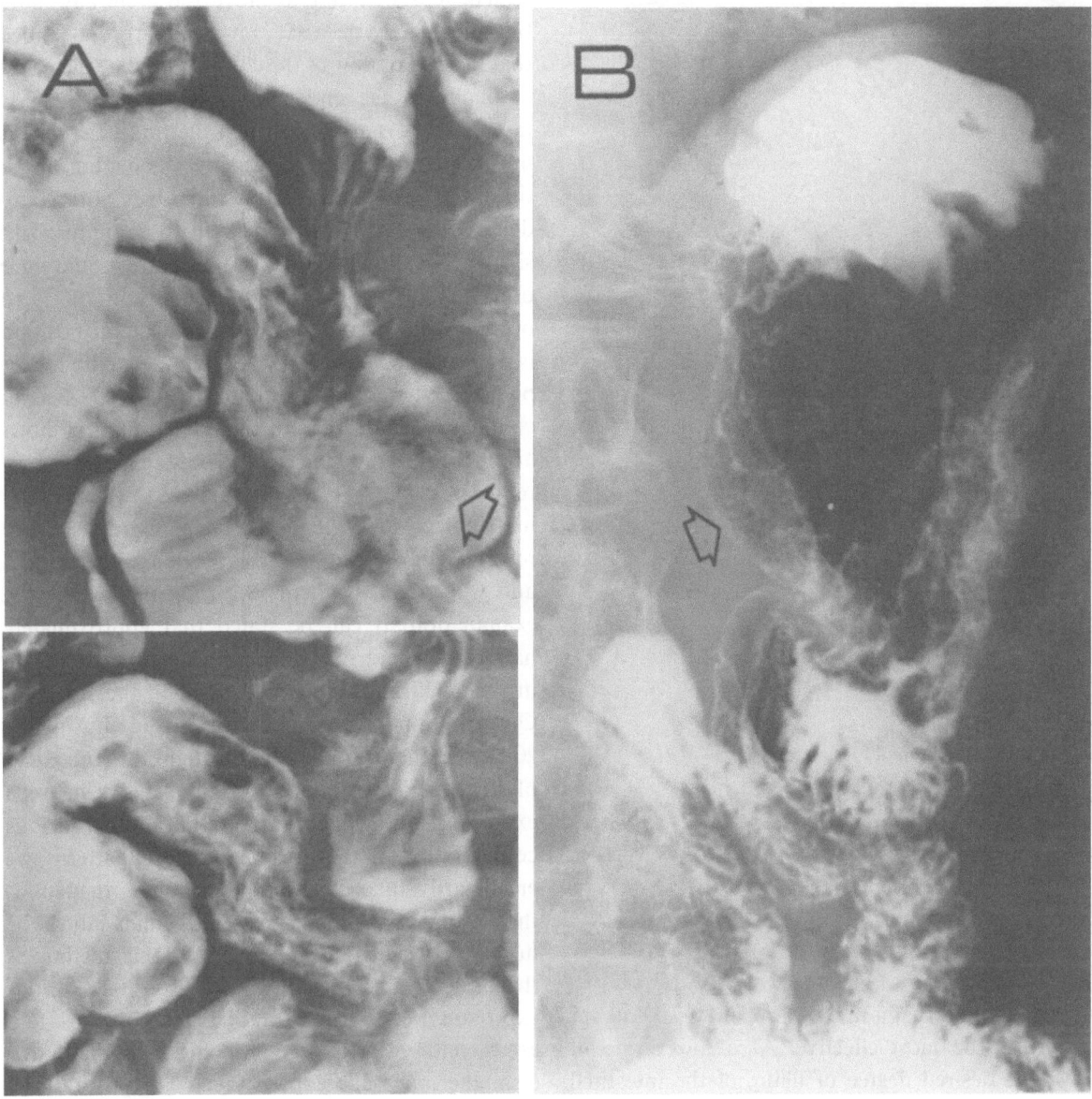

Fig. 7.15
A. Filling defects of approximately the same size as in fig. 7.14 caused by lymph follicles.
B. Similar filling defects due to colonies of Candida albicans in a patient who has undergone a BII partial gastrectomy.

Fig. 7.14
A. Antifoaming characteristics of the contrast fluid in this convolution of intestinal loops are insufficient.
B. An extremely irritating foam develops after air insufflation.

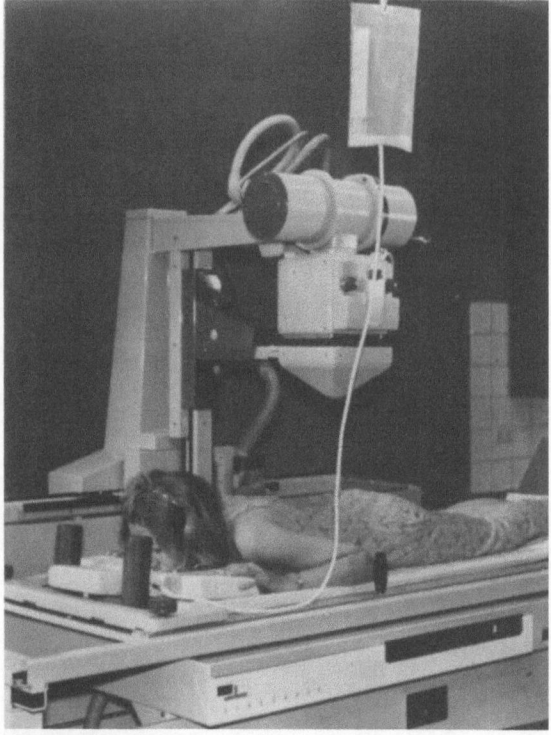

Fig. 7.16
Our infusion system used for enteroclysis.
1. Extended Bilbao-Dotter tube.
2. Plastic connecting piece (available in various sizes and models).
3. Bag and tube 2 m long, also plastic and available in diverse models.
4. Hook which can be adjusted in height via a rope and a pulley mounted on the ceiling.

We have found that a rate of flow of 80–100 ml per minute is the most effective. At a lower rate of flow, the desired degree of filling of the intestinal loops cannot be achieved. Furthermore because there is less stretching of the intestinal wall, peristaltic movement is not as strong and transit then takes longer. A higher rate of flow includes the considerable risk of reflux into the stomach which greatly retards the transit time. In 50% of the cases, the cecum is reached in 6–10 minutes when a contrast medium dosage of 600 ml is administered at the above-mentioned optimum rate of flow.

The easiest method is to administer the contrast fluid while the patient is in a prone position. In this position the intestinal loops remain in a well-ordered group longer and relative projection with both the common Bucky table and the telecommand apparatus is better. If the patient is slightly nau-

seated, it is wise not to move the table any more than absolutely necessary; it is also recommended that the rate of flow of the contrast fluid be increased gradually to the maximum value during the first minute. This is also true when the tip of the tube is not in the most distal part of the duodenum. If the tip of the tube lies in the proximal half of the duodenum it is better for the patient to lie on his right side during administration of the contrast fluid since otherwise reflux into the stomach is quite likely to occur. A disadvantage of the right lateral position is of course that x-rays of the jejunum can no longer be taken after administration of the first 200–300 ml contrast medium. Loss of these early films is, however, less objectionable than increasing the chance of reflux into the stomach by turning the patient on his stomach or back for these photographs. Once reflux occurs, it can as a rule no longer be averted and will gradually increase during the rest of the examination. It can be stated that approximately half of the fluid not yet administered will end up in the small intestine and the rest in the stomach. Gastric emptying can be improved by giving 20–30 cc metoclopramide through the tube and placing the patient on his right side in between exposures. To facilitate interpretation of suspicious configurations in the intestinal mucosal patterns, we customarily take our survey exposures in pairs – the second x-ray being 10–30 seconds after the first. A considerable advantage of this method is that the diverse intestinal loops on the various exposures retain their mutual relationships and are therefore easy to recognize and compare. However, the mucosal folds on the two exposures will appear quite different since they fall in different phases of contraction. If after an initial dose of 600 ml the cecum is not yet reached, a second dose is administered immediately or several minutes later at the most. If the cecum has almost been reached or a confusing clump of ileal loops has developed in the pelvis minor, it is better to give only 300 ml. If the contrast medium still has a long way to go to reach the cecum and superposition of the intestinal loops is not too pronounced, then the second dosage should be 600 cc. As a rule we dilute the second dosage of barium suspension somewhat, mainly because it is easier to see through 2 or 3 superimposed loops when the s.g. is lower (fig. 7.17). Dilution of course means that the viscosi-

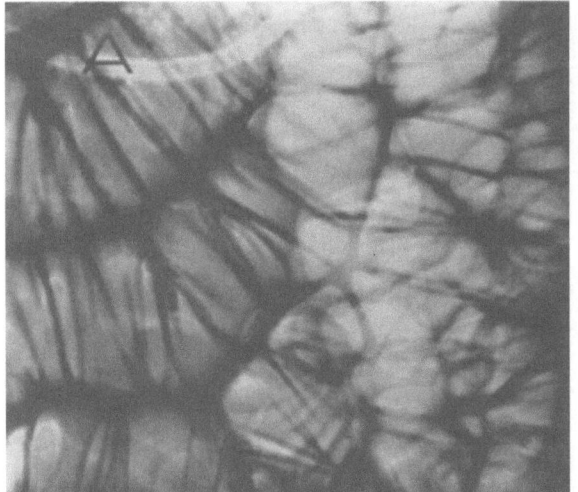

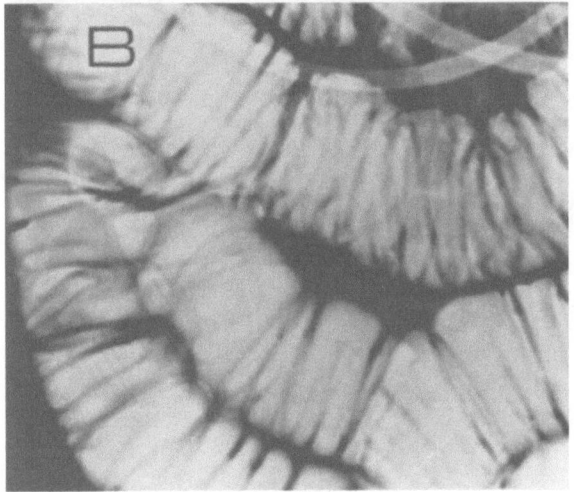

Fig. 7.17
Filling of the proximal jejunal loops with a contrast fluid of lower s.g. (A). The contrast fluid in the more distal loops still has a high s.g. (B).

greatly reduced peristalsis due to fatigue of the overloaded and probably already atrophied smooth musculature. Only when the cecum has almost been reached can a dose of 2 cc metoclopramide be administered intravenously without objection since in this case the period of action (about 10 minutes) is sufficient to complete the examination before atony develops. The entire examination is carried out under intermittent fluoroscopy and spot films are taken using compression. If a telecommand apparatus is not available and the Bucky table is used, it is better to wait until the cecum has been reached, as seen on the survey exposures, before making spot films – not only of the last ileal loops but of course of all the other loops of the small intestine. For a standard examination of the small intestine without conspicuous abnormalities, our routine procedure is to take the following films:

2 × 24/30 of the proximal jejunum after 300 ml;
2 × 35/35 of the entire abdomen after 600 ml;
2 × 35/35 of the entire abdomen after the cecum
    has been reached;
4–6 spot films (2–3 × 24/30).

If the case is without complications, the total length of the examination is 15–30 minutes including duodenal intubation; the total exposure time is 3–5 minutes.

6. Administration of water after the barium suspension

As in the colon examination, mucosal patterns are an essential part of the examination of the small intestine, especially for evaluation of inflammatory diseases. The cobblestone appearance and swollen folds in fig. 7.18 give the mucosa a conspicuous spiculated appearance; on the survey exposures, they could easily have been overlooked by a less experienced observer. On the other hand it is often very difficult to identify small abnormalities of the mucosa in intestinal loops which coincide or have contracted. Because of the superposition of the posterior and anterior walls of the usually twisted intestinal loops, the thin layer of barium coating the mucosal folds often produces a maze of curved lines. Better filling of the intestine causes a greater

ty of the barium solution is reduced; as a result the bag of contrast fluid must be placed closer to the table since otherwise the rate of flow will become too high and reflux to the stomach may occur, eventually followed by nausea and vomiting.

If during the first infusion of 600 cc contrast medium, it is noted that peristalsis in the intestine is particularly slow, then it is recommended that, depending upon the weight of the patient, 20 or 30 cc metoclopramide be added to the second dose of 600 cc. It is not wise to administer this drug intravenously since the period of action is then much shorter; furthermore there can be a subsequent fairly long period, lasting 30–60 minutes, of

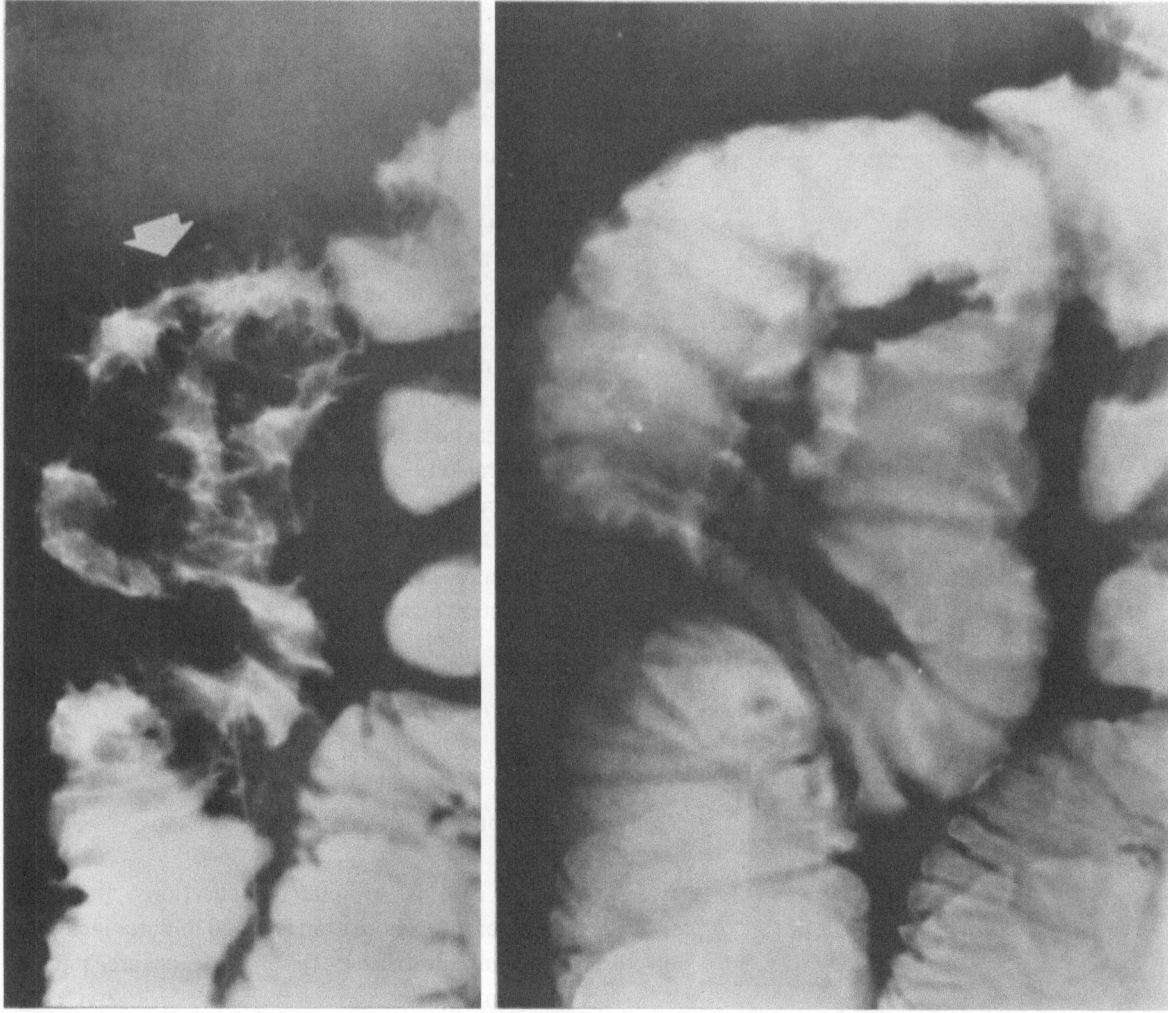

Fig. 7.18
Recurrence of Crohn's disease after an ileocecal resection. The cobblestones and swollen mucosal folds are clearly visible when the intestinal loops are only moderately filled, but are difficult to see when the loops are well-filled.

Fig. 7.19
Several examples of abnormalities in the small intestine which are seen most clearly when the loops are well-filled.
A.   Local ulceration in Crohn's disease.
B.   Atrophy of the mucosa as a result of celiac disease.
C.   Yersinia EC infection.
D.   Appendicular infiltration.
E.   Aspecific ulceration.
F–G.   Metastasis of melanoma.

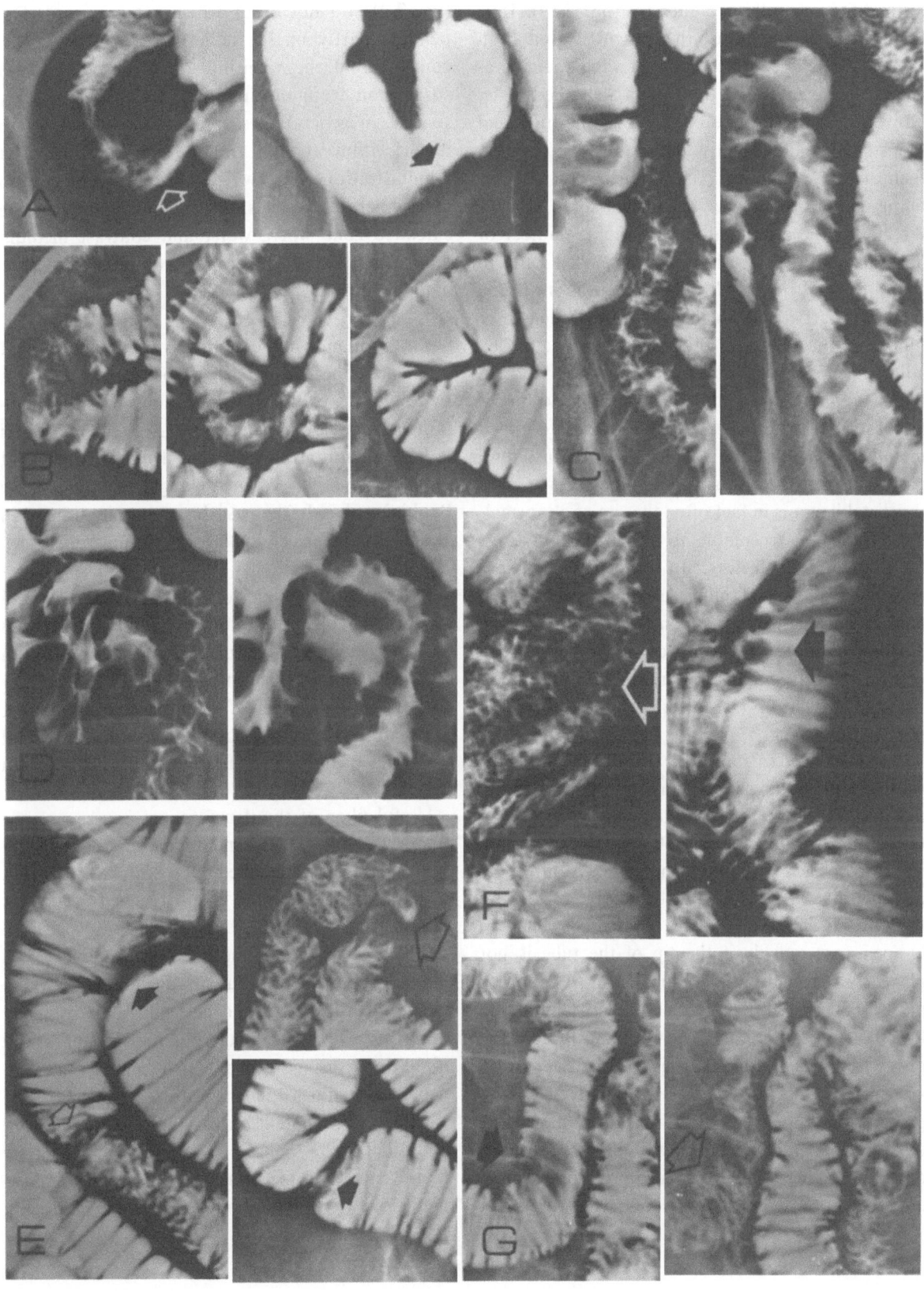

degree of stretching of the folds; as a result they lie in a more or less circular configuration and abnormalities are easier to identify (fig. 7.19). It is therefore recommended that each examination should, if possible, include at least a few roentgenograms of the intestinal loops in a well-filled state. However, a high degree of filling of the intestinal loops also means that it is more difficult to project them freely by means of compression. Greater filling should therefore be carried out towards the end of the examination and after a number of films have been made of the partially filled loops in order to avoid the problem of superposition. In the proximal part of the small intestine, the degree of filling of the loops is regulated fairly easily by adjusting the rate of flow of the contrast fluid. In the distal part of the ileum, however, this no longer applies; instead the degree of filling is determined mainly by the ease with which the contrast fluid passes through Bauhin's valve to the cecum. Since the distal ileum is in fact often the site of abnormalities, it is not acceptable to simply acknowledge these disrupting factors. In most cases a very reasonable degree of filling of the important last part of the small intestine can still be obtained by exerting pressure on the region of Bauhin's valve with a blunt compressor and also forcing the contrast column in a distal direction as quickly as possible.

The best way to force the contrast column onwards is to administer 600 ml or more of water through the tube. Since water has a very low viscosity, a rate of flow of 150–200 ml per minute can easily be achieved in this manner. It is, however, possible that the patient, not being able to tolerate this rate of flow, will become nauseated. This can happen very quickly if the tip of the tube is not placed far enough into the duodenum. As soon as nausea develops, the infusion bag should be lowered so that the rate of flow will again decrease or the flow even stops. If the viscosity of the barium suspension meets the requirements established in the preceding sections, then this water infusion will not only give better x-rays of the well-filled distal loops of the small intestine but will also produce excellent double contrast films of the jejunum (fig. 7.20). The

irritating large differences in density seen when double contrast exposures are taken with air (fig. 7.21) do not occur when water is used. Depending partly on the adhesive properties of the contrast fluid, the water infusion flushes the barium suspension from the intestinal wall fairly quickly so that in general these roentgenograms must be taken within about 1 minute. In addition after administration of the water infusion, disintegration of the barium suspension develops rapidly in the extended zone where water and contrast medium mix so that one is forced to discontinue the examination (fig. 7.22).

Several common indications for administration of water after the barium suspension are:

In colitis, the contents of the colon mix with secretions induced by infectious diseases and are found in large quantities in the distal ileum as a result of reflux from the cecum through an inadequate Bauhin's valve. In the past this contamination often led to the incorrect diagnosis: 'reflux ileitis' (fig. 7.23).

In fig. 7.24 the cobblestones in the distal ileum did not become obvious until this segment had been flushed clean. In the event of disturbed motility in the intestine due to neurological disorders, damage due to the toxic effect of some drugs, scleroderma or amyloidosis, residue of food consumed several days previously can be found in the distal ileum (fig. 7.25).

Useful films of the ileum can of course only be made when the contamination in this part of the intestine has been removed. Quite often if the ileum is not empty, the cecum is not reached even after administration of 1200 ml barium suspension. Administration of even more barium could lead to a persistent obstipation due to dehydration in the colon, at least in diseases accompanied by disturbed motility. As a rule we avoid giving more than 1200 ml barium suspension; a supplementary infusion of 600, sometimes 1200 ml water can then be quite effective. Since there is already more than sufficient dilatation of the loops in these cases, nausea must be prevented and the infusion is therefore administered slowly at a rate of about 80 ml per minute.

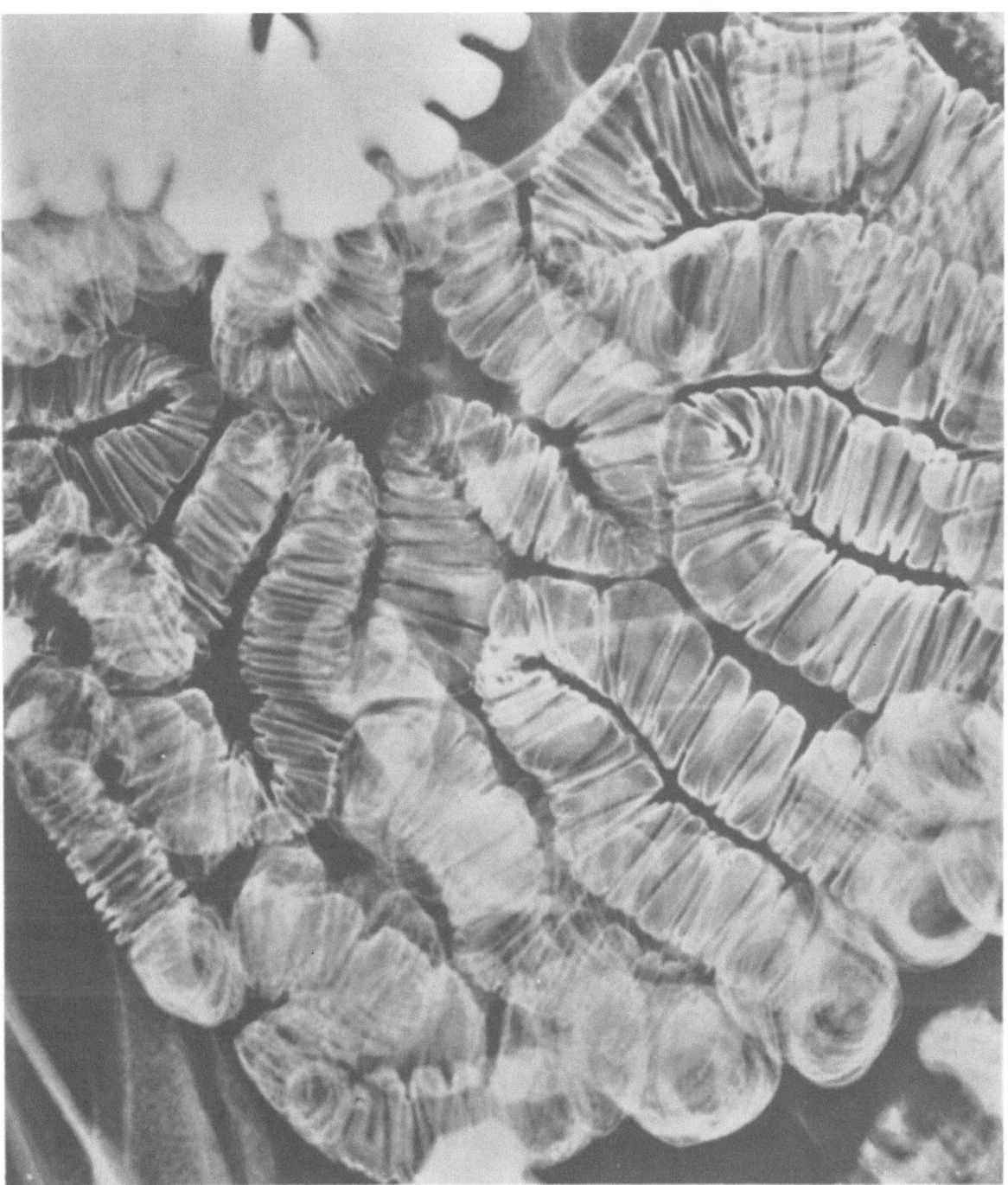

Fig. 7.20
Double contrast exposures of a jejunum after water is administered. A thin film of contrast fluid remains on the mucosa for 15–30 seconds.

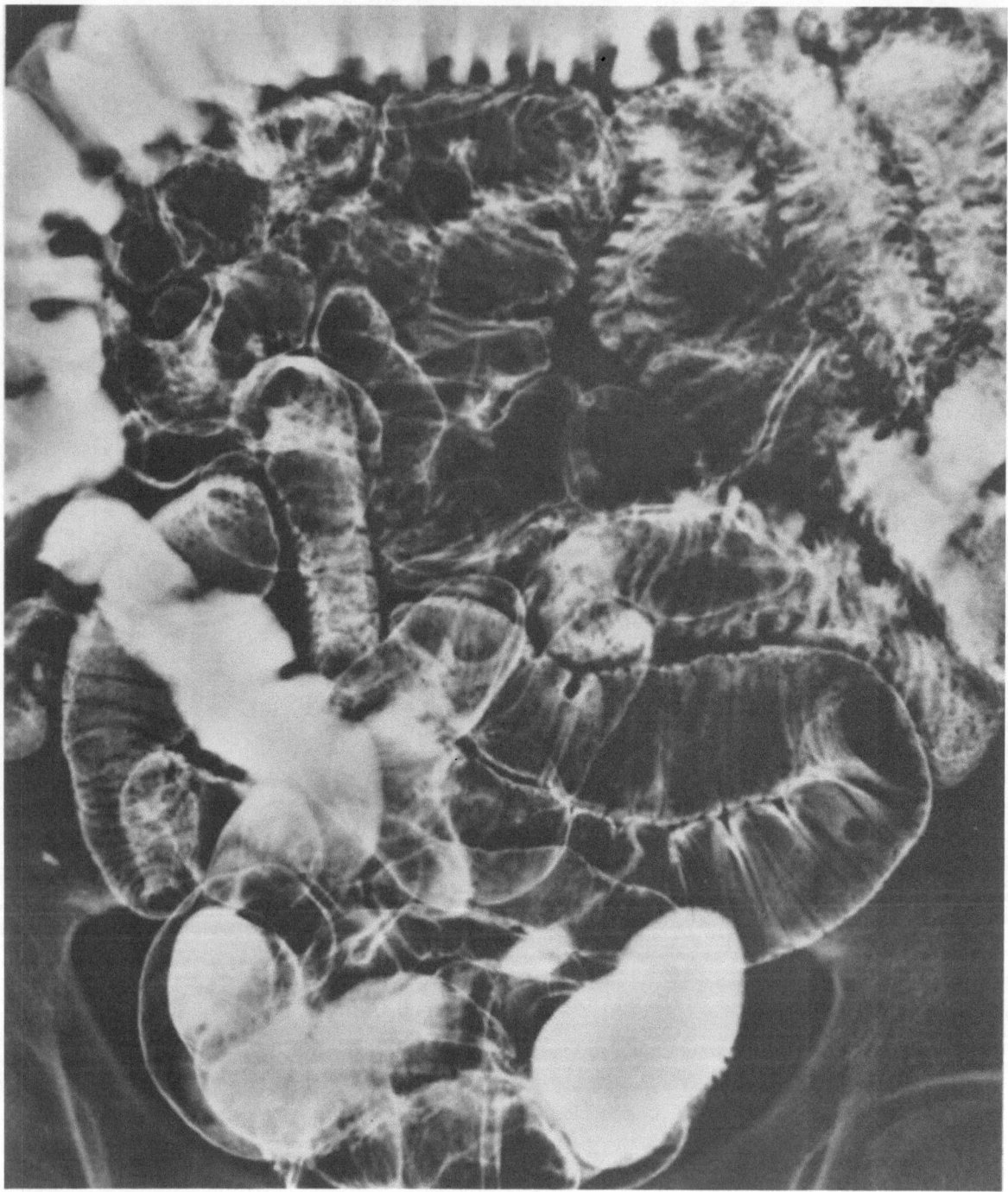

Fig. 7.21
The contrast differences are considerably greater and therefore irritating on double contrast exposures taken after air is administered instead of water. The time available for taking the x-rays, however, is much longer.

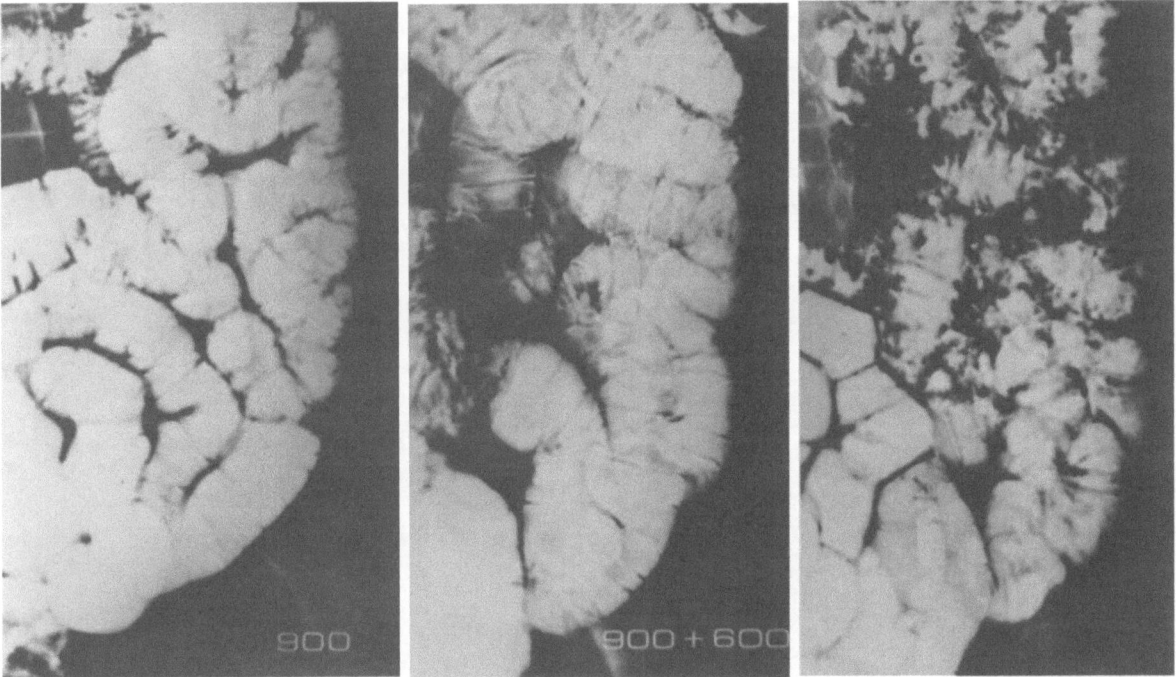

Fig. 7.22
Disintegration of contrast fluid by mixing with an excess of water (flocculation).

In addition to disturbed motility or a contaminated ileum as a result of an inadequate Bauhin's valve, the cecum is often not reached after administration of 1200 ml barium suspension in cases of mechanical obstruction caused by shriveled skip lesions or tumors. In such cases too, which are often accompanied by a manifest or incipient ileus, enteroclysis is extended to include slow water infusions. If after administration of a total fluid dosage of $2\frac{1}{2}$ liters the obstruction has not yet been reached, which sometimes does occur, no further fluid is administered and further developments are awaited as in a conventional examination. Our experience has shown that free projection of the intestinal loops by means of the compression technique can cause insurmountable problems when the dosage exceeds $2\frac{1}{2}$ liters, and sometimes even sooner, so

that a worthwhile contribution to anatomical diagnostics is no longer possible. In some cases, the maximum permissible fluid dosage for enteroclysis depends of course partly on what the patient's heart and kidneys can tolerate; this should be determined in consultation with the attending physician.

For various reasons rectal filling of the colon with contrast medium is not always possible. By means of the method described above, enteroclysis can give very worthwhile roentgenograms of the colon. This can even be supplemented if necessary with air double contrast exposures via rectal insufflation or through the tube. The procedure for such an examination of the colon is as follows: after 900–1200 ml barium suspension has been introduced

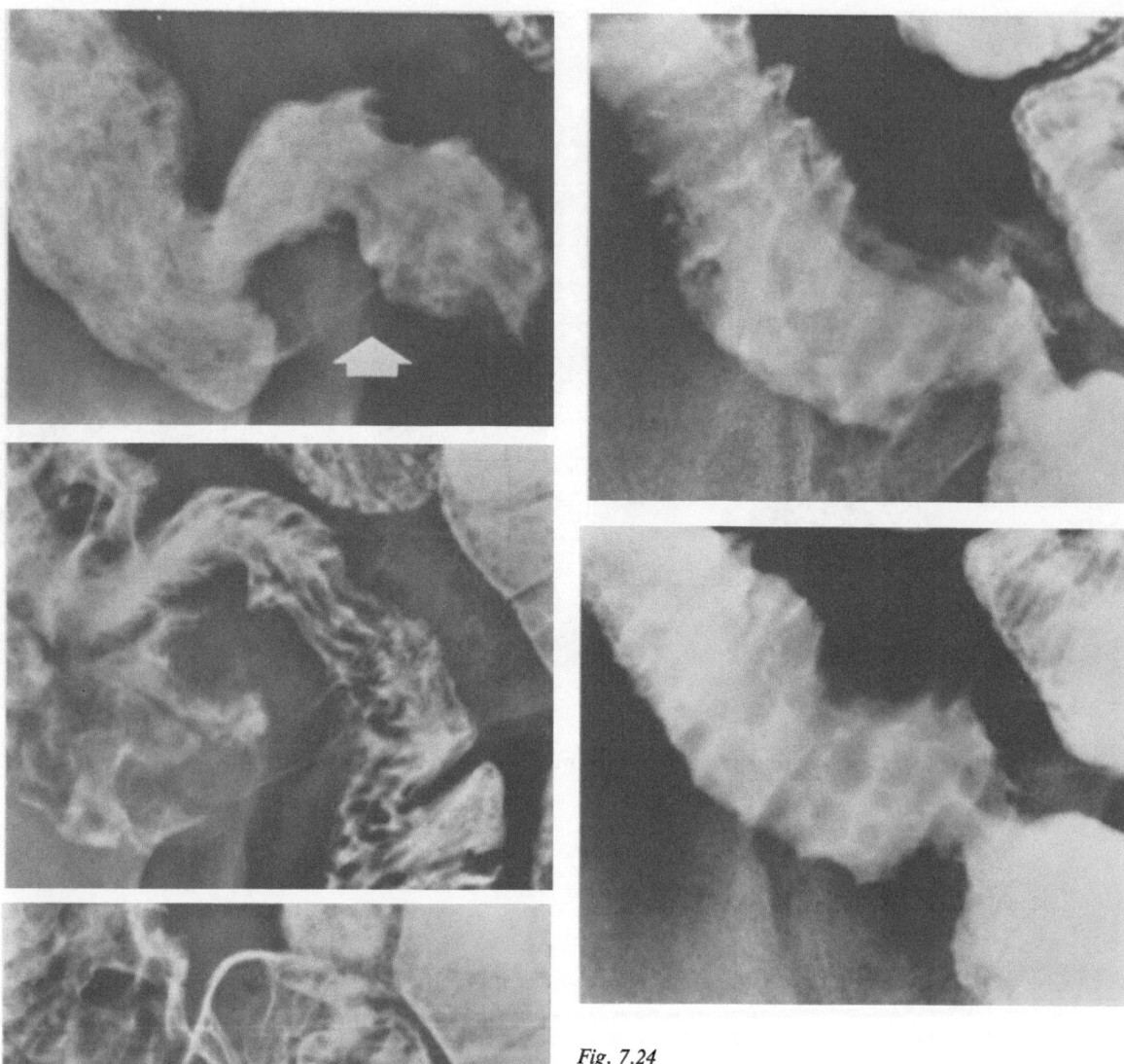

Fig. 7.24
Swollen mucosal folds and cobblestones in Crohn's disease which were only clearly visible after the contamination in this loop was flushed away.

Fig. 7.23
Misleading pattern of a so-called 'reflux ileitis' in ulcerative colitis (→) which disappears after the distal ileum is flushed clean with a large dose of contrast medium.

into the small intestine through the duodenal tube and x-rays have been taken, the entire contrast dosage is forced into the colon by means of an equally large water infusion. The small intestine can in this way be flushed clean in several minutes so that residual barium in the jejunum or ileum will not interfere with the colon films (fig. 7.26).

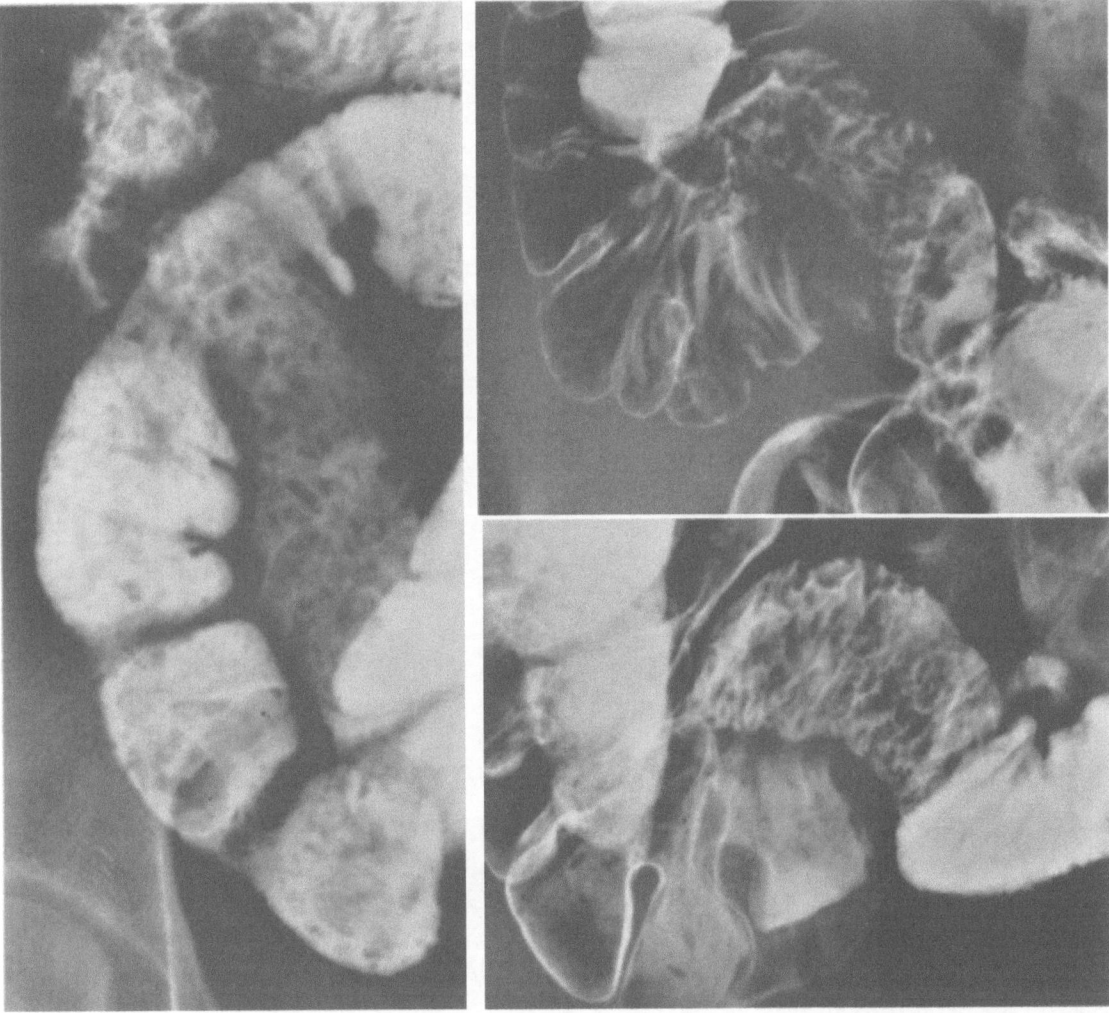

Fig. 7.25
Evaluation of the mucosa in the ileum in a patient with drug-induced atony of the bowel is only possible after the food residue has been forced out of the colon.

Fig. 7.26
Examples of the survey exposures of the colon after the jejunum is flushed clean with water. Useful reproduction of the mucosa in the colon is then generally no problem at all (pp. 96–97).

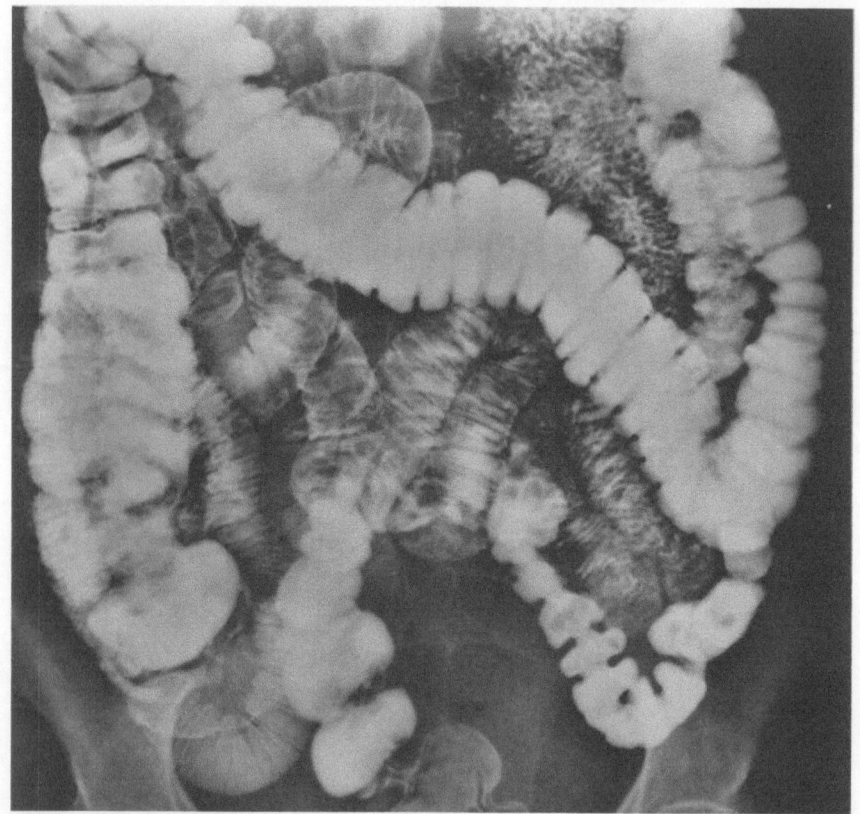

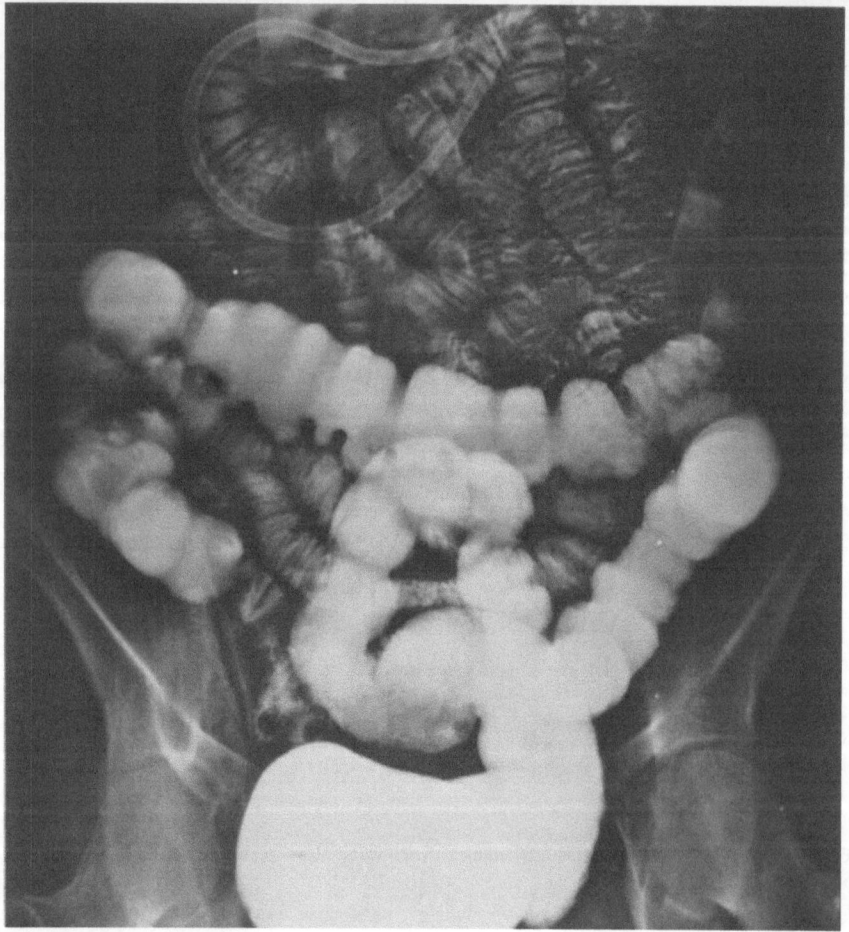

Fig. 7.26

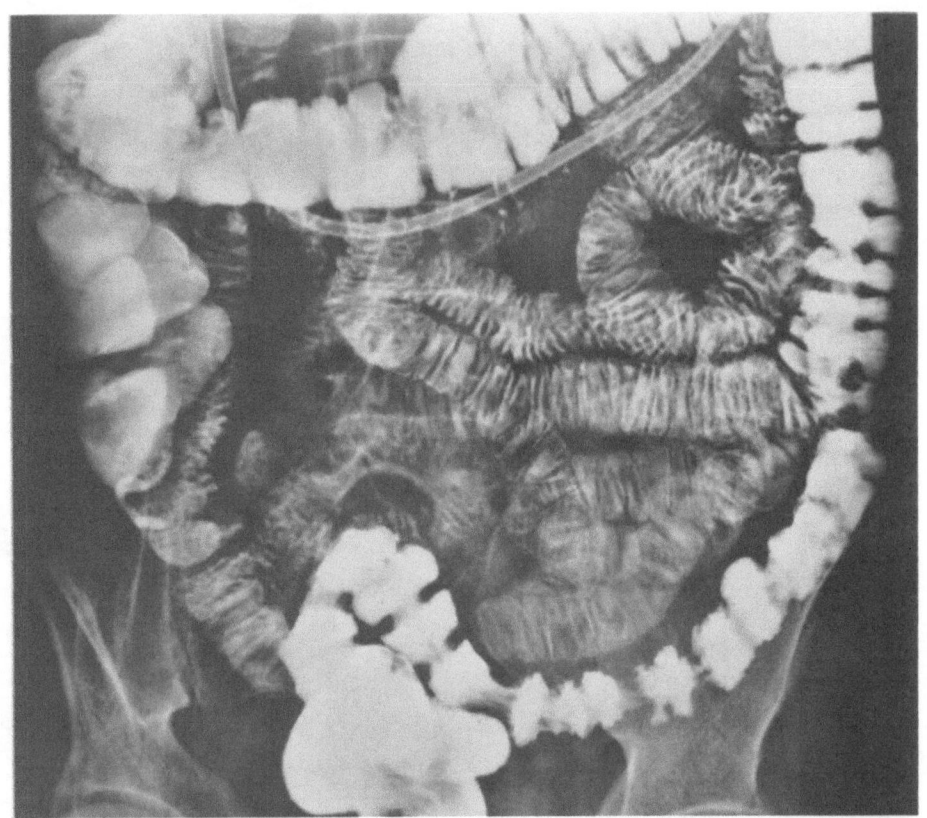

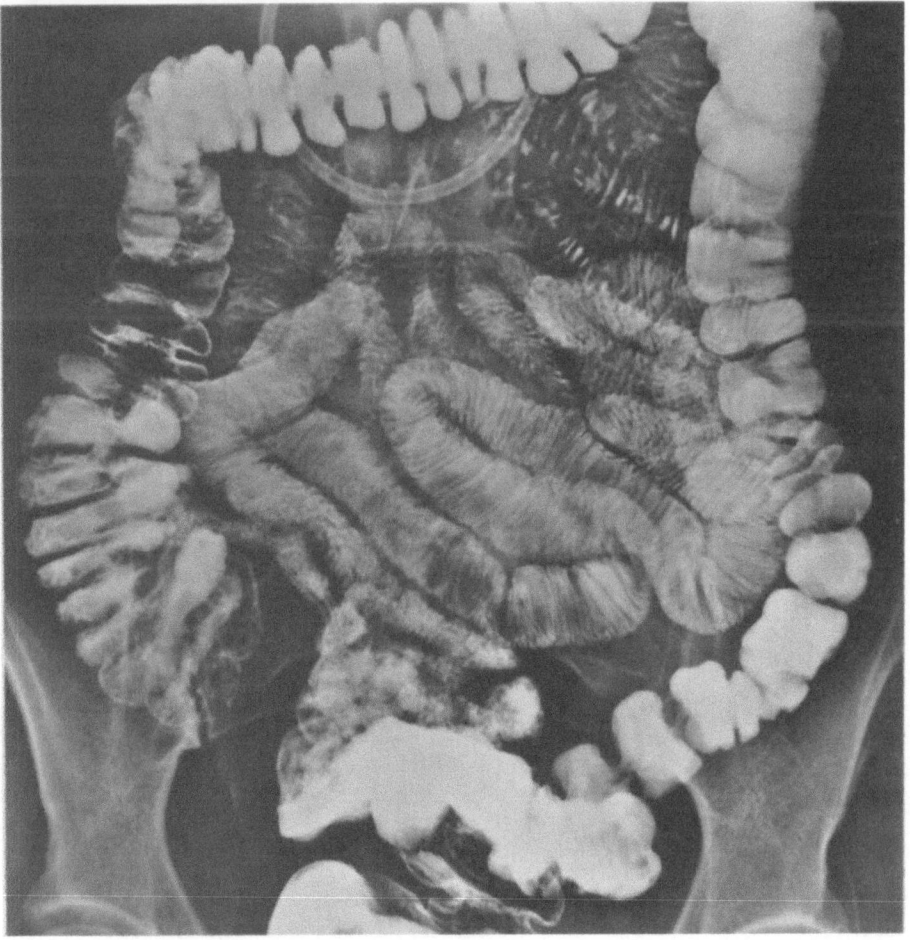

Fig. 7.26

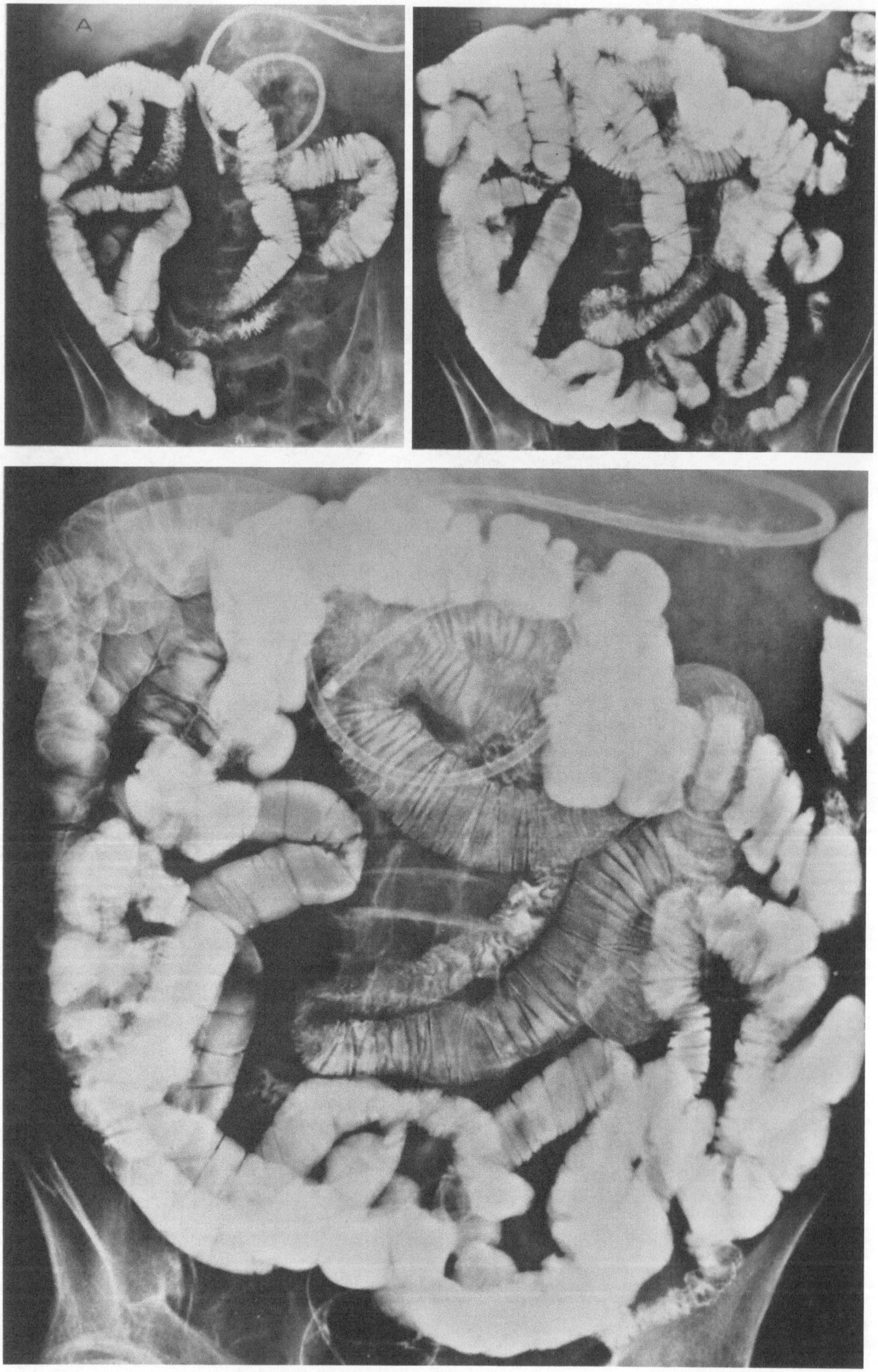

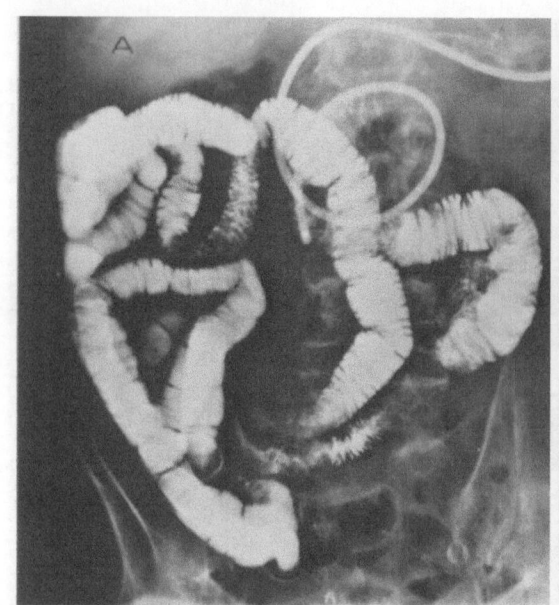
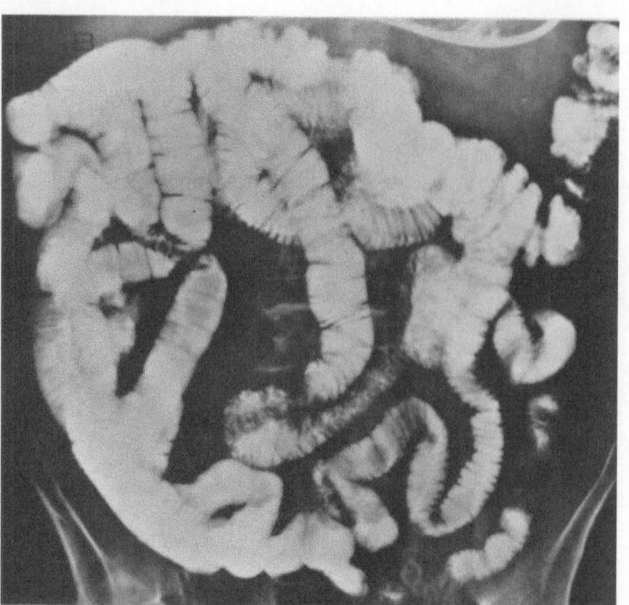

A relatively rare indication for administration of water after the contrast medium infusion is when the cecum and the distal ileum are difficult to find as a result of a congenital anomaly. By filling the small intestine with water, the colon becomes more clearly visible against this background (fig. 7.27).

In summary, administration of water after the barium suspension is indicated in the following cases:

1. to obtain a better degree of filling of the distal ileum after the cecum has been reached.
2. to obtain filling of the distal ileal loops when the contrast column has almost reached the cecum. One could in this case also give an additional 300 cc contrast fluid but water is cheaper!
3. flushing of the distal ileum when it is contaminated with food residue or by reflux from the colon as a result of an inadequate Bauhin's valve.
4. filling of the rest of the small intestine after 1200 ml barium suspension has already been administered and the cecum is not yet reached. In general this occurs in the event of a functional or mechanical obstruction.
5. for double contrast films of the jejunum, filling with water is greatly preferred over filling with air. One disadvantage is, however, that there is very little time available to take the films.
6. if it is necessary to examine the colon with contrast medium administered orally, the entire small intestine can be flushed clean with water in 5–10 minutes. The barium suspension used for enteroclysis is then used again for the colon examination.
7. position of the ascending colon and the distal ileum cannot be identified.

7. Administration of air after contrast fluid

Often in very slender individuals the ileal loops may already have clumped together in the pelvis minor after administration of 600 ml contrast fluid or even less. Since this part of the abdominal cavity is not accessible for compression, special measures must be taken to force the mass of ileal loops out of the pelvis minor. The drawing in fig. 7.28 shows that if the patient lies on his stomach in a slight Trendelenburg position, the heavy barium-filled ileal loops are most likely to drop spontaneously in the direction of the navel and the posterior abdominal wall. The result is, however, often disappointing. The next step is to try filling the bladder with water, the rectosigmoid with air or both. For hygienic reasons, we believe that filling the bladder with water through a catheter is not very desirable; moreover this procedure costs more time than rectal air insufflation. One might consider asking leptosome patients to hold their morning urine. We feel, however, that this causes the patient considerable discomfort; in addition it could have an adverse effect on the motility of the small intestine via the autonomous nervous system. Furthermore for the reasons discussed previously it is recommended that the patient evacuate just before the examination to be sure that the colon is as empty as possible. Selective emptying of the colon without emptying the bladder would be extremely difficult and we object to this approach for that reason. Filling only the rectosigmoid with air often turns out to be sufficient to project the deep-lying ileum freely (fig. 7.29).

In general this method is also useful when the cecum is located deep within the pelvis minor

---

Fig. 7.27
Positional anomaly of the small intestine: the ascending colon is difficult to find.
A. Filling of the jejunal loops in the right half of the abdomen.
B. Now the ileal loops are also filled and parts of the colon are visible in the upper left quadrant. The cecum, usually located either in the lower right quadrant or high up under the liver, is not visible here.
C. After the jejunum is filled with water, the cecum and the ascending colon are visualized clearly on the right side.

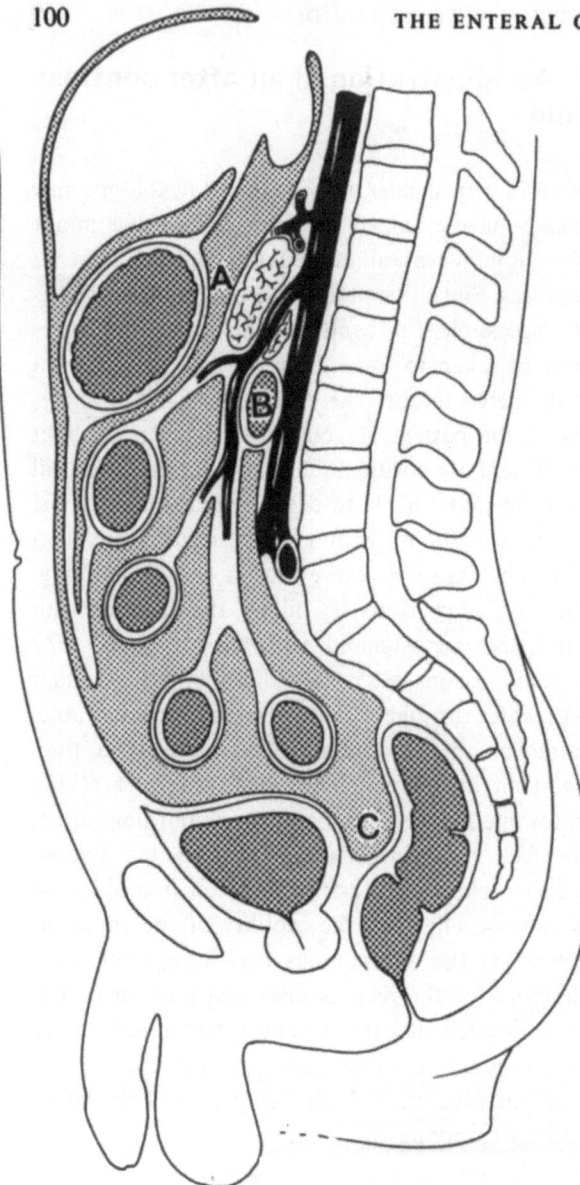

Fig. 7.28
Lateral cross-section of the abdominal cavity.
A. Via the foramen of Winslow or an opening in the transverse mesocolon, the jejunal loops may end up behind the stomach in the bursa omentalis.
B. The duodenum can be pinched between the aorta and the superior mesenteric artery.
C. By filling the bladder and the rectum, the ileal loops are forced out of the pelvis minor.

(fig. 7.30). In these cases it is better to administer so much air rectally, that the cecum is also filled.

If necessary, the lowest part of the cecum can also be filled with air and even, via reflux through Bauhin's valve, the distal ileal loops. Rectal air insufflation of the distal ileal loops can be necessary when oral air insufflation takes too long as in diseases accompanied by greatly reduced motility of the small intestine. If peristalsis is normal, oral air insufflation of the tangle of ileal loops is certainly the best and the quickest way to increase the chance of evaluating the mucosal patterns in this section. Air is administered intermittently through the duodenal tube with the insufflation balloon; at the same time the expression on the patient's face must be observed closely. When the air is administered too rapidly, sensations of pain due to cramps are immediately visible on the face. The total amount of air to be administered can be estimated at about 1 liter. The air causes pronounced local stretching

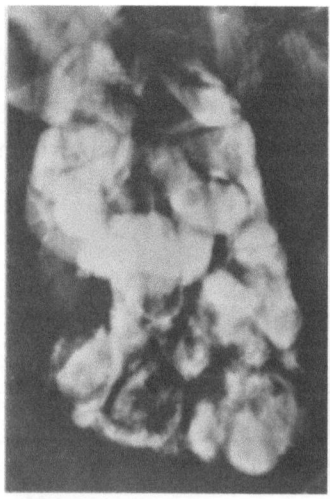
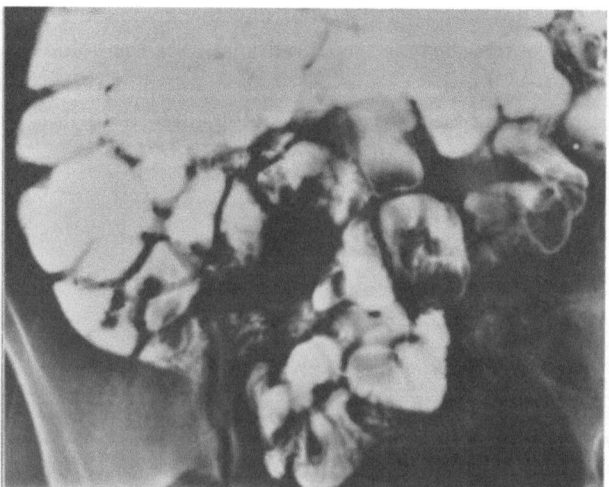

Fig. 7.29
Rectal air insufflation with the patient in the prone position is often sufficient for free projection of the ileal loops in the pelvis minor.

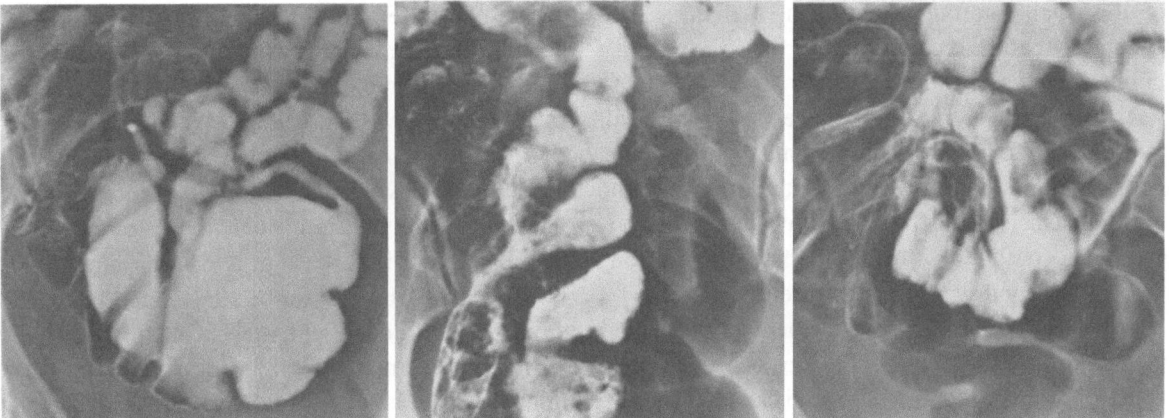

Fig. 7.30
Filling the rectosigmoid with air, and if necessary continuing insufflation until the cecum is also filled with air, is a good method for forcing the deep-seated ileocecal segment out of the pelvis minor.

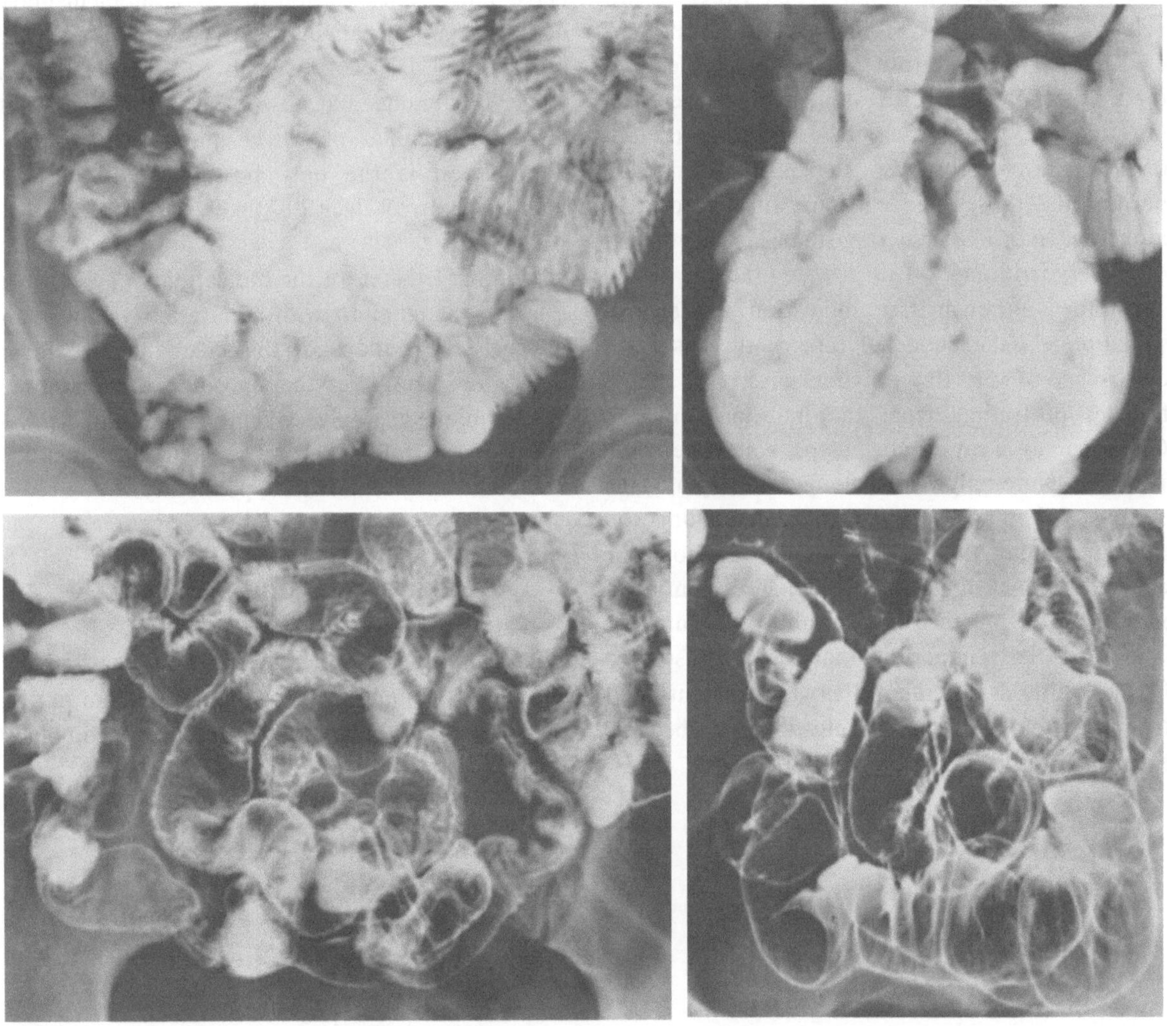

Fig. 7.31
Two examples of free projection of the ileal loops in the lower abdomen and the pelvis minor using air insufflation through the duodenal tube. The patient is in the prone position.

of the small intestine resulting in such an active peristalsis that the cecum is often reached within one minute. Each and every time it is an experience to watch the rush of air through the meters of small intestine and to note at the same time that this active peristalsis does not influence the rate of flow of the barium suspension in the small intestine. In fact it even appears that as a result of the passage of air, the flow of contrast fluid is retarded.

When the air reaches the segment of the ileum located in the pelvis minor, the loops can be forced apart by means of compression and can be projected almost separately (fig. 7.31).

Although the double contrast examination with air is without a doubt exceedingly useful for examining tangled intestinal loops either in the pelvis minor or due to adhesions, it has become evident that there are not many other indications for this technique. Because the loops of the small intestine are greatly twisted, large contrast differences develop between the parts filled with barium and those filled with air; furthermore the numerous more or less ring-shaped shadows are often very irritating.

Another although rare indication for air insufflation via the duodenal tube is the suspected occurrence of very tiny polypoid masses or lymph follicles protruding from the intestinal mucosa. On the survey x-rays these polyps, sometimes only 1 mm long, are only visible along the margin of the contrast column; on air double contrast films, on the other hand, they can be seen throughout the entire intestinal loop (fig. 7.32). To examine a patient for the presence of such subtle abnormalities it is particularly important that the contrast fluid foam as little as possible; otherwise differentiation from gas bubbles in the intestine can become exceedingly difficult or even impossible.

The exposure time for the x-ray must be short because of the large quantity of air in the exposed area. Quite often double contrast films are mistakenly taken with a low tube voltage. We have found that this is only admissible when a solitary freely projected loop is involved. Evaluation of double contrast films with air is easiest when the intestinal loops contain only a little barium and when air insufflation is carried out during the last stage of the examination. If during enteroclysis it appears that a mass of intestinal loops has formed in the pelvis minor or if it is known or becomes clear that adhesion has occurred, it is not wise to decide too quickly to give a second dose of contrast fluid; it is better to wait or to give metoclopramide.

When a mass of ileal loops is discovered in the pelvis minor, the decision to give a supplementary dosage of water can be disastrous. The mass will only become larger as a result and usually can no longer be untangled at all – even a belated attempt to use air insufflation will be unsuccessful. A new examination is the only possible solution after such an incorrect decision (fig. 7.33).

In summary therefore the indications for a double contrast examination with air are fairly limited in enteroclysis. If loops of the small intestine form clumps as a result of their position or adhesions, this technique can be very helpful; it should also be considered if follicular or polypoid abnormalities of the mucosa are a distinct possibility.

8. Compression technique

When it appears that neither rectal nor oral air insufflation is enough to force the distal ileum out of the pelvis minor for adequate projection, a combination of these two methods can be attempted.

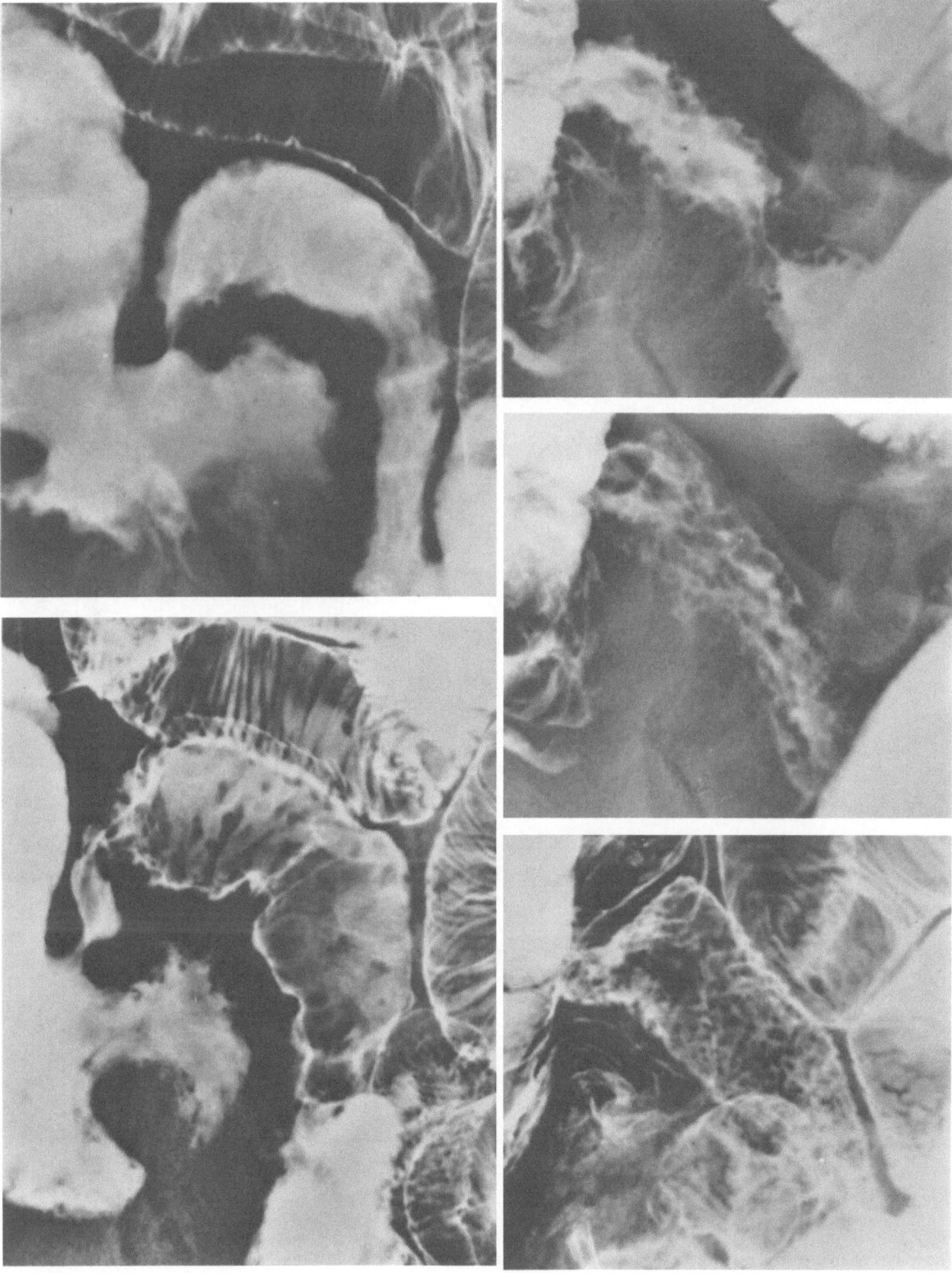

Fig. 7.32
Two examples of lymph follicles in the distal ileum which are clearly visible on the double contrast exposures but could not or barely be seen when the loop was filled with barium only.

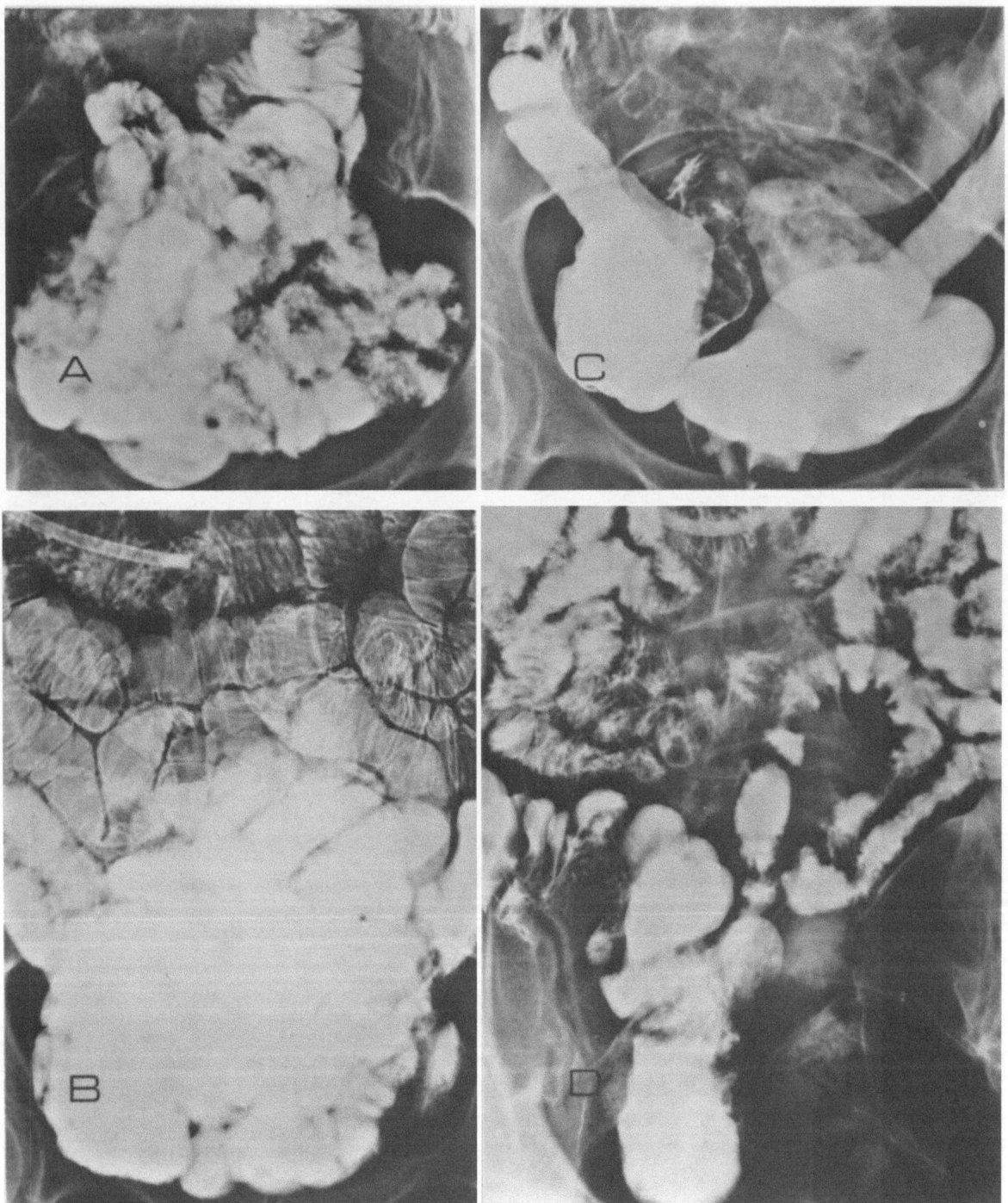

Fig. 7.33
The results of an incorrect decision as to procedure during the course of the examination. There is a clump of ileal loops in the pelvis minor (A). Because the cecum has not yet been reached, water was administered. Figure B shows the results of this decision. Although the reasoning was in principle correct, this step was apparently undertaken without consideration of the problems which could be expected during free projection of the distal ileum since a previous colon examination (fig. C) had already indicated that the ileocecal segment was deep-seated. Fig. D shows the survey exposures obtained after 2 cc metoclopramide was administered intravenously, on the basis of the original situation seen in fig. A, and air was insufflated rectally. Air insufflation via the duodenal tube would serve no purpose.

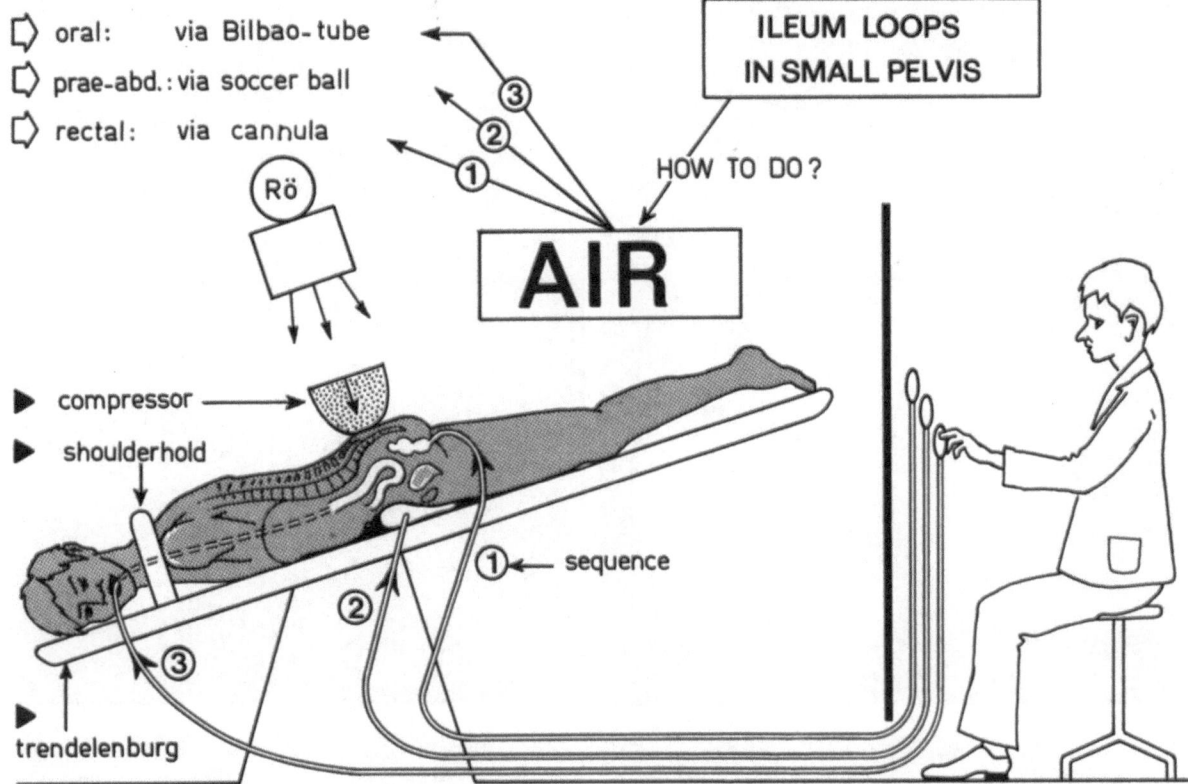

oral: via Bilbao-tube
prae-abd.: via soccer ball
rectal: via cannula

ILEUM LOOPS
IN SMALL PELVIS

HOW TO DO?

AIR

▶ compressor
▶ shoulderhold
▶ trendelenburg

① ← sequence

Fig. 7.34
Position of the patient during the combined insufflation and special compression technique. The sequence of steps is usually as follows:
1. Place the balloon under the lower abdomen.
2. Rectal air insufflation.
3. Air insufflation via the duodenal tube.
4. Fill the balloon between the patient and the table with air.
5. Compression on the dorsal side of the patient.
6. If necessary, direct roentgen rays along craniocaudal axis.

This combined air insufflation, as well as the subsequent application of compression, can be divided into a number of steps as follows (fig. 7.34):

1. the patient lies on his stomach in a slight Trendelenburg position. Between the lower abdomen and the table, just above the symphysis, is an empty inner tube of a soccer ball which is connected by a long tube to an insufflation balloon. In this way, in spite of the prone position, compression can be exerted on the intestinal loops from the abdominal side. However, the balloon is not blown up until air has been administered rectally at least (see 2) and often also orally (see 3).

2. a cannula in the rectum is connected by a long tube to a second insufflation balloon. One almost always begins with rectal air insufflation since it takes less time than 'oral' insufflation and causes the patient the least discomfort.

3. air is administered orally through the Bilbao-Dotter tube which is connected to a third insufflation balloon.

4. pressure can be exerted on the dorsal side of the patient by means of an electric or manually operated compressor or a tourniquet as used in intravenous pyelography.

Careful execution of this technique, which after some practice only costs several minutes, gives the results seen in fig. 7.35.

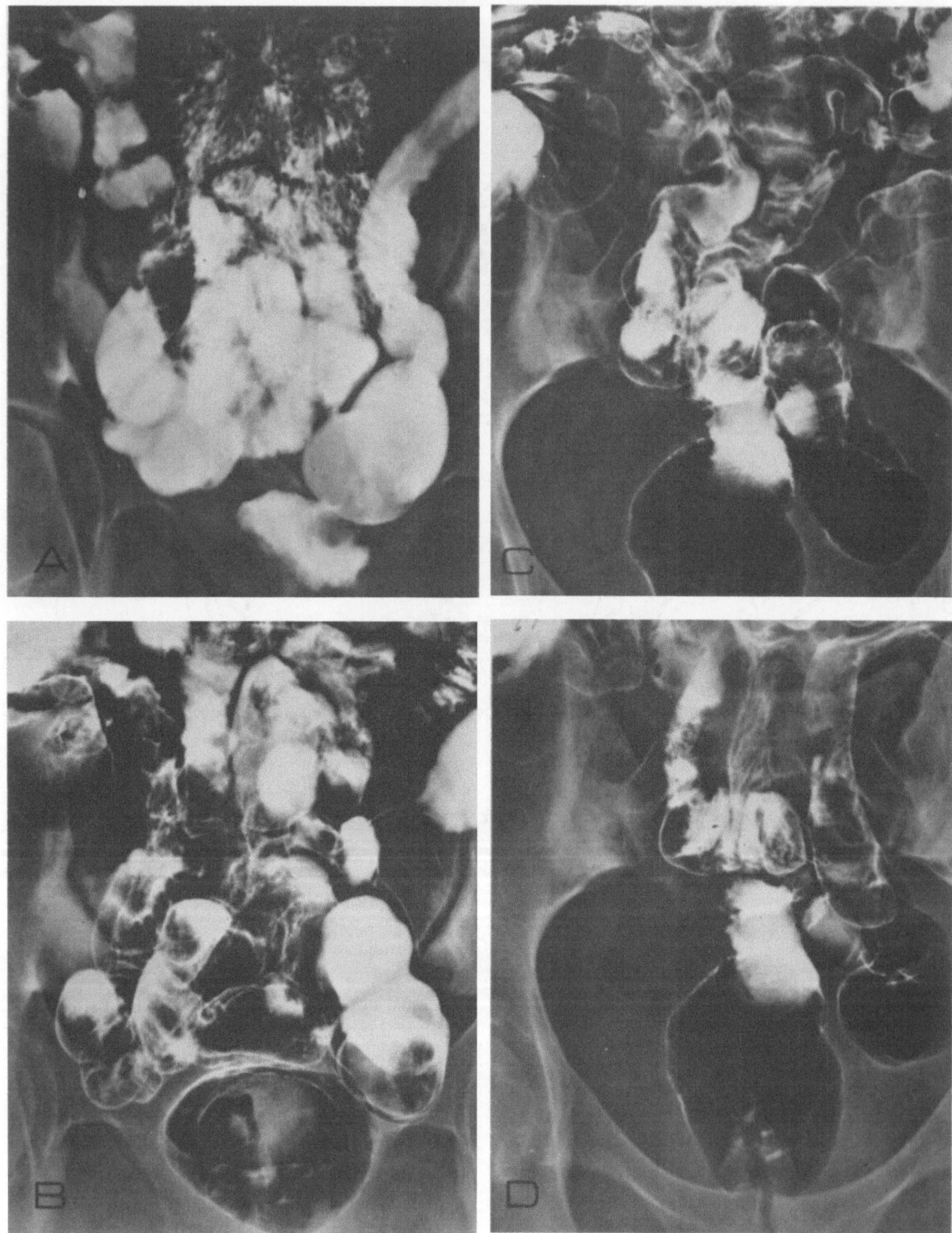

Fig. 7.35
Two examples of the results obtained with the special compression technique and combined air insufflation.
Patient 1: figures A–D.
Patient 2: figures E–F.

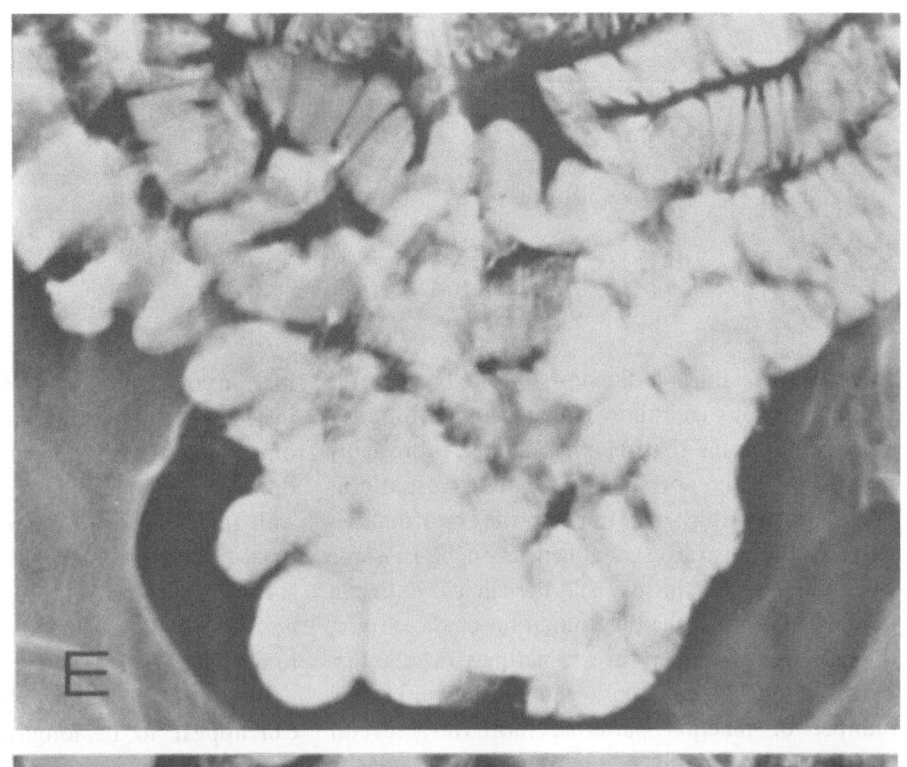

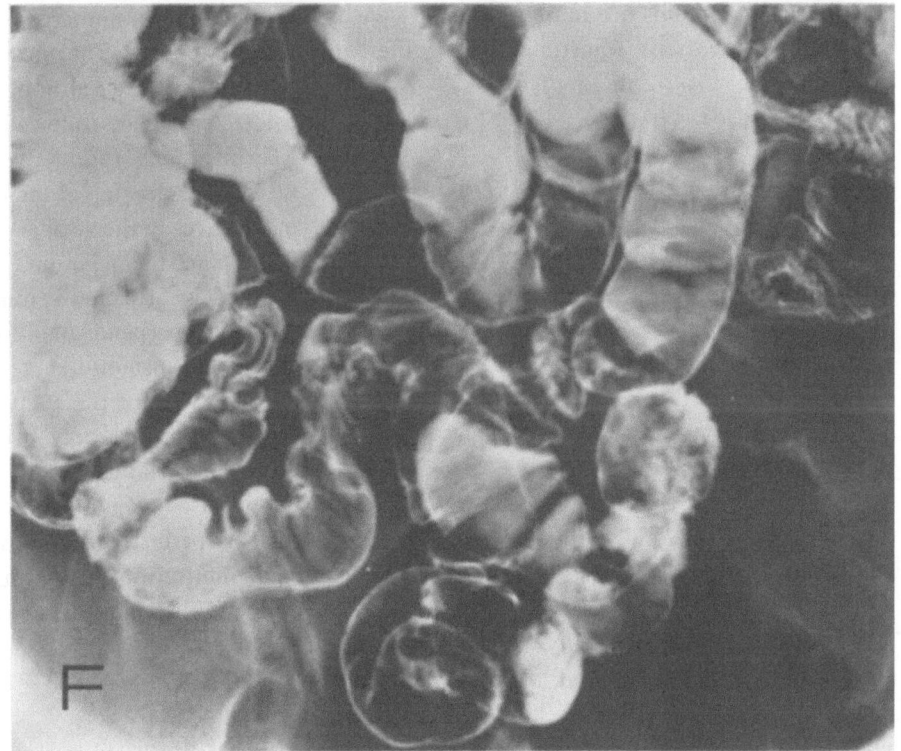

VIII

BASIC SIGNS OF ABNORMALITY

In order to establish a diagnosis on the basis of the roentgenograms and fluoroscopic examination, it is above all essential that the physician be thoroughly familiar with the normal roentgenological patterns and their variations; only then can the abnormalities seen on the x-rays be identified as such. In some cases, the patient's history and the clinical data can be quite useful for the determination of the correct diagnosis; in fact they are sometimes even indispensable since the mucosa shows only a limited number of reaction patterns; moreover, several radiological symptoms are not specific and can be encountered in various, sometimes quite different, diseases.

1. Changes in the mucosal pattern

Changes in the shape of the folds of Kerkring can be subdivided into three main categories:

1. the original shape of the fold is still easily recognized,
2. the original shape cannot be recognized, and
3. there is evidence of destruction.

a. SWELLING AND EDEMA

The most common abnormality although certainly not the most easily recognized, at least when only slight, is edema or mucosal swelling. On the other hand this diagnosis is also quite often established incorrectly when the coarse folds are a consequence of a misleading pattern (see chapter VIII-7).

Edematous swollen folds are found in diseases which are associated with protein deficiency and hypoalbuminemia as in inflammatory processes and disturbed protein synthesis, among others. The margins of each fold then do not always lie parallel – instead the folds can assume a somewhat biconvex omega-like (Ω) shape whereby the base of the fold does not change. The thickness of the intestinal wall increases only slightly or not at all (fig. 8.1 KLMN). In Whipple's disease and lambliasis the surface of these folds can be covered with tiny nodular swellings which bulge out into the intestinal lumen (see p. 216).

In the distal ileum, where the mucosal folding can appear to be longitudinal, the swollen folds become more numerous and begin to follow a twisting course. The mucosal relief appears somewhat disordered, although the continuity of the folds can still be followed, for instance in yersinia EC infections (fig. 8.2vw). In Crohn's disease ulcerations develop at the bottom of deep longitudinal grooves in the swollen mucous membrane of the ileum and the jejunum. The continuity of these grooves is broken by numerous deep ulcerations which lie perpendicular to the longitudinal folds, causing a cushion-like relief – the so-called cobblestone pattern (fig. 8.3). This cobblestone relief, a result of a markedly swollen mucosal surface, is, however, certainly not specific to Crohn's disease but is also encountered in many other disorders such as periarteritis nodosa (fig. 8.4), lymphoreticular infiltration in the mucosa (fig. 8.5) and even after repositioning of an intussusception (fig. 8.6).

Fig. 8.1 →

Four patients with edematous swollen folds due to hypoalbuminemia.

K. only swollen folds, no thickening of the intestinal wall.

L. swollen folds and thickening of the intestinal wall.

M. biconvex or omega-shaped folds but no thickening of the intestinal wall. The patient has Crohn's disease of the colon.

N. omega-shaped folds and thickened wall in the bowel of a patient with celiac disease.

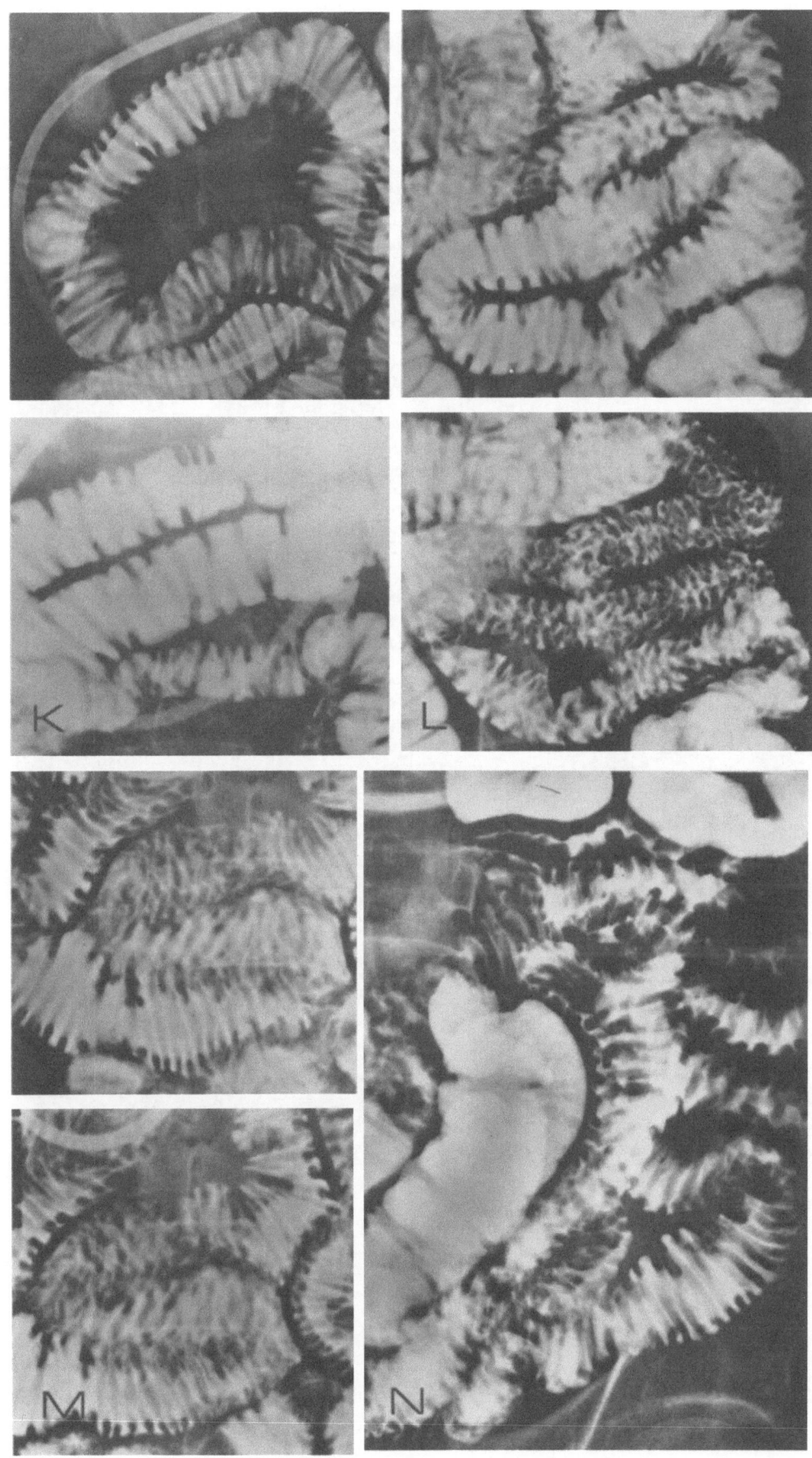

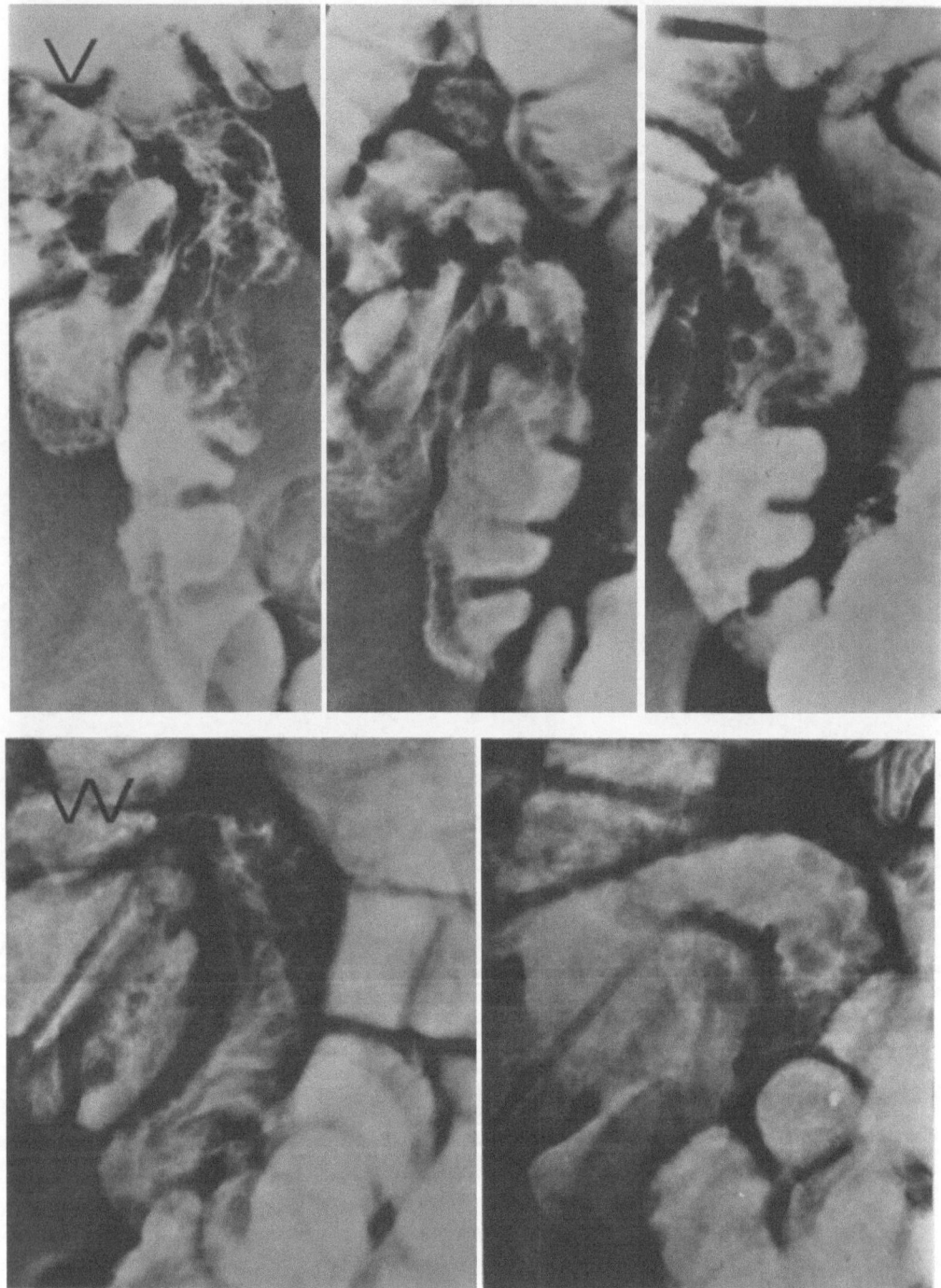

Fig. 8.2 vw.
Thick folds with twisting in the distal ileum, due to yersinia EC infection.

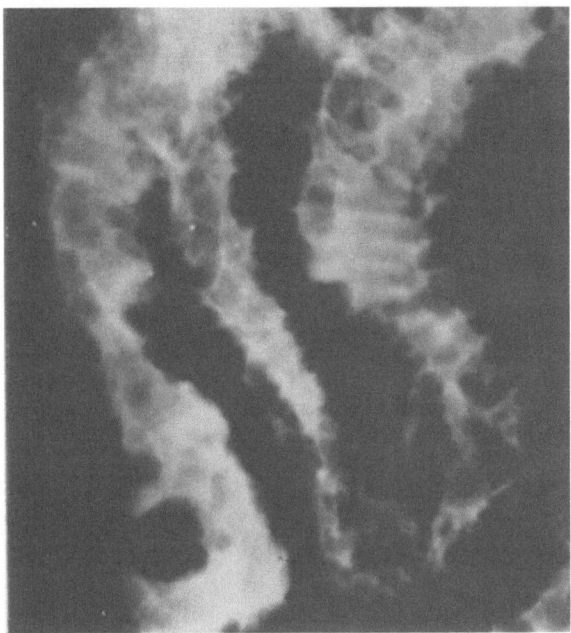 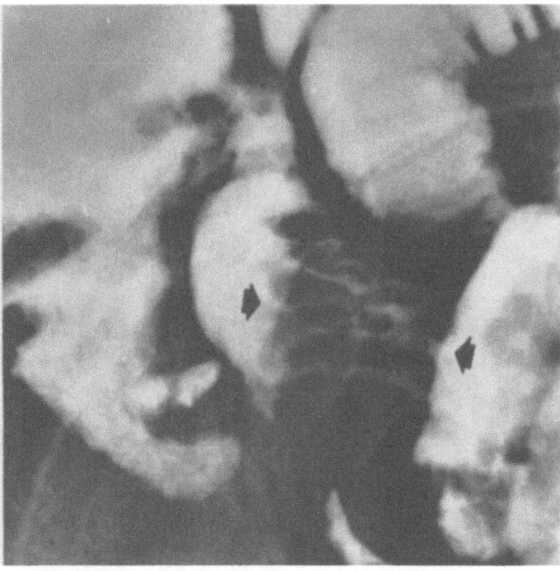

Fig. 8.3
So-called cobblestone relief in Crohn's disease caused by longitudinal and transverse grooves in the edematous swollen mucosal surface.

Fig. 8.4
Cobblestone pattern in the distal ileum as a result of periarteritis nodosa.

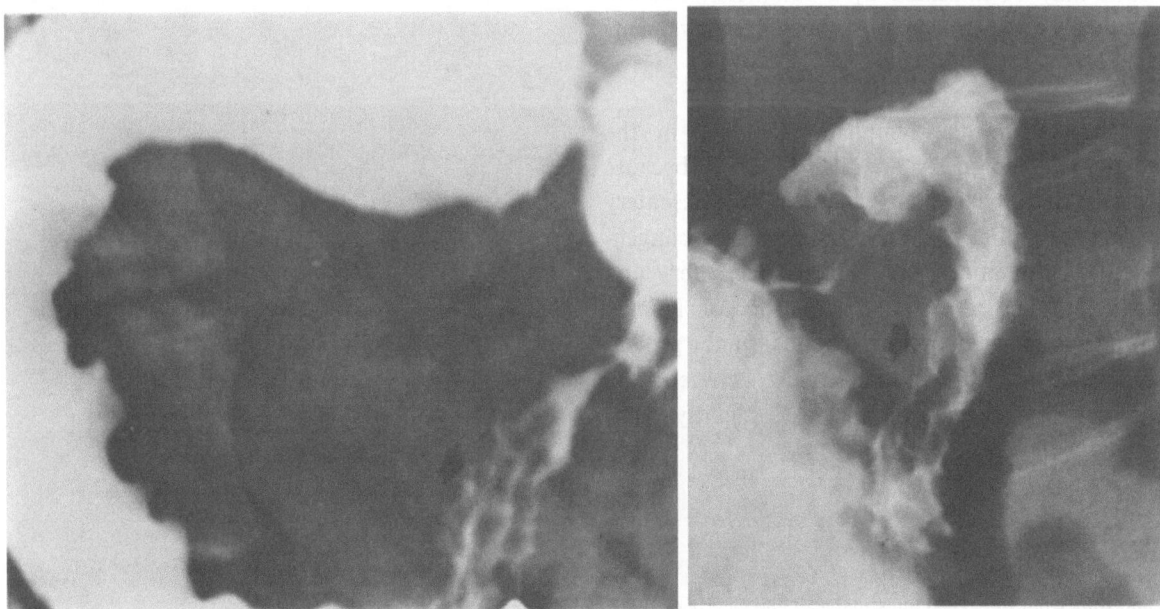

Fig. 8.5 Cobblestone pattern in the duodenum due to a lymphoreticular malignancy.

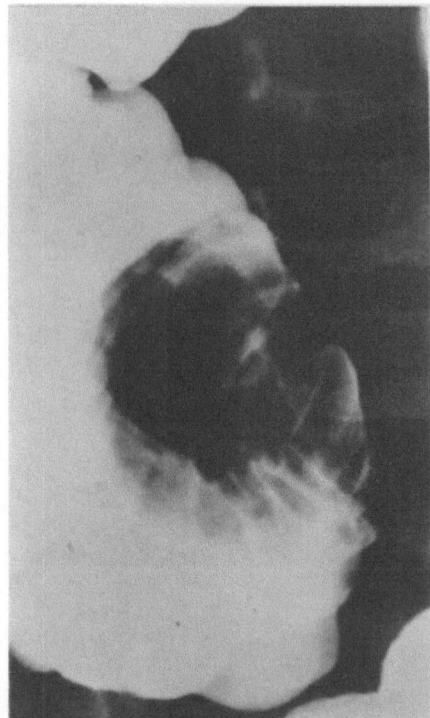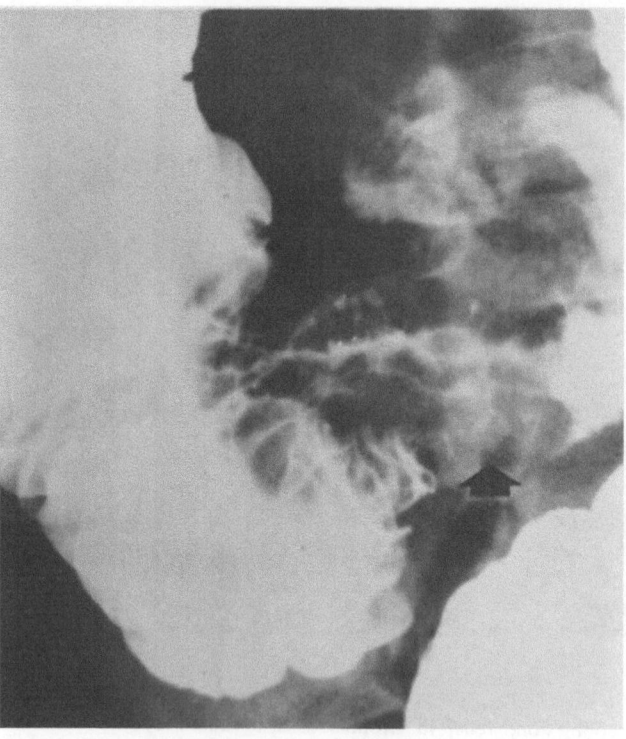

Fig. 8.6 Cobblestone relief in the distal ileum and edematous swollen Bauhin's valve after repositioning of an ileocolic intussusception.

Because the folds of Kerkring are thinner and farther apart in the ileum than in the jejunum, a slight edematous swelling of this part of the intestine may be indicated by a completely smooth intestinal wall with decreased peristaltic movements (fig. 8.7).

In lymphedema the lymphatic channels in the mucosa and submucosa are dilated, usually because drainage is impeded somewhere in the mesentery or the paralumbar region. The cause can be congenital, the lymphatic channels in the mesentery and the extremities are then hypoplastic, or it may result from an inflammatory process, tumor growth or irradiation fibrosis. The space between two adjacent intestinal loops increases slightly as a

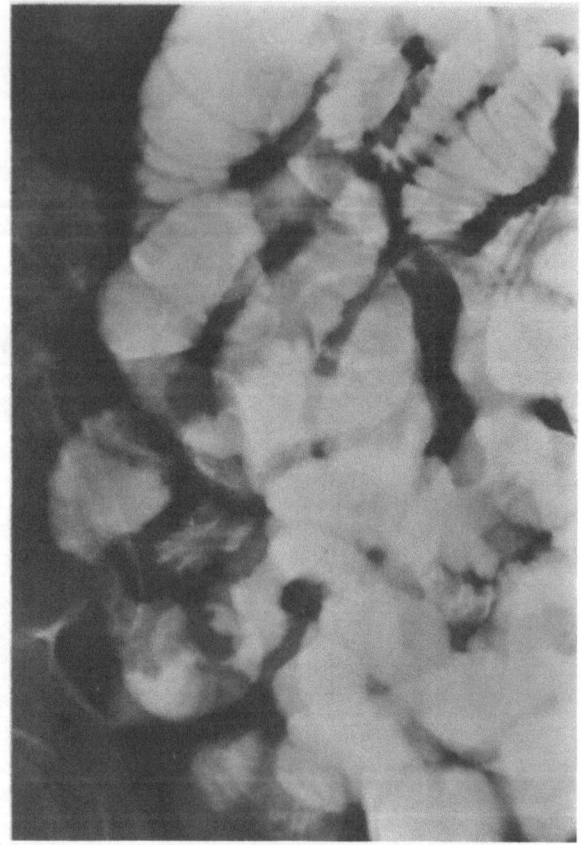

Fig. 8.7
Rigid somewhat thickened intestinal wall and clearly outlined smooth mucosal surface in the ileum as a result of a lymphoreticular malignancy.

result of the edematous swelling of the intestinal wall; the lumen is usually somewhat dilated. The mucosal folds become thicker and shorter; the space in between clearly decreases. As a result the mucosal surface in the jejunum can even appear spiculated and may be compared with a coarsely toothed saw (fig. 8.8). When there is lymphedema, the swollen intestine appears somewhat stiff and tube-like; on the x-rays as well as under fluoroscopy it is obvious that the contractions are impeded and less frequent. Lymphedema is accompanied by considerable leakage of serum albumin from the digestive tract. Histologically little or no inflammatory reaction is seen – in contrast, in regional enteritis the lymphatic channels are dilated and there is also an obvious inflammatory reaction.

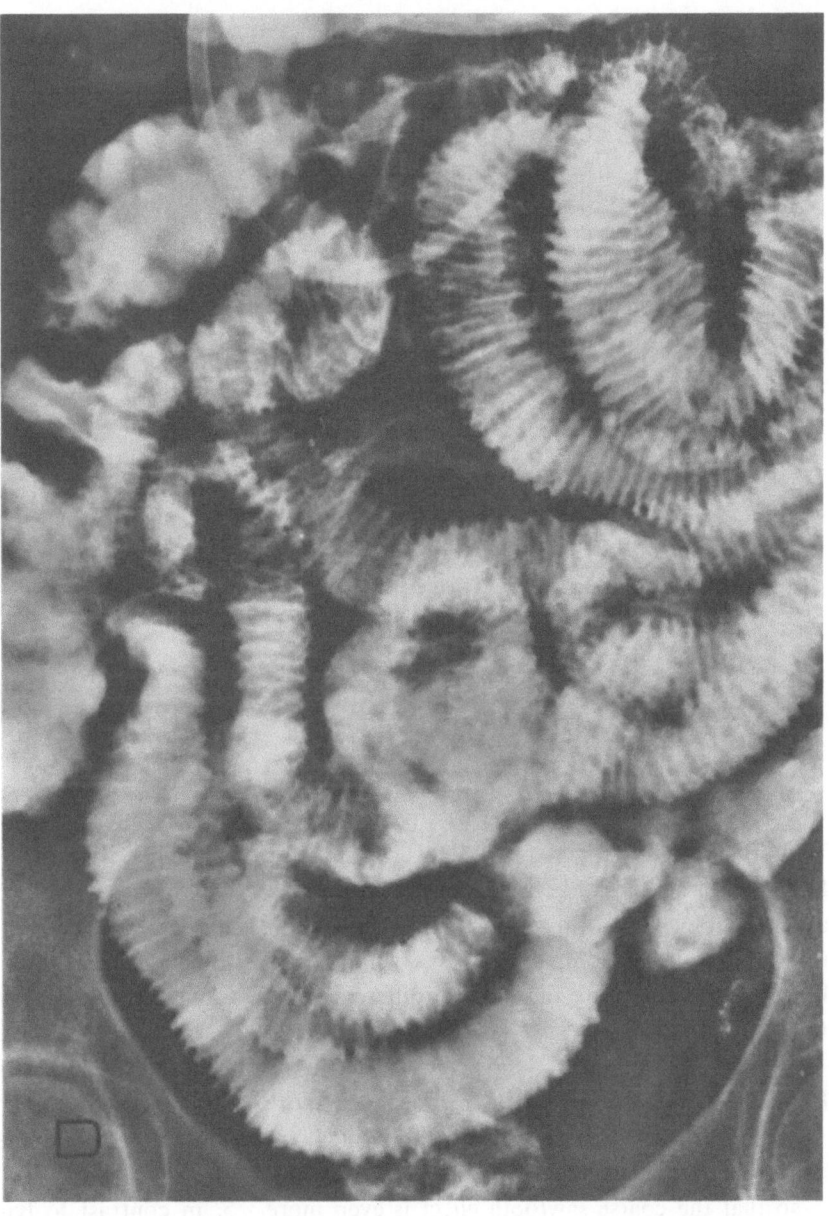

Fig. 8.8
D. Post-irradiation lymphedema. Because this edema has developed in a much shorter time than a congenital lymphedema, the mucosal folds are thicker, the wall of the intestine is more rigid and therefore there is less peristaltic activity.

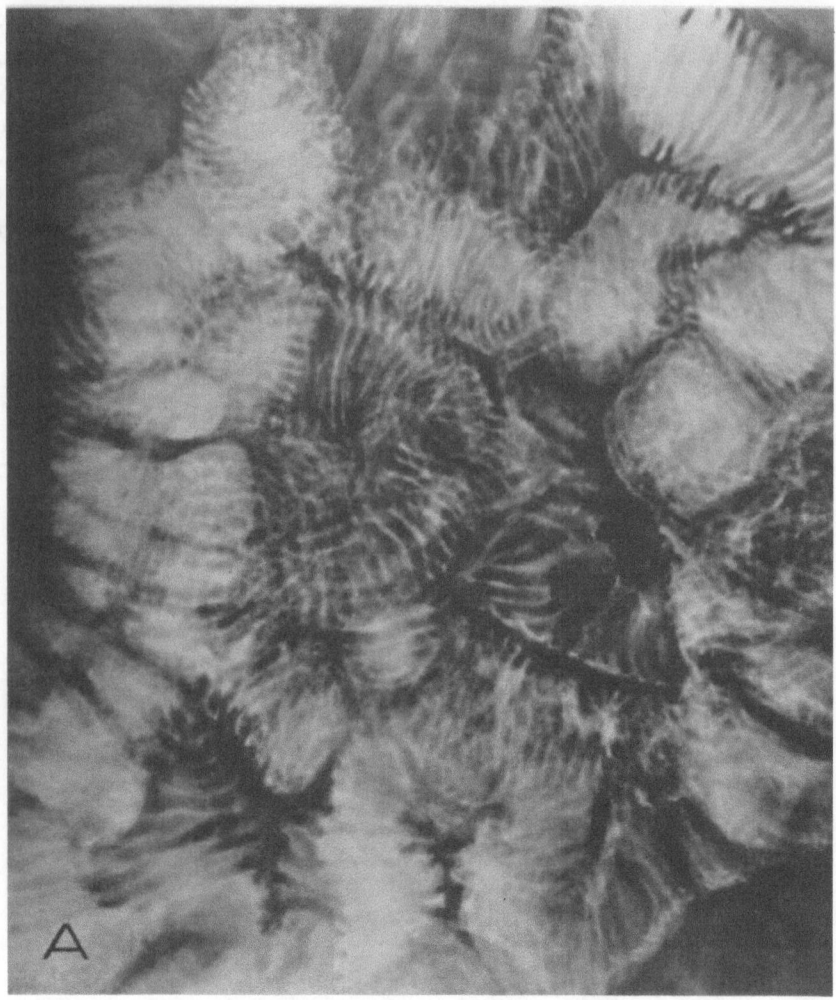

Rigidity and reduced peristalsis, thickened mucosal folds and larger spaces between the intestinal loops are also associated with vascular disorders of the intestinal wall. In comparison with lymphedema, however, the following radiological differences are found:

1. thickening of the folds is as a rule much more prominent, the spaces between the folds are smaller and very pointed and the folds are wider so that the coarse sawtooth effect is even more pronounced than in lymphedema (fig. 8.9D), which develops more gradually.
2. because multiple hematomas are found in the mucosa, the swollen fold relief often appears highly irregular; in addition multiple swellings which bulge out into the intestinal lumen may be visible (fig. 8.9E).
3. the intestinal wall may be markedly thicker than in lymphedema so that the spaces between the loops appear on the x-ray to be larger and, as a result of the hematomas, can vary greatly in shape and size.
4. the intestinal lumen is often narrower instead of dilated.
5. in contrast to lymphedema a vascular accident and celiac disease (fig. 8.9F) affect only a restricted segment of the intestine varying in length from 25 to 50 cm.

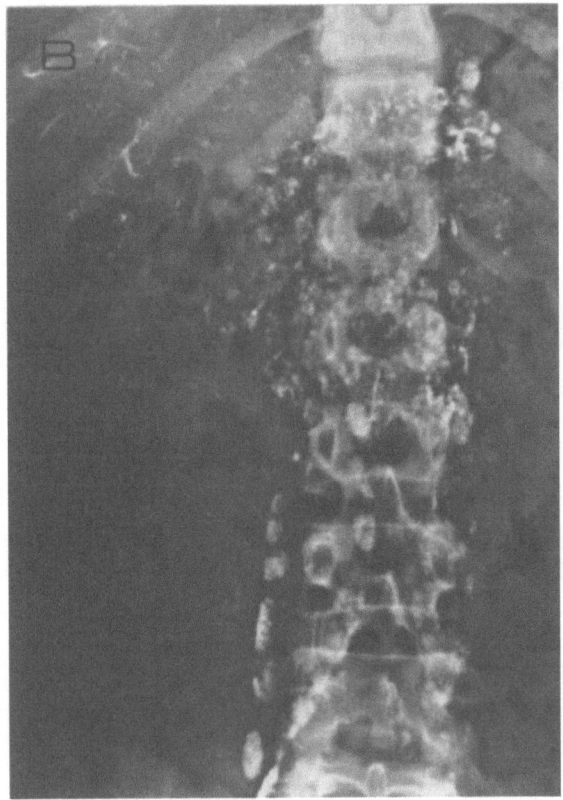

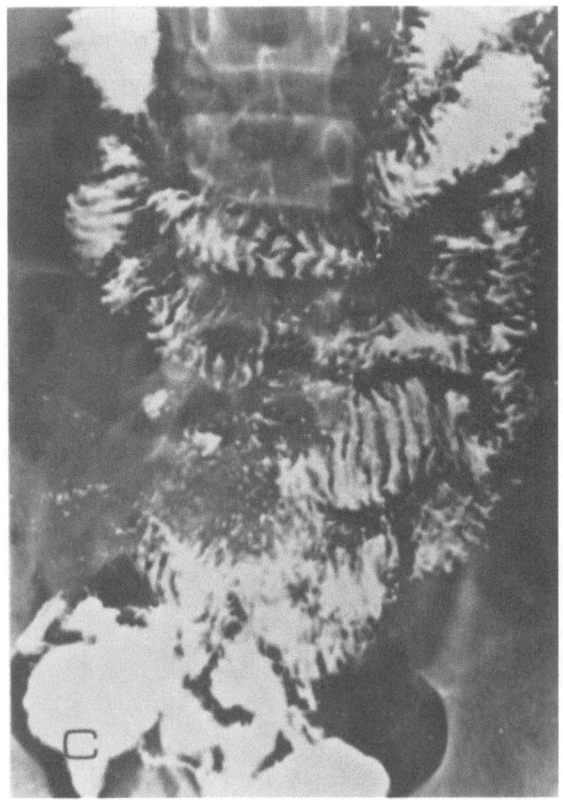

←

Fig. 8.8

A. Lymphedema of a congenital origin. It may be difficult to differentiate this pattern from certain forms of celiac disease (fig. 8.62). In celiac disease, however, there is an increased motility and if there is no hypoalbuminemia or secondary infection, then the mucosal folds are not thickened.

Fig. 8.8

B. Lymphography, showing a congenital hypoplasia of the lymphvessels. There is also a hypoplasia of the lymphvessels in the legs.

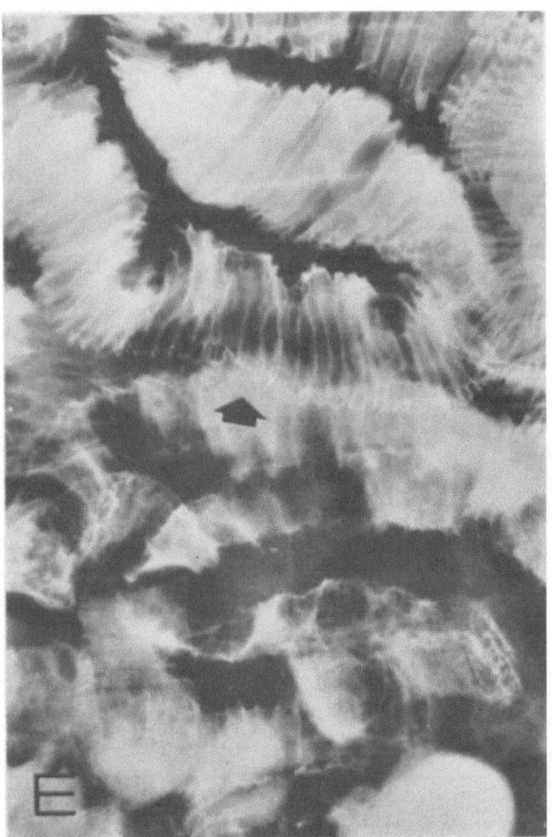

Fig. 8.8

C. Conventional examination of the patient in fig. 8.8A.

Fig. 8.8

E. Pronounced edema and clearly thickened wall of the intestine in a case of lymphoreticular malignancy.

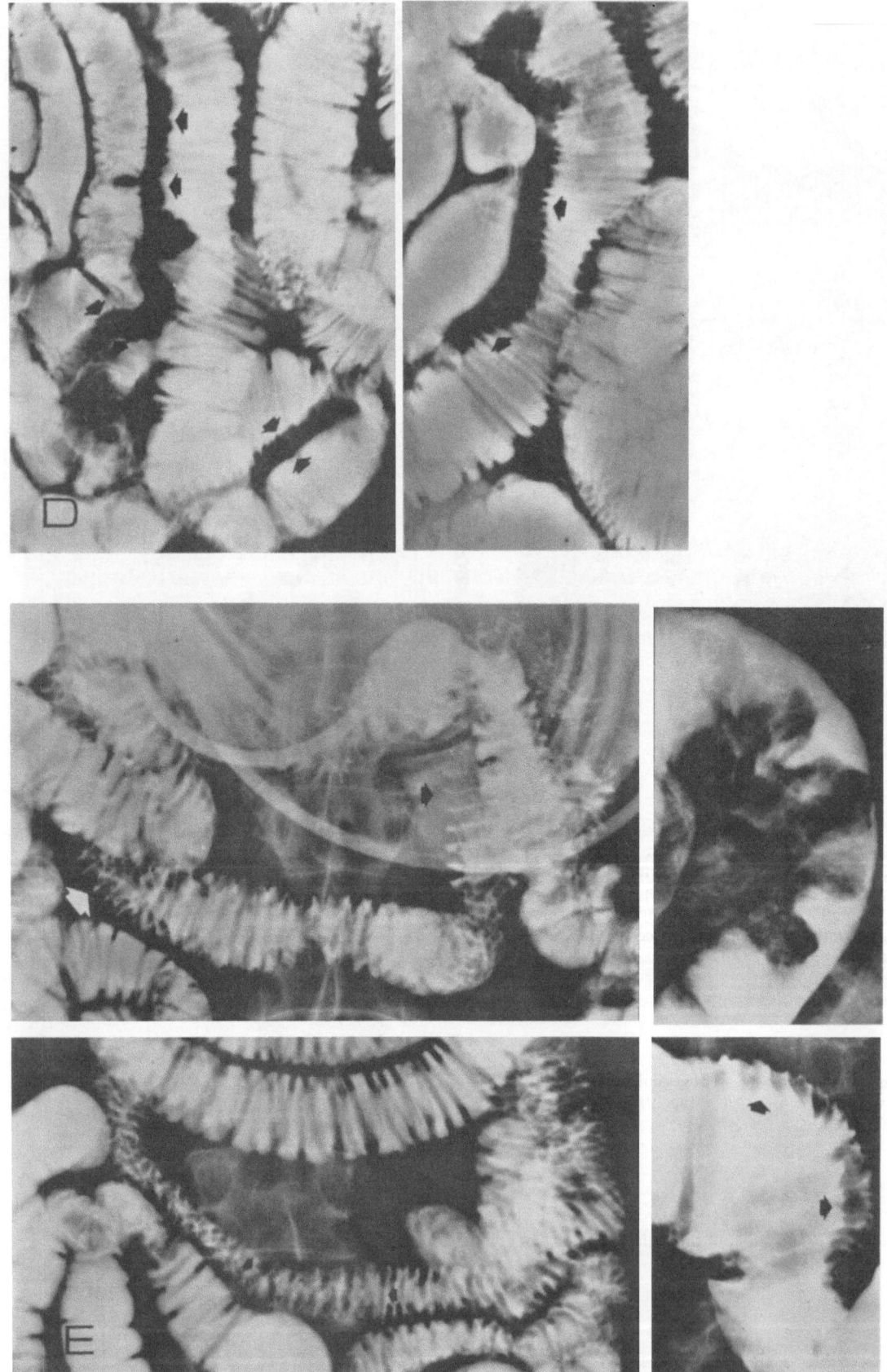

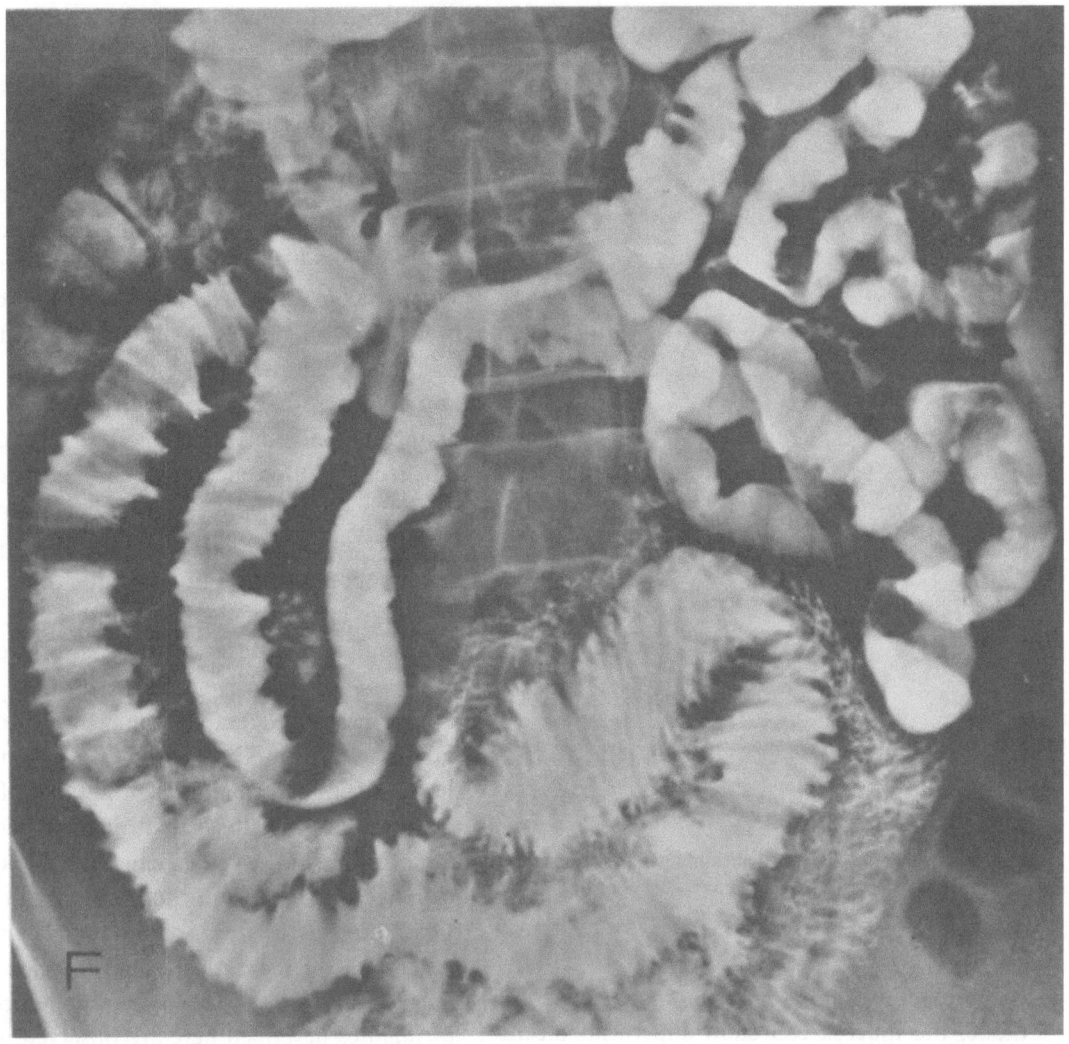

Fig. 8.9
F.   Broad mucosal folds in celiac disease and thickened intestinal wall due to a concomitant paratyphoid infection.

Fig. 8.9
D.   Exceedingly swollen mucosal folds in the jejunum as a result of ischemia. Pronounced swelling of the intestinal wall.

Fig. 8.9
E.   When anticoagulant therapy is too drastic, mucosal bleeding can cause very thick mucosal folds (left) and multiple swellings which bulge out into the intestinal lumen (right).

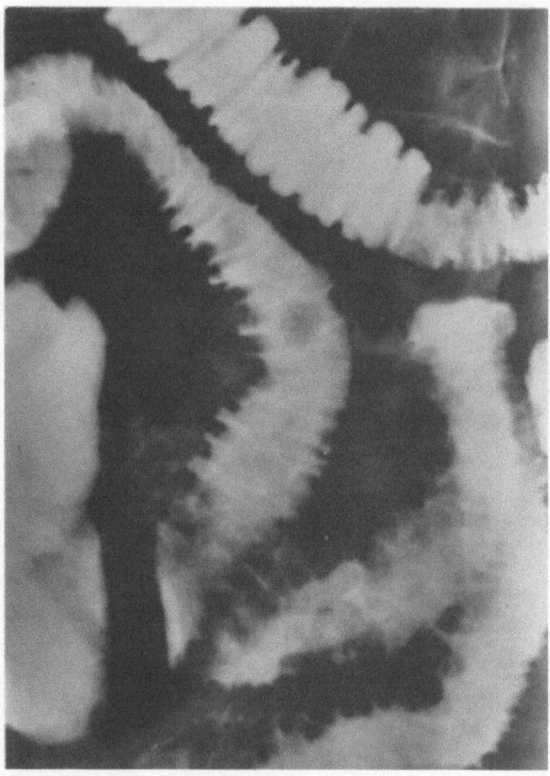

Fig. 8.10
Swollen mucosal folds, thickened intestinal wall and superficial ulcerations in radiation enteritis.

6. as a result of inflammatory phenomena in necrotic tissue, the mucosa can show superficial ulcerations (fig. 8.10) and the intestinal wall may contain gas (fig. 8.11P). It is obvious that these gas accumulations will often have ragged contours in contrast to the misleading patterns of gas sometimes seen (fig. 8.11Q). Moreover, if the gas pattern is misleading, the adjacent mucosal folds appear quite normal.

b. ATROPHY

Atrophy of the mucosal folds is a common although somewhat incorrect term used in all those cases when the fold relief has partly or completely disappeared leaving a more or less smooth intestinal wall. Most cases, however, do not involve a true atrophy but instead a destruction of the mucosal surface as a result of an inflammatory process or disturbed circulation.

In the ileum where the folds are thinner, shorter and also less numerous than in the jejunum, such a process will lead sooner, as well as more often, to a smooth mucosal surface than in the jejunum. The most frequent cause of a smooth ileal wall is a very superficial 'reflux ileitis' (fig. 8.12F) in conjunction with a ulcerative colitis. In those cases of Crohn's disease whereby the inflammatory process is fairly superficial, a completely smooth wall can sometimes develop in the small intestine after several years (see page 193). These patients often also show abnormalities due to Crohn's disease in the cecum or throughout the entire colon so that differentiation from a cured ulcerative colitis can cause considerable difficulties. However, in Crohn's disease the segment of atrophied ileum is often significantly longer than in ulcerative colitis (fig. 8.12G). A moderate anoxia of the intestinal wall, for example as a result of a diffuse vasculitis, also leads in some cases to an extensive abnormality of the same nature in the ileocecal region which is difficult to differentiate from Crohn's disease in particular. If the entire colon or mainly the right half of the colon and a large or small segment of the adjacent ileum are atrophied, then this can also be caused by prolonged intoxication due to certain laxatives (fig. 8.12H). It is strange that the cecum in these patients is dilated rather than shriveled as in the cases mentioned above. When therefore the abnormalities described here are observed, it is essential that the history be taken with care. Finally the mucosal folds can disappear when the circulation is disturbed due to a functional disturbance or a diffuse process in the intestinal wall, such as for instance an amyloidosis or a superficial lymphoreticular malignancy. In lymphoma the intestinal wall is obviously thickened; in amyloidosis this thickness may vary greatly and the colon may also be involved.

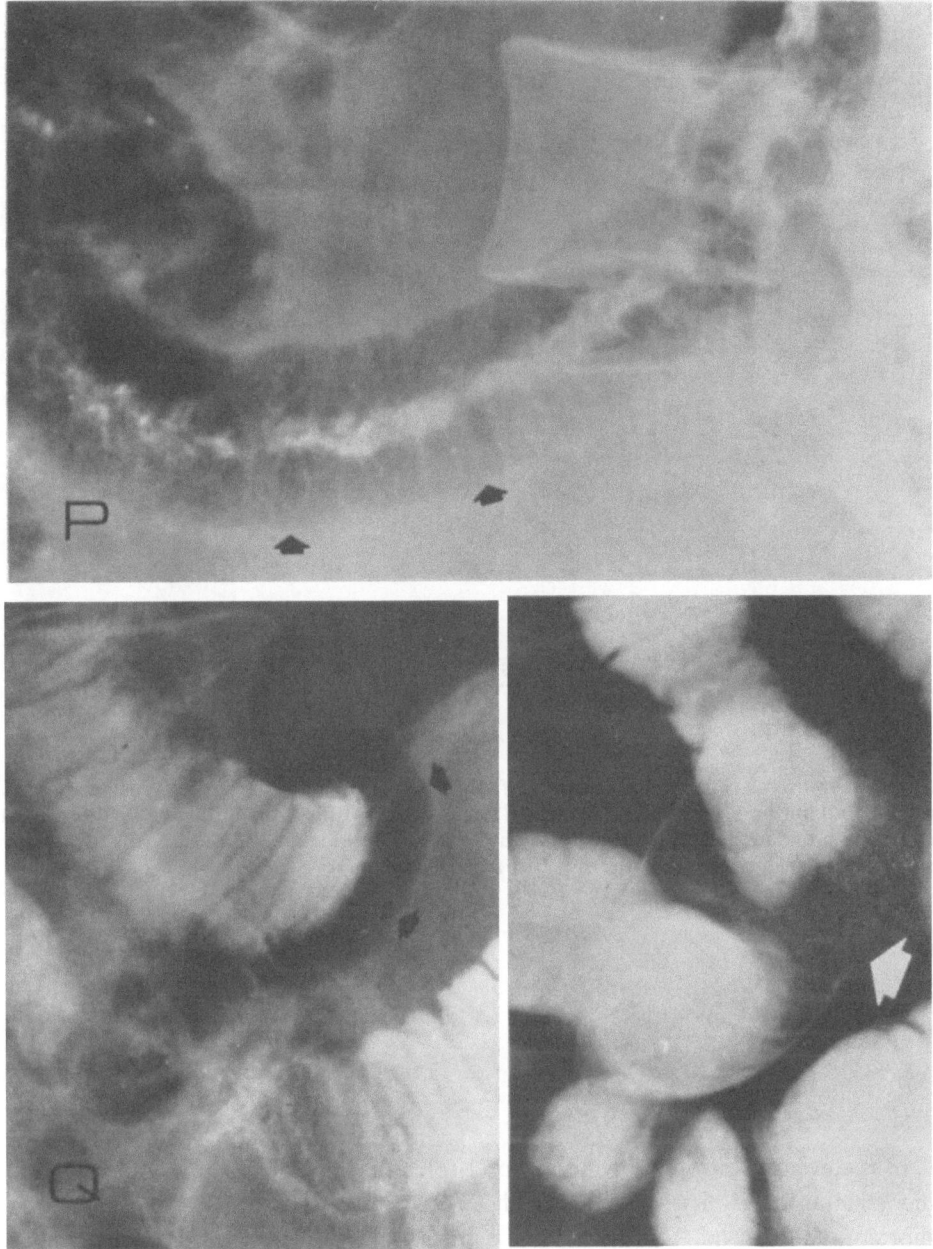

Fig. 8.11
P. Gas in the intestinal wall due to necrosis in a case of thrombosis of the superior mesenteric vein. The contours of these gas configurations are often ragged.
Q. Misleading pattern of gas in the small intestine with sharply defined margins.

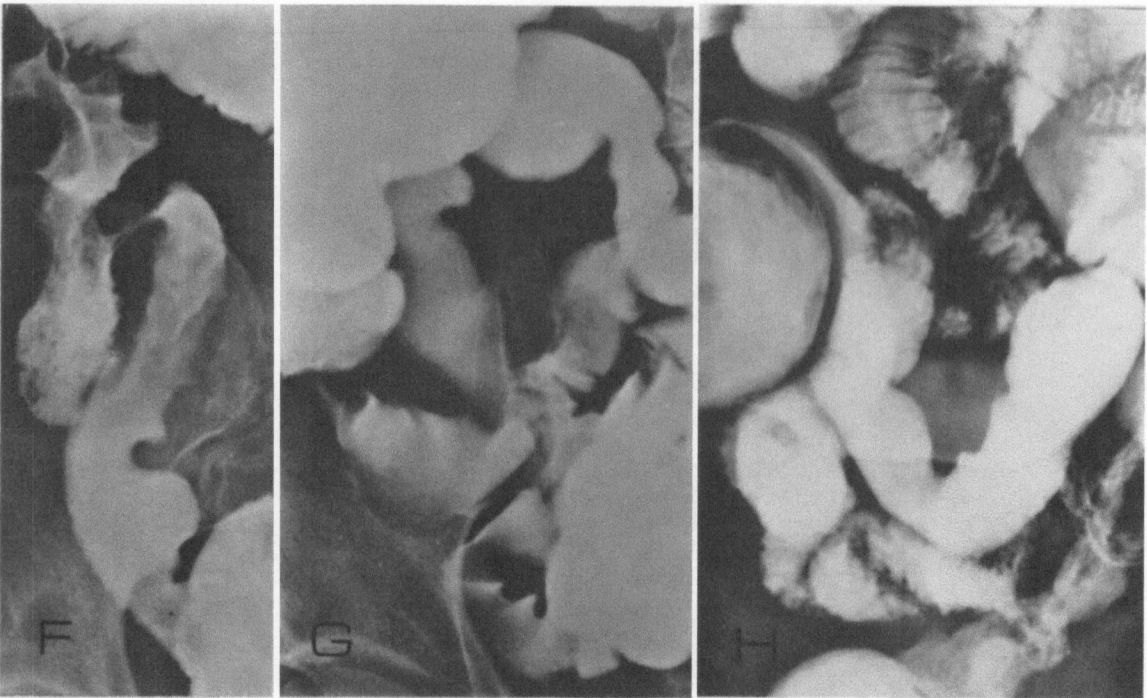

Fig. 8.12

F.   Colitis with reflux ileitis. That segment of the ileum containing the atrophied mucosa is usually only about 15 cm long.
G.   Smooth mucosal surface in the ileum and cecum 30 years after Crohn's disease in the ileocecal region was cured.
H.   Quite pronounced atrophy of the mucosa in the ileocecal region as a result of the chronic use of drugs. The cecum is highly dilated, which is not the case after an ileocolitis.

In the event of atrophy of the mucosal folds in the jejunum it is first noted that they become shorter and that the transition to the intestinal wall has become more rounded. In celiac disease (see chapter XII), there is no dilatation of that part of the jejunum containing the atrophied folds; furthermore the distance between the folds increases (fig. 8.13). If there are no complications then this superficial obliteration of the folds or true atrophy is not accompanied by thickening of the intestinal wall. A thickened intestinal wall can, however, be seen in amyloidosis whereby the folds in the jejunum become highly irregular due to the numerous deposits; in other cases the mucosal folds are only broadened and flatter and assume a more or less undulating course (fig. 8.14).

c. ABNORMAL COURSE

When otherwise completely healthy mucosal folds enclose a triangular plateau without fold relief, then this can only be caused by a triple junction in the small intestine. This must be the omphalo-mesenteric duct – even if the large or small sack-like mouth of this Meckel's diverticulum is not visible on the available exposures (fig. 8.15). Theoretically a duplication could also cause a triple junction configuration of the fold relief of the intestinal mucosa. It has been shown, however, that as a rule this abnormality develops as a so-called duplication cyst which causes a smoothly defined bulge into the lumen of the intestinal loop or a compression effect on the outside. We have also

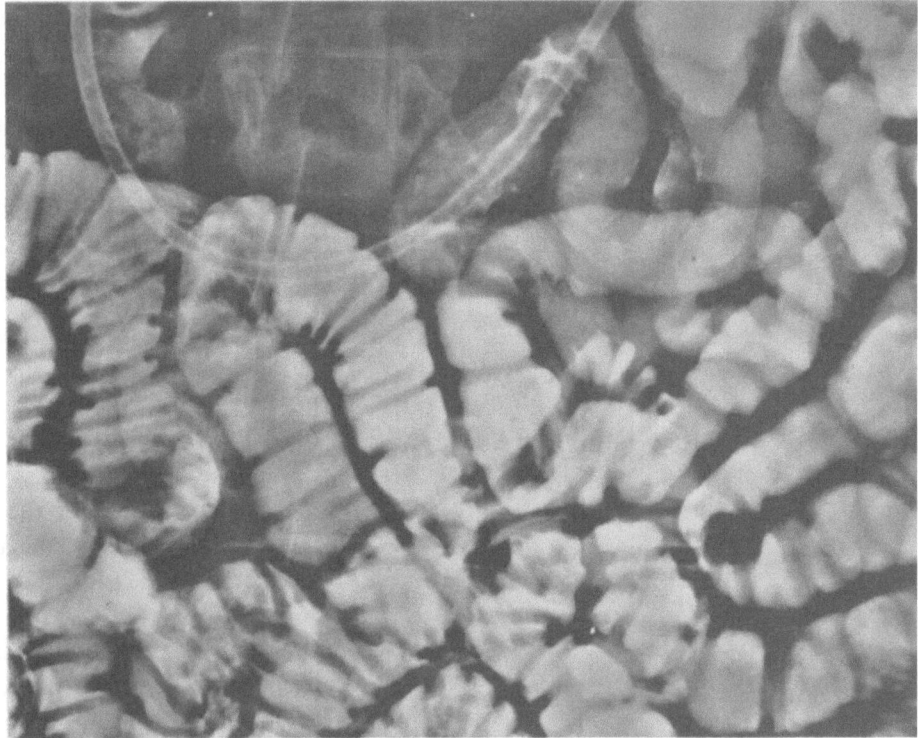

Fig. 8.13
Atrophy of the mucosal folds in the jejunum in celiac disease. The folds are shorter than normal and are farther apart; the transition from fold to intestinal wall is more rounded than normal. Broadening of the folds and thickening of the wall of the intestine are probably due to a hypoalbuminemia.

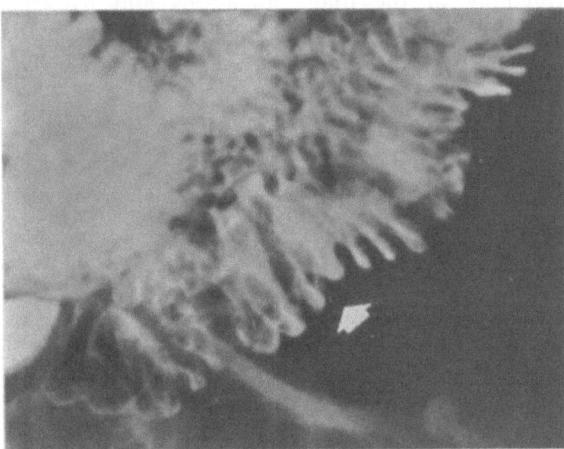

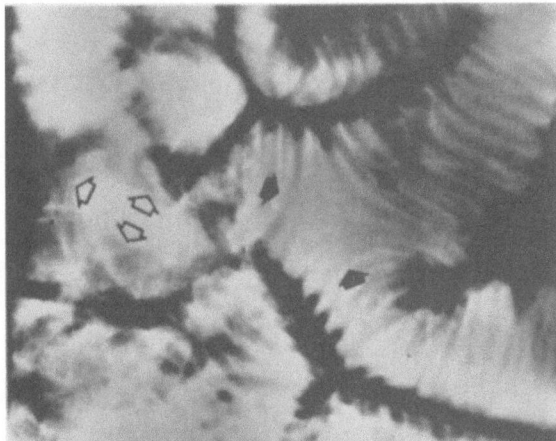

Fig. 8.14
Slightly undulant course or broad and highly irregular folds with a marked thickening of the intestinal wall in amyloidosis.

Fig. 8.15
Triangular configuration in the mucosal pattern at the mouth of the omphalomesenteric duct (Meckel's diverticulum).

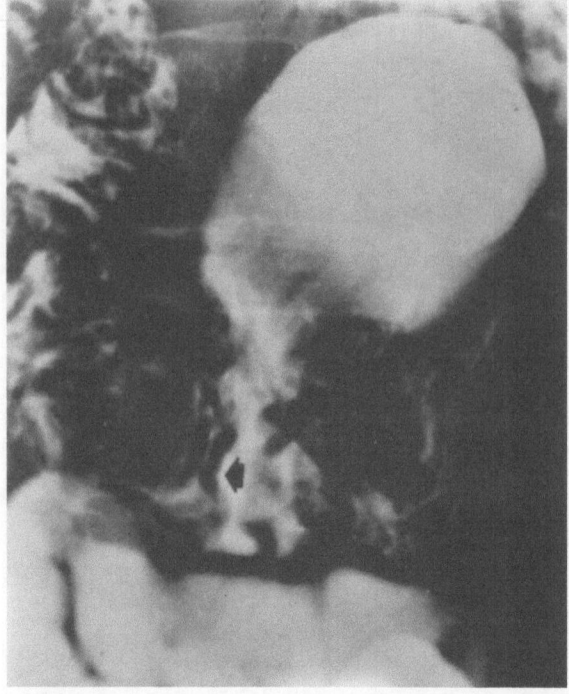

Fig. 8.16
Mucosal pattern at the mouth of a normal diverticulum.
The mucosal folds of the intestine extend into the neck of the
diverticulum (→).

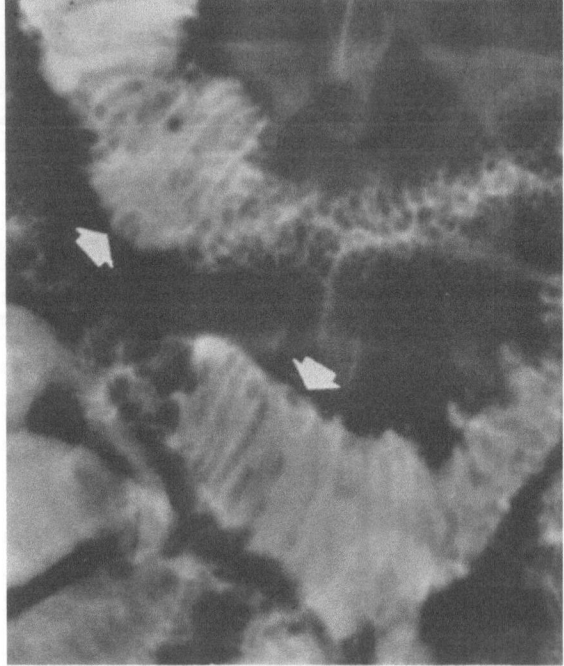

Fig. 8.17
Mucosal folds terminate abruptly at the plateau of a healed
superficial ulceration in Crohn's disease.

never seen a triple plateau between the mucosal folds at the mouth of a diverticulum (fig. 8.16).

In a mucosal surface with ulcerations, the folds of Kerkring can completely disappear locally. When the inflammatory process is arrested by treatment, the pock-marked surface of these flat ulcers can show a fairly smooth outer zone with such a fine granular surface that it is barely or not visible on the x-rays. The mucosal folds which are still intact terminate abruptly – sometimes more or less gradually – at the plateau of the healed ulcer (fig. 8.17). Later the fibrous tissue which is formed during the healing process shrivels, thus reducing the original surface of the ulcer. The still intact mucosal folds then assume a radial course with the ulcer on one side (fig. 8.18).

One long segment of the small intestine containing irregularly broadened mucosal folds and an intestinal wall which is also irregularly thickened are indicative, if there are no signs of destruction, of deposits such as those seen in primary amyloidosis (fig. 8.14).

Local absence of mucosal folding together with an obvious thickening of the intestinal wall, recognized as a bulge in the lumen or an enlargement of the space between adjacent intestinal loops, suggests tumor growth (fig. 8.19). If the sites are multiple, then leukemia or a reticuloendothelial tumor should be considered. Total destruction of the mucosal pattern, pronounced local stretching of the folds, adhesions and irregular spacing between the intestinal loops indicate a malignant tumor only (fig. 8.20).

2. Lymph follicles – nodules – polyps

Under pathological conditions, lymph follicles about 2 mm in diameter, common in the distal ileum of children and sometimes even young adults, are also found in older adults in other parts of the small intestine, in particular in the distal half of the jejunum and the proximal half of the ileum.

In congenital or acquired protein synthesis disorders accompanied by an IgA of IgM deficiency, the mucous membrane in the small intestine can be covered with 1–3 mm hyperplastic nodular lymph follicles arising from the lamina propria (fig. 8.21); sometimes they are also seen in the colon. Although it has appeared that more than half of these cases of so-called dysgammaglobulinemia are accompanied by lambliasis, the latter probably cannot be considered as an etiological factor in this so-called lymphoid nodular hyperplasia.

The small intestine is then often highly irritated so that adequate filling with contrast fluid is extremely difficult. The mucosal folds are fairly thin instead of thickened and lie close together (fig. 8.22).

Very small nodular elevations in the mucosa of the duodenum and proximal jejunum combined with a fairly coarse fold relief and moderate dilatation of the intestinal lumen can occur in Whipple's disease. In such cases the nodular aspect is due to villi which are so swollen that they are visible to the naked eye during endoscopic examination of the mucous membrane (fig. 8.23). On the x-ray these swollen villi must be distinguished from small gas bubbles which can develop when the contrast fluid does not contain enough anti-foaming agent (fig. 8.24).

Multiple, stalked or sessile filling defects in the contrast column, many of them much more than 2 or 3 mm long, can be attributed to the rare forms of familial polyposis but in other cases they may be indicative of a lymphoreticular malignancy. In polyposis they occur more frequently in the stomach and especially in the colon than in the small intestine. Histologically they are found to be adenomas (Gardner's syndrome) or hemartomas (Peutz-Jeghers syndrome) (fig. 8.25).

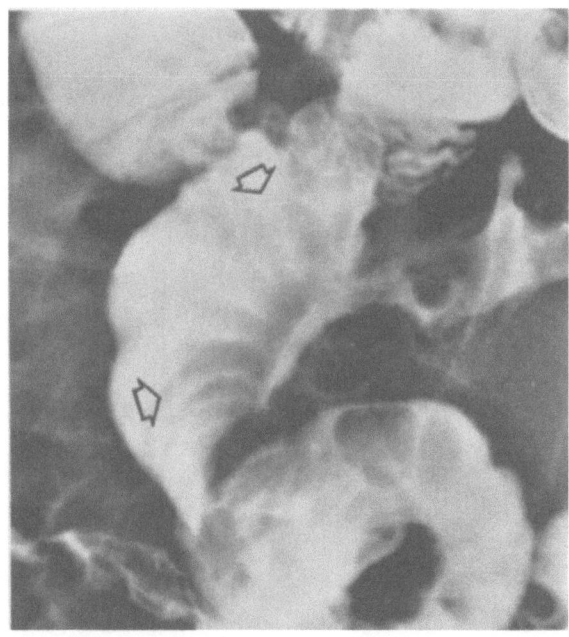

Fig. 8.18
More or less concentric course of the mucosal folds is directed toward the site of the ulceration in the intestinal wall.

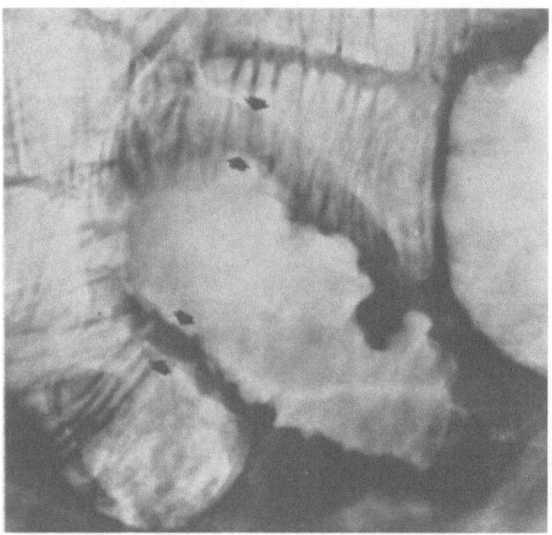

Fig. 8.19
Thickening of the intestinal wall and local absence of mucosal folds due to tumorgrowth.

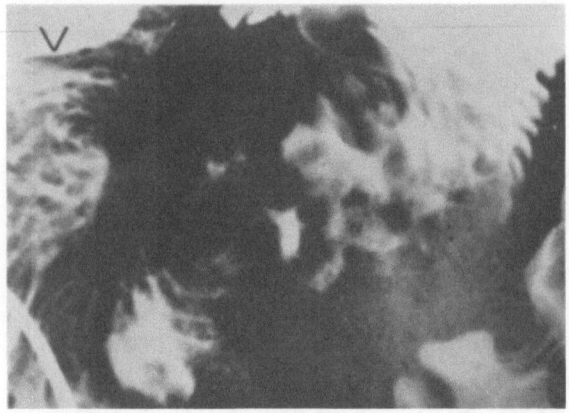

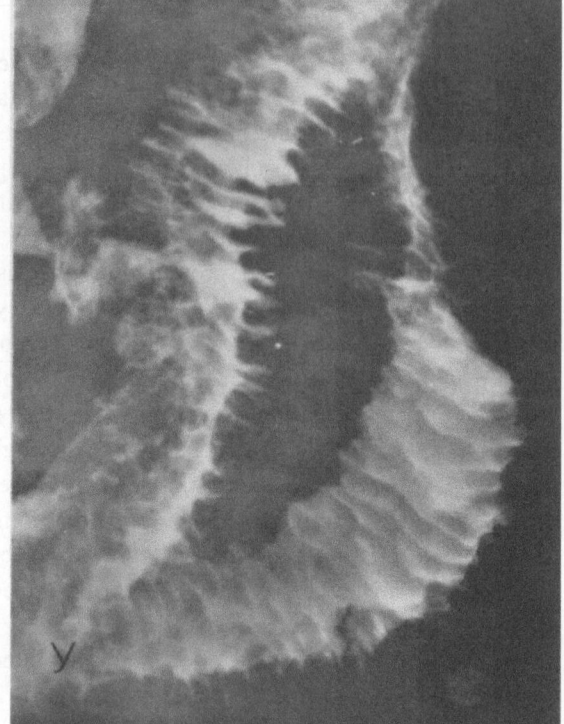

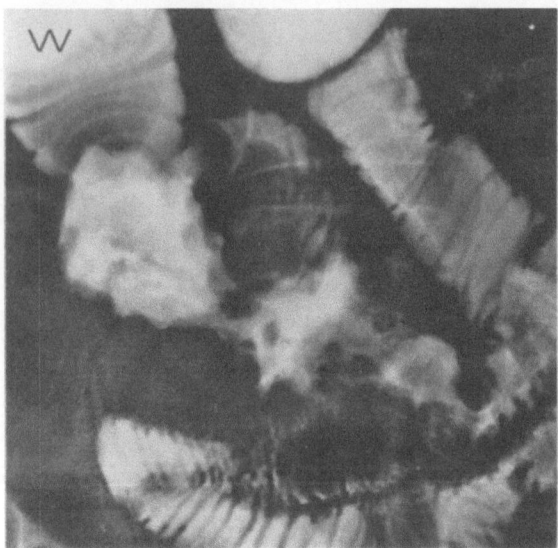

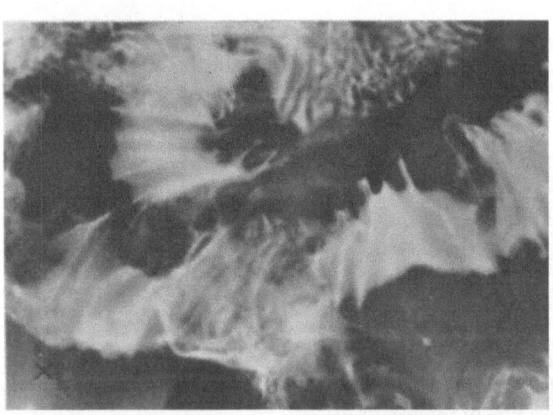

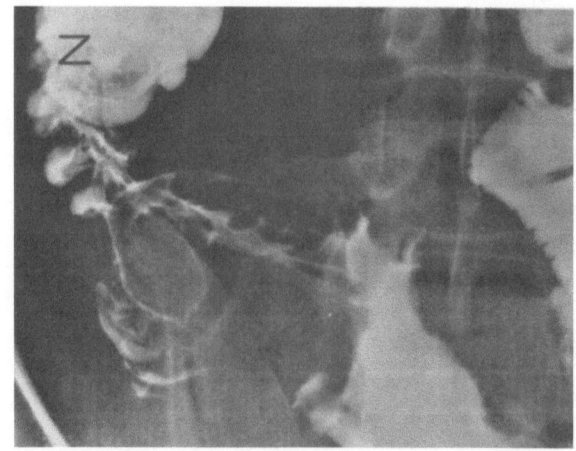

Fig. 8.20
Total destruction or completely irregular course of the mucosal folds in the event of a tumor. v. adenocarcinoma. w. lymphosarcoma x. malignant lymphoma Y. liposarcoma. z. reticulumcellsarcoma.

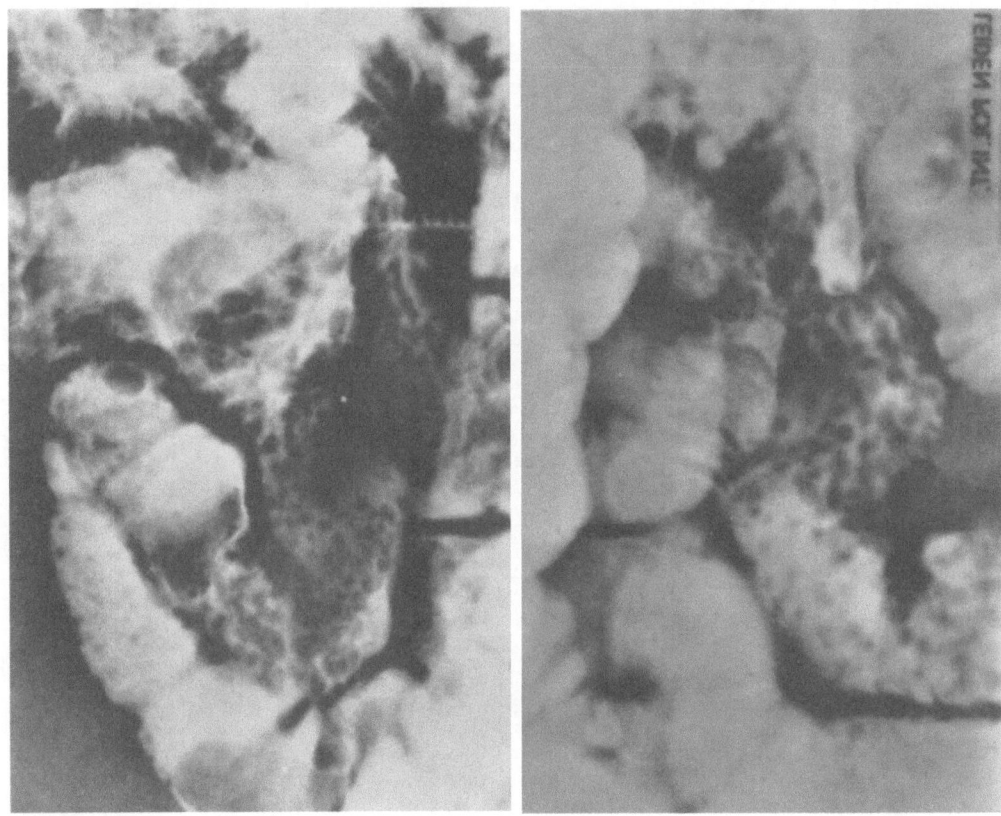

Fig. 8.21
Lymphoid nodular hyperplasia. Multiple filling defects in the contrast fluid, 1–3 mm across.

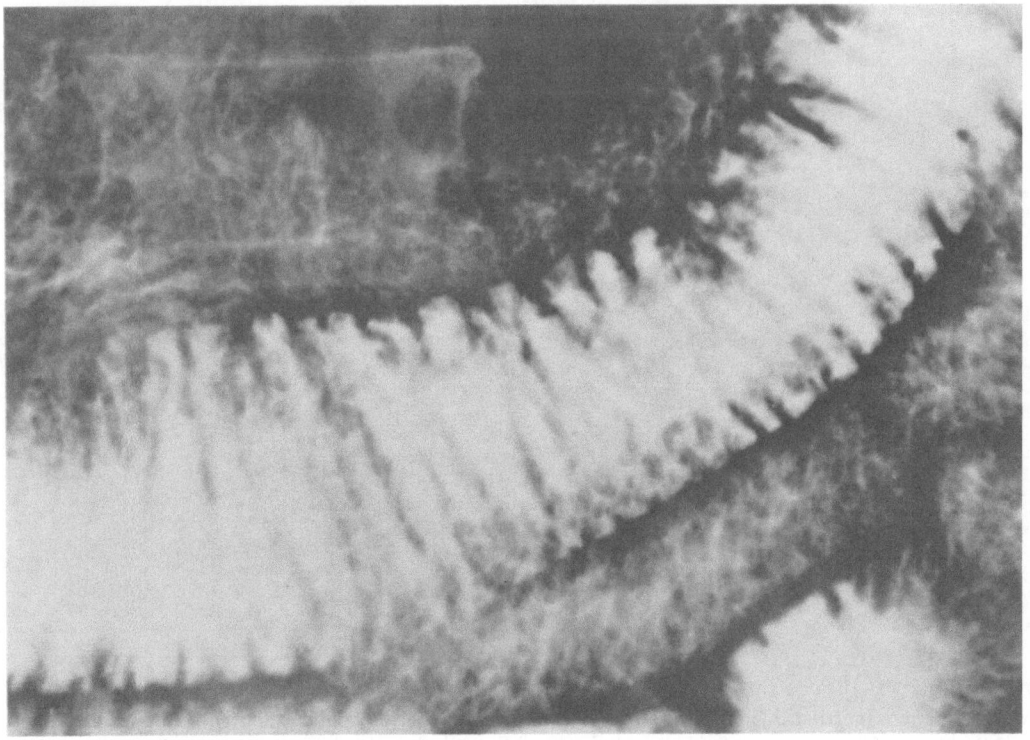

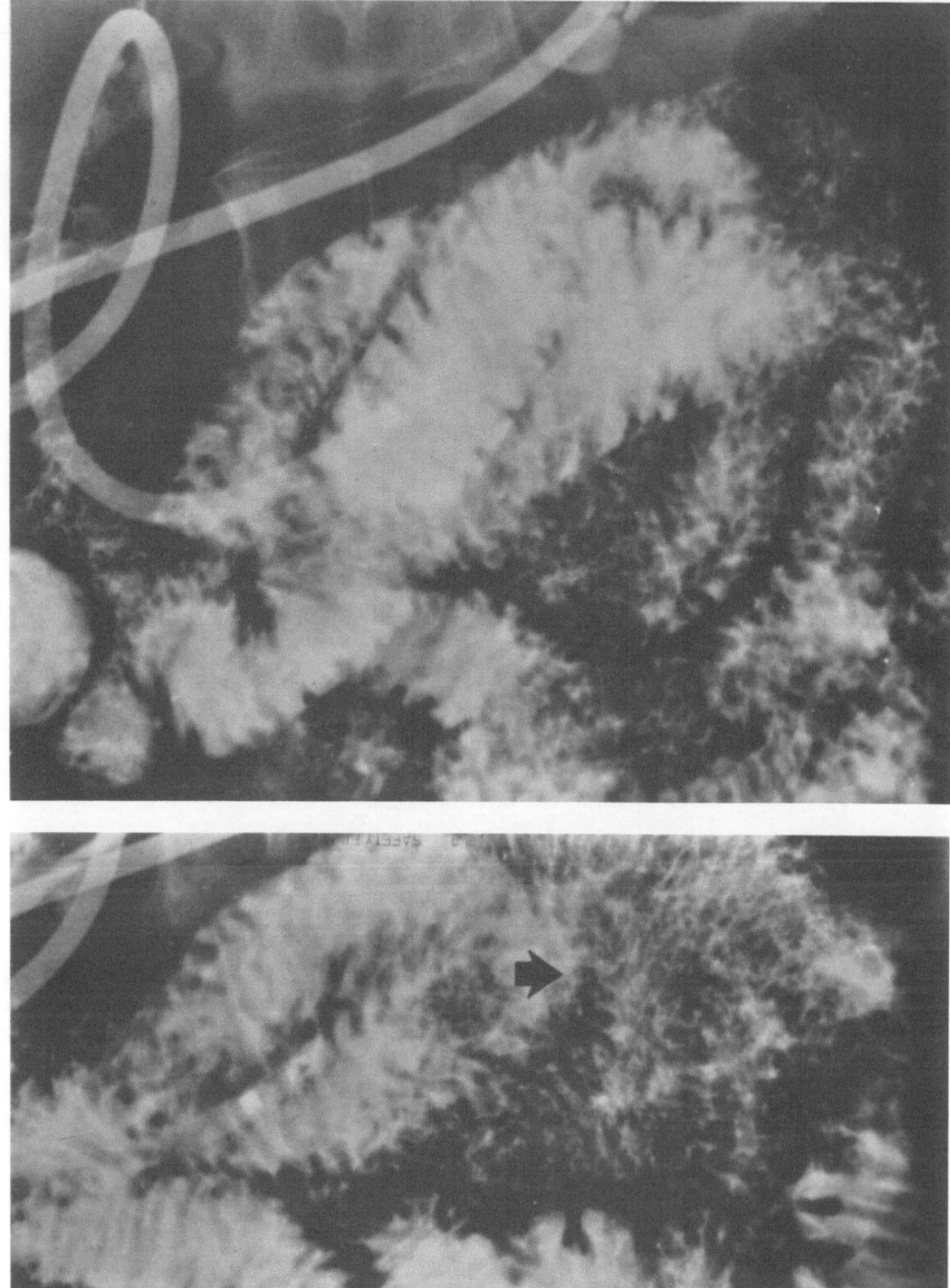

Fig. 8.22
Mucosal pattern in irritated jejunum of a patient infected with Giardia lamblia (upper). Rapid disintegration after 1 minute (right) although 900 ml contrast fluid was administered through the tube (lower).

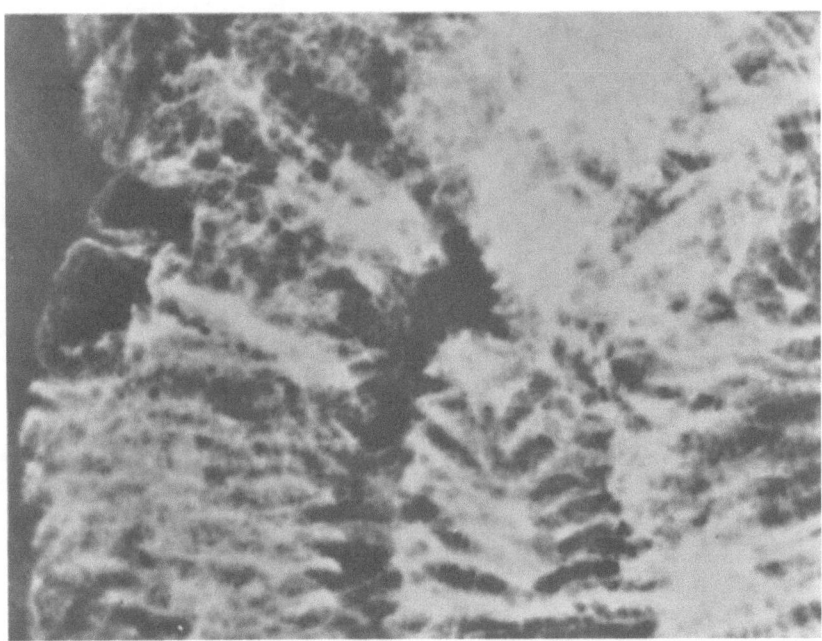

Fig. 8.23
Foamy aspect in the jejunum due to abnormal swelling of the villi in a patient with Whipple's disease.

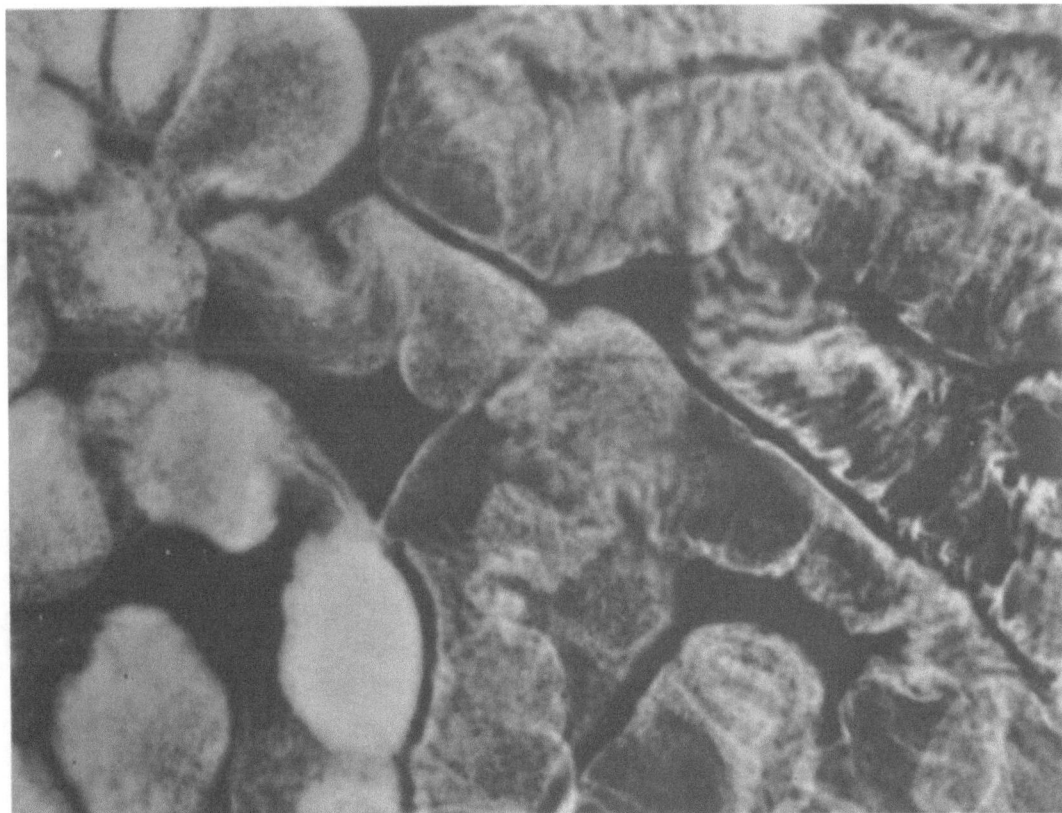

Fig. 8.24
Gas bubbles in the contrast fluid, which are the same size as the villi in fig. 8.23, are due to foaming of the barium suspension. The margins of the contrast column are not interrupted by the bubbles as in 8.23.

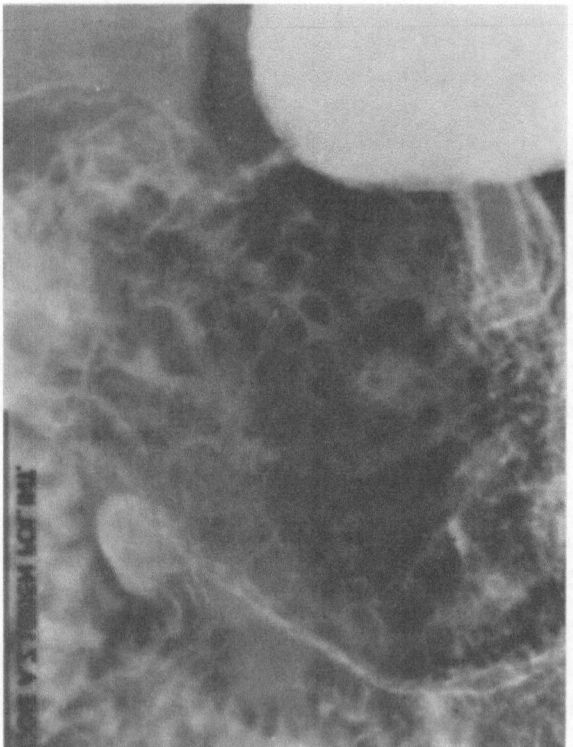

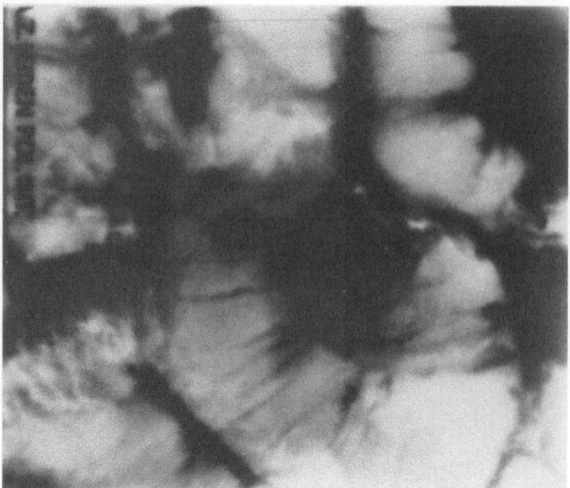

Fig. 8.25
Polypoid or nodular filling defects in the contrast fluid in a patient with familial polyposis. If the filling defects in the small intestine are numerous and much smaller than the one seen here, differentiation from a lymphoid nodular hyperplasia is not really possible on strictly radiological grounds.

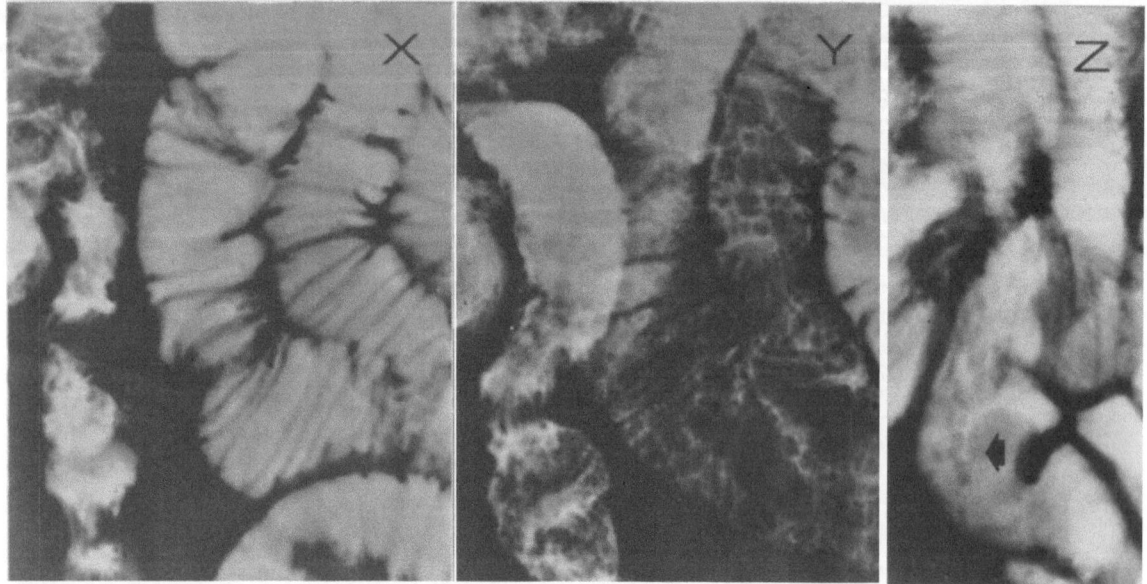

Fig. 8.26
Filling defects 2–3 mm across in the contrast fluid due to gas bubbles (the same loops in x and y). Highly similar to lymph nodules (z).

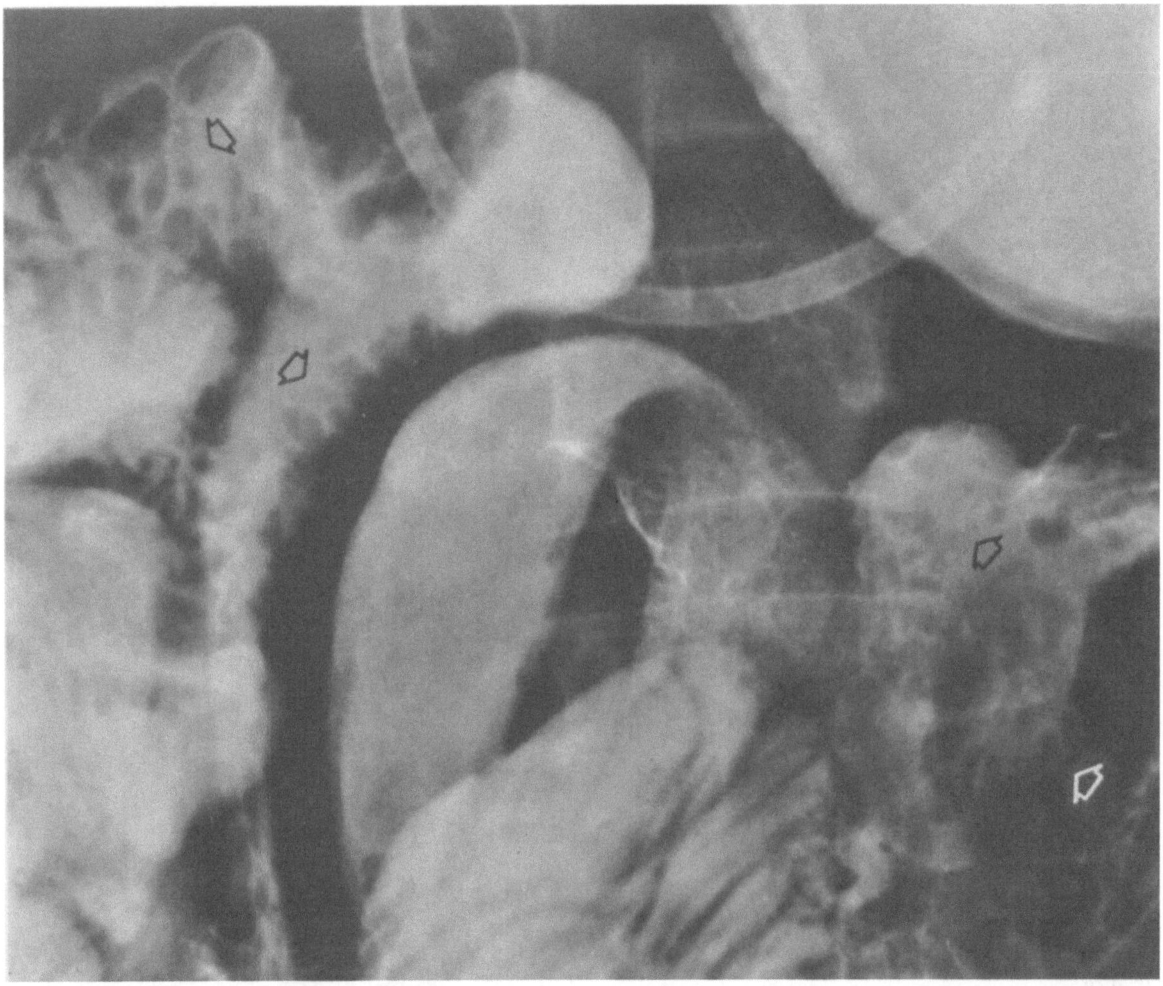

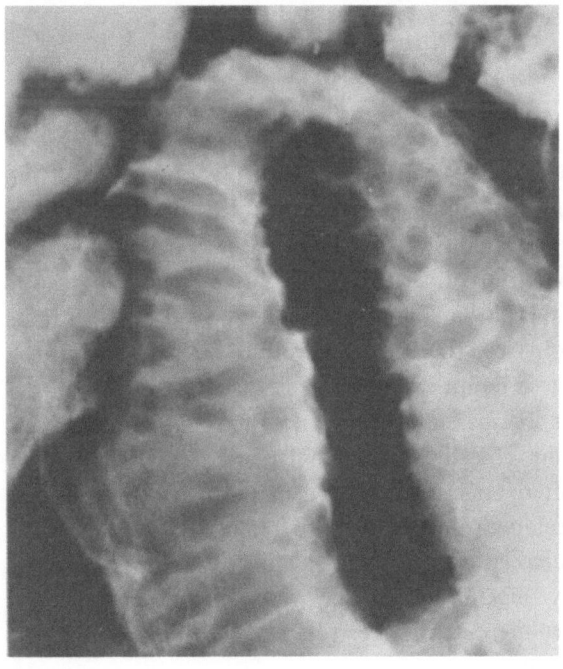

It is of course particularly important that the small nodules or polyps described here are not mistaken for multiple gas bubbles of the same size in the contrast fluid. Although not always valid (→), it may help to remember that gas bubbles lie very close together and do not interrupt the contour of the intestinal mucosa (fig. 8.26). Follicles or polyps are usually farther apart and when they lie along the margin of the contrast column, it can sometimes be seen that they interrupt the contour.

Fig. 8.27
Round, oval or elongated clarifications in the contrast fluid caused by residual mucosal folds in an otherwise atrophied mucosal surface in Crohn's disease.

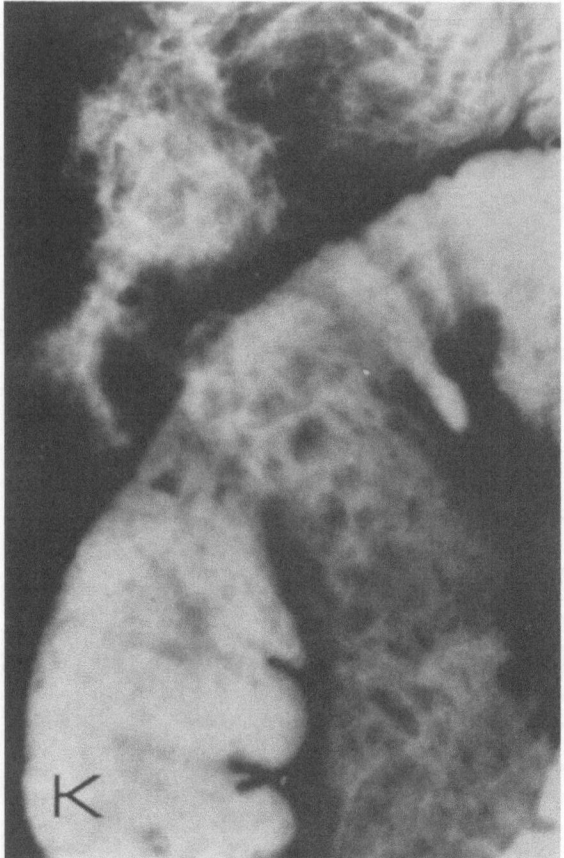

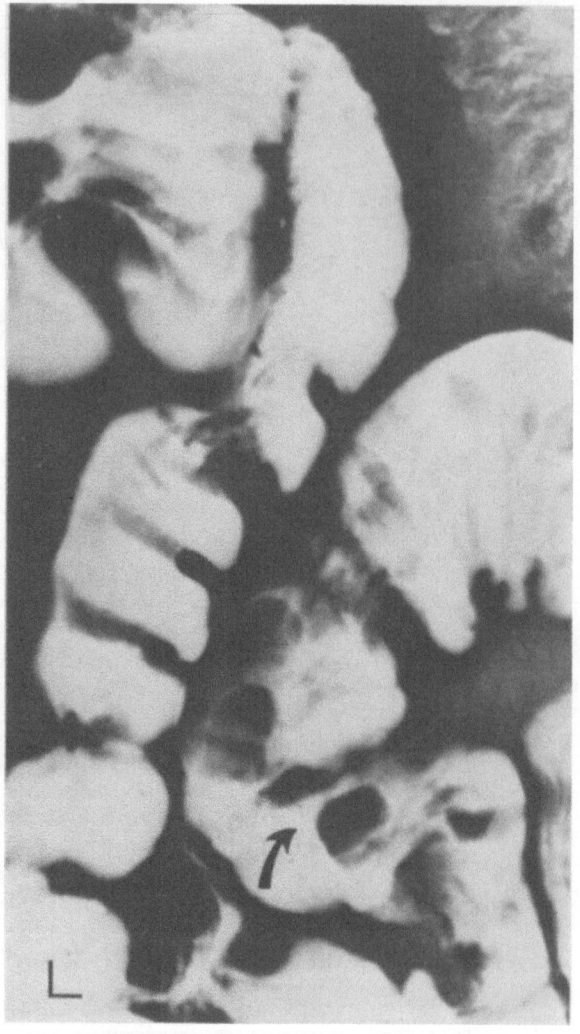

Fig. 8.28

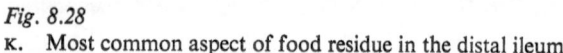

K. Most common aspect of food residue in the distal ileum.

L. Filling defects resembling fruit pits.

Finally, very small nodules along the margins of a well-filled loop should not be confused with the serrated regular puckers in the mucosa due to contractions of the muscularis (see page 14). Somewhat larger, usually slightly ovoid, nodular elevations in an ulcerative mucosal surface without folds can be seen in Crohn's disease. Sometimes these lumps are widespread and have a broad base at the intestinal wall. Like the larger cobblestones and so-called pseudopolyps in the colon, they often consist of the edematous swollen mucosal residue from an otherwise totally destroyed mucosal surface (fig. 8.27). Since a mucosal surface destroyed by ulceration can be very smooth during the healing process, correct classification can be difficult.

3. Foreign bodies and filling defects in the contrast fluid

The s.g. of the foreign body is usually lower than that of the barium suspension; it is therefore visible as a filling defect in the contrast fluid. The most frequently encountered foreign body is without a doubt undigested food residue. Food residue is seen almost exclusively in the distal half of the ileum since transit is most likely to be disturbed in this section because the cecum is so often full. Food residue can also be found when the patient has eaten shortly before the radiological examination, gastric emptying is mechanically impeded or there is disturbed motility (see page 304). This type of foreign body usually causes a conglomeration of relatively small bright spots in the barium suspension (fig. 8.28KL), but sometimes, for example,

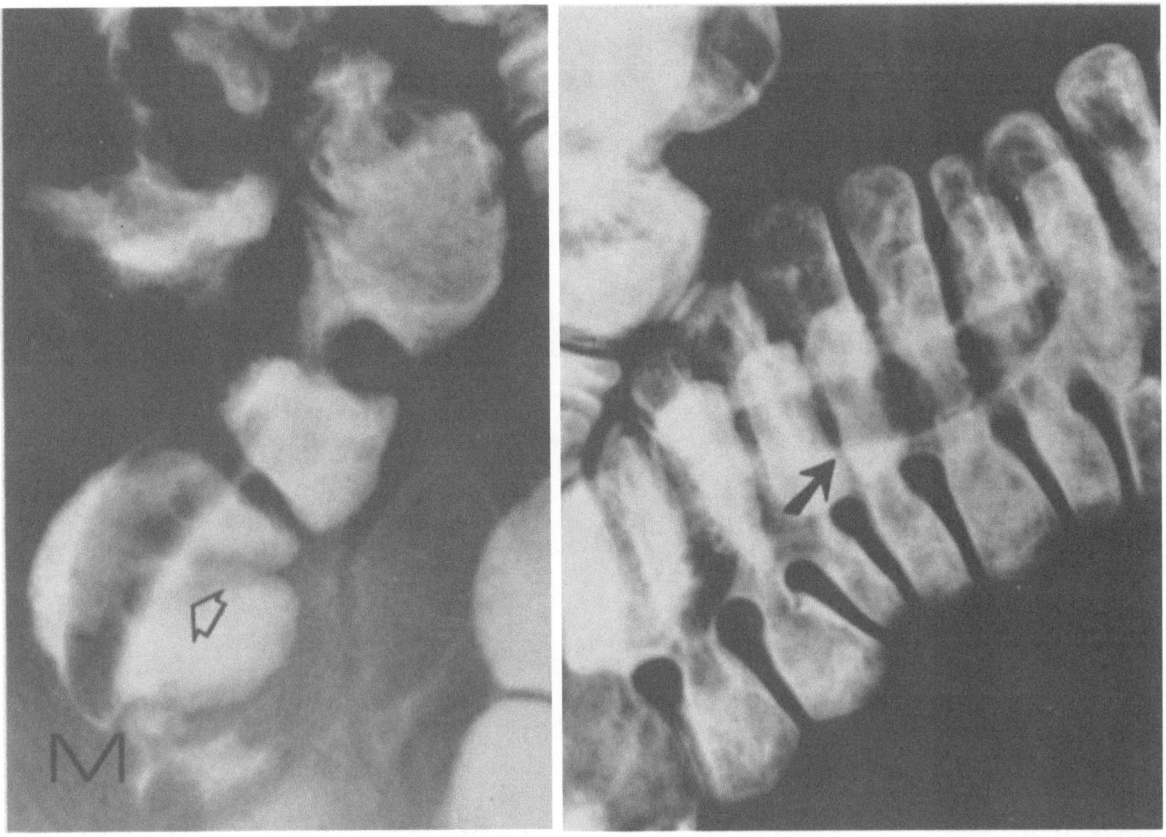

Fig. 8.28 M.   Undigested bean.

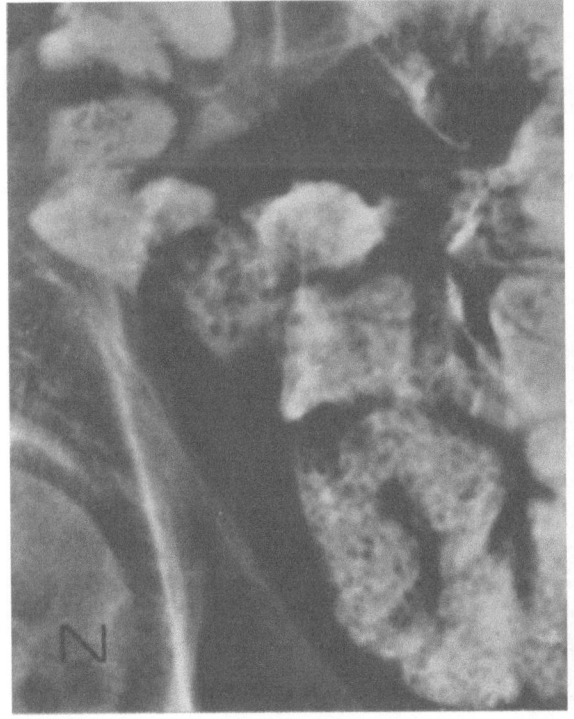

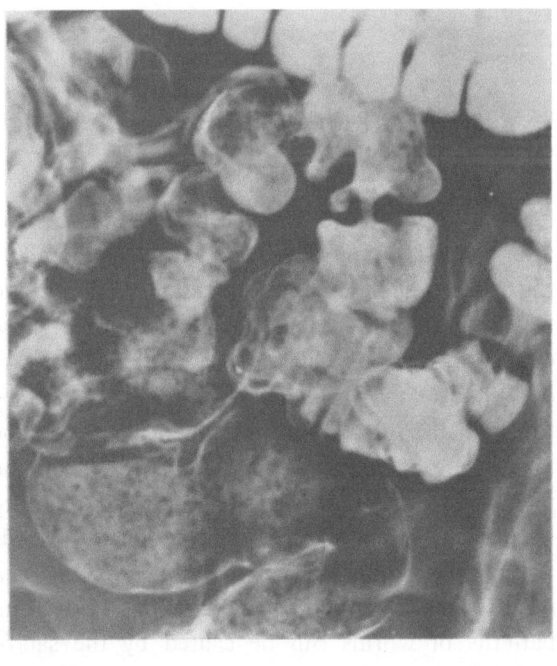

Fig. 8.28 N.   Round filling defects due to undigested rice.

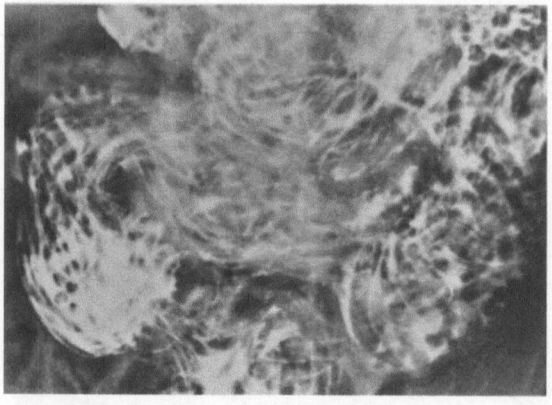

1

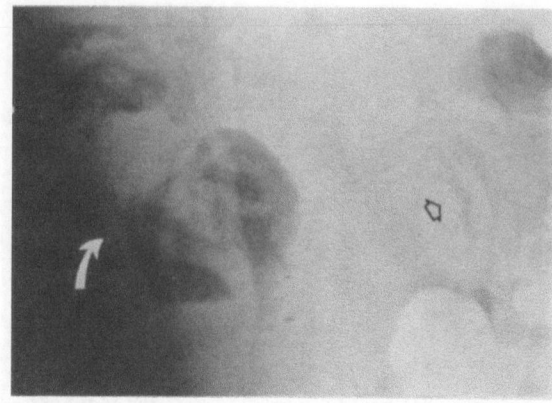

2

3

Fig. 8.29 (1–5)
Several examples of filling defects in the contrast fluid
caused by Ascaris or tape worms. The worms are sometimes
seen as a tangled mass; in other cases they are even visible on
a survey exposure of the abdomen.

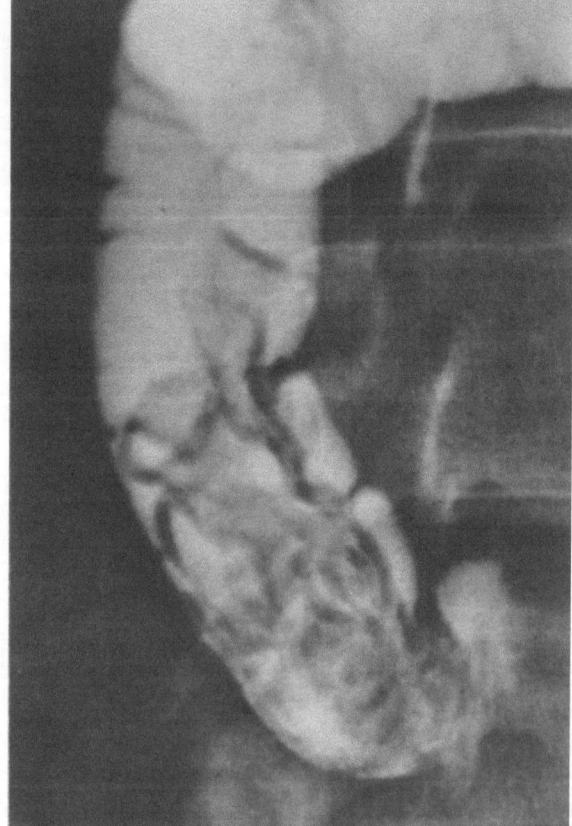

an undigested bean pod can also produce a sharply
defined filling defect and then it will be necessary
to examine the feces carefully for several days (fig.
8.28M). The pattern caused by the food residue
after rice has been eaten is particularly misleading
(fig. 8.28N). These filling defects are small and
round and have to be differentiated from those
caused by lymph follicles or air bubbles. In rare
cases one or more elongated filling defects will be
found in the intestinal loops which are caused by
tapeworms or round worms (fig. 8.29). Then the
intestine often also exhibits enhanced motility
locally – sometimes there is even a tendency towards
flocculation of the contrast medium, probably as a
result of a likewise enhanced secretion. Misleading
patterns of worms can be caused by the sacro-
iliac joint, threads of mucus and superposition of
mucosal folds in other intestinal loops (fig. 8.30).

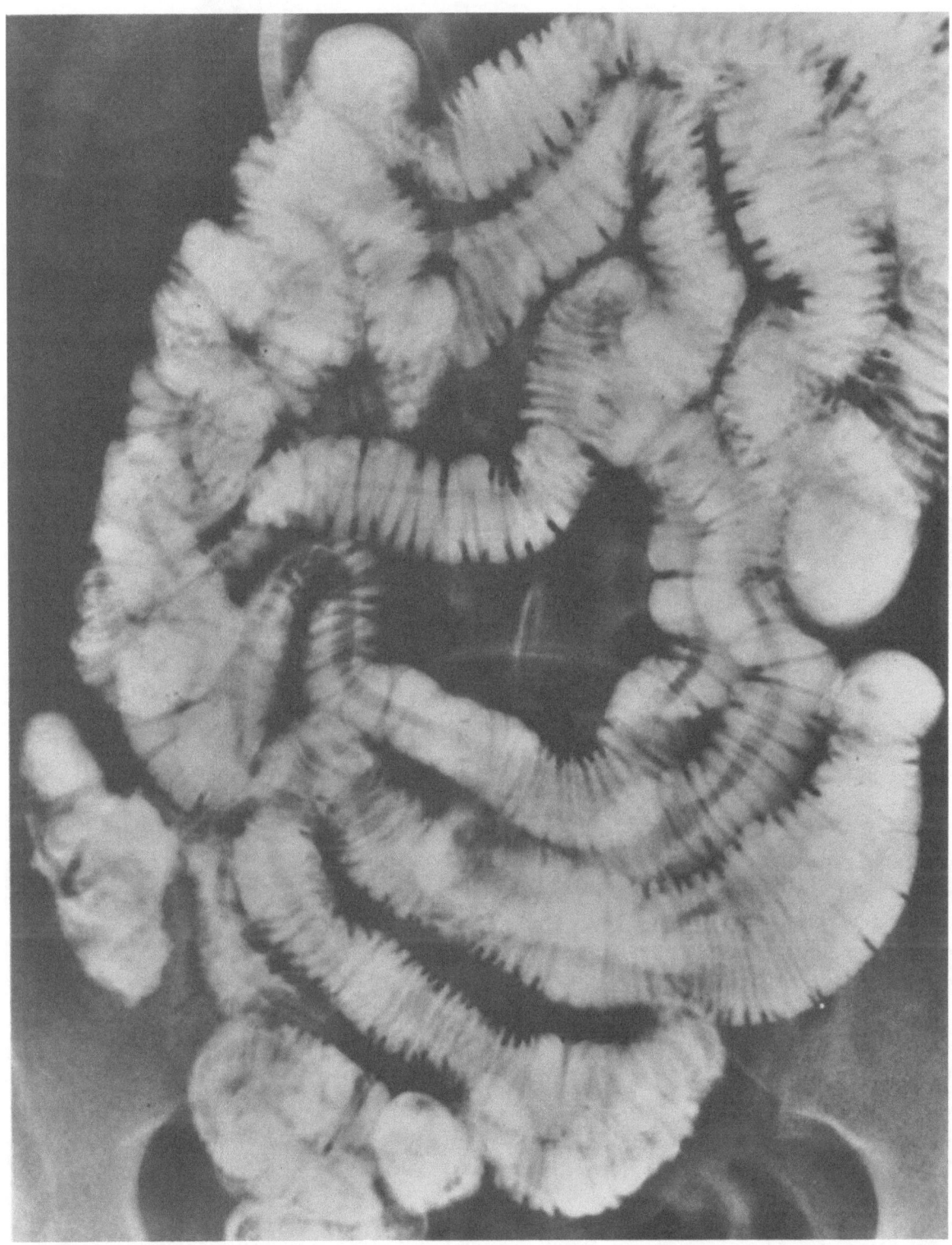

4

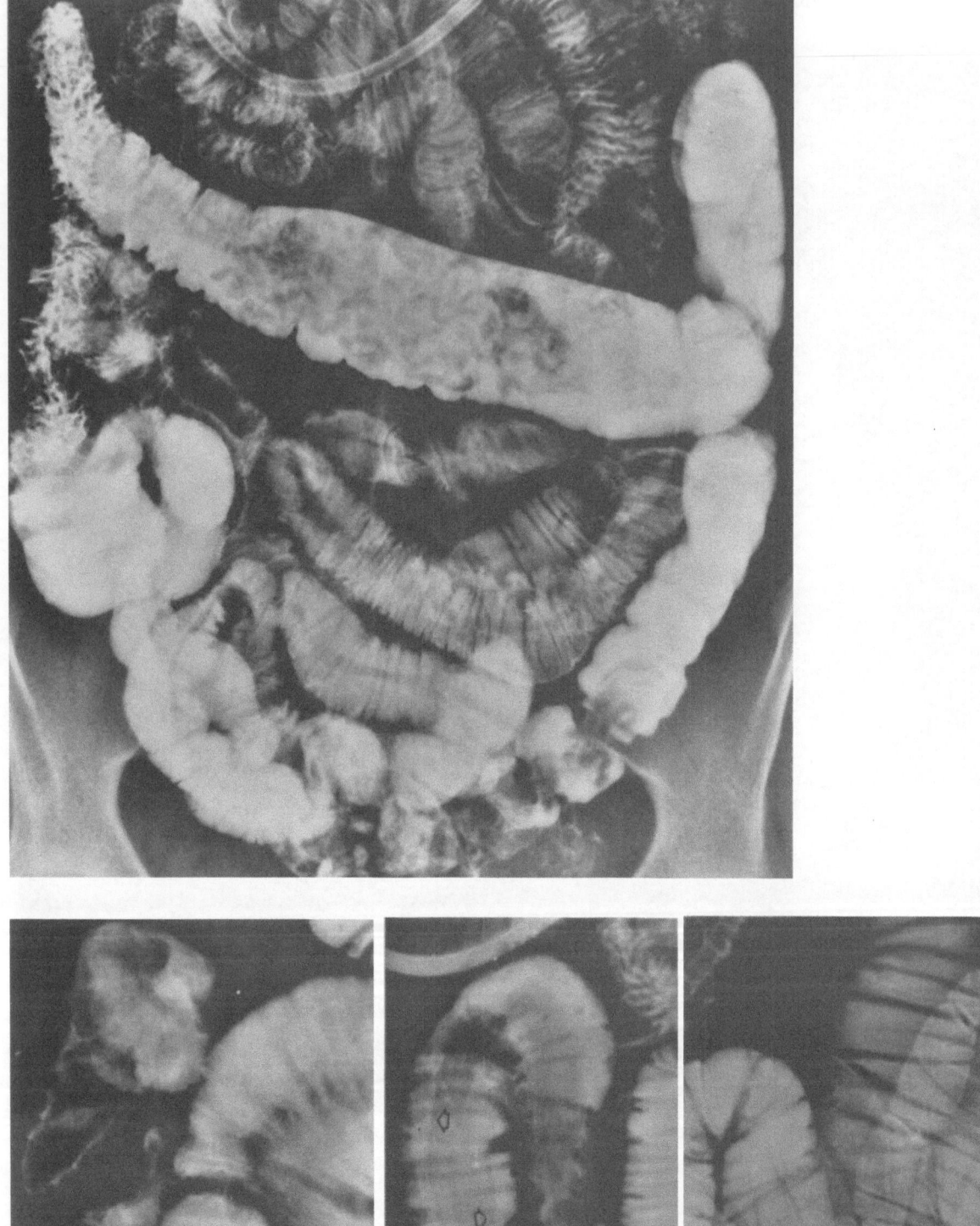

5

Fig. 8.30
Misleading pattern of worms caused by sacro-iliac joint, threads of mucus and mucosal folds in other intestinal loops.

4. Ulcerations

It is very difficult to recognize superficial ulcerations in the small intestine – even more so than in all other parts of the digestive tract. Their presence can in fact only be demonstrated indirectly since the mucosal relief is more or less destroyed and the surface irregularly defined (fig. 8.31). Locally the intestinal wall is somewhat thicker and stiff and is not affected by peristalsis. In this initial stage ulcer craters can seldom or never be demonstrated, unless they are obviously very deep (→). Differentiation between extensive and rather superficial inflammatory processes and a lymphoreticular malignancy is of course difficult and often is only possible several months later on the basis of a follow-up examination. In the case of an inflammatory process, the abnormalities have as a rule obviously changed, and usually improved; in a lymphoreticular malignancy, they have increased or are practically unchanged.

If there are small mucosal infiltrates then differentiation is based predominantly on the consideration that the relationship between the depth and the surface distribution is different for an infiltrate and a malignancy. An inflammatory process will spread out over the surface whereas the difference between growth in depth and growth in width will be much less pronounced in a tumor. Clinically, too, differentiation may be possible: a tumor can exist for some time without symptoms so that a radiological examination is in fact never carried out in such an early stage of development. On the other hand in spite of the fact that there are only minor radiological abnormalities, inflammatory processes can be preceded by months of vague complaints.

Finally it is statistically much more likely that the abnormalities are due to an inflammatory process rather than a tumor; this factor can also play a role in establishing the probable diagnosis. As soon as the ulcers become larger or acquire a more or less mushroom-like shape, radiological recognition is not difficult (fig. 8.32). It must be noted that it is easier to discover these ulcers when they are located along the margin of the contrast column; on the other hand, however, they can sometimes be overexposed so that they are barely visible. In Crohn's disease, if the ulcers are surrounded by a zone of cobblestone-like mucosal swelling and are viewed en face, they may appear identical to metastases of melanoma or other tumors with necrosis in the center (fig. 8.33). Although the differential diagnosis will seldom be a problem in this respect, these small granulomas with ulcer craters can in no way be considered specific for Crohn's disease since they can also be encountered in other inflammatory processes; we have for instance observed them in yersinia EC infections. We have occasionally been confronted with a misleading pattern somewhat similar to that of an aphthous ulcer (fig. 8.34). Comparison of the same intestinal loop during other stages of contraction soon provided the answer. In addition to very local penetrating ulcer craters in granulomatous inflammatory processes, deep elongated ulcers can also develop between the folds of edematous swollen mucosa when the circulation of blood and lymph is disturbed. Moreover, these fissure-shaped ulcers can also not be considered specific, as in the case of the above-mentioned aphthous ulcers, although in practice on the basis of statistical evidence it will be seen that they usually indicate Crohn's disease.

Split-like ulcers between the folds of the edematous swollen mucosa can also penetrate deep into all layers of the wall of the small intestine; they extend in a longitudinal as well as a transverse direction and cause the characteristic irregular stripe (fig. 8.35R) or cushion-like cobblestone pattern (fig. 8.35S) which is seen in Crohn's disease. Because of the greater number of mucosal folds in the jejunum, the cobblestones in the proximal small intestine (fig. 8.35T) are much more pronounced than in the ileum where the folds are relatively scarce. It is often difficult to obtain a sharp pattern at the site of an ulcerative surface since the intestinal wall is coated with purulent mucus which is not easily flushed off (fig. 8.31).

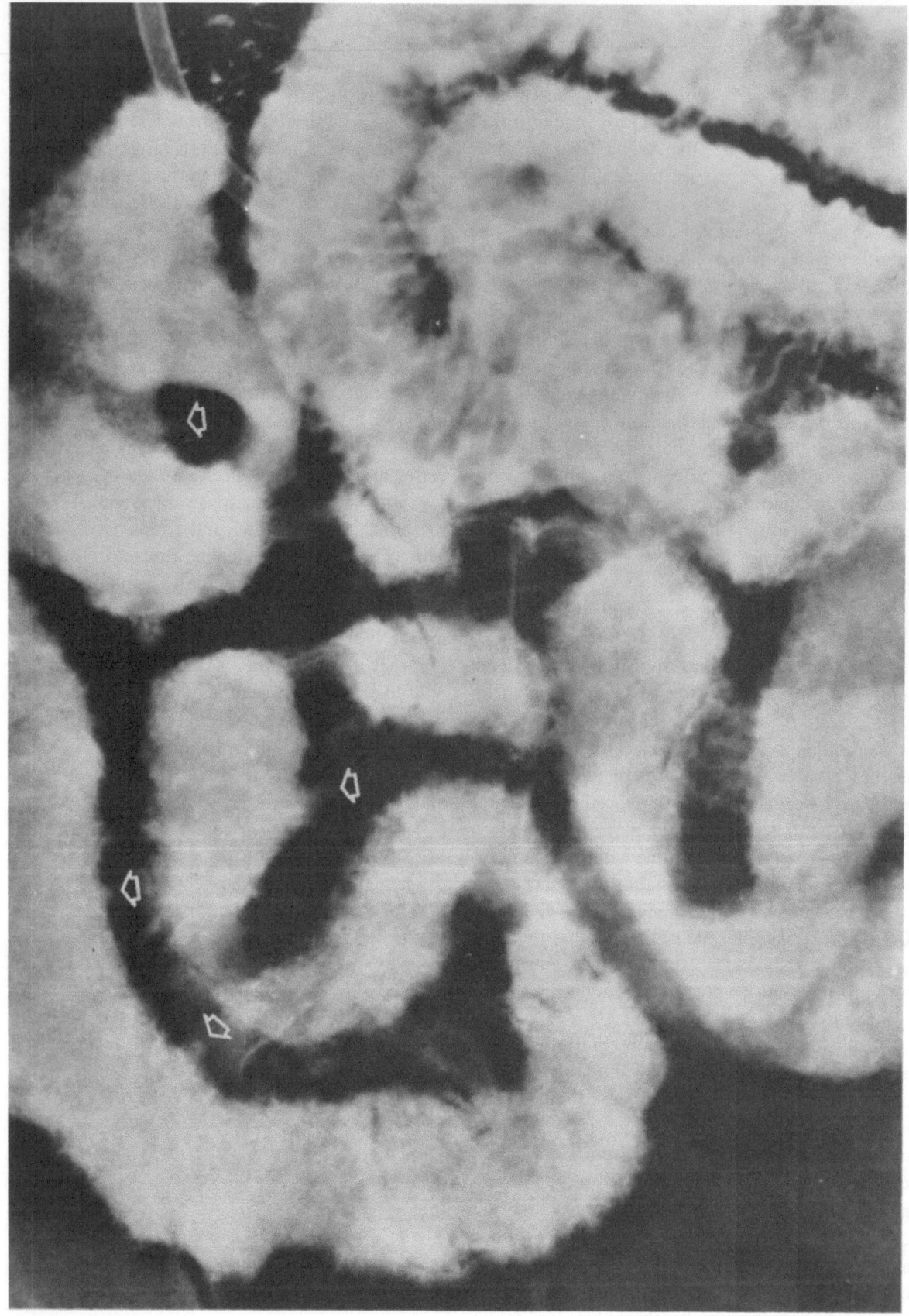

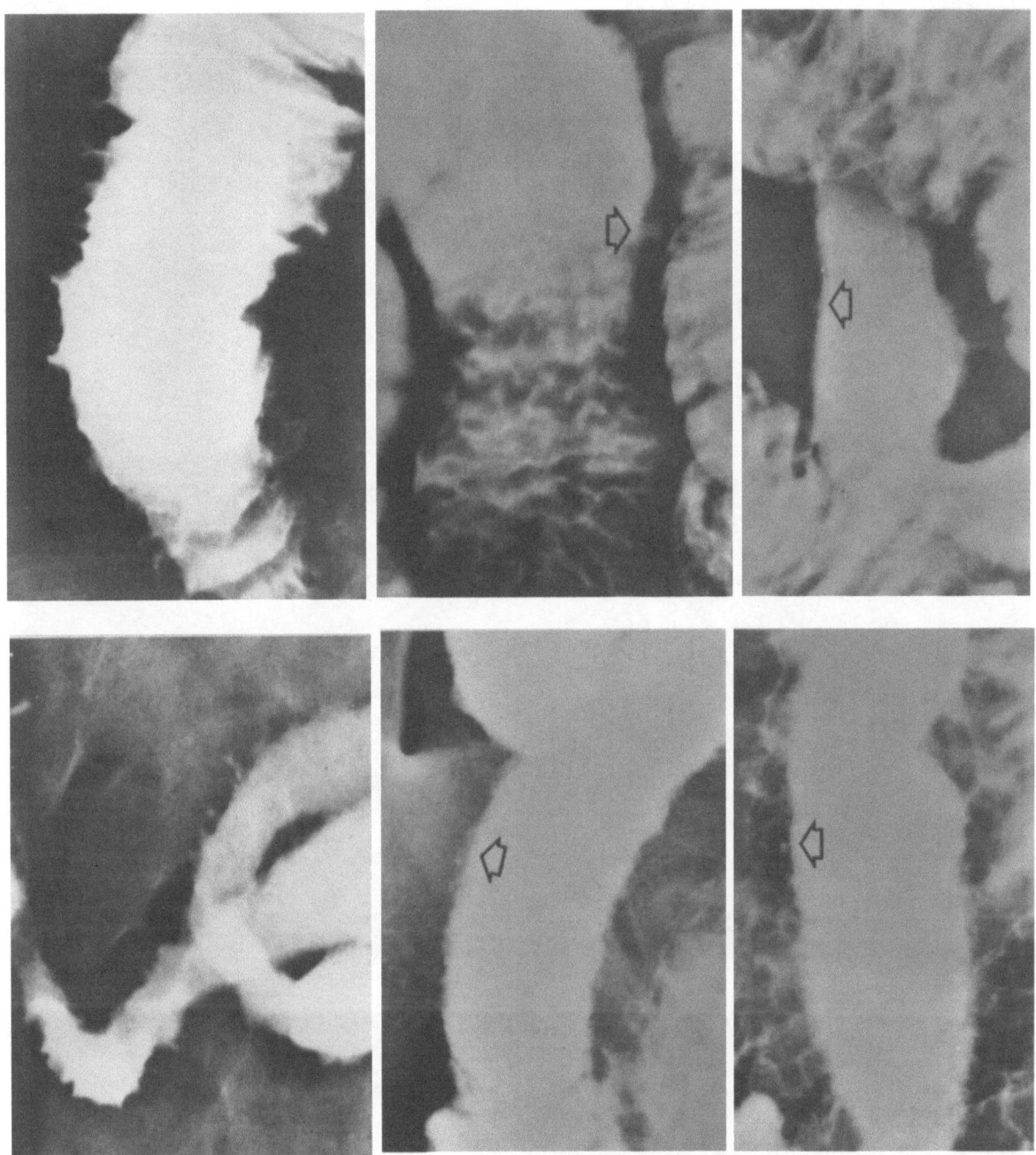

Fig. 8.32
Ulcers in Crohn's disease, some of them mushroom-shaped (→).

←

Fig. 8.31
Locally stiff and thickened wall of the small intestine due to an inflammatory process. A very long section of the contrast column has ragged margins. Deep ulcerations are observed most easily along the margin of the intestine (→). If the film density is too high, they can no longer be seen because of overexposure. Vaguely defined intestinal wall due to purulent secretion on an ulcerative mucosal surface.

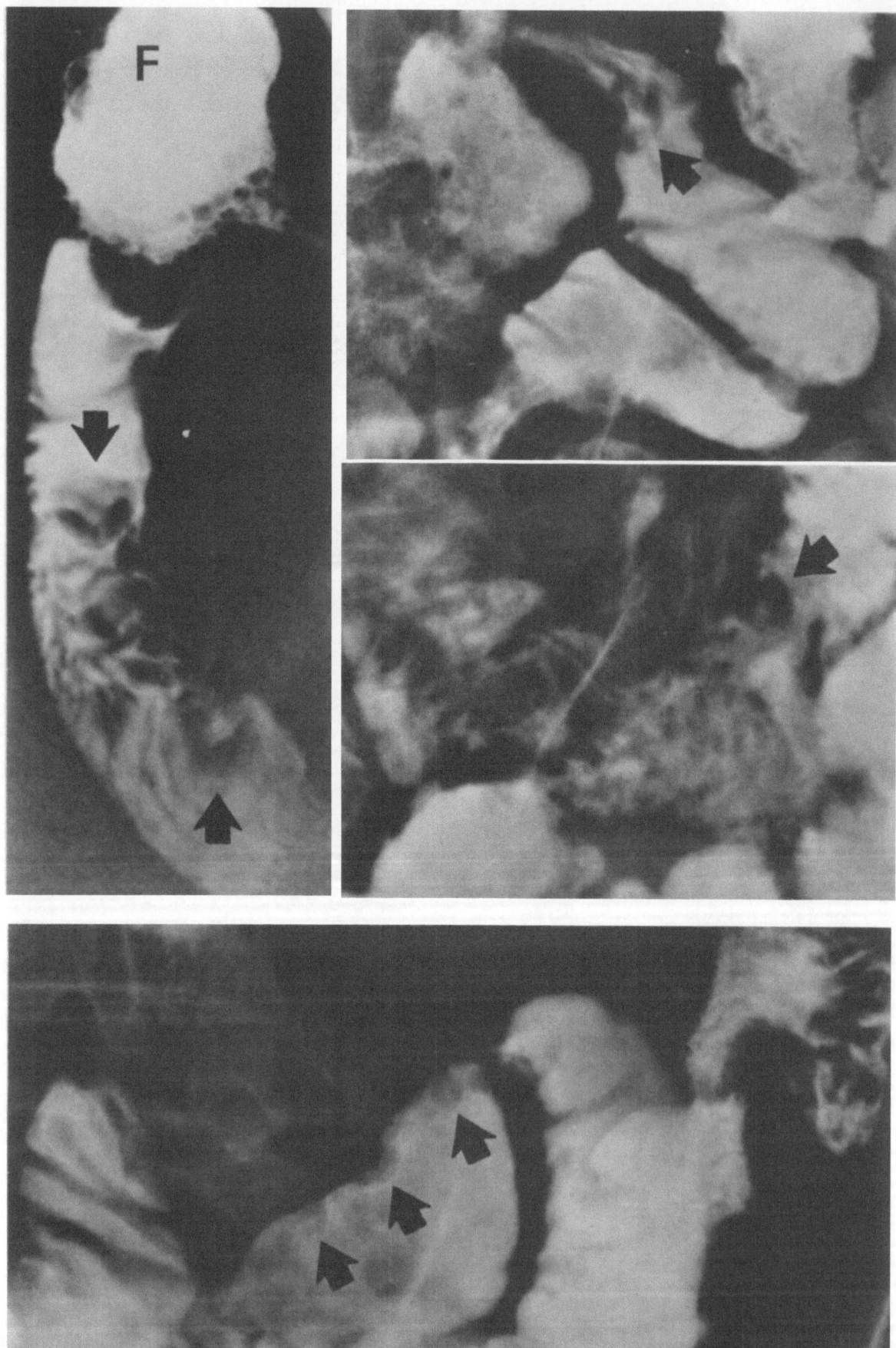

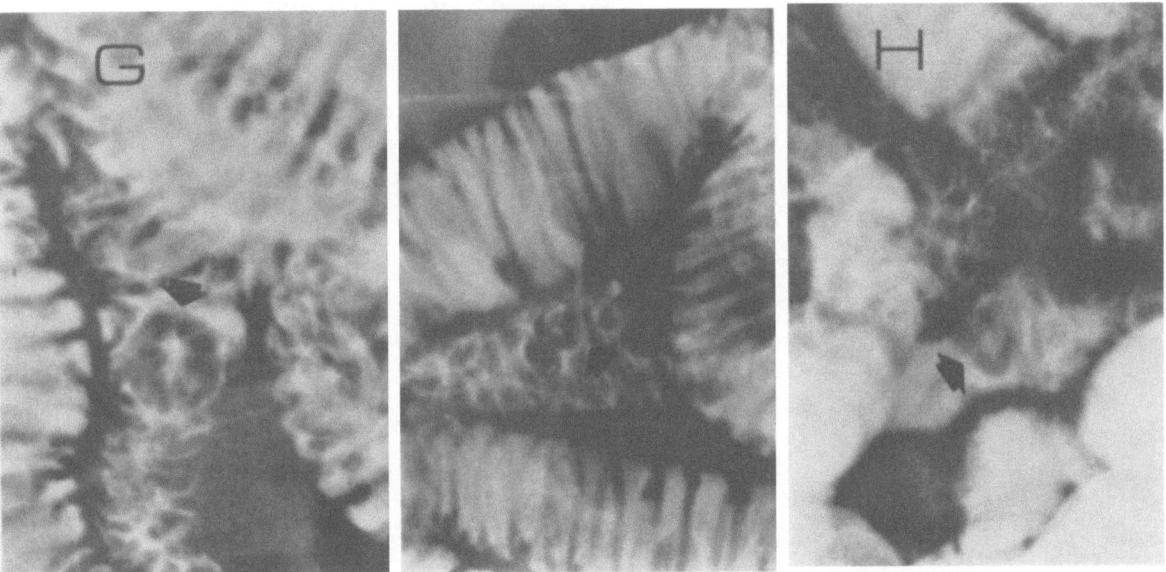

Fig. 8.33
Crater-shaped ulcers in the center of 4–8 mm inflammatory granulomas in Crohn's disease (F). Similar granulomas are seen in other inflammatory processes. The x-ray closely resembles those of metastasis of melanoma (G) or reticulumcellsarcoma (H) with central necrosis.

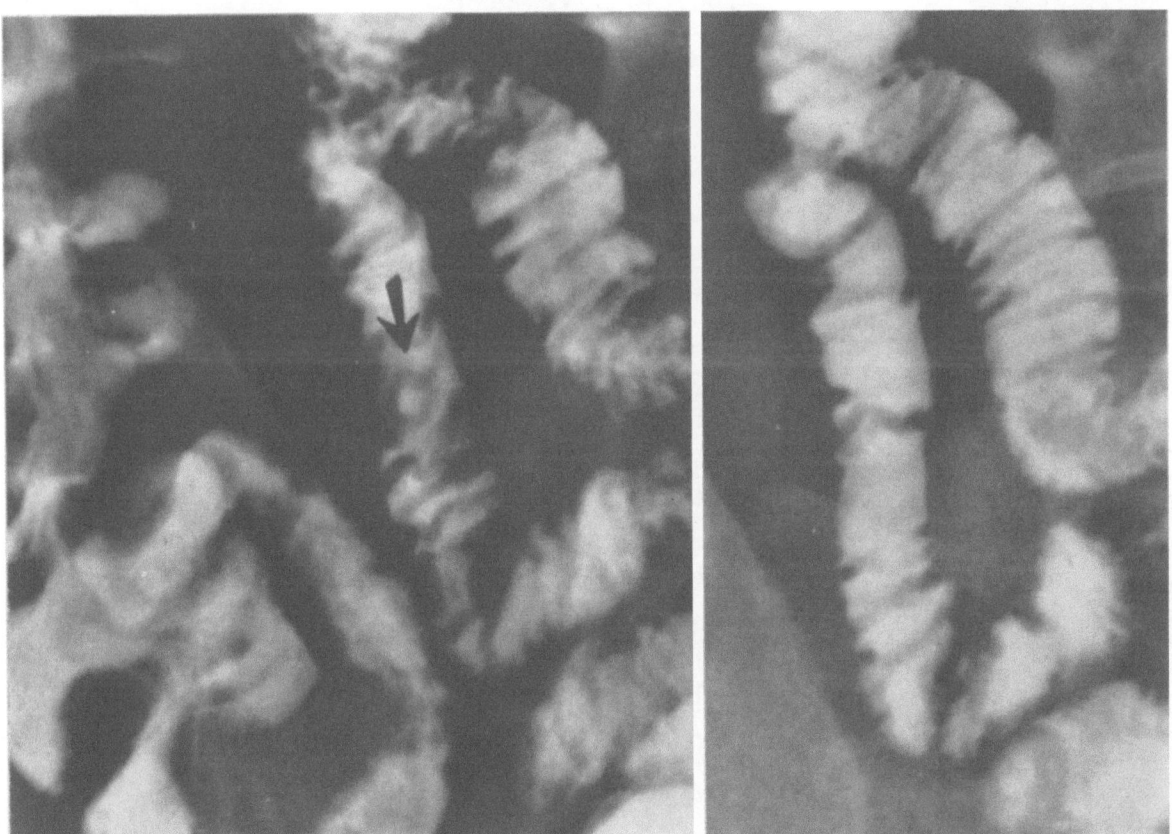

Fig. 8.34
Misleading pattern of an aphthous ulcer (→).

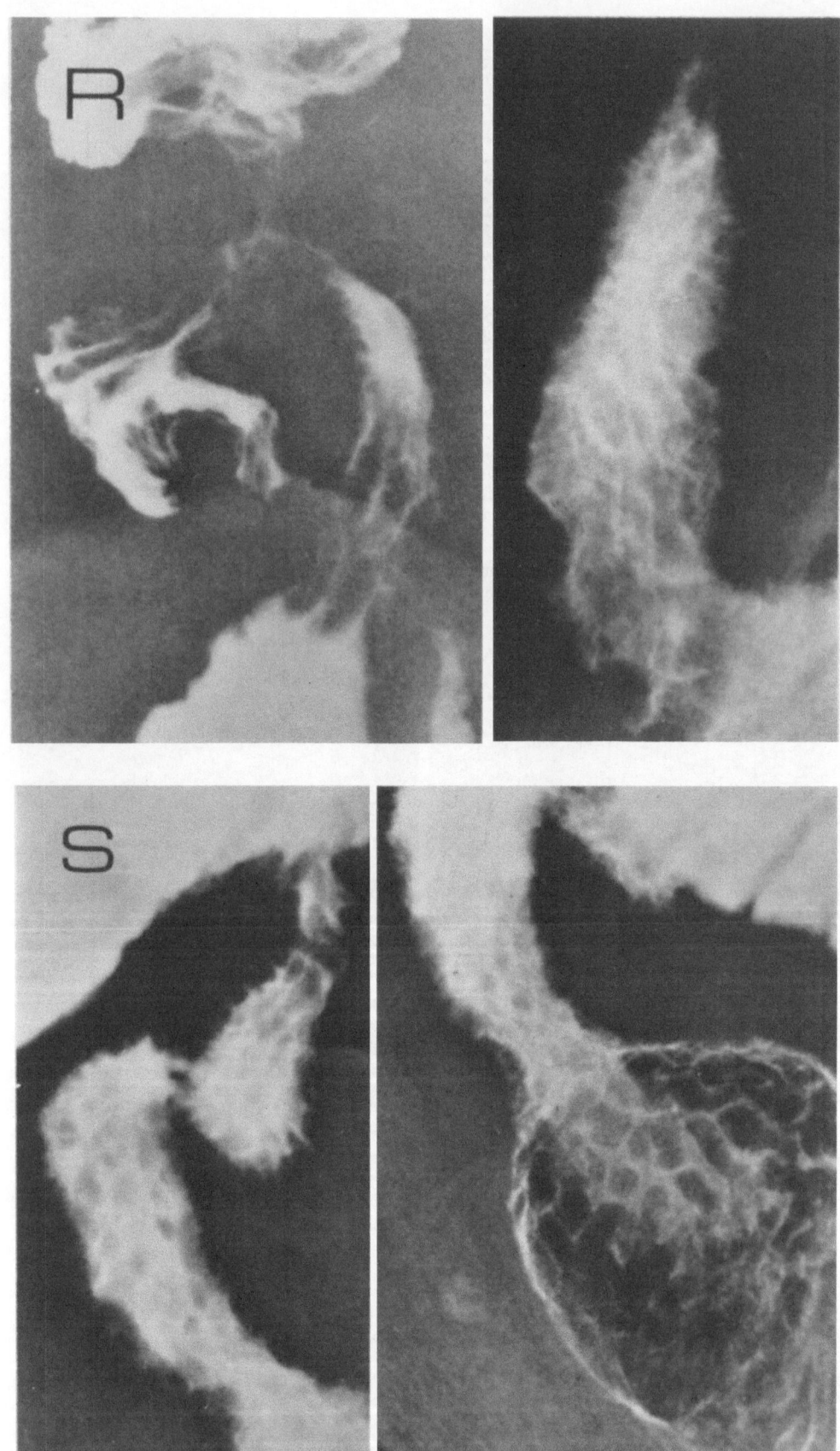

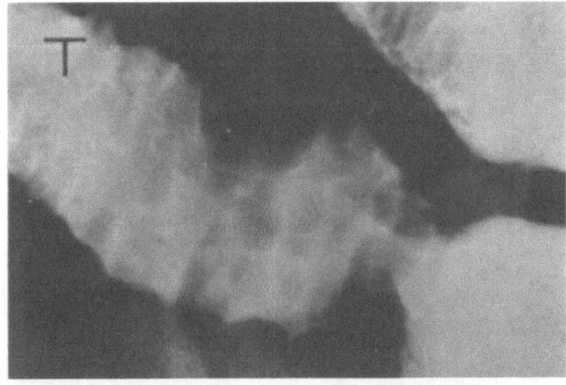

fig. 8.37: Meckel's diverticulum with a large ulcer, extended infiltration, adhesions, growths and fistula formation between the adjacent intestinal loops.

· In other cases solitary ulcers, either specific (see fig. 9.9, page 178), or aspecific (fig. 8.36), may cause only irregular mucosal relief in a segment one to several centimeters long without any indication of a crater, so that differentiation from local tumor growth is practically impossible.

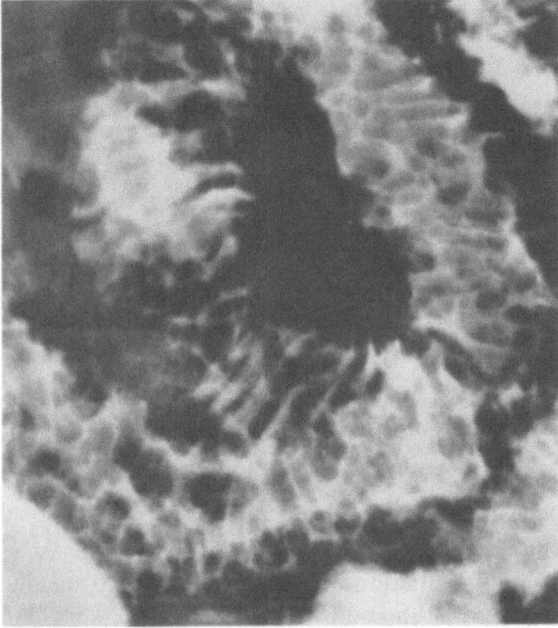

Fig. 8.35
Irregular stripe (R) or cobblestone-like (s, T) patterns in Crohn's disease.

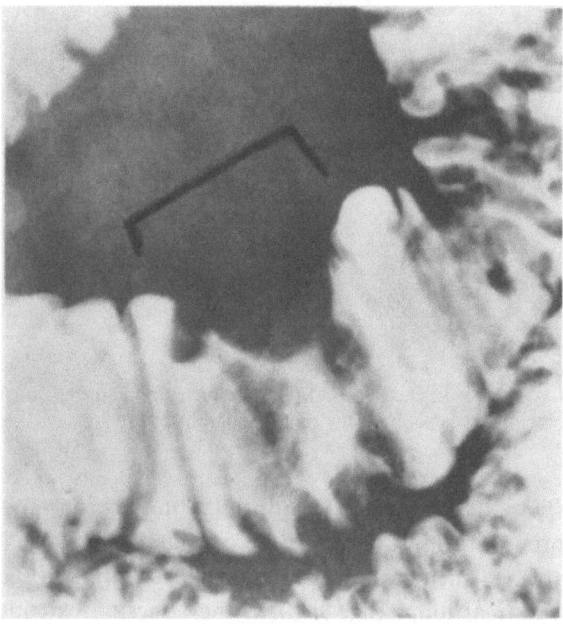

Fig. 8.36
Aspecific ulceration in the jejunum which closely resembles a skip lesion in Crohn's disease or tumor growth.

5. Deformation of the intestine

If the ulcerations are located predominantly on one side of the intestinal wall, usually the mesenterial side, the opposite wall of the bowel will sometimes show spastic contractions. Not only the diagnosis of the very small ulcer can be difficult but also that of very large ulcers. Often the segment containing the large ulcer will show extensive abnormal infiltrations and erratically defined filling defects so that it is impossible to identify the normal anatomy as well as the presence of an ulcer crater. An example of this is seen in

a. ADHESIONS

It is seldom possible to demonstrate adhesions or fusion of intestinal loops with survey films alone. The finding of two intestinal loops which appear to lie close together in the same manner on all x-rays has turned out to be useless as a sign of adhesions. Many times we have seen that it is possible to force the two apparently fused loops apart by using compression. If two intestinal loops are truly fused then this should also be clearly visible on the

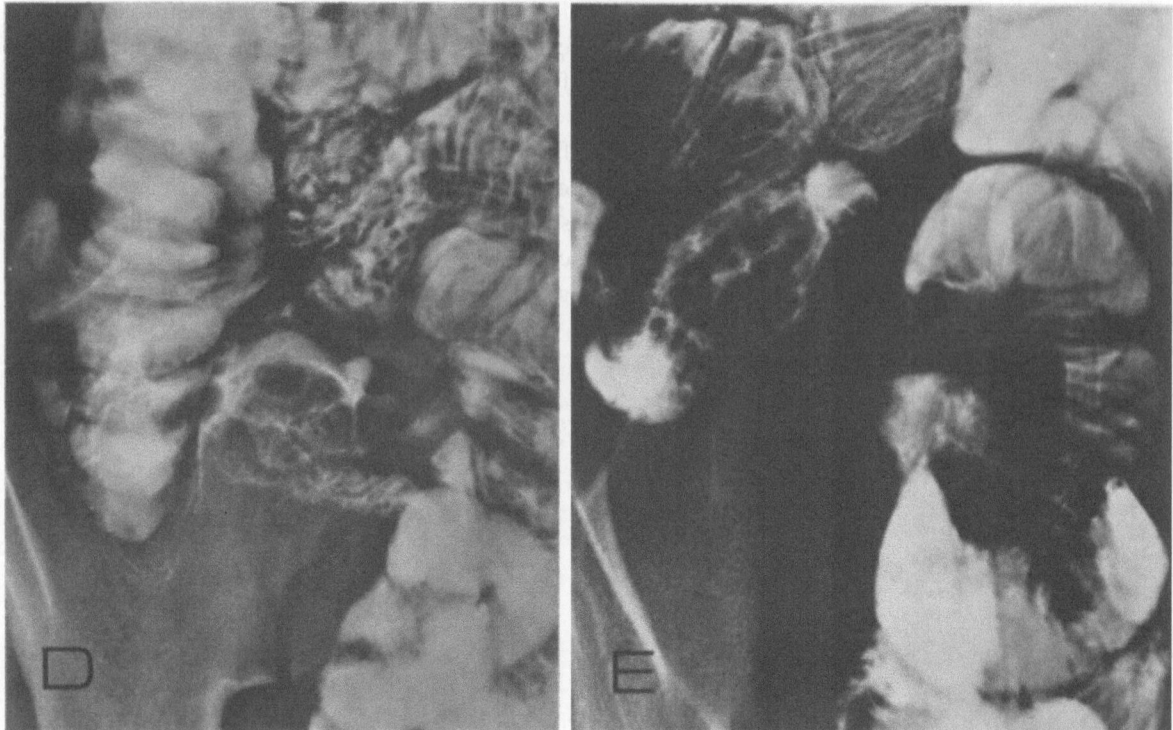

Fig. 8.37
Large ulcer in the ileocecal region which upon surgery turned out to be an ulcerating Meckel's diverticulum. This was not recognized as such on the roentgenogram. x-ray E was taken 2 months after x-ray D.

spot photographs taken during compression; this procedure must therefore be considered indispensable. In such cases we see tent-shaped bulges in the intestinal loops (fig. 8.38); if the adhesion extends over a somewhat longer distance the termination of the plane of contact of the two intestinal loops is rather abrupt or sharply angular (⌣). The mucosal pattern in intestinal loops which have fused with surrounding tissue is always intact, but during dilatation of the loop, induced for example by air insufflation, a very local slightly serrated or wrinkled contour can be seen at the site of the adhesion which is due to- the fact that the intestinal wall there cannot stretch with the rest of the wall (➡). Adhesions rarely cause any restriction of the passage of the contrast fluid. .

b. FISTULAS

The differentiation between a bulge due to an adhesion and one caused by a fistulous tract is rarely difficult. A fistulous tract is a very long canal which often follows a tortuous course and is irregularly defined; as a rule it does not broaden at the junction with the intestinal loop but passes through as a narrow opening or wide canal. There is often an infiltrate in the neighbourhood and the mucosal relief at the site where the fistulous tract originates has changed pathologically. Since fistulous tracts are often very narrow, it is only possible to visualize them when the contrast fluid is still very thin and there is as yet no increase in the viscosity due to dehydration. Careful projection in order to distinguish them from

Fig. 8.38   ⟶
Several examples of adhesion and fusion of adjacent intestinal loops. The tent-shaped bulges in the intestinal loops are seen consistently on all x-rays; in addition certain sections of the intestinal loops cannot be forced apart by compression. Short planes of contact between 2 intestinal loops or 1 loop and the surrounding tissue are indicated by arrows.

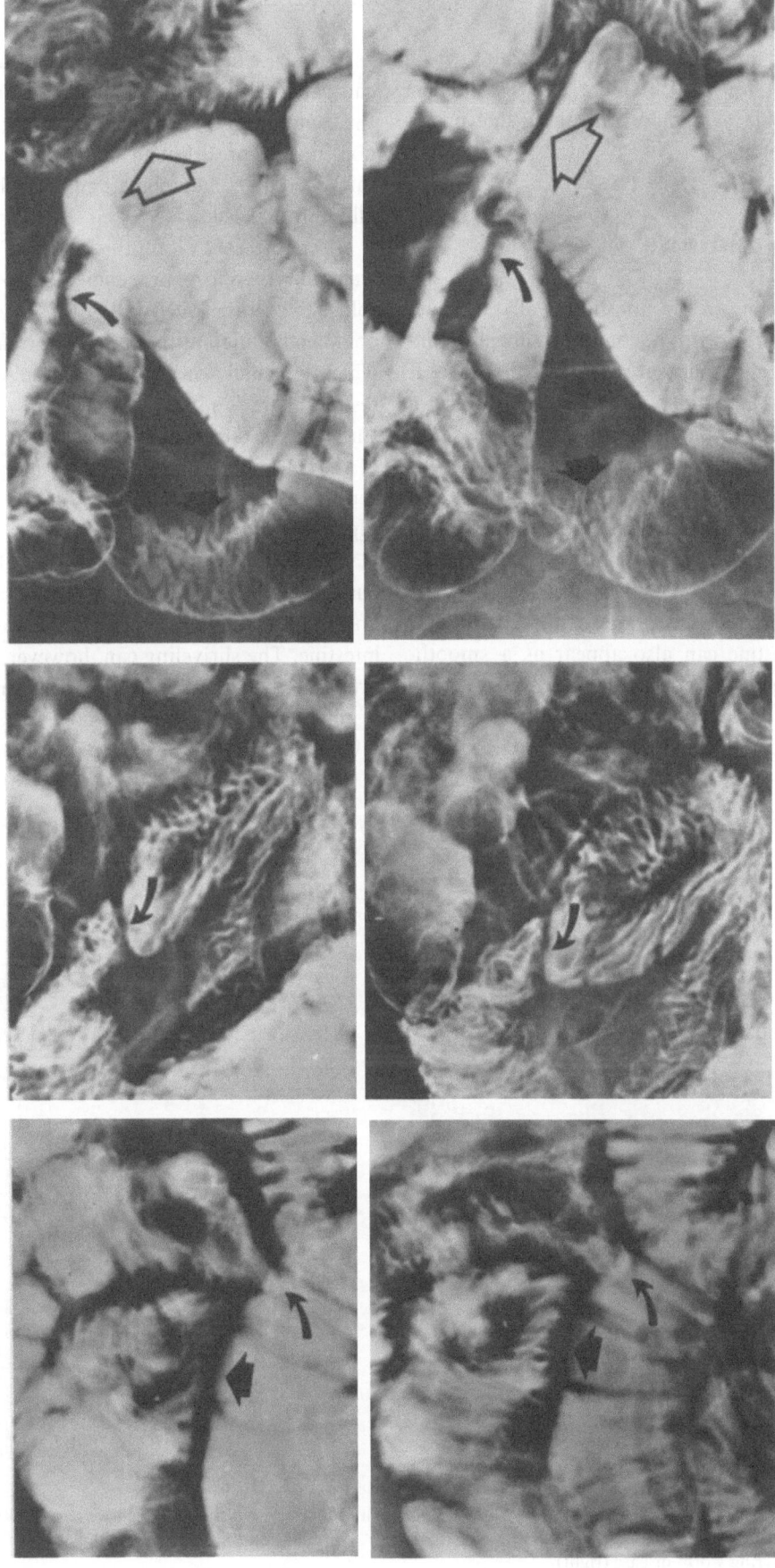

adjacent intestinal loops and underexposure with a low tube voltage ($\pm$ 80 kV) are also essential in order to be able to demonstrate these fine canals (fig. 8.39).

C. FIBROSIS AND SHRIVELING

Fibrotic shriveling of the intestinal wall can cause circular strictures with a completely healthy intestine and normal mucosal relief on either side. If the stricture is about 0.5 cm long, then either a healed ulcer of aspecific origin (fig. 8.40k) or shriveling as a result of carcinoid (fig. 8.40L) must be considered in particular. In Crohn's disease when a skip lesion has healed with the formation of fibrosis or after a cured ischemia with secondary ulceration, the stenosis is as a rule somewhat longer (fig. 8.40m). In some cases an adenocarcinoma of the small intestine can also appear as a smooth-walled circular stenosis (fig. 8.40n). However, then the transition between the stenosis and the healthy small intestine is biconvex and not nozzle-shaped

as in the case of a healed ulcer. In addition the tumor can cause a small space-occupying process outside the stenosis; in the event of shriveling this generally does not occur although here, too, the wall can be thickened due to an increase in muscular and especially fibrotic tissue.

Ulcers directed along the length of the intestinal wall and therefore perpendicular to the mucosal folds, as so often seen in Crohn's disease, heal in a completely different manner. At the site of the ulcer which is usually on the mesenterial side of the intestine, there is plaque-like fibrosis with secondary shriveling so that the mucosal folds on the other side of the intestinal lumen acquire a more or less concentric course directed toward the healed ulcer (fig. 8.41p). In other cases we can find sclerotic plaques in the intestine (fig. 8.41q). A highly similar pattern can be seen in the rare case of metastasis of a linitis plastica of the stomach in the wall of the small intestine. The shriveling can, however, be much less pronounced here or even practically missing. As a result of shriveling on one side, so-called pseudo-diverticula can also develop. They sometimes have a

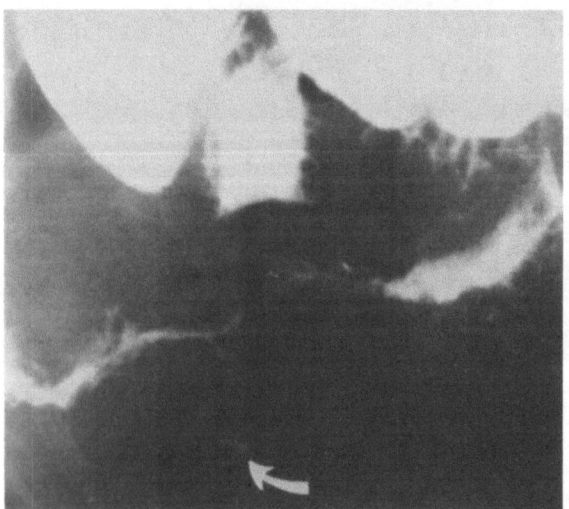
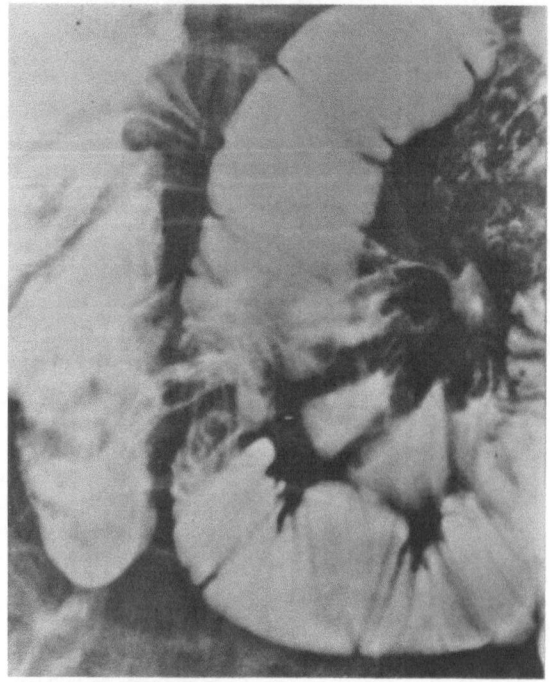

Fig. 8.39
Thin fistulous tracts can best be demonstrated with a contrast fluid of low viscosity and high s.g. and are visualized most clearly with a low tube voltage and also a low film density (left). A combination of adhesion and a fistulous tract in a patient suffering from herring worm disease (right).

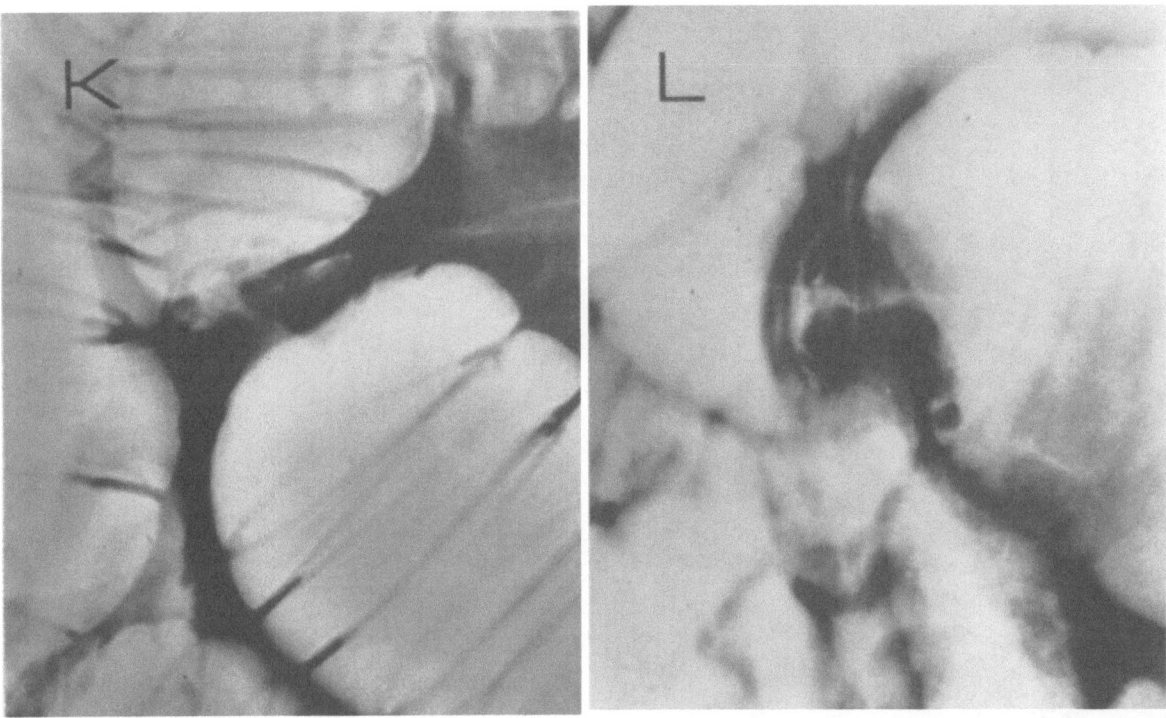

Fig. 8.40
Stenosis in the small intestine, 0.5 to 1 cm long, as a result of an aspecific ulceration (K) and a carcinoid (L). In both cases fibrosis is pronounced.
Stenoses in the small bowel more than 1 cm long due to a skip lesion in Crohn's disease (M) and an adenocarcinoma (N).

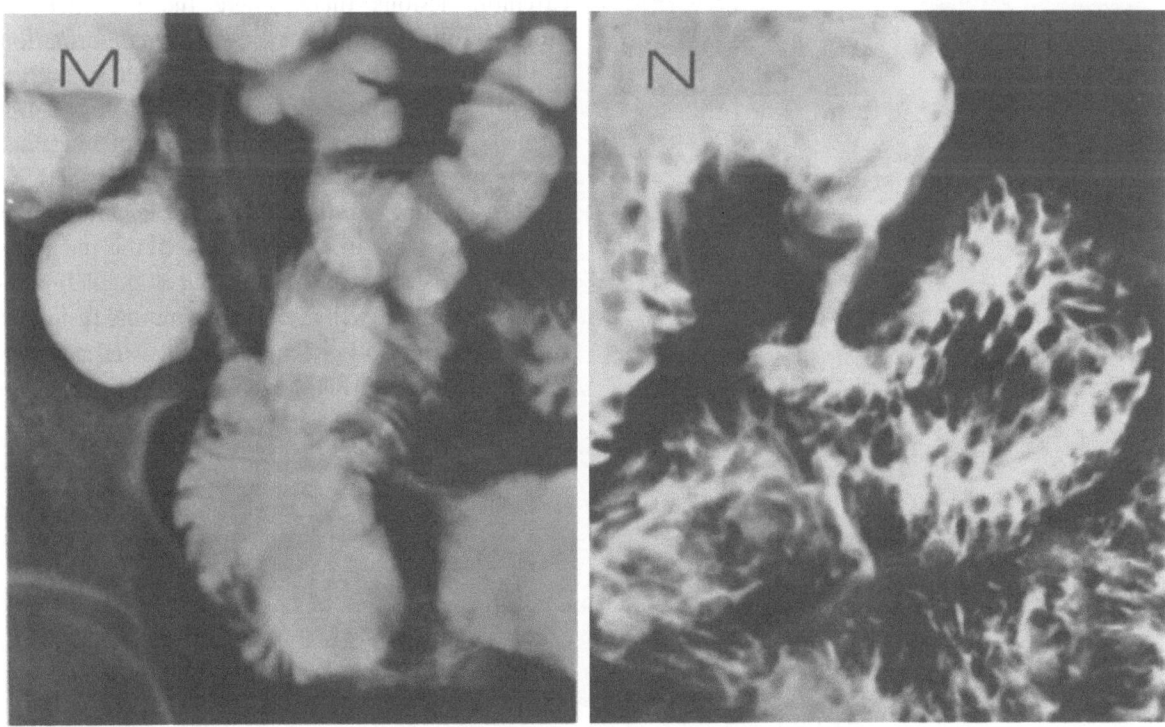

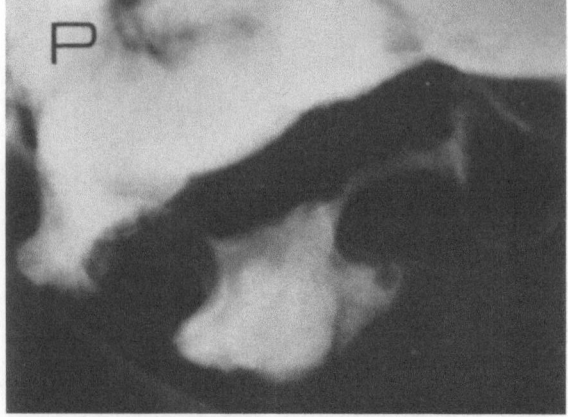

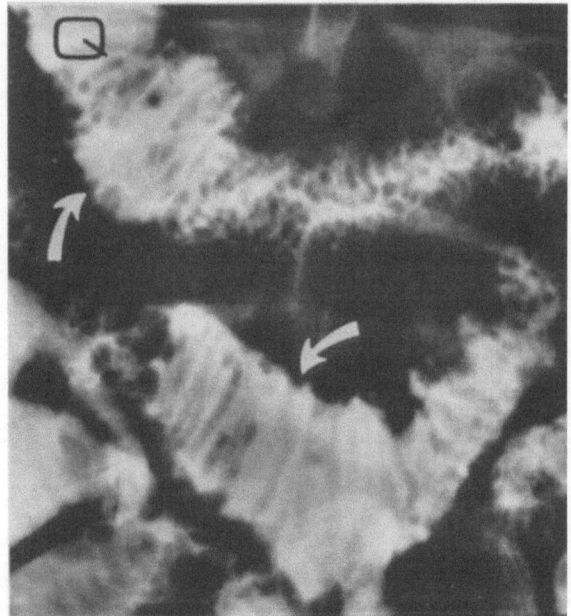

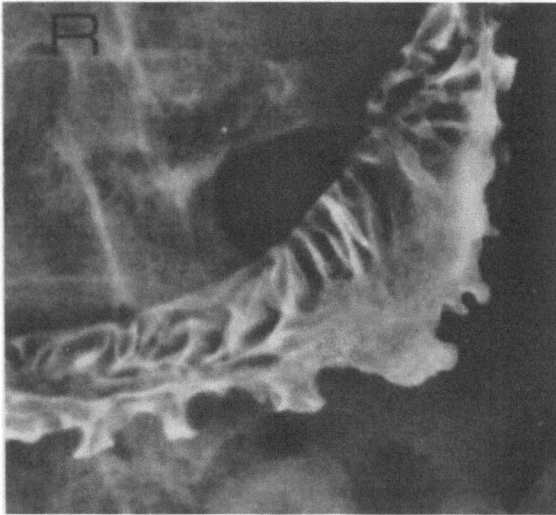

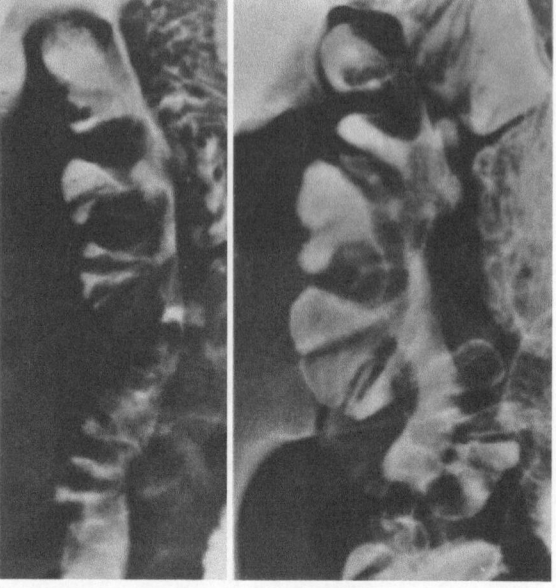

Fig. 8.42
Pseudo-diverticula in the intestine opposite stretched, shriveled longitudinal ulcerations develop as a result of spastic or partially fibrotic constrictions and vary in shape and size.

very broad base at the intestinal wall and may change continuously in size and shape during the various stages of the examination (fig. 8.42). Fibrosis due to carcinoid lesions there where the mesentery is attached to the intestine causes marked deformation of the intestinal lumen, sometimes with strictures, which is called kinking in the literature (fig. 8.43). Surgical anastomoses for the purpose of intestinal resection generally do not cause such deformations of the intestine so that this obvious alternative diagnosis need not be considered when this phenomenon is observed (fig. 8.44). Kinking or angulation of intestinal loops as well as extensive mutual fusion or adhesions can also be seen in so-called retractile or sclerosing mesenteritis, a rare disorder which is

Fig. 8.41
P. Concentric course of mucosal folds due to asymmetric shriveling as a result of an ulceration on one side of the intestine.
Q. Plaque without mucosal relief in the intestine, not yet shriveled.
R. The same pattern can be seen in the colon.

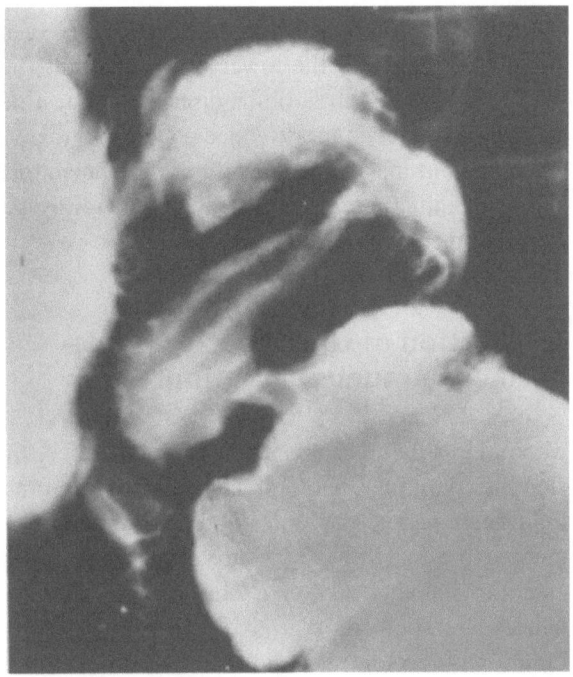

Fig. 8.43
Sudden changes in the caliber of the lumen and direction of
the longitudinal axis of the intestine as a result of shriveling
at a carcinoid site (so-called kinking).

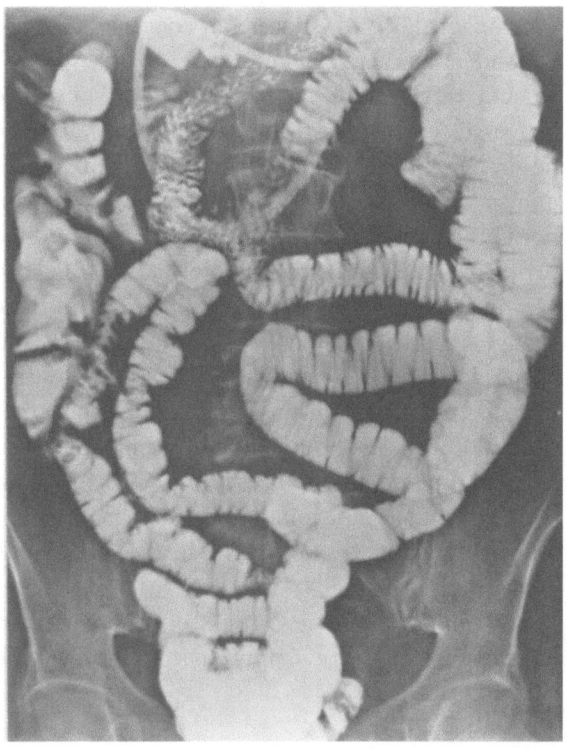

Fig. 8.45
Large empty spaces in the middle of the abdomen in pyknics,
possibly caused not only by a short and fatty mesentry but
partly also by intra-abdominal autocompression by a voluminous greater omentum when the patient is in the prone
position.

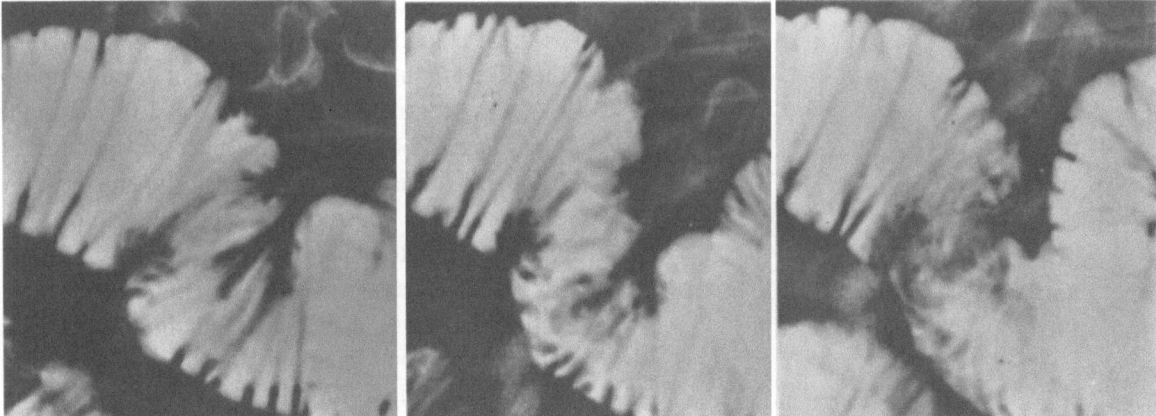

Fig. 8.44
Relatively stenotic area at a surgical anastomosis in the jejunum, made visible by stretching of the intestine. Moderately
disordered mucosal pattern.

accompanied by pronounced fatty degeneration and post-infectious shriveling of the mesentery.

As a result of the pronounced shortening and increased thickness of the mesentery, there are then only a few intestinal loops in the center of the abdomen which sometimes follow a more or less taut polycyclic convex course extending outwards to the periphery. The decreased lumen of the intestine can vary in size. It is striking that in spite of all of these changes the mucosal relief is still relatively unchanged. The space between the separate intestinal loops is sometimes obviously greater; this phenomenon although less pronounced can sometimes also be seen in obese patients possibly due in part to an intra-abdominal autocompression of the intestinal loops in the prone position caused by the voluminous greater omentum (fig. 8.45).

In Crohn's disease, as a result of the increase in mesenterial fat, large empty spaces between the

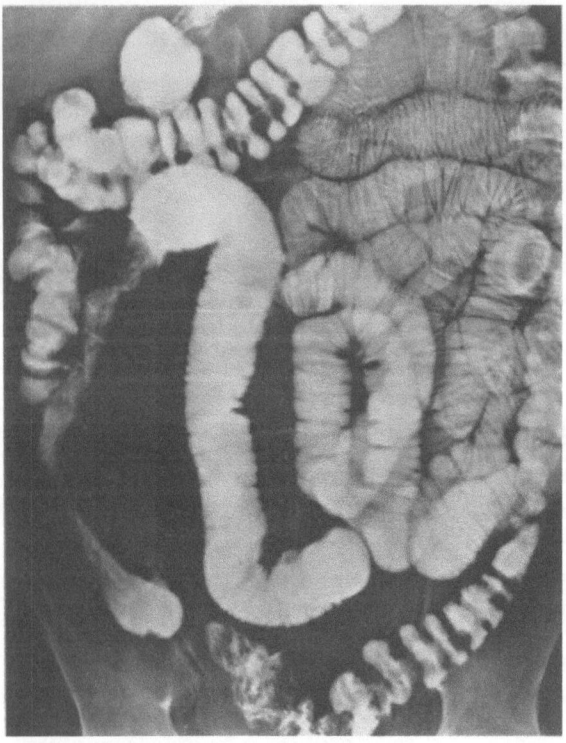

Fig. 8.46
Large empty spaces in the lower right quadrant in a patient with Crohn's disease due to fatty degeneration and shriveling of the mesentery, an extensive layer of fat around the involved intestine and in some cases also due to infiltration abnormalities. No indications of an infiltrate could be found in this patient.

intestinal loops may sometimes also be seen, usually of course in the lower right quadrant (fig. 8.46). If, however, in Crohn's disease the intestinal loops also follow a taut extended course and there is a varying but marked narrowing of the lumen, then this is definitely accompanied by an obviously abnormal mucosal pattern.

6. Dilution of the contrast fluid – haziness – mucus secretion

Maximum adhesion to the mucosa and therefore the sharpest patterns are obtained when the contrast fluid flows past a 'dry' intestinal wall. Addition of glucose products or other substances with hyperosmotic characteristics or a high caloric value enhances secretion of digestive juices and mucus. Dilution of the contrast fluid then occurs so that the specific gravity is decreased and contrast is reduced, which of course means a reduction in the apparent sharpness of the pattern. This is clearly demonstrated by comparing two examinations of the same patient carried out within a few days of one another. Fig. 8.47D shows a jejunum x-ray when 40 g glucose was added to the 600 ml barium suspension; fig. 8.47E shows the same without any additives in the barium suspension. It is obvious that the differences which are already clearly visible here would have been even greater if both examinations had been carried out in the conventional manner.

When the intestinal wall is coated with mucus which is not immediately flushed off by a contrast fluid with a lower viscosity, the outer margins of the contrast column are also in fact less sharp. Within the layer of mucus there is a gradual decrease in the s.g. of the contrast fluid from 1.25 to 1.0. The vague reproduction of the intestinal mucosa which results from this decrease in s.g. and can be enhanced by dilution of the contrast fluid and by a decrease in sharpness due to hypermotility of the intestinal wall is called 'haziness' in the literature (fig. 8.48).

If the viscosity of the mucus coating is very high, which can occur in inflammatory processes, it is often impossible to flush it from the intestinal wall, in spite of the administration of large amounts of contrast fluid, and the patterns remain vague (fig. 8.36). Under normal circumstances it can sometimes also be seen that the difference in viscosity between

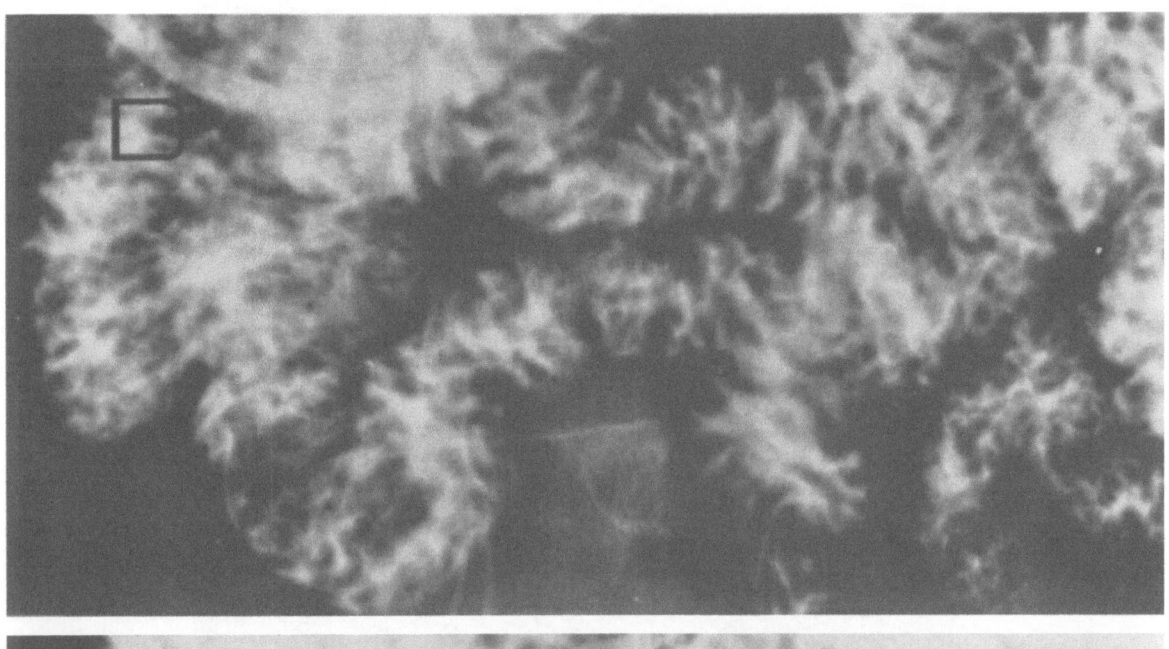

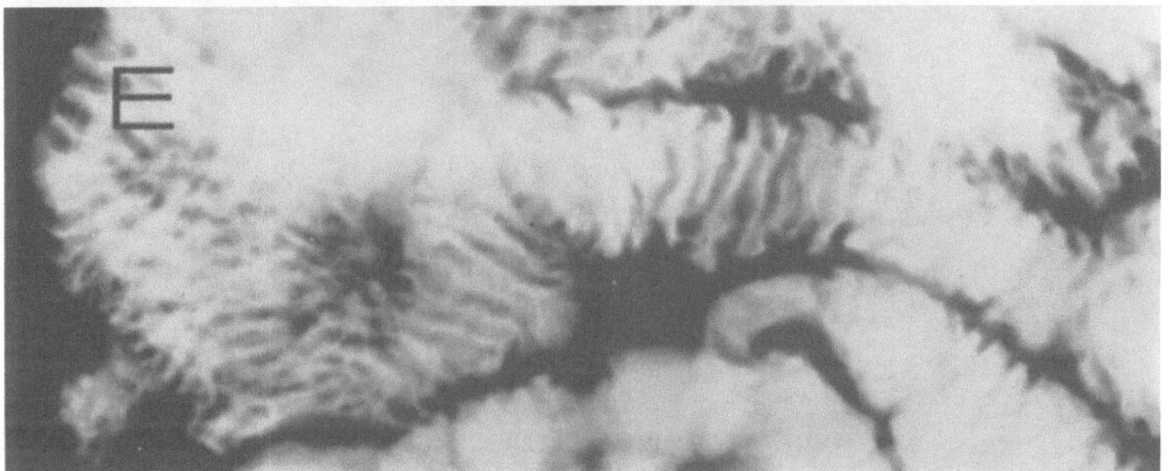

Fig. 8.47
Spot films of the jejunum of same patient as seen in fig. 7.13.
D. Glucose added to the contrast fluid.
E. Repeat examination without glucose.

the barium suspension and mucus is so great that mixing does not occur; the mucus then remains visible as poorly defined threads which are carried off distally in toto (fig. 8.49).

In other cases, for instance in the event of mechanical obstructions, the intestinal wall is not coated with mucus; instead large quantities of watery fluid are found in the intestinal lumen. There is complete mixing, right up to the intestinal wall, of the barium suspension and the thin fluid in the intestine so that the specific gravity of the former decreases but the sharp delineation of the intestinal wall is still retained.

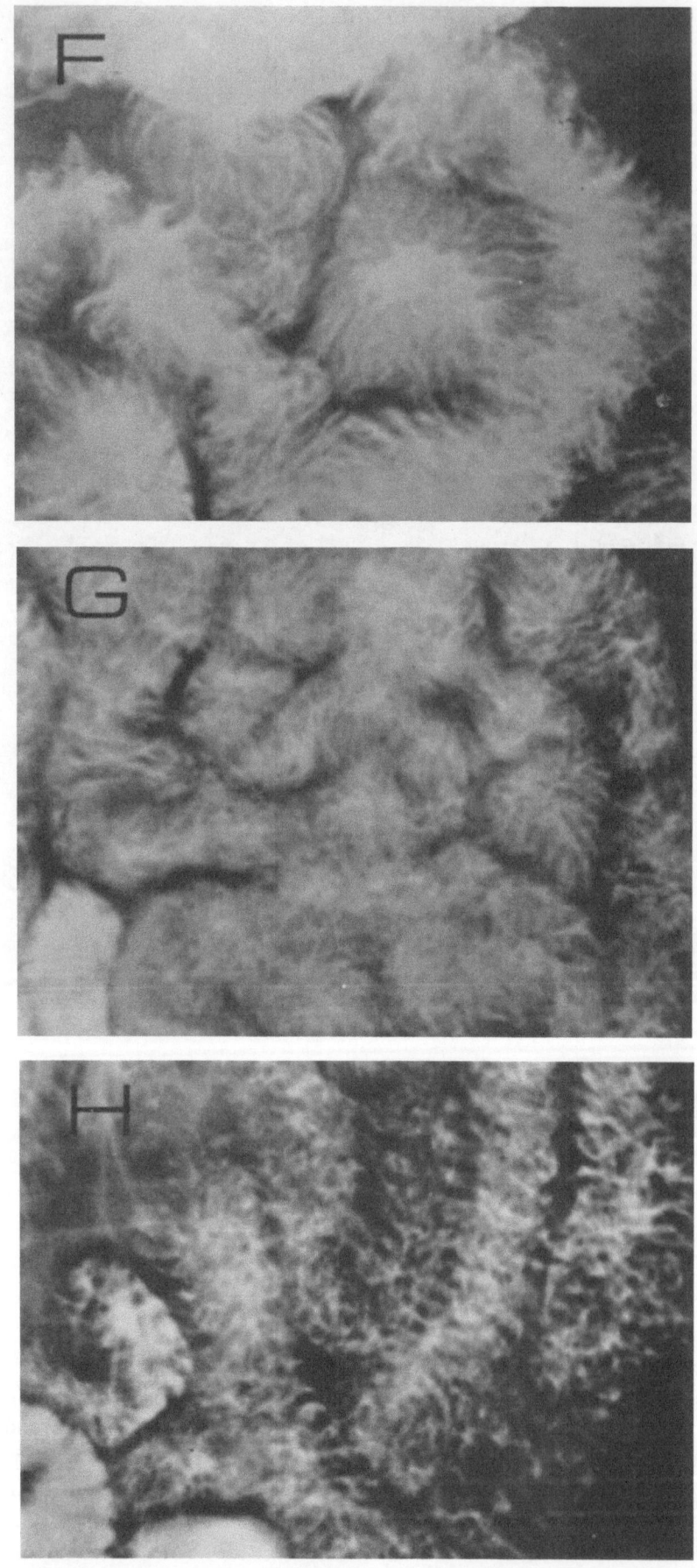

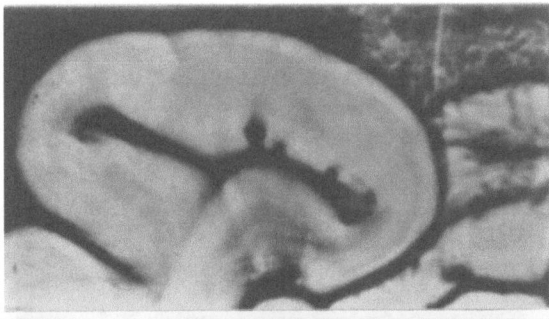

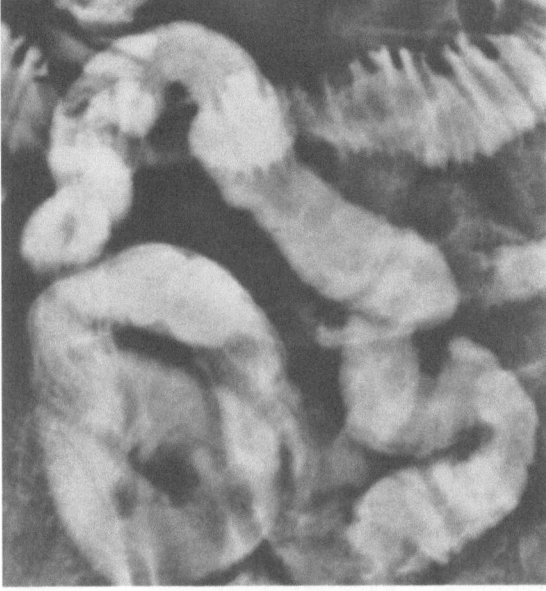

Fig. 8.49
The viscosity of threads of mucus is often higher than that of the contrast fluid so that direct mixing does not occur and poorly defined thread-like filling defects extending along the length of the intestine are seen.

7. Disintegration and misleading patterns

Flocculation of the contrast fluid is a phenomenon which is still seen regurlarly in a conventional follow-through examination, at least in cases of severe malabsorption, even when the most stable barium suspension is used. As soon as flocculation occurs, anatomical representation of the intestinal mucosa has become an illusion and the radiological examination should be terminated (fig. 8.50). In an adequately executed enteroclysis examination, flocculation of the contrast fluid is never encountered within the period required for the actual examination, even in cases of severe malabsorption. If, however, a water infusion is administered after the contrast medium infusion, flocculation may occur at the end of the contrast column where the water column and the barium suspension meet and mix (fig. 7.22). The same phenomenon can occur at the beginning of the contrast column under certain circumstances (fig. 8.51). The first quantity of barium suspension administered has after all the most intense contact with the contents of the intestine. Local enhanced secretion of digestive juices or heightened mucus production as well as fluid absorption or dehydration due to disturbed resorption of hyperosmotic food particles can sometimes cause disintegration of the first 50 or 100 cc barium suspension. However, the small quantity of disintegrated contrast fluid is quickly forced onwards by the rapidly flowing fresh barium suspension. This disintegration of the contrast fluid is of course only observed when there is sufficient penetration of the contrast fluid by the roentgen rays; it can be masked entirely by underexposure (fig. 4.8). A contrast medium which has flocculated is much more viscous than an intact barium suspension and is no longer able to retain

←

Fig. 8.48
Contrast column with vague margins due to a combination of movement of the intestinal wall caused by hypermotility and dilution of the contrast fluid caused by hypersecretion or disturbed resorption of fluids (F and G). With the infusion technique this vagueness or haziness is of course less pronounced (H) (same patient).

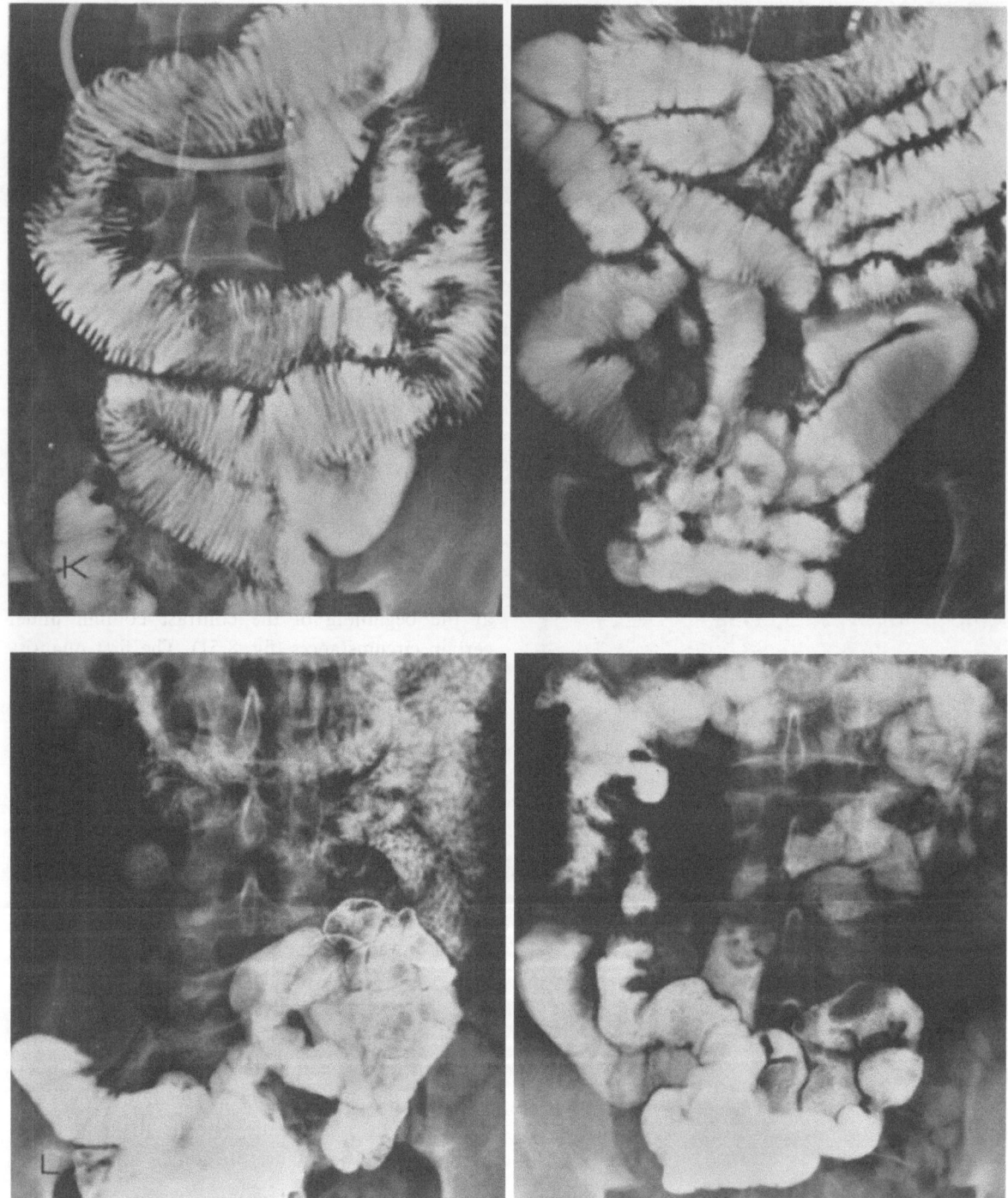

Fig. 8.51
Disintegration of the barium suspension can sometimes also occur at the beginning of the contrast column. Because of the increase in the viscosity of the contrast medium, it is no longer possible to obtain a good reproduction of the mucosal folds (R). At the same location but several minutes later, disintegration is less and vague impressions of the mucosal folds can already be seen (s). Still later the disintegrated contrast fluid has moved distally and the fresh completely intact barium suspension gives a normal reproduction of the fold relief (T).

⟶

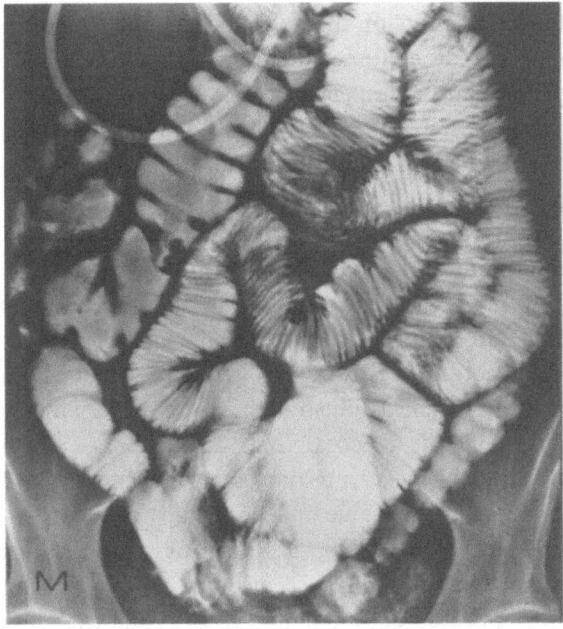

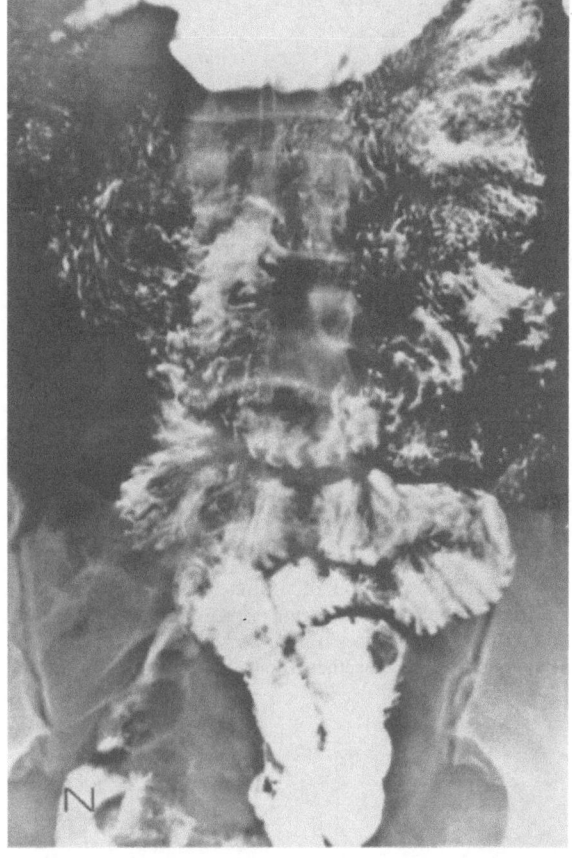

Fig. 8.50

KM. Enteroclysis films of the small intestine of two patients with a clinical malabsorption syndrome.

LN. The films of the conventional examination carried out one week earlier showed clear disintegration of the contrast medium so that a true reproduction of the intestinal mucous membrane could no longer be obtained.

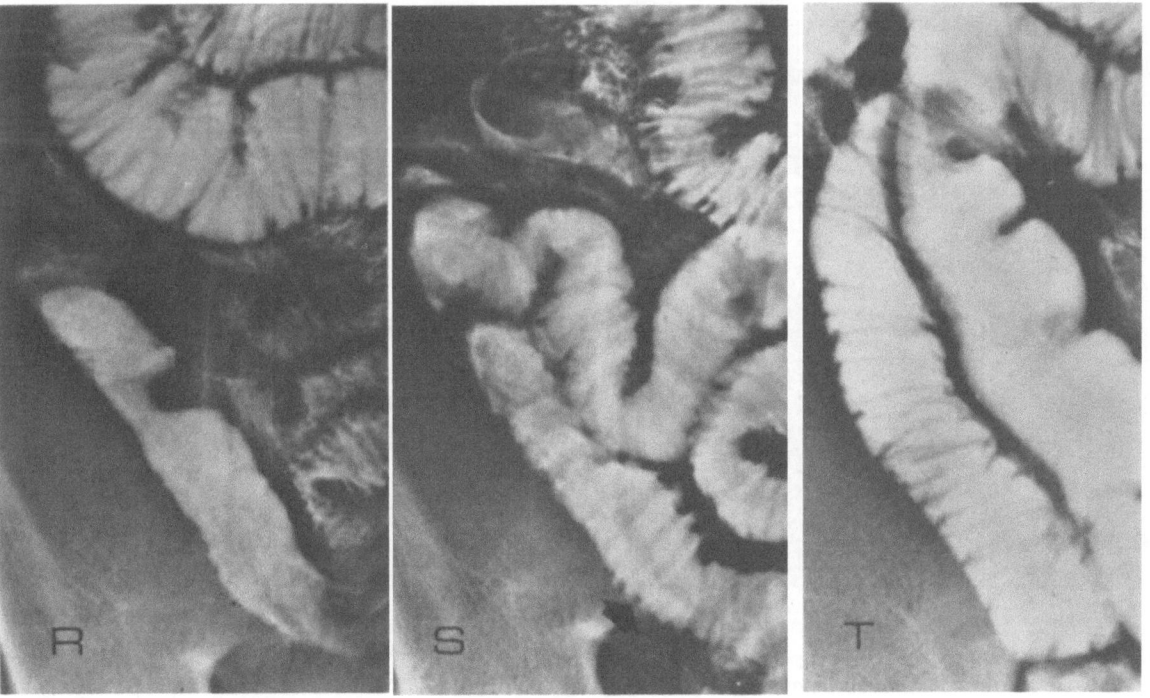

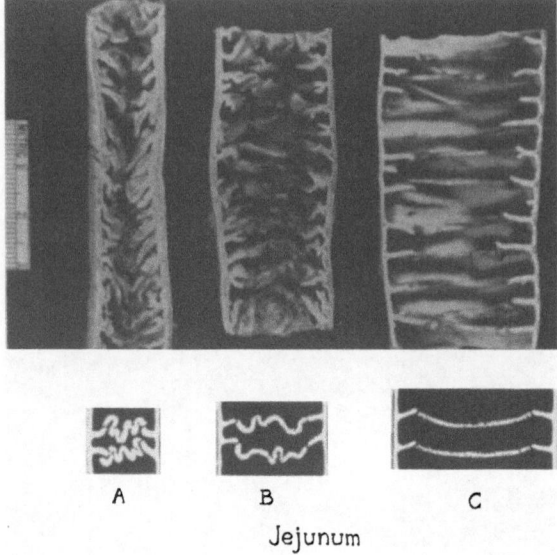

Fig. 8.52
Schematic representation of a stretched and a contracted intestinal loop. Stretched mucosal folds probably cause thinner clarification lines on the x-ray than those which are more or less folded together (Sloan 1953).

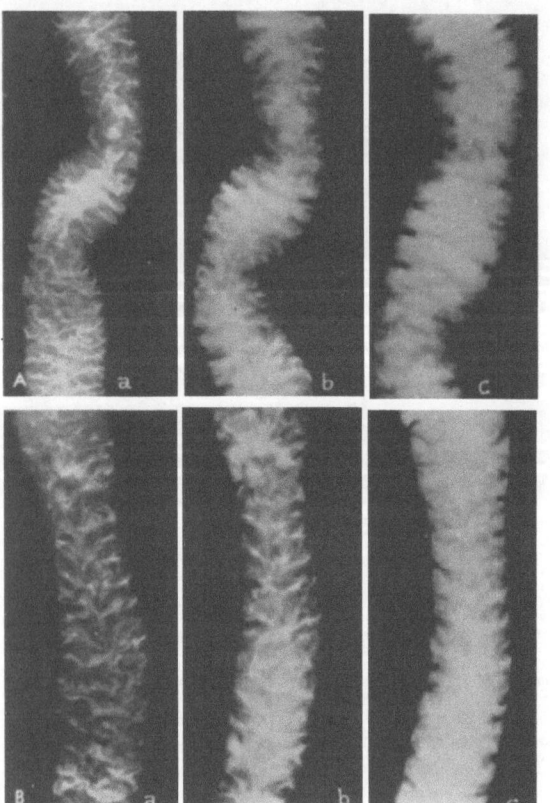

Fig. 8.53
Sloan's experiments in vitro showing that mucosal folds appear coarser when the intestinal loops are moderately filled with contrast fluid than when the loops are well-filled.

the impression of the folds of the soft intestinal mucosa. Never forget therefore that disintegration of the barium suspension leads to apparent coarsening of the fold relief (fig. 4.9). Failure to recognize this symptom will lead to thoroughly incorrect conclusions.

In the proximal part of the jejunum this tendency to reproduce the mucosal folds more coarsely than they in fact are is enhanced when there is only moderate filling of the intestinal loops because of hypermotility. The drawing in fig. 8.52 and the in vitro experiment illustrated in fig. 8.53 already show that the mucosal folds appear coarser in a moderately filled intestine than in a well-filled intestine. This same phenomenon can be encountered in vivo. Fig. 8.54P shows mucosal folds in the jejunum which seemed to be very coarse; they appeared quite different in a second examination taken after hypotonia had been induced (fig. 8.54Q). Endoscopic examination and biopsy studies revealed no abnormalities. In our opinion, which is supported by our experience, the coarse mucosal patterns in Whipple's disease which are mentioned so often in the literature are also mainly due to an artifact – at least in most cases. In practice an increased tendency toward flocculation and hypermotility often coincide leading to an accumulation of unfavourable factors. Evaluation of the shape of the mucosal folds should therefore not be based on the patterns obtained at the beginning nor at the end of the contrast column, and certainly not if it is obvious that the contrast fluid has lost its original structure. In exceptional cases, for instance after irradiation of the lower abdomen, we can see quite local and randomly situated spots of disintegrated barium suspension in the middle of the contrast column soon after the infusion is terminated (fig. 8.55). It should now be apparent that local abnormalities of an inflammatory nature or local enhanced secretion must be involved. For evaluation of the mucosal patterns therefore, it is better to use the films taken during the infusion, and preferably those towards the end of the series.

When an examination has to be prolonged for any reason, changes in the structure of the contrast fluid can also occur in the distal ileum where dehydration leads to thickening of the barium suspension. One then sees a crackle pattern con-

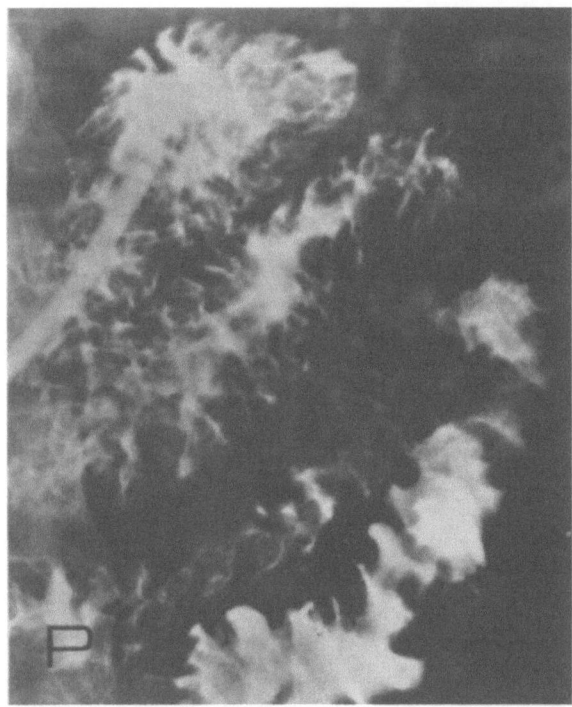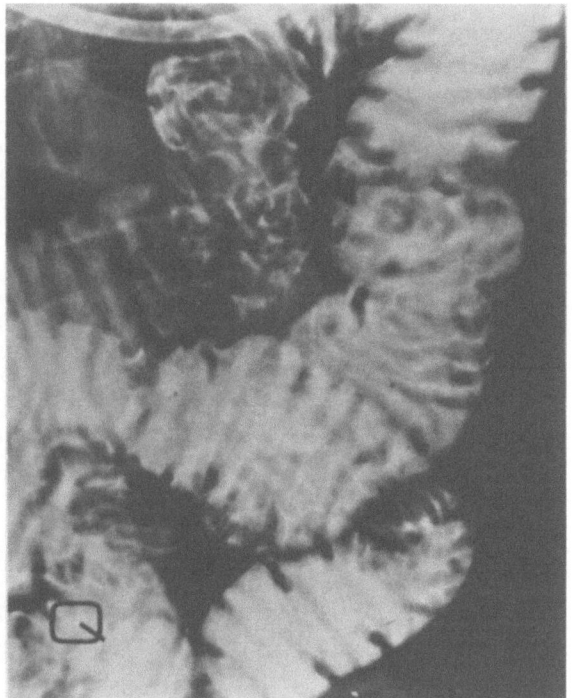

Fig. 8.54
These mucosal folds in the jejunum were judged definitely too coarse (P). Before the repeat examination, a hypotonic agent was administered. The folds are now seen to be completely normal (Q).

sisting of haphazardly arranged thin bright lines throughout the barium column (fig. 8.56). These lines can probably be ascribed to residual fold impressions of the more proximal loops where the contrast fluid was less thick only a short time before. As a result of the kneading action in the intestine, these lines become haphazardly arranged; they are so thin because they no longer contain folds. An argument in favor of this theory is the fact that often such lines lie perpendicular to the longitudinal axis of the intestine and terminate in a fold impression which is still just visible at the margin.

If during an adequately executed enteroclysis examination the structure in the distal ileum is grainy or inhomogeneous, then each of the following causes should be considered:

1. beginning of the contrast column (fig. 8.51);
2. food residue as a result of atony of the small intestine due to chronic use of tranquillizers, sedatives or antispasmodics (fig. 8.28);
3. the stomach was not empty;
4. reflux of the contents of the cecum due to an inadequate Bauhin's valve in ulcerative colitis (fig. 7.23).

8. Malabsorption

In the past a great deal has been written about malabsorption, and today it is still the subject of an occasional article. For older radiologists it is probably the diagnosis most frequently encountered in the course of their career, since in the past the contrast medium very often flocculated. In fact malabsorption does accompany 50–100 disorders of

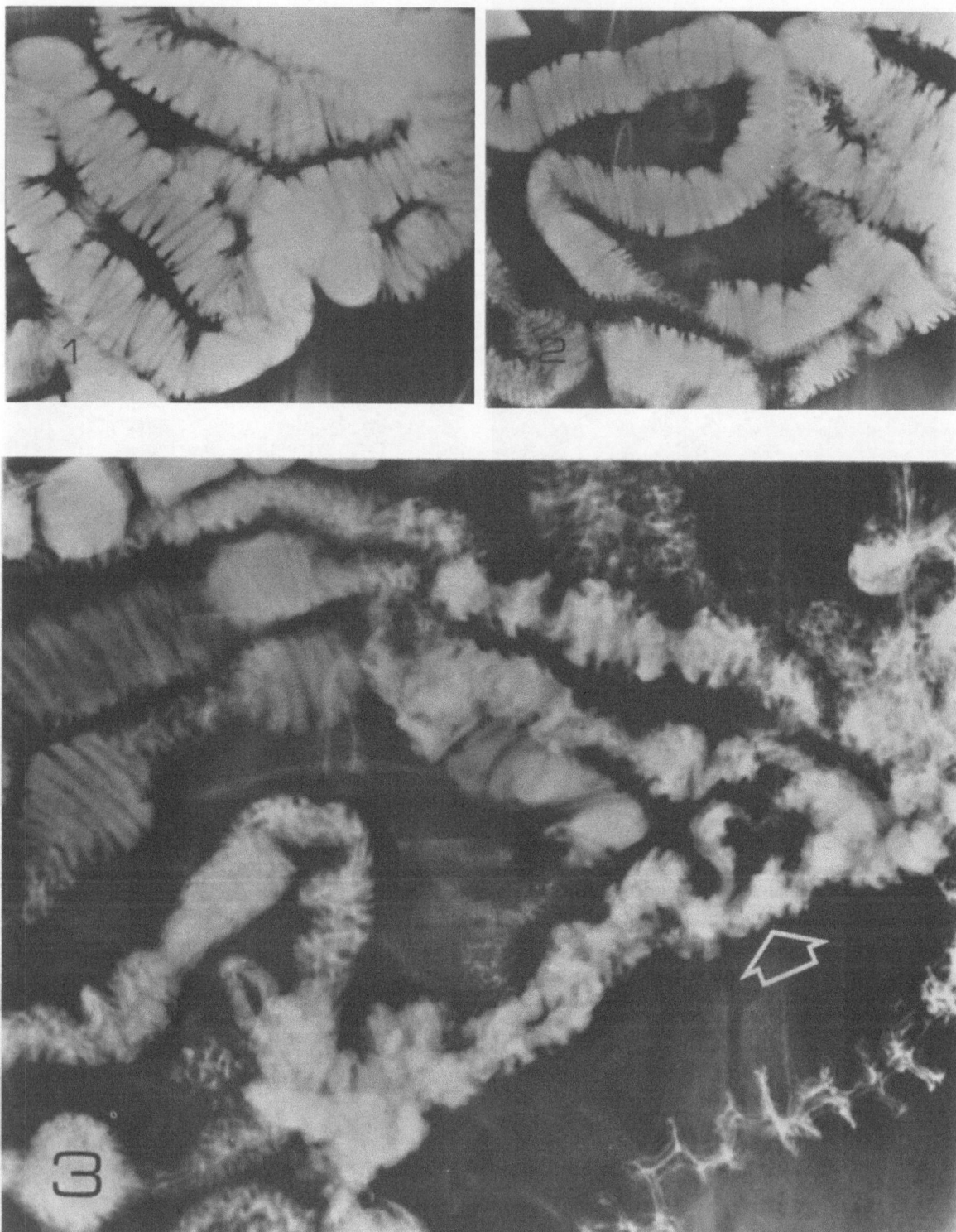

Fig. 8.55
Quite local spasticity of the intestine and disintegration of the barium suspension in the middle of the contrast column, soon after the infusion was terminated. Three x-rays taken at 2-minute intervals. The cause of these abnormalities in this patient remained unknown.

the small intestine so that this diagnosis was without a doubt seldom incorrect. One wonders therefore why radiodiagnosis of the small intestine is regarded with such disfavor. If desired, malabsorption can be subdivided into three categories which with a little effort could include practically all existing disorders of the small intestine:

1. disturbed digestion of food, irrespective of whether this is caused by a bacterial infection or a deficiency of digestive juices or enzymes.
2. disturbed food transport either because transit is too rapid or too slow or because the intestine is too short after repeated resections.
3. truly disturbed resorption of the partially digested food particles as a result of various disorders which more or less damage the intestinal mucosa or, as in edema, impede its function.

Radiology can only offer an extremely modest contribution to the differentiation between the many diseases with the malabsorption syndrome. In a number of cases, radiological differential diagnosis in in principle not possible because there are only histological and biochemical abnormalities of the mucous membrane of the small intestine without macroscopic abnormalities. There remain, however, many diseases with malabsorption for which a morphological examination can be highly valuable. This applies for:

1. diseases with gross anatomical abnormalities:
   anastomoses, fistulas, blind loops;
   strictures, adhesions;
   diverticula.
2. diseases with local, usually rather gross, mucosal abnormalities:
   leukemia, Hodgkin's disease, lymphosarcoma;
   intramural bleeding;
   local edema due to venous congestion (e.g. thrombosis) or lymphatic obstruction (irradiation).
3. diseases with more general mucosal abnormalities:
   edema due to: lymphangiectasis,
                 allergic reactions,
                 protein-losing enteropathy;
   amyloidosis, Whipple's disease, scleroderma.

For some of these diseases, the radiologist is the only one who can provide the correct diagnosis. However, with the conventional methods of examination still in use, he often cannot even make a differential diagnosis and must suffice with the report that malabsorption probably exists. This opinion is based on the observation of flocculation as well as the eventual disintegration into segment clumps of the barium meal in the small intestine. This conclusion incidentally is seldom important since the referring specialist is usually already aware of the malabsorption syndrome on the basis of other evidence. As soon as flocculation occurs, every

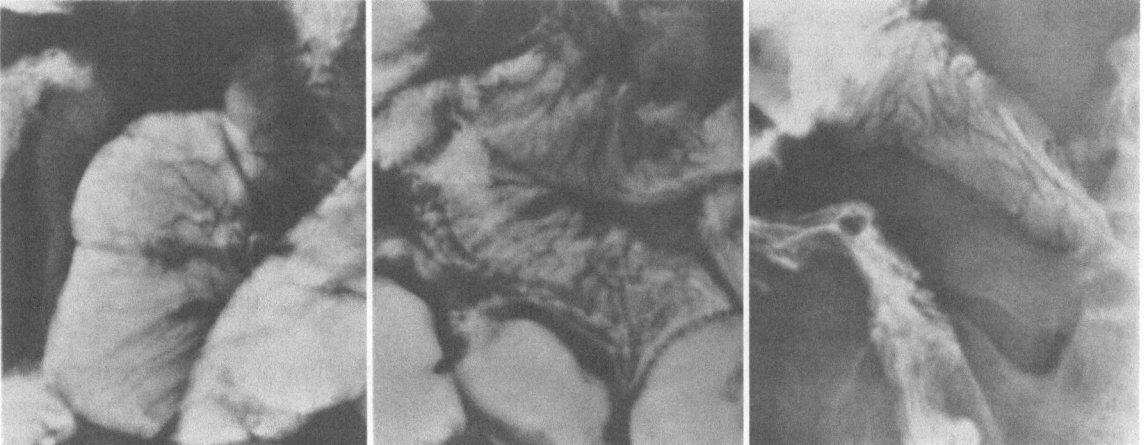

Fig. 8.56
Crackle-like configuration of bright lines in the contrast fluid in the distal ileum. We have seen these lines as yet only in the ileum; presumably they are caused by residual fold impressions in a thickened barium suspension.

morphological evaluation of the small intestine becomes impossible, because there is no longer any relationship between the margins of the contrast column and those of the intestinal mucous membrane.

The flocculation is usually irreversible and the flocculi continue to grow in size until segments are formed. In addition, when the rate of transit of the contrast fluid through the small intestine is slow, this clump formation is further promoted in the distal ileum by the absorption of fluids from the intestine. In the colon, segmentation of the barium column is the natural end of every normal passage through the small intestine. When various methods of examination as well as the results obtained with diverse brands of contrast media are observed, it then becomes apparent that the development of flocculation is also highly dependent upon both of these factors. As a result, one radiologist will observe flocculation frequently and the other only when there is a serious malabsorption. The highly illogical situation then arises that a radiologist can only interpret the small intestine examination of a colleague to a limited degree. Even if there are signs of a pronounced and relatively early flocculation on the x-ray film of a patient with a known malabsorption, he will not be able to express his opinion about the severity of this malabsorption. It is therefore obvious that in the roentgenologic findings an observed flocculation and segmentation must be reported such that faulty conclusions will not be drawn. In fact, this means that each radiologist builds up experience exclusively for himself based on the use of one specific contrast medium for one specific method of examination; this experience cannot be transferred to someone else. Should he change one or both of these aspects, then he has lost his experience in this respect and he must start again.

Actually flocculation of the contrast medium, which has for the most part been overcome in the past several years, can be caused by many factors which have nothing to do with the clinical concept of resorption. Clinical malabsorption therefore cannot be demonstrated on x-rays but must instead be identified by means of feces examination.

For the radiological examination of the small intestine in babies in particular, which fortunately is a rare necessity, the physician should realize that an optimum examination technique is essential to obtain useful results. Babies only several months old are fed almost entirely on milk products; therefore there is a high lactic acid content in the small intestine which greatly enhances flocculation. In these infants the tendency towards flocculation is so exceptionally strong that the natural rate of flow of the contrast medium through the stomach and pylorus is almost never fast enough to prevent it, even when a very large dose is administered. This is illustrated in fig. 6.2A; this x-ray of an eight-month-old baby was made after 400 ml barium suspension, s.g. = 1.15, was administerd at a rate of 80 ml per minute by infusion. Since it was not possible to insert the tube to Treitz's ligament, reflux of the barium suspension into the stomach occurred and the tip of the tube ended up in the stomach again. Although another 200 ml barium suspension as well as several ml metoclopramide were given before the tube was removed, the natural rate of gastric emptying was too slow to prevent flocculation. The second x-ray (fig. 6.2B), taken only several minutes later, shows total flocculation whereas the mucosal pattern was clearly visible on the first x-ray.

Hypersecretion of mucus or digestive juices in the small intestine, a phenomenon which leads to flocculation and segmentation in a conventional examination, is accorded too much diagnostic significance by many; it can be distinguished in an enteroclysis examination by the following:

1. disintegration of the contrast fluid over a fairly large segment at the beginning of the contrast column.
2. dilution of the contrast fluid so that the s.g. is decreased and the intestinal loops appear more transparent.
3. there may be signs of 'haziness'.
4. rapid disintegration of the barium suspension at the end of the contrast column, thus after termination of the flow of contrast medium. This can be determined easily by taking several residual films after the actual examination is completed, for instance 15 or 30 minutes later.

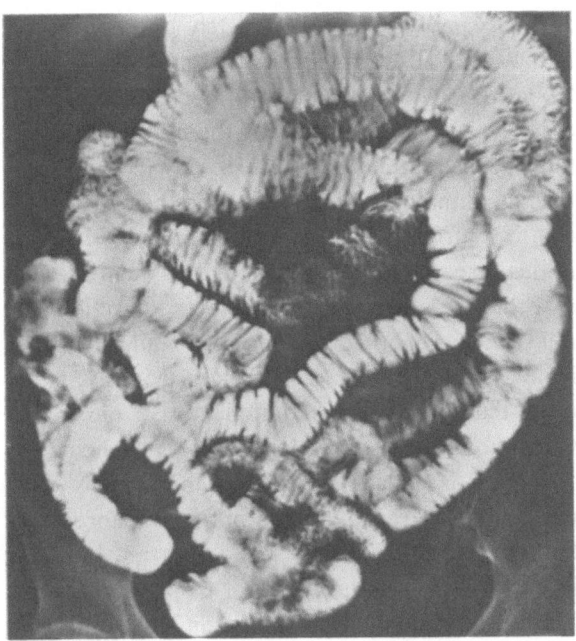

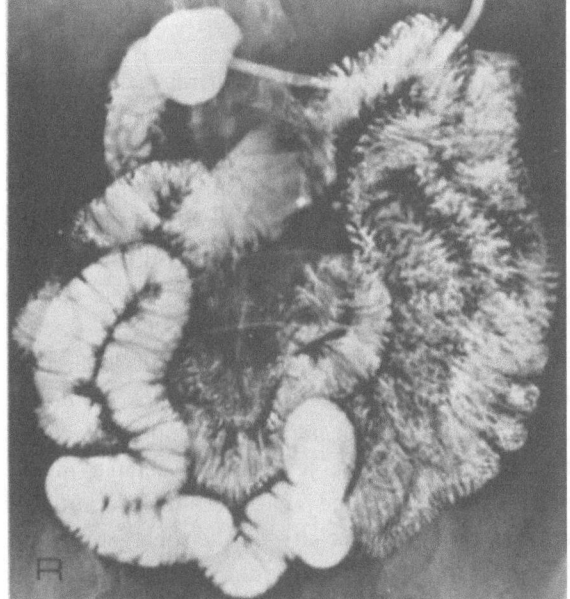

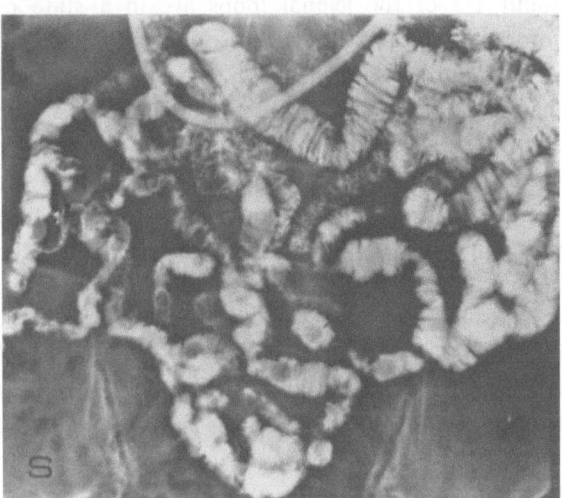

Fig. 8.57
In normal patients about 1/3 of the loops visualized on a survey exposure are in a state of contraction.

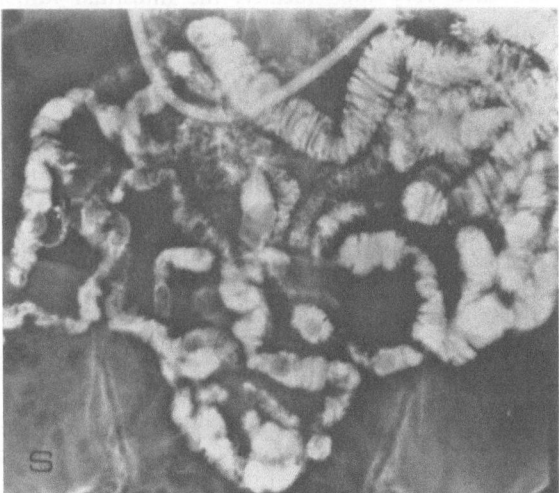

Fig. 8.58
In the event of hypermotility of the intestine, about 2/3 of the loops (R) and sometimes even more (S, T) are in a state of contraction and the diameter of the intestine is usually somewhat smaller than normal.

9. Motility

The enteroclysis technique, whereby the rate of flow of the contrast fluid is the same for all patients, has enabled us to compare the ability of various patients to expel this fluid stream in a distal direction. We have found that if peristalsis is normal the cecum is reached in 6–10 minutes and the amount of contrast fluid required is 600–900 ml. During fluoroscopy it is noted that peristalsis is most active in the jejunum, particularly in the proximal half. Furthermore when these peristaltic movements are abnormal, whether overactive or diminished, this is easiest to see in the jejunum. A change in the motility of the intestine is easily established not only under fluoroscopy but also on the roentgenograms. On the survey films taken during the enteroclysis examination, it appears that in normal patients about 1/3 of the jejunal loops are in a state of contraction (fig. 8.57). In cases of so-called 'intestinal hurry' the cecum is reached in much less than 6 minutes and sometimes less than 600 ml contrast fluid are required. Moreover, on the x-rays it can be seen that the intestinal loops are on the average several mm narrower than normal and that now 2/3, and sometimes even more, of the jejunal loops are in a state of contraction (fig. 8.58).

Although by far less common than a general intestinal hurry which involves the entire small intestine and often also the colon, a very local hyperperistalsis can sometimes be seen on the roentgenograms as well as during fluoroscopy. The tone of the musculature of the intestinal wall is then also very high locally; the intestinal lumen is narrow and the folds of Kerkring lie together producing an exceedingly fine feathered pattern (fig. 8.59).

This type of local spasticity can be encountered for example in cases of parasitosis, allergic reactions to food substances, adjacent carcinoids and inflammatory processes. A very local hyperperistalsis also occurs in those diseases which are accompanied by a slight anoxia such as minute or moderate vascular occlusions, intermittent herniation and after local radiotherapy.

Often local stimulation of the intestine is also accompanied by an enhanced mucus production in the same region; this can be seen on the x-rays as a very local clump formation in the contrast fluid (fig. 8.55).

A local spasticity of a completely different nature is the so-called 'string sign' in Crohn's disease (fig. 8.60P). Here the intestinal wall is greatly thickened as a result of hypertrophy of the musculature; the mucous membrane has been totally destroyed by the inflammatory process and has become an ulcerating surface. There is no question of peristalsis in this case; the involved intestinal segment exists as a whole in a prolonged state of contraction and relaxes only slightly every once in a while. This then is not a true stenosis, as believed previously; moreover, the prestenotic dilatation is also missing. It will be obvious that the chance of visualizing the string sign is considerably greater in the contraction phase than during a dilatation. The fluoroscopic findings can therefore be very important in establishing the true nature of these apparent stenosis. More prolonged contractions of an entire intestinal segment are rare in the jejunum, especially when no other abnormalities can be demonstrated in the intestinal wall or the mucosa (fig. 8.60Q). The reverse, decreased motility and a somewhat larger average diameter of the intestinal lumen, is seen even more often than intestinal hurry (see also chapter XII). It takes much longer for the contrast medium to reach the cecum and the amount required is also considerably greater. On the x-ray it is obvious that only a few loops are in a state of contraction (fig. 8.61). If the decrease in or even absence of peristaltic movements and the dilatation are only local or if the dilatation shows sacculations, the possibility of scleroderma must also be considered, even if none of the abnormalities characteristic of this disease are found in the esophagus and even if no ectodermal abnormalities can be discerned.

Fig. 8.59
Three examples of local spasticity of the intestine with feathery mucosal folds.   ➔

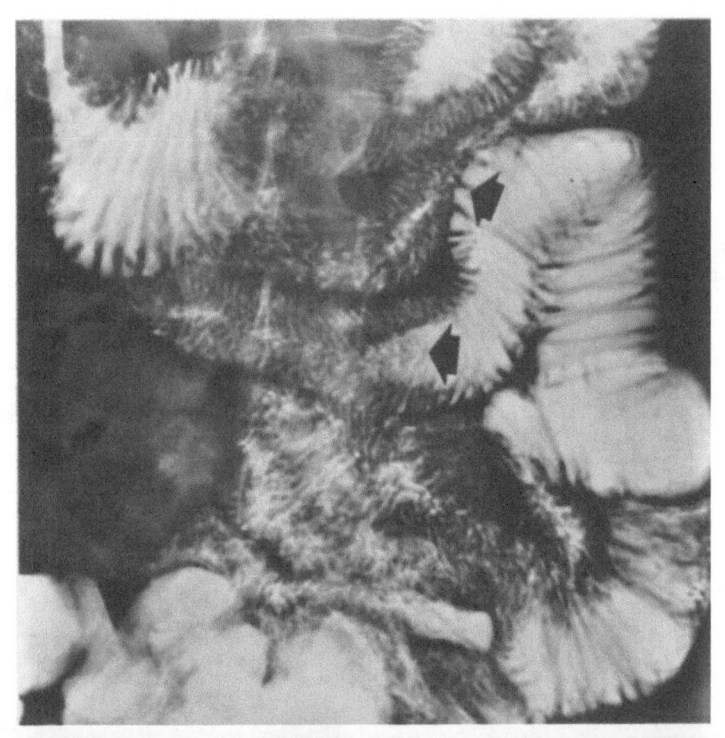

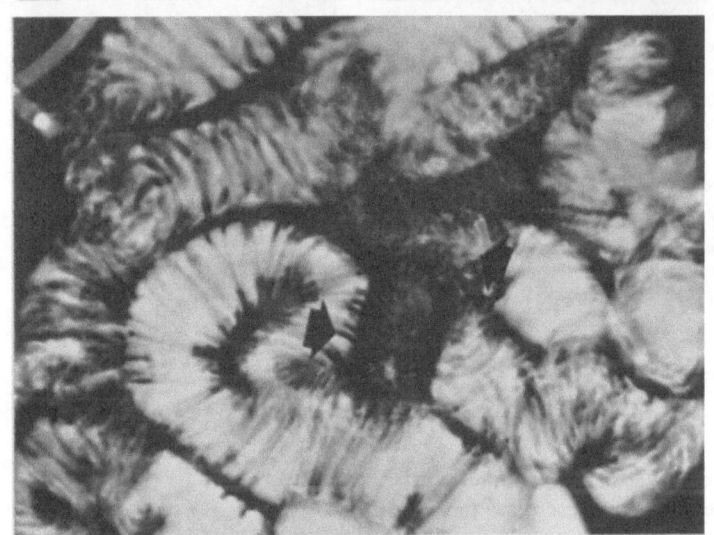

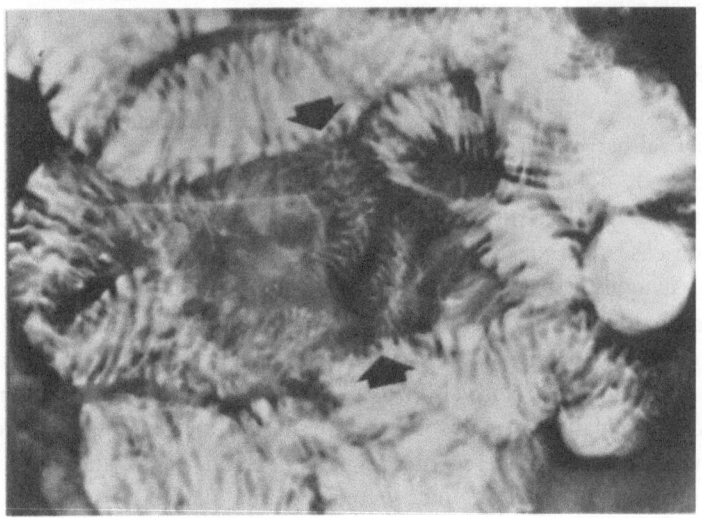

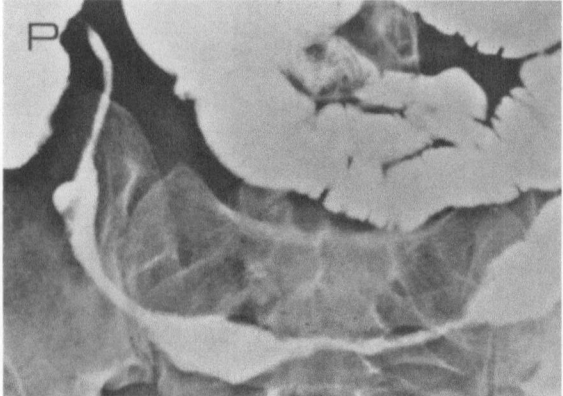

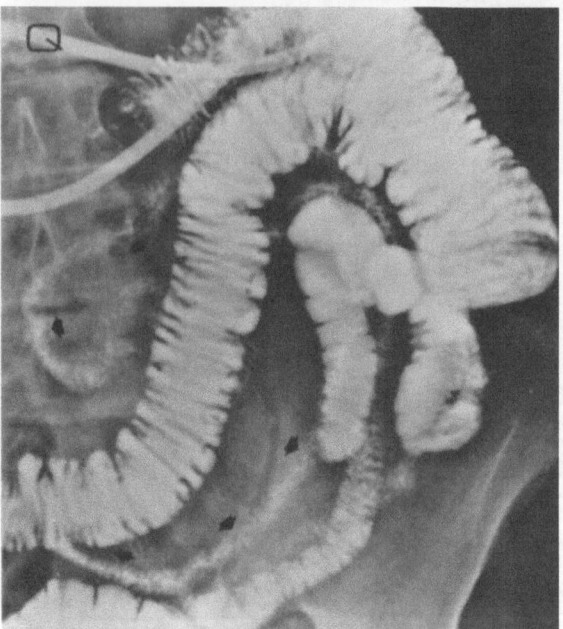

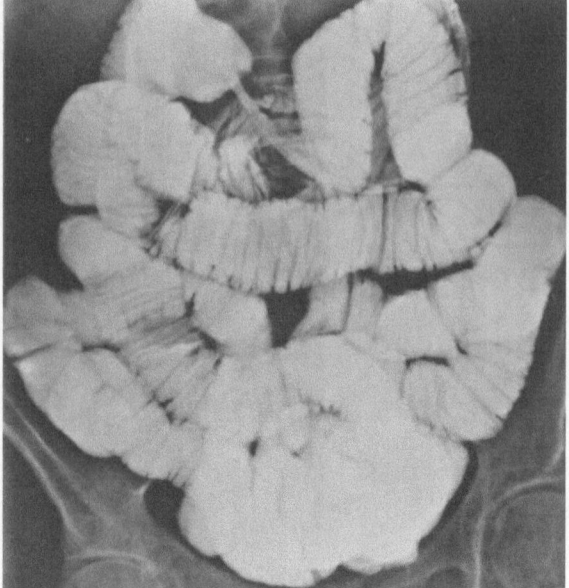

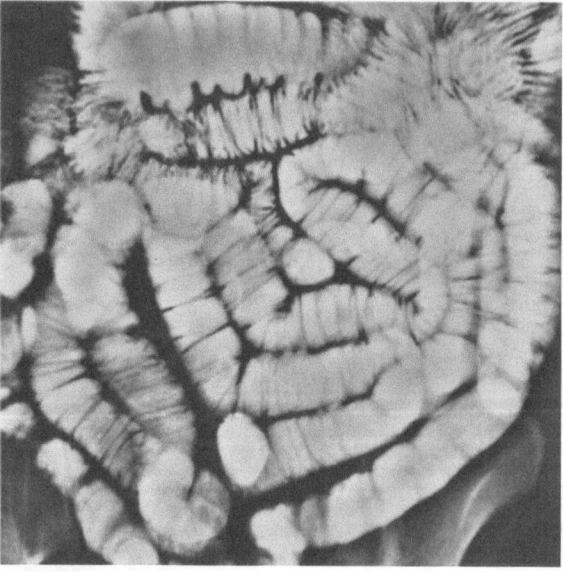

Fig. 8.60

P. Local spasticity or 'string sign' in Crohn's disease.
Q. Spasms of an entire intestinal segment are rare in the jejunum. No abnormalities of the mucosa or intestinal wall could be seen in this patient. Etiology unknown.

Fig. 8.61

In hypomotility of the intestine, very few loops are in a state of contraction and in addition the lumen of the intestine is clearly dilated. Both patients had used vagotonics for years.

It will be clear that decreased peristalsis and dilated intestinal loops, as well as a highly contractile intestine and a narrow caliber, will as a rule occur together. This is, however, not true in Whipple's disease, pancreatogenic steatorrhea (fig. 8.62) and in particular in certain cases of celiac disease (see page 316) when there is a highly active peristalsis and obviously dilated intestinal loops. In celiac disease, this causes a very characteristic x-ray pattern (fig. 8.63) which is observed almost exclusively with enteroclysis since total flocculation usually occurs when the contrast medium is administered orally. We have found that intestinal hurry is only accom-

panied by a small caliber when the hyperperistalsis is either neurogenic or humoral in origin.

If, on the other hand a true malabsorption exists, that is ·a diminished resorption of food substances, then the hyperperistalsis is found together with a dilated lumen. This hyperperistalsis is probably due to an increase in the intestinal contents which in turn is a result of the absorption of fluid from the intestinal wall and the enhanced secretion of intestinal juices.

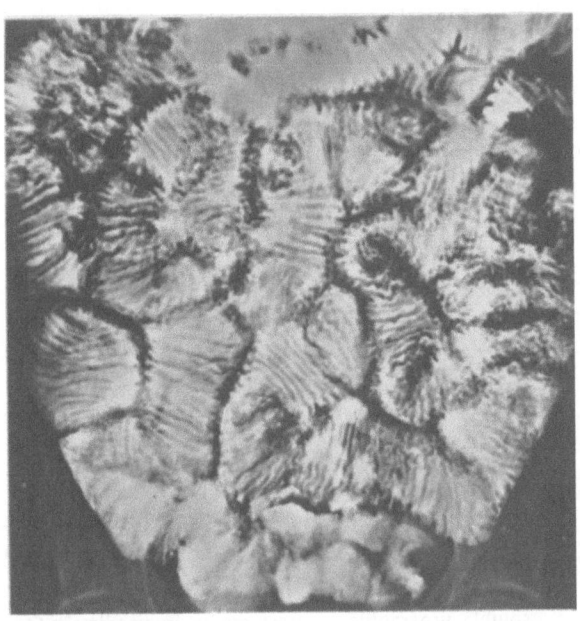

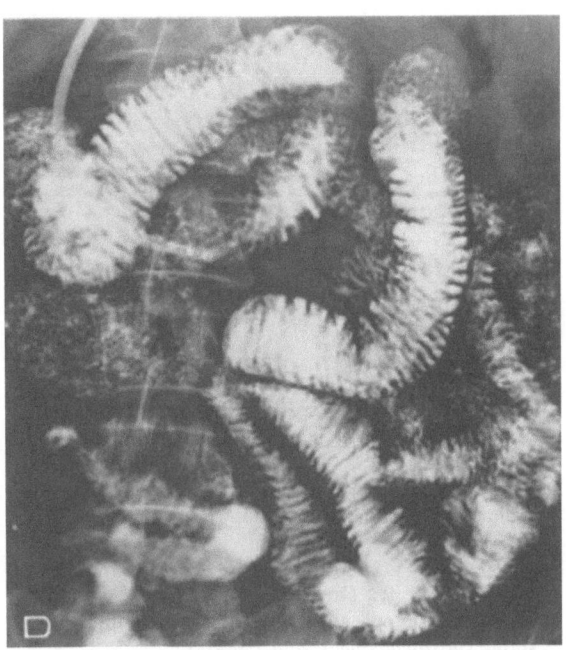

Fig. 8.63
Pattern characteristic of certain cases of celiac disease.
Increased motility and obviously dilated loops.

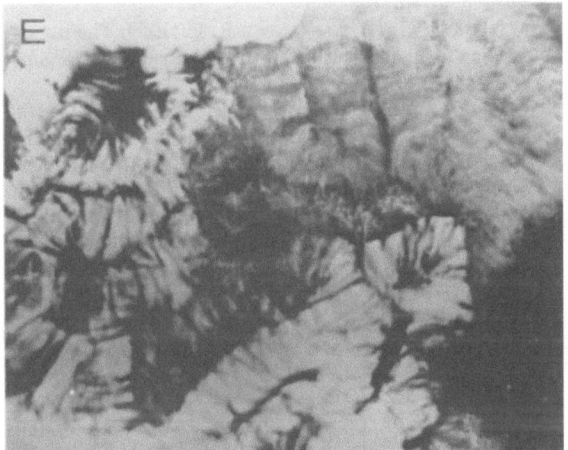

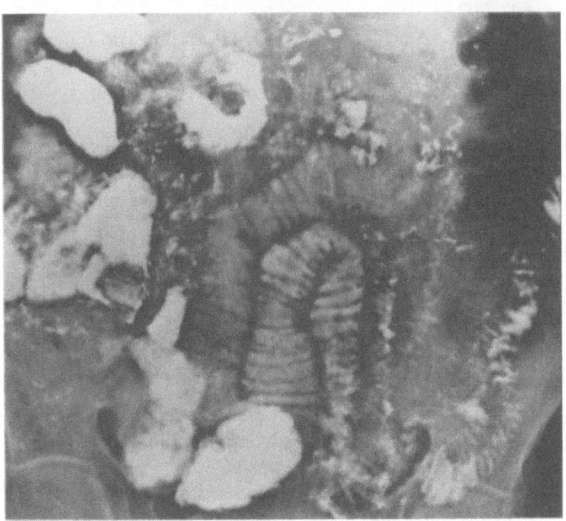

Fig. 8.62
Hypermotility of the intestine accompanied by a dilated
lumen in pancreatogenic steatorrhea (D). The conventional
examination of the same patients showed only dilution and
marked flocculation of the contrast fluid (E).

Bibliography chapter I-VIII

1. ABBOTT O.; PENDERGRASS E. P. (1936) Intubation studies of the human small intestine. *Amer. J. Roentg. 35*, 289–299.
2. ADAM, A. (1932) Kontrastmittel und Innenwanddarstellung des Verdauungstraktes. *Fortschritte R. 45/4*, 385–396.
3. ADLERSBERG D.; MARSHAK R. H.; COLCHER H.; DRACHMAN S. R.; FRIEDMAN A. I.; WANG C. I. (1954) The roentgenologic appearance of the small intestine in sprue. *Gastroenterology 26/4*, 548–581.
4. ADOLPH W.; TAPLIN G. V. (1950) Use of micropulverized barium sulfate in x-ray diagnosis. A preliminary report. *Radiology 54/6*, 878–883.
5. ALEXANDER G. H.; ALEXANDER R. E. (1950) The use of gastric mucin as a barium suspension medium. *Radiology 54/6*, 875–877.
6. ALISTER MC. W. H.; ANDERSON S.; BLOOMBERG G. R.; MARGULIS A. R. (1963) Lethal effects of tannic acid in the barium enema. Report of three fatalities and experimental studies. *Radiology 80/5*, 765–773.
7. AMENT M. E.; RUBIN C. E. (1972) Relation of Giardiasis to abnormal intestinal structure and function in gastrointestinal immunodeficiency syndromes. *Gastroenterology 62*, 216–226.
8. ANDERSON Ch. M.: ASTLEY R.; FRENCH J. M. and GERRARD J. W. (1952) The small intestine pattern in coeliac disease. *Brit. J. Radiol. 25*, 526–530.
9. ARDRAN G. M.; FRENCH J. M.; MUCKLOW E. H. (1950) Relationship of the nature of the opaque medium to small intestine radiographic pattern. *Brit. J. Radiol. 23*, 697–702.
10. ARENS R. A.; MESIROW S. D. (1937) Gastric mucosal relief. A modified sedimentation method, using a colloidally suspended bariumsulphate. *Radiology 29*, 1–11.
11. ASTLEY R.; FRENCH J. M. (1950) The small intestine pattern in normal children and in coeliac disease. Its relationship to the nature of the opaque medium. *Brit. J. Radiol. 24*, 321–330.
12. BARCLAY A. E. (1938) The practical importance of mechanics in digestion. *Amer. J. Roentg. 40*, 325–334.
13. BARDEN R. P.; THOMPSON W. D.; RAVDIN I. S.; FRANK I. L. (1938) The influence of the serum protein on the motility of the small intestine. *Surg. Gynec. Obstet. 66/5*, 819–821.
14. BEERSTECHER H. J. P. (1973) *De ileo-rectale anastomose bij de chirurgische behandeling van colitis ulcerosa.* Thesis, Leiden.
15. BENDICK A. J. (1954) *Diagnostic advances in gastrointestinal roentgenology.* New York.

16. BERGER G. (1968) Erfahrungen über die Verwendung von Visotrast in der Kinderklinik. (In der Magen-Darm-Diagnostik bei Kindern). *Dtsch. Gesundh.-Wes. 23/8*, 356–360.
17. BERKOVITS L.; JAVOR T. (1965) Über die Untersuchung des Dünndarms mit Enteramin. *Fortschritte R. 103/1*, 60–62.
18. BERMAN C. Z.; AVNET N. L. (1960) The use of water soluble urographic contrast media in paediatric G.I. studies. *Brit. J. Radiol. 33/386*, 92–97.
19. BILBAO M. K.; FRISCHE L. H.; DOTTER CH. T.; RÖSCH J. (1967) Hypotonic duodenography. *Radiology 89*, 438–443.
20. BOURDON R.; HUMMEL J. (1956) Basis de la radiologie du grêle. *J. Radiol. Electr. 37/3–4*, 210–215.
21. BOUSLOG J. S. (1942) The normal stomach and small intestine in the infant. *Radiology 39*, 253–260.
22. BOUSLOG J. S. (1937) The gastro-intestinal tract in children. *Radiology 28*, 683–692.
23. BRAECKMAN P. (1947) Over suspensies met bariumsulfaat. *Pharm. Weekblad 49/50*, 709–719.
24. BROWN F. O. (1959) On routine barium examination of the small bowel. *Lancet 2*, 530–533.
25. BROWN G. R. (1963) High-density barium-sulfate suspensions; an improved diagnostic medium. *Radiology 81/5*, 839–846.
26. BUFFARD P. (1952) Le diagnostic des tumeurs de l'intestin grêle est-il possible dans le pratique radiologique quotidienne? *J. Radiol. Electr. 33/1–2*, 64–66.
27. BUFFARD P.; CROZET L. (1952) Zur Dünndarmallergie. *Fortschritte R. 76/4*, 497–507.
28. BUGYI B. (1955) Praktische Beiträge zur röntgenologischen Untersuchung der Verdauungsorgane. *Röntgenblätter 8/4*, 107–111.
29. BULATAO E.; CARLSON A. J. (1924) Contributions to the physiology of the stomach. Influence of experimental changes in blood sugar level on gastric hunger contractions. *Amer. J. Physiol. 69*, 107–115.
30. BURHENNE J. H.; VOGELAAR P.; ARKOFF R. S. (1966) Liver function studies in patients receiving enema's containing tannic acid. *Amer. J. Roentg. 96/2*, 510–518.
31. BUSSCHER G. DE (1950) Étude radiologique du grêle au cours de diverses affections. *Acta gastroent. belg. 13/4*, 295–350.
32. CALDWELL W. L.; FLOCH M. H. (1963) Evaluation of the small bowel barium motor meal with emphasis on the effect of volume of barium suspensions ingested. *Radiology 80/3*, 383–391.
33. CALDWELL W. L.; SWANSON V. L.; BAYLESS TH. M. (1965) The importance and reliability of the roentgen-

ographic examination of the small bowel in patients with tropical sprue. *Radiology 84/2*, 227–240.

34. CAMERON A. L. (1938 II) Primary malignancy of the jejunum and ileum. *Ann. of Surg. 108*, 203–220.

35. CHAMBERLIN G. W. (1939 II) The roentgen anatomy of the small intestine. *J. Amer. med. Ass. 113*, 1537–1541.

36. CLURE MC. C. W.; REYNOLDS L.; SCHWARTZ C. O. (1920) On the behavior of the pyloric sphincter in normal man. *Arch. int. Med. 26*, 410–423.

37. COLE, and collaborators (1932) Findings observed in the gastro-intestinal tract. *Radiology 18*, 886–941.

38. CROHN B. B.; GINZBURG L.; OPPENHEIMER G. D. (1932) Regional ileitis. A pathologic and clinical entity. *J. Amer. med. Ass. 99/16*, 1323–1329.

39. CROWLEY R. T.; JOHNSTON CH. G. (1946) Physiological principles in intestinal obstruction. *Surg. Clin. N. Amer.* 1427–1439.

40. CUMMACK D. H. (1969) *Gastro-intestinal X-ray diagnosis.* Livingstone, Edinburgh.

41. CUMMINS A. J.; ALMY T. P. (1953) Studies on the relationship between motility and absorption in the human small intestine. *Gastroenterology 23*, 179–190.

42. DEUCHER W. G. (1949) Über die Variabilität der Dünndarmschleimhaut. *Radiol. clin.* (Basel) *18/1*, 265–272.

43. DINER W. C. (1968) Small intestinal edema in cirrhosis; its disappearance with diuresis. *Radiology 91*, 792–794.

44. DONATO H.; MAYO JR. H. W.; BARR L. H. (1954) The effect of peroral barium in partial obstruction of the small bowel. *Surgery 35/5*, 719–723.

45. EMBRING G.; MATTSSON O. (1968) Barium contrast agents. *Acta radiol. 7/NS diagn. 3*, 245–256.

46. EMBRING G.; MATTSSON O. (1966) An improved physiologic contrast medium for the alimentary tract. *Acta radiol. 4/NS*, 105–109.

47. EPSTEIN B. S. (1957) The use of a water soluble contrast medium (Hypaque) for gastrointestinal roentgenography. *J. Amer. med. Ass. 165*, 44–46.

48. ETTINGER A. J. H. (1949) Small intestinal pattern in sprue and similar deficiency diseases. *Amer. J. Roentg. 61/5*, 658–670.

49. FABIAN M.; LAKOS A.; FEHER I. (1966) Passagebeschleunigende Methoden zur röntgenologischen Untersuchung des Darmtraktes. *Röntgenblätter 19/1*, 58–64.

50. FIGIEL S. J.; FIGIEL L. S. (1964) Tumors of the terminal ileum. Diagnosis by retrograde filling during barium enema study. *Amer. J. Roentg. 91*, 816–818.

51. FISCHER A. W. (1925) Uber die Röntgenuntersuchung des Dickdarms mit Hilfe einer Kombination von Lufteinblasung und Kontrasteinlauf. ('Kombinierte Methode'). *Archiv klin. Chir. 134*, 209–269.

52. FLACH A. (1949) Vergleichende Untersuchungen über die Viscosität, Oberflächenspannung und Grenzflächenspannung verschiedener Kontrastmittel. *Röntgenblätter 2/6*, 303–310.

53. FLOCH M. H.; CALDWELL W. L.; SHEEHY T. W. (1962) A histopathologic basis for the interpretation of small bowel roentgenography in tropical sprue. *Amer. J. Roentg. 87/4*, 709–716.

54. FORSSELL G. (1923) Studies of the mechanism of movement of the mucous membrane of the digestive tract. *Amer. J. Roentg. 2*, 87–104.

55. FORSSELL G. (1939) Role of autonomous movements of the gastrointestinal mucous membrane in digestion. *Amer. J. Roentg. 41*, 145–165.

56. FOUBERT F.; ROBERT F. (1951) Intérêt d'un nouveau support de produit de contraste dans le radiodiagnostic digestif: la Carboxy-Méthyl-Cellulose. *J. Radiol. Electr. 32*, 925.

57. FRAZER A. C.; FRENCH J. M.; THOMPSON M. D. (1949) Radiographic studies showing the induction of a segmentation pattern in the small intestine in normal human subjects. *Brit. J. Radiol. 22/255*, 123–136.

58. FRENCH J. M. (1950) Further studies in the radiology of the small intestine. *Gastroenterologia* (Basel) *76/6*, 343–345.

59. FRIEDENBERG M. J.; ALISTER MC. W. H.; MARGULIS A. R. (1962) Roentgen study of the small bowel in adults and children with neostigmine. *Amer. J. Roentg. 88/4*, 693–701.

60. FRIEDMAN J. (1954) Roentgen studies of the effects on the small intestine from emotional disturbances. *Amer. J. Roentg. 72*, 367–379.

61. FRIEDMAN J.; RIGLER L. G. (1950) A method of double-contrast roentgen examination of the small intestine. *Radiology 54*, 365–379.

62. FRIK K.; BLÜHBAUM TH. (1928) Eine neue Anwendungsart der Kolloide in der Röntgendiagnostik. *Fortschritte R. 38/6*, 1111–1120.

63. FRIMAN-DAHL J. (1954) The administration of barium orally in acute obstruction; advantages and risks. *Acta Radiol. 42*, 285–295.

64. FURNEMONT E. (1966) L'utilisation du Sorbitol dans l'exploration radiologique du tractus intestinal. *Acta gastroent. belg. 24/8–9*, 779–790.

65. GERSHON-COHEN J.; SHAY H. (1939) Barium enteroclysis. A method for the direct immediate examination of the small intestine by single and double contrast techniques. *Amer. J. Roentg. 42/3*, 456–458.

66. GERSHON-COHEN J.; SHAY H.; FELS S. S. (1940) The relation of meal temperature to gastric motility and secretion. *Amer. J. Roentg. 43/2*, 237–242.

67. GERSHON-COHEN J.; SHAY H.; FELS S. S. (1938) Experimental studies on gastric physiology in man. The influence of osmotic pressure changes of salt and sugar solutions on pyloric action and gastric emptying in the normal and operated stomach. *Amer. J. Roentg. 40*, 335–343.

68. GERSHON-COHEN J.; SHAY H. (1937) Experimental studies on gastric physiology in man. A study of pyloric control. The rôle of milk and cream in the normal and in subjects with quiescent duodenal ulcer. *Amer. J. Roentg. 38*, 427–446.

69. GIANTURCO C. (1950) Fast radiological visceral survey. *Radiology 54*, 59–64.

70. GIRAND M.; BRET P.; PINET F.; ROCHE P. (1951) L'examen radiologique du grêle par transit accéléré. *J. Radiol. Electr. 32/7–8*, 583–595.

71. GLASER F. H.; KÖLLING H. L. (1967) Beitrag zur peroralen Magen-Darm-Diagnostik mit Bariumsulfat-Amidotrizoat-Gemischen. *Radiol. diagn.* (Berl.) *8*, 13–22.

72. GOIN L. S. (1952) Some obscure factors in the production of unusual small bowel patterns. *Radiology 59/2*, 177–184.

73. GOLDEN R. (1951) Advances in gastro-enterological radiology 1937–1950. *Brit. J. Radiol. 24*, 237–245.

74. GOLDEN R. (1959) Technical factors in the roentgen examination of the small intestine. *Amer. J. Roentg. 82/6*, 965–972.

75. GOLDEN R. (1959) *Radiologic examination of the small intestine.* second ed. Lippincott, Philadelphia.

76. GOLDEN R. (1941) Abnormalities of the small intestine in nutritional disturbances. *Radiology 36*, 262–286.

77. GOLDEN R. (1950) Some clinical problems in small intestinal physiology. *Brit. J. Radiol. 23*, 390–409.

78. GOOD A. (1963) Tumors of the small intestine. *Amer. J. Roentg. 89*, 685–705.

79. GREENSPON E. A.; LENTINO W. (1960) Retrograde enterography. A new method for the roentgenologic study of the small bowel. *Amer. J. Roentg. 83/5*, 909–919.

80. GRIER T.; MILLER; KARR W. G. (1936) Intubation studies of the human small intestine. The influence of variations in the reaction and the motility of the stomach contents on the reaction and the motility of the intestinal contents. *Amer. J. Roentg. 35*, 300–305.

81. GRYBOSKI J. D.; SELF T. W.; CLEMENT A.; et al. (1968) Selective immunoglobulin A deficiency and intestinal nodular lymphoid hyperplasia: Correction of diarrhea with antibiotics and plasma. *Pediatrics 42*, 833–837.

82. HAFTER ERNST (1973) *Praktische Gastroenterologie.* Thieme, Stuttgart.

83. HANAFEE W.; WEINER M. (1967) External guided passage of an intestinal intubation tube. *Radiology 89*, 1100–1102.

84. HARRIS P. D.; NEUHAUSER E. B. D.; GERTH R. (1964) The osmotic effect of water soluble contrast media on circulating plasma volume. *Amer. J. Roentg. 91/3*, 694–698.

85. HECHT G. (1934) *Heubners Handbuch der experimentellen Pharmakologie 8*, 97. Springer, Berlin.

86. HEITZMAN R. E.; BERNE A. S. (1961) Roentgen examination of the cecum and proximal ascending colon with ingested barium. *Radiology 76*, 415–421.

87. HENDERSON N. P. (1944) The value of the opaque enema and its modifications. *Brit. J. Radiol. 17*, 140–149.

88. HENDERSON S. G. (1942) The gastrointestinal tract in the healthy newborn infant. *Amer. J. Roentg. 48*, 302–335.

89. HIGHMAN J. H. (1964) Urinary excretion as a sign of intestinal perforation. *Brit. J. Radiol. 37*, 697–700

90. HIRSCH J.; AHRENS E.; BLANKENHORN D. H. (1956) Measurement of the human intestinal length in vivo and some causes of variation. *Gastroenterology 31*, 274–285.

91. HODGES F. J.; RUNDLESS R. W.; HANELIN J. (1947) I. Roentgenologic study of the small intestine. Neoplastic and inflammatory diseases. *Radiology 49*, 587–602.
II. Roentgenologic study of the small intestine. Dysfunction associated with neurologic diseases. *Radiology 49*, 659–673.

92. HODGSON J. R.; HOFFMAN H. N. II; HUIZENGA K. A. (1967) Roentgenologic features of lymphoid hyperplasia of the small intestine associated with dysgammaglobulinemia. *Radiology 88*, 883–888.

93. HOLT J. F.; LYONS R. H.; NELIGH R. B.; NOE G. K.; HODGES F. J. (1947) x-ray signs of altered alimentary function following autonomic blockade with tetraethylammonium. *Radiology 49/5*, 603–610.

94. HOLZKNECHT G. (1931) *Handbuch der theoretischen und klinischen Röntgenkunde.* Wien.

95. HOWARTH F. H.; COCKEL R.; ROPER B. W.; HAWKINS C. F. (1969) The effect of metoclopramide upon gastric motility and its value in barium progress meals. *Clin. radiol. 20*, 294–300.

96. HUDAK A. (1951) Le transit accéléré du grêle. *Radiol. clin.* (Basel) *20/3*, 148–154.

97. HÜPCHER N. (1961) Het gebruik van bariumsulfaat-suspensies, in het bijzonder tylosebarium in de tractus digestivus. *J. belge Radiol. 44/2*, 161–169.

98. JAMES W. B.; HUME R. (1968) Action of metoclopramide on gastric emptying and small bowel transit time. *Gut 9*, 203–205.

99. JANOWER M. L.; ROBBINS L. L.; TOMCHIK F. S.; WEYLMAN W. T. (1965) Tannic acid and the barium enema. *Radiology 85/5*, 887–894.

100. JEFFRIES G. H.; WESER E.; SLEISINGER M. H. (1964) Progress in gastroenterology. Malabsorption. *Gastroenterology 46*, 434–466.

101. JOHNSTON C. G.; RAVDIN I. S. (1935, I) Action of glucose on emptying of stomach. Effect of varying concentrations in both normal stomachs and after various gastric operations. *Amer. Surg. 101*, 500–505.

102. JOLLASSE (1907) Zur Motilitätsprüfung des Magens durch Röntgenstrahlen. *Fortschritte R. 11*, 47–53.

103. JONES G. E.; CHALECKE W. E.; DEC J.; SCHILLING J. A.; RAMSEY G. H.; ROBERTSON H. D.; STRAIN W. H. (1947) Jodinated organic compounds as contrast media for radiographic diagnosis. Studies on tetraiodophthalimidoethanol as a medium for gastrointestinal visualization. *Radiology 49/2*, 143–151.

104. KAESTLE (1907) Bolus alba und Bismutum subnitricum, eine für die röntgenologische Untersuchung des Magen-Darmkanals brauchbare Mischung. *Fortschritte R. 11*, 266–271.

105. KANTOR J. L. (1939) The roentgendiagnosis of idiopathic steatorrhea and allied conditions. Practical value of the 'Moulage sign'. *Amer. J. Roentg. 41/5*, 758–778.

106. KAUFMANN H. J. (1969) *Progress in Pediatric Radiology-* Vol. 2, Gastro-intestinal Tract. S. Karger, Basel.

107. KHILNANI M. T.; KELLER R. J.; CUTTNER J. (1969) Macroglobulinemia and steatorrhea: Roentgen and pathologic findings in the intestinal tract. *Radiol. Clin. N.A. 7*, 43–55.

108. KING C. E.; ARNOLD L. (1922) The activities of the intestinal mucosal motor mechanism. *Amer. J. Physiol. 59*, 97–121.

109. KIRSH I. E. (1956) Motility of the small intestine with non-flocculating medium; A review of 173 roentgen examinations. *Gastroenterology 31*, 251–260.

110. KIRSH I. E.; SPELLBERG M. A. (1953) Examination of small intestine with carboxymethylcellulose. *Radiology 60*, 701–707.

111. KNOEFEL P. K.; DAVIS L. A.; PILLA L. A. (1956) Agglomeration of barium sulfate and roentgen visualisation of the gastric mucosa. *Radiology 67/1*, 87–91.

112. KNOX R. (1919) *Radiography and radio-therapeutics.* E. and C. Black Ltd., London.

113. KORPASSY B.; HORVAI R.; KOLTAY M. (1951) On the absorption of tannic acid from the gastrointestinal tract. *Arch. int. Pharmacodyn. 88*, 368–377.

114. KUNZ B.; LEMM M.; HAUBACH D. (1965) Die Verwendung von „Visotrast 370" in der Magen-Darm Diagnostik. *Dtsch. Gesundh.-Wes. 20/13*, 593–595.

115. LAFONTAINE A. (1965) Danger de l'acide tannique utilisé en lavement. *J. belge Radiol. 48/5*, 551–555.

116. LAREN MC. J. W. (1960) *Modern trends in diagnostic radiology. Third series. Examination of the small bowel* by W. G. Scott Harden 84–87. Butterworths, London.

117. LÄSER S. (1966) Verbesserungen der Eigenschaften von

Bariumsulfatsuspensionen für die Magen-Darm-Passage durch Zusatz von Polysaccharidlösungen. *Schweiz. med. Wschr. 96/19*, 633–638.

118. LAWS J. W.; NEALE G. (1966) Radiological diagnosis of disaccharidase deficiency. *Lancet II*, 139–143.

119. LAWS J. W.; PITMAN R. G. (1960) The radiological investigation of malabsorption syndromes. *Brit. J. Radiol. 33*, 211–228.

120. LAWS J. W.; SHAWDON.H.; BOOTH C. C.; STEWART J. S. (1963) Correlation of radiological and histological findings in idiopathic steatorrhea. *Brit. med. J. May*, 1311–1314.

121. LEB A. (1951) Eine Röntgen-Digestionsprüfung. Die Röntgenuntersuchung des resezierten Magens mit Eiweiss- und Fett- Bariumkernen. *Fortschritte R. 75*, 106–116.

122. LEDOUX-LEBARD G. (1968) Histoire de la radiologie du tube digestif. *Gaz. med. Fr. 75/2*, 209–216.

123. LEHNER H. H.; MÄRKI W.; ZIMMER E. A. (1948–49) Ueber ein neues Barium-Kontrastmittel, zugleich ein Beitrag zur Prüfung solcher Substanzen. *Gastroenterologia* (Basel) *74/4*, 193–208.

124. LENZ H. (1962) Weitere Untersuchungen zur Funktionsanalyse der Dünndarmperistaltik. *Fortschritte R. 97/2*, 147–159.

125. LENZ H. (1962) Die Segmentationsbewegungen des Ileums im Röntgenkinobild. *Fortschritte R. 97/2*, 159–168.

126. LENZ H.; KREPPEL E. (1965) Röntgenkinematographische Untersuchungen über das Verhalten der Dünndarmmotorik bei der Katze unter Prostigmin, Pilocarpin und Arecolin. *Fortschritte R. 102/3*, 268–277.

127. LESSMAN F. P.; LILIENFELD R. M. (1959) Gastrografin as water soluble medium in roentgenexamination of the G.I. tract. *Acta radiol. 51/3*, 170–178.

128. LETTERS K.; GAUL M. (1951) Neue Untersuchungen zur Charakterisierung von Röntgenkontrastmittel für Magen und Darm. *Fortschritte R. 74/2*, 229–234.

129. LIERE E. J. v.; NORTHUYS D. W.; CLIFFORD S. J. (1946) The effect of glucose on the motility of the stomach and small intestine. *Gastroenterology 7*, 218–223.

130. LÖNNERBLAD L. (1951) Transit time through the small intestine. A roentgenologic study on normal variability. *Acta radiol.* suppl. 88.

131. LUMSDEN K.; TRUELOVE S. C. (1965) *Radiology of the digestive system*. Blackwell, Oxford.

132. LURA A. (1951) Radiology of the small intestine, Enema of the small intestine with special emphasis on the diagnosis of tumours. *Brit. J. Radiol. 24/281*, 264–271.

133. MAGNUSSON W. (1931) On meteorism in pyelography and on the passage of gas through the small intestine. *Acta radiol. 12*, 552–561.

134. MANECKE H.; SCHMIDT F. W. (1962) Die Magen-Darm-Passage mit Karion. *Fortschritte R. 97/2*, 142–146.

135. MARETIC Z.; HOMADOVSKI K.; RAZBOJNIKOV S.; BRECEVIC V. (1957) Barium poisoning. Ein Beitrag zur Kenntnis von Vergiftung mit Barium. *Med. Klin. 52/45*, 1950–1953.

136. MARGULIS A. R. (1967) Some new approaches to the examination of the gastro intestinal tract. *Amer. J. Roentg. 101*, 265–286.

137. MARGULIS A. R.; MANDELSTAM P. (1961) The use of parenteral neostigmine in the roentgen study of the small bowel. *Radiology 76*, 223–229.

138. MARGULIS A. R.; BURHENNE H. J. (1967) *Alimentary tract roentgenology*. C. V. Mosby Company, St. Louis.

139. MARSHAK R. H. (1961) Roentgen findings in lesions of the small bowel. *Amer. J. dig. Dis. 6*, 1084–1114.

140. MARSHAK R. H.; LINDNER A. E. (1970) *Radiology of the small intestine*. Saunders, Philadelphia.

141. MARSHAK R. H.; LINDNER A. E. (1966) Malabsorption syndrome. *Seminars Roentg. 1/2*, 138–177.

142. MARSHAK R. H.; KHILNANI M.; ELIASOPH J.; WOLF B. S. (1967) Intestinal edema. *Amer. J. Roentg. 101/2*, 379–387.

143. MARSHAK R. H.; WOLF B. S.; COHEN N.; JANOWITZ H. D. (1961) Proteinlosing disorders of the gastrointestinal tract: Roentgen features. *Radiology 77/6*, 893–905.

144. MARSHAK R. H.; WOLF B. S.; ADLERSBERG D. (1954) Roentgenstudies of the small intestine in sprue. *Amer. J. Roentg. 72*, 380–400.

145. MARSHAK R. H.; FRIEDMAN A. J.; WOLF B. S.; CROHN B. B. (1951) Roentgen findings in ileo-jejunitis. *Gastroenterology 19/3*, 383–408.

146. MARSHAK R. H.; HAZZI CH.; LINDNER A. E.; MAKLANSKY D. (1975) The small bowel in immunoglobulin deficiency syndromes.

147. MARSHAK R. H.; RUOFF M.; LINDNER A. E. (1968) Roentgen manifestations of Giardiasis. *Am. J. Roentgenol. 104*, 557–560.

148. MARTEL W.; HODGES F. J. (1959) The small intestine in Whipple's disease. *Amer. J. Roentg. 81/4*, 623–636.

149. MATTSSON O.; PERMAN G.; LAGERLÖF H. (1960) The small intestine transit time with a physiologic contrast medium. *Acta radiol. 54*, 334–344.

150. MELLINK J. H. (1961) Radiophysical aspects of the use of contrast substances in radiodiagnosis. *J. belge Radiol. 44/2*, 107–126.

151. MENVILLE L. J.; ANÉ J. N. (1932) An x-ray study of the passage of different foodstuffs through the small intestine of man. *Radiology 18*, 783–786.

152. MILLER R. E.; BRAHME F. (1969) Large amounts of orally administered barium for obstruction of the small intestine. *Surg. Gyn. Obst. 129/6*, 1185–1188.

153. MILLER R. E.; MILLER W. J. (1966) Inflammatory lesions of the small bowel. Complete reflux small bowel examination. *Amer. J. Gastroent. 45*, 40–49.

154. MILLER R. E. (1965) Barium sulfate suspensions. *Radiology 84/2*, 241–251.

155. MILLER R. E. (1965) Complete reflux small bowel examination. *Radiology 84/3*, 457–463.

156. MORETON R. D.; YATES CH. W. (1950) The double-contrast study of the colon. A comparative study of barium sulfate preparations. *Radiology 54*, 541–547.

157. MORI P. A.; BARRETT H. A. (1962) A sign of intestinal perforation. *Radiology 79/3*, 401–407.

158. MORRISON B. O.; HALEY T. J.; PAYZANT A. R.; GENTNER G. A.; PAGON-CARLO J. (1959) Use of Hypaque as contrast medium in G.I. examination. *Amer. J. Gastroent. 31/4*, 398–407.

159. MORTON J. L. (1961) Notes on a small bowel examination. *Amer. J. Roentg. 86/1*, 76–85.

160. MÜLLER J. H. A. (1968) Die Röntgendiagnostik des Dünndarms mit Neostigmin. *Dtsch. Gesundh.-Wes. 23/9*, 391–397.

161. MUNTEAU E. (1951) Experimentelle Grundlagen einer röntgenologischen Eiweiss Digestionsprüfung. *Radiol. Austr. 4*, 187–199.

162. MURRAY J. P. (1966) Buscopan in diagnostic radiology of the alimentary tract. *Brit. J. Radiol. 39/458*, 102–111.

163. NAUMANN W. (1948) *Funktionelle Dünndarmdiagnostik im Röntgenbild.* Thieme, Stuttgart.

164. NELSON S. W.; CHRISTOFORIDIS A. J. (1967) The use of barium sulfate suspensions in the study of suspected mechanical obstruction of the small intestine. *Amer. J. Roentg. 101*, 367–378.

165. NELSON S. W.; CHRISTOFORIDIS A. J.; ROENIGK W. J. (1965) Dangers and fallibilities of jodinated radiopaque media in obstruction of the small bowel. *Amer. J. Surgery 109*, 546–559.

166. NICE CH. M. (1963) Roentgenographic pattern and motility in small bowel studies. *Radiology 80*, 39–45.

167. OSBORN ANNE G.; FRIEDLAND GERALD W. (1973) A radiological approach to the diagnosis of small bowel disease. *Clin. Radiol. 24*, 281–301.

168. PAJEWSKI M.; ITZCHAK Y.; PROFIS A. (1970) The double contrast examination of the small intestine. Preliminary communication of a new technique. *Clin. radiol. 21*, 83–86.

169. PANSDORF H. (1937) Die fraktionierte Dünndarmfüllung und ihre klinische Bedeutung. *Fortschritte R. 56*, 627–634.

170. PATTERSON D. E.; RAD M.; DAVID R.; BAKER S. J. (1965) Radiodiagnostic problems in malabsorption. *Brit. J. Radiol. 38/447*, 181–191.

171. PAULSON MOSES (1969) *Gastroenterologic medicine.* Lea and Febiger, Philadelphia.

172. PENDERGRASS E. P. (1936) The small intestine. *J. Amer. med. Ass. 107/23*, 1859–1861.

173. PENDERGRASS E.; RAVDIN I. S.; JOHNSTON C. G.; HODES P. J. (1936) The effect of foods and various pathologic states on the gastric emptying and the small intestinal pattern. *Radiology 26*, 651–662.

174. PEREZ C. A.; FRIEDENBERG M. J. (1967) Comparison of carboxy-methyl-cellulose, tannic-acid and no additive in barium examinations of the colon. *Amer. J. Roentg. 99/1*, 98–105.

175. PESQUERA G. S. (1929) A method for the direct visualization of lesions in the small intestines. *Amer. J. Roentg. 22/3*, 254–257.

176. PIRK F.; STÁHLAVSKA A.; CERNÁ M. (1967) Vergleich der Eigenschaften einiger Bariumkontrastmittel verschiedener Herkunft. *Radiol. diagn.* (Berl.) *8/6*, 773–780.

177. PIRK F.; VULTERINOVÁ M. (1964) The x-ray picture of the small intestine and impaired absorption. *Radiol. clin.* (Basel) *33/4*, 249–267.

178. POCK-STEEN O. C.; LORENZEN J. (1968) Gluten-intolerance and food allergy. Clinical signs and radiological changes of the small intestine. *Radiol. clin.* (Basel) *37/2*, 65–78.

179. PORCHER P.; CAROLI J. (1957) Un accélérateur inattendu du transit intestinal (grêle et colon). *Arch. Mal. Apper. dig. 46/7–8*, 663–665.

180. PORTIS S. A. (1941) The clinical significance of the roentgenological findings of the small intestine. *Radiology 37*, 289–293.

181. PREGER L.; AMBERG J. R. (1967) Sweet diarrhea. Roentgen diagnosis of disaccharidase deficiency. *Amer. J. Roentg. 101/2*, 287–295.

182. PRÉVÔT R. (1940) Ergebnisse röntgenologischer Dünndarmstudien unter besonderer Berücksichtigung der Morphologie. *Fortschritte R. 62/2*, 341–388.

183. PYGOTT F. (1958) *Modern trends in gastroenterology.* Butterworth, London.

184. PYGOTT F.; STREET D. F.; SHELLSHEAR M. F.; RHODES C. J. (1960) Radiological investigation of the small intestine by small bowel enema technique. *Gut 1*, 366–370.

185. RAIFORD TH. S. (1931) Tumors of the small intestine. Their diagnosis, with special reference to the x-ray appearance. *Radiology 16*, 253–270.

186. REIDELL H. (1937) Vergleichende Untersuchungen an Magen-Darmkontrastmitteln. *Fortschritte R. 56*, 653–662.

187 REINHARDT K. (1960) Untersuchungen über den Wert einer Sorbitolbeimischung zum Bariumbrei für die Röntgendarstellung des Darmtraktes. *Fortschritte R. 92*, 78–84.

188. REINHARDT J. F.; BARRY W. F. (1962) Scleroderma of the small bowel. *Amer. J. Roentg. 88/4*, 687–692.

189. REYNOLDS L.; MACY I. G.; HUNSCHER H.; OLSON M. B. (1940) The gastro-intestinal response of average, healthy children to test meals of barium in milk, cream, meat and carbohydrate media. *Amer. J. Roentg. 43/4*, 517–532.

190. RICE R. P.; ROUFAIL W. M.; REEVES R. J. (1967) The roentgen diagnosis of Whipple's disease (Intestinal lipodystrophy). *Radiology 88*, 295–301.

191. RIEDER H. (1904–05) Beiträge zur Topographie des Magen-Darmkanals beim lebenden Menschen, nebst Untersuchungen über den zeitlichen Ablauf der Verdauung. *Fortschritte R. 8*, 141–172.

192. ROBBINS L. L. (1969) *Goldens Diagnostic Radiology* – Section 5 – Digestive Tract. The Williams and Wilkins Company, Baltimore.

193. ROBINSON D.; LEVENE J. M. (1958) Oral Renografin: A new contrast medium for gastrointestinal tract. *Amer. J. Roentg. 80*, 79–81.

194. ROSEN R. S.; JACOBSON G. (1965) Visible urinary tract excretion following oral administration of water-soluble contrast-media. *Radiology 84/6*, 1031–1032.

195. RUBIN R. J.; OSTRUM B. J.; DEX W. J. (1960) Watersoluble contrast media. Their use in the diagnosis of obstructive gastrointestinal disease. *Arch. Surg. 80*, 495–500.

196. SACK G. M. (1963) Die orale Schnellpassage des Darms. *Fortschritte R. 99/3*, 337–342.

197. SCHATZKI R. (1943) Small intestinal enema. *Amer. J. Roentg. 50/6*, 743–751.

198. SCHÖNBAUER E. (1955) Mitteilung über die Verwendung von Baridol in der Magen-Darmdiagnostik. *Röntgenblätter 8*, 8–15.

199. SCOTT-HARDEN W. G.; HAMILTON H. A. R.; MC CALL SMITH S. (1961) Radiological investigation of the small intestine. *Gut 2*, 316–322.

200. SEARS A. D.; HAWKINS J.; KILGORE B. B.; MILLER J. E. (1964) Plain roentgenographic findings in drug induced intramural hematoma of the small bowel. *Amer. J. Roentg. 91*, 808–813.

201. SEIJSS R. (1961) High kV technique for gastro-intestinal diagnosis. *Röntgenblätter 14/2*, 54–56.

202. SHAY H.; GERSHON-COHEN J. (1934–6) Experimental studies in gastric physiology in man. A study of pyloric control. The rôles of acid and alkali. *Surg. Gynec. Obstet. L VIII*, 935–955.

203. SHEHADI W. H. (1963) Studies of the colon and small intestines with water-soluble jodinated contrast media. *Amer. J. Roentg. 89/4*, 740–751.

204. SHEHADI W. H. (1960) Orally administered watersoluble jodinated contrast media. *Amer. J. Roentg. 83*, 933–941.

205. SHIMKIN P. M.; WALDMAN T. A.; KRUGMAN R. L. (1970) Intestinal Lymphangiectasia. *Amer. J. Roentgenol. 110*, 827–841.

206. SHUFFLEBARGER H. E.; KNOEFEL P. K.; TELFORD J.; DAVIS L. A.; PIRKEY E. L. (1953–5) Some factors influencing the roentgen visualization of the mucosal pattern of the gastrointestinal tract. *Radiology 61*, 801–805.

207. SIDAWAY M. E. (1964) Use of water-soluble contrast medium in paediatric radiology. *Clin. radiol. 15/2*, 132–138.

208. SIELAFF H. J. (1970) Die Radiologische Diagnostik der Dünndarmerkrankungen. *Therapiewoche 20*, 3207–3215.

209. SINCLAIR D. J.; BUIST T. A. S. (1966) Instrumental and technical notes. Water contrast barium enema using methyl cellulose. *Brit. J. Radiol. 39/459*, 228–232.

210. SLEISENGER M. H.; FORDTRAN J. S. (1973) *Gastrointestinal Disease*. Saunders, Philadelphia.

211. SLOAN R. D.; BROCK J. W.; FANT W. M. (1961) Nonstrangulating distal ileal obstruction. The rôle of hydration. An experimental study correlating pathologic and radiologic findings. *Radiology 76*, 407–414.

212. SLOAN R. D. (1957) The mucosal pattern of the mesenteric small intestine; an anatomic study. *Amer. J. Roentg. 77/4*, 651–669.

213. SNELL A. M.; CAMP J. D. (1934) Chronic idiopathic steatorrhea. Roentgenologic observations. *Arch. int. Med. 53*, 615–629.

214. SÖVÉNYI E.; VARRÓ V. (1959) Uber eine neue Methode zur Röntgenuntersuchung des Dünndarms. *Fortschritte R. 91/2*, 269–270.

215. SPENCER R. P. (1961) Microvilli and intestinal surface area: An evaluation. *Gastroenterology 41*, 313–314.

216. STACY G. S.; LOOP J. W. (1964) Unusual small bowel diseases. Methods and observations. *Amer. J. Roentg. 92/5*, 1072–1079.

217. STECKEN A.; RICHTER K.; WEISS U. (1961) Zur Kontrastmitteldarstellung des Magen-Darm-Traktes. Ergebnisse von 117 Untersuchungen mit Gastrografin und Gastrografin-Bariumsulfat Gemischen. *Fortschritte R. 95/2*, 172–188.

218. STEINBACH H. L.; BURHENNE J. (1962) Performing the barium enema: Equipment, preparation and contrast medium. *Amer. J. Roentg. 87*, 644–654.

219. SUSSMAN M. L.; WACHTEL E. (1943) Factors concerned in the abnormal distribution of barium in the small bowel. *Radiology 40*, 128–138.

220. SWISCHUK L. E.; WELSH J. D. (1968) Roentgenographic mucosal patterns in the 'malabsorption syndrome'. A scheme for diagnosis. *Amer. J. dig. Dis. 13/1*, 59–78.

221. TACHEV T.; HADJIDEKOV G.; NEDKOVA-BRATANOVA N;. IJANEV S. (1967) Radiologic stigmata of allergic enteropathies. *Acta gastroent. belg. 30/3*, 209–224.

222. THORNER R. S. (1955) The effect of exclusion of the bile upon gastrointestinal motility. *Amer. J. Roentg. 74*, 1096–1122.

223. TOSCH R. (1961) Untersuchungen über die Resorption von J 131 markiertem Gastrografin aus dem Magen-Darm kanal. *Fortschritte R. 95/2*, 189–192.

224. TRUELOVE S. C.; REYNELL P. C. (1972) *Diseases of the Digestive System*, Blackwell. Oxford.

225. UNDERHILL B. M. L. (1955) Intestinal length in man. *Brit. med. J. 4950*, 1243–1246.

226. VEST B.; MARGULIS A. R. (1962) Roentgen diagnosis of postoperative ileus-obstruction. *Surg. Gyn. Obst. 115*, 421–427.

227. WEEL J. G. A. v.; WOUTERS J. O. (1963) Het meten van röntgencontraststoffen 'in vitro' door middel van röntgen-stralen. *J. belge Radiol. 46/5*, 481–489.

228. WEIGEN J. F.; PENDERGRASS E. P.; RAVDIN I. S.; MACHELLA T. E. (1952) A roentgen study of the effect of total pancreatectomy on the stomach and small intestine of the dog. *Radiology 59*, 92–102.

229. WEINTRAUB S.; WILLIAMS R. G. (1949) A rapid method of roentgenologic examination of the small intestine. *Amer. J. Roentg. 61*, 45–55.

230. WELTZ G. A. (1937) Der kranke Dünndarm im Röntgenbild. *Fortschritte R. 55*, 20–40.

231. WILSON J. P. (1967) Surface area of the small intestine in man. *Gut 8*, 618–621.

232. WOOLDMAN E. E. (1938) Barium sulphate suspension in colloidal Aluminium hydroxyde. An improved contrast medium for the roentgenographic diagnosis of gastrointestinal lesions. *Amer. J. Roentg. 40*, 705–707.

233. WOLF B. S.; FAEGENBURG D. H. (1963) Progress in gastroenterology. *Gastroenterology 44*, 886–899.

234. WOLF B. S. (1959) Functional aspects of gastro-intestinal radiology. *Surg. Clin. N. Amer. 39/5*, 1431–1449.

235. YOUMANS W. B. (1944) The intestino-intestinal inhibitory reflex. *Gastroenterology 3*, 114–118.

236. ZASLON J.; PORTNER J. H.; COHEN E. A.; KREMENS V.; BERGER S. M. (1961) Complete small intestinal obstruction in the absence of positive roentgen findings. *Amer. J. Gastroent. 35/2*, 122–126.

237. ZBORALSKE F.; BESSOLO R. J. (1967) Metastatic carcinoma of the mesentery and gut. *Radiology 88*, 302–310.

238. ZBORALSKE F.; HARRIS P. A.; RIEGELMAN S.; RAMBO O. N.; MARGULIS A. R. (1966) Toxity studies on tannic acid administered by enema. Studies on the retention of enemas in humans. Review and conclusions. *Amer. J. Roentg. 96/2*, 505–509.

239. ZIMMER E. A. (1954) Die Röntgenologie des Dünndarms. *Gastroenterologia* (Basel) 70, 113–171.

240. ZIMMER E. A. (1948–49) Barium 'Wander'. A new contrastmedium with special advantages in examination of the gastro-intestinal tract. *Gastroenterologia* (Basel) 74/4, 208–224.

241. ZIMMER E. A. (1951) Radiology of the small intestine. Studies on contrastmedia for the x-ray examination of the gastro-intestinal tract. *Brit. J. Radiol. 24*, 245–251.

242. ZOLLNER S. (1937) Physiologische Schwankungen in der Motorik des Dünndarms. *Fortschritte R. 56*, 644–649.

BIBLIOGRAPHY

IX

INFLAMMATION AND INFLAMMATORY-LIKE DISEASES

1. General

Inflammatory processes in the wall of the small intestine can be due to or enhanced by various, highly divergent factors. Several of these are:

1. Direct action on the intestinal mucosal membrane of chemicals or toxins produced by bacteria.
2. Impaired arterial or venous circulation in the involved intestinal segment; intramural bleeding as a result of an abdominal blunt trauma; a greatly prolonged coagulation time. Both embolic processes and thrombosis or intramural hematomas can lead to necrosis of the intestinal wall.
3. Ulcerations can also develop in mucosa swollen as a result of lymphedema. Lymph drainage can be disturbed by a number of causes such as tumorous growth, inflammatory processes or fibrotic shriveling. Although rare, congenital lymphedema can also occur.
4. Stimulation of the mucosa by parasites not normally found in the intestine.
5. Lowered resistance of the intestinal mucosal membrane as a result of a marked atrophy of the folds of Kerkring can also lead to an increased susceptibility to harmful agents.

If the wall of the small intestine is inflamed, it will appear upon examination to be red and swollen. Roentgenologically one or more of the following phenomena may be observed during the transit examination:

1. The intestine is highly irritated and numerous contractions in rapid succession will be observed. Locally the transit time is greatly accelerated so that antispasmodics must be used in order to obtain an x-ray of the involved loops in a sufficiently well-filled state. Prolonged spasms in intestinal segments with an otherwise normal mucosal pattern, such as can be observed during the colon examination, seldom occur in the small intestine (fig. 8.60Q). In Crohn's disease, however, we can see spastic contractions extending over a length of 5 to 15 cm. On the roentgenogram, the barium in the involved intestinal segment then sometimes appears to be as thin as a thread. In the loops where this so-called 'string sign' is observed, the mucosal surface has already become highly ulcerous. Pathological-anatomical examination has revealed that under the ulcerous mucosa there is an obviously thickened muscular layer which without a doubt causes these spasma. If the flow of contrast fluid is sufficiently abundant, then under prolonged fluoroscopy the shorter periods of relaxation can also be observed. That we are concerned with a temporary spasm and not a manifest stenosis can be concluded from the fact that there is no sign of an obvious prestenotic dilatation in these cases.
2. As a result of the edematous swelling of the mucosa, the diameter of the lumen of an inflamed intestinal loop can be somewhat smaller than normal during the rest phase. The affected intestinal loops then also show a certain degree of rigidity: they more or less stretch across the abdomen and the number of loops in the affected area has clearly decreased.
3. As a result of multiple ulcerations the normal mucosal pattern can be completely or partially disturbed over a large or small area, sometimes even completely destroyed.
4. A deep necrosis involving all layers of the in-

testinal wall can lead easily to the formation of fistulas or adhesion to adjacent intestinal loops. Gas can be found in the intestinal wall and even in the portal vein; it is caused by gas-producing bacteria or enters from the lumen of the intestine. These accumulations of gas in the intestinal wall are first visible on the roentgenogram as 1–3 mm thin straight or ring-shaped shadows with a somewhat ragged margin along both sides. As a result of the cleavage of the intestinal wall into its layers, these strips of gas often have a sort of fibrillar structure similar to that of muscle bundles. If the gas accumulation is larger, then of course the clarifications are wider but the ragged margins remain as well as the thin offshoots along the edges of these gas shadows.

5. The mucosal surface can appear coarsely nodular or cushion-like. Sometimes these polypous formations are more or less spread out over the mucosal surface: in such cases they are the sites of inflammatory infiltration or nodules of lymphatic tissue. In other cases, for instance Crohn's disease, the cushion-like mucosal swellings obviously lie adjacent to one another and are separated by deep longitudinal and transverse grooves so that a more or less regular pattern resembling cobblestones is seen. Ulcerations often develop in the depths of the grooves as a result of or enhanced by local circulatory disorders.

6. On the x-rays, the spaces between the intestinal loops can be obviously increased in the inflamed region. These wider spaces can be due to thickening or fatty degeneration of the intestinal wall, shriveling of the mesentery or an inflammatory infiltrate.

7. On the mesenteric side of the intestine there may be impressions in the intestinal lumen which are caused by thickening of the mesentery and enlargement of the glands within the mesentery.

A superficial inflammatory process in the mucosa of the small intestine can heal without radiologically visible scarring. If, however, the inflammatory process is not limited to the surface but is transmural in character, which is in fact the case in Crohn's disease, then the mucosa can be completely destroyed and there is no longer any chance

of recovery of the fold relief. In such an intestine we will find areas, corresponding more or less to these sites, in which the fold relief has completely disappeared. Such foldless plaques can also be due to metastases of a linitis plastica from the stomach. In spite of the great similarity radiologically between these two very different diseases, differentiation will in practice never be difficult when the patient is examined further and the history is carefully taken. If a previous examination has revealed a wide-spread inflammatory process, then on a later roentgenogram there will be an extensive area with no circular mucosal folds at all.

Due to the transmural character of the inflammation, the deep-seated muscular layers will be replaced by connective tissue so that the intestine becomes dilated and shows no peristalsis at all. As a result of the passive collapse of these completely atonic loops, only coarse longitudinal folds will be seen which are formed by the entire intestinal wall and not only the mucosa, as in an intact intestine. During the roentgenological examination, it is noted that the contrast fluid flowing in the distal direction is passively propelled through these loops. In our clinic, this phenomenon which is so characteristic of complete atony of the mucosal membrane and the muscular layers has acquired the name 'bike tire phenomenon' in view of the similarity to the inner tube only.

Ulcers in the intestinal wall heal with the formation of fibrous tissue. As a result of the shriveling of this connective tissue, circular strictures may ultimately develop which cause more or less pronounced stenoses.

2. Crohn's disease

In 1932 when most of the inflammatory processes in the small intestine were ascribed to tuberculosis, the internist Crohn and his associates identified a disease which they called regional ileitis because they thought at that time that it would only develop in the terminal ileum. We now know that this disease can involve the entire digestive tract from the mouth to the anus; moreover, at least radiologically it cannot be distinguished from tuberculosis. Today almost every internist and radiologist believe that Crohn's disease has spread considerably in the past few years, although it is difficult to determine with any certainty whether this should be attributed solely or in part to the greatly improved clinical and radiological diagnostic methods in use today. In any event it has been established that regional enteritis or ileitis is definitely now one of the most common diseases of the small intestine. A precise estimate of the frequency is difficult but it is known that one out of every 10.000 Dutchmen is being treated in a University Hospital for this disease. It can certainly be assumed that an equal number is being treated elsewhere.

Of course the question which logically follows is: were some of the cases diagnosed in the past as tuberculosis in fact Crohn's disease? In the numerous publications of the 19th and early 20th centuries, the clinical and in particular the pathological and histological descriptions were so detailed that it has become apparent that the answer is probably yes!; in a number of cases it has now even been established definitely. The earliest of this series of publications is that of Morgagni in 1769; in 1920 Tietze collected some 281 literature references to cases of tb which probably were not tuberculosis. On the grounds of the publications which have appeared so far, Crohn's disease appears to occur mainly in western and northwestern European countries and in the northeastern part of North America, with a possible predisposition for the Jewish race. There is no clear predilection for sex; occasionally a hereditary relationship can be established. The disease is seen predominantly in young adults between 15 and 40 years of age, is less common in older adults and only rarely occurs in children under 10 years of age. It is not surprising that for a long time the disease was called terminal ileitis because it is this part of the intestine which is involved in 4 out of 5 patients. In about 1/5 of these cases the wall of the cecum is also thickened and inflamed so that in fact one could speak of an ileocecal infection.

In general it can be stated that about 1 out of every 10 patients has Crohn-like abnormalities in the colon when the small intestine does not appear to be involved. On the average these patients are somewhat older than the patients with a localization in the small intestine. It has never been established with any certainty how often the abnormalities characteristic of ulcerative colitis occur in the small intestine. It is known that the radiological abnormalities of some of the patients being treated for a probable Crohn's disease are very similar to those of an ulcerative colitis. In the latter case the ulceration are collar-button shaped and are fairly superficial. Sometimes there are even no indications of cobblestones, deep longitudinal ulcerations, fistulization, skip lesions or strictures (fig. 9.1M). Upon remission of Crohn's disease, there remains

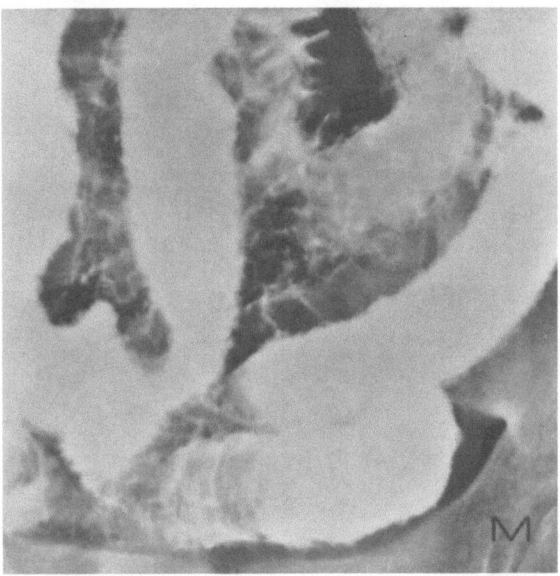

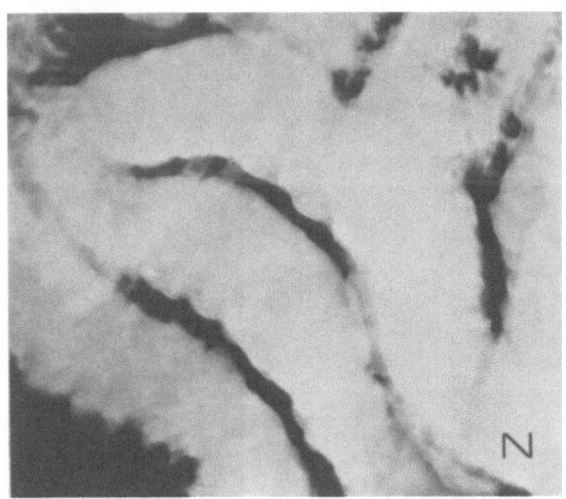

Fig. 9.1

M. Superficial more or less merging ulcerations in Crohn's disease slightly similar to the mucosal abnormalities in the colon in a case of ulcerative colitis. There are only a few cobblestones, no skip lesions and no healthy segments.

N. One year later the ulcerations have disappeared and the intestinal wall is more or less smooth with no visible mucosal relief.

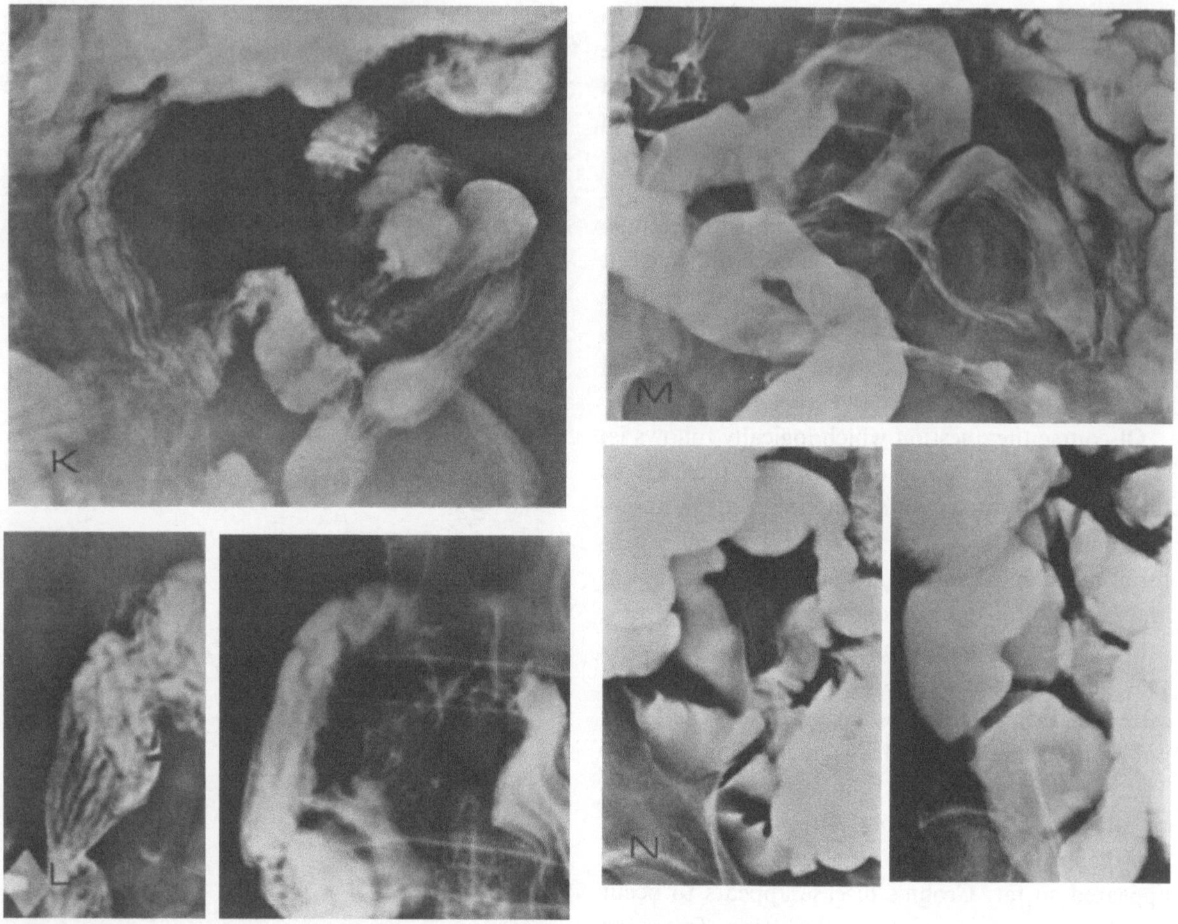

Fig. 9.2
Four examples of atrophied mucosa after Crohn's disease with longitudinal folds when the intestine is inadequately filled: the so-called bike tire phenomenon.

K. proximal jejunum.
L. distal duodenum.
M. proximal ileum.
N. distal ileum.

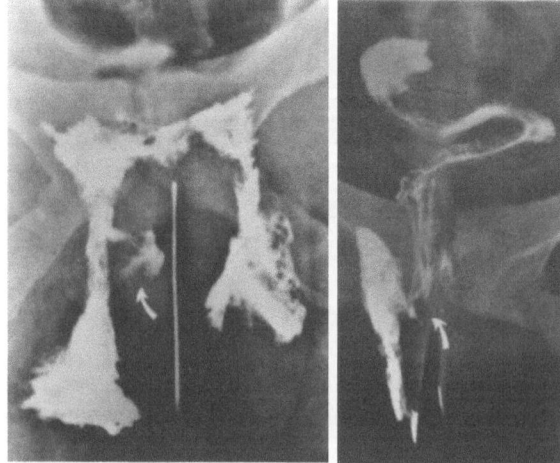

Fig. 9.3
Right-sided ischiorectal fistula in Crohn's disease. At the time the abnormalities in the small intestine were minimal (see fig. 9.9W); now (4 years later) they have become extensive.

a smooth flaccid thin intestinal wall which shows no peristalsis (fig. 9.1N). If the intestinal loop is only moderately filled then the 'bike tire' phenomenon (see page 172) will be observed (fig. 9.2).

In addition to the primary lesion in the small intestine, a mucosal abnormality is also found in 1 out of every 10 patients in the anorectal region. In this same region anal fissures, right-sided ischiorectal fistulas (fig. 9.3) and abscesses (fig. 9.4) can precede the appearance of the intestinal lesions by many months, sometimes even years. If these fistulas are filled very carefully then it is often

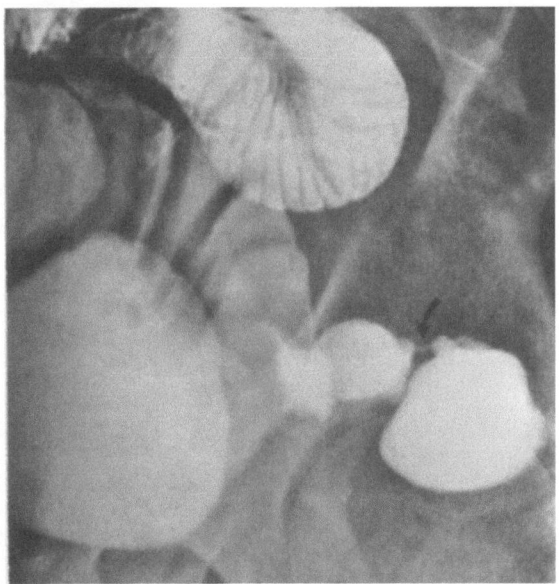

Fig. 9.4
Abscess in Douglas' pouch in Crohn's disease which communicates via a fistulous tract with the highly dilated ileum.

possible to demonstrate a communication between these canals and the rectum, usually just inside the sphincter muscle of the anus. In another 10% of the patient material Crohn abnormalities are not encountered in the distal ileum but more proximal in the digestive tract. In one-half of these cases they involve the remaining part of the ileum (fig. 9.5); the other half are localized in the jejunum (fig. 9.6), duodenum (fig. 9.7) or stomach (fig. 9.8) with a relative frequency of about 6:3:1, respectively. Prodromic indications of Crohn's disease occur not only in the mucosal membrane of the anus but also

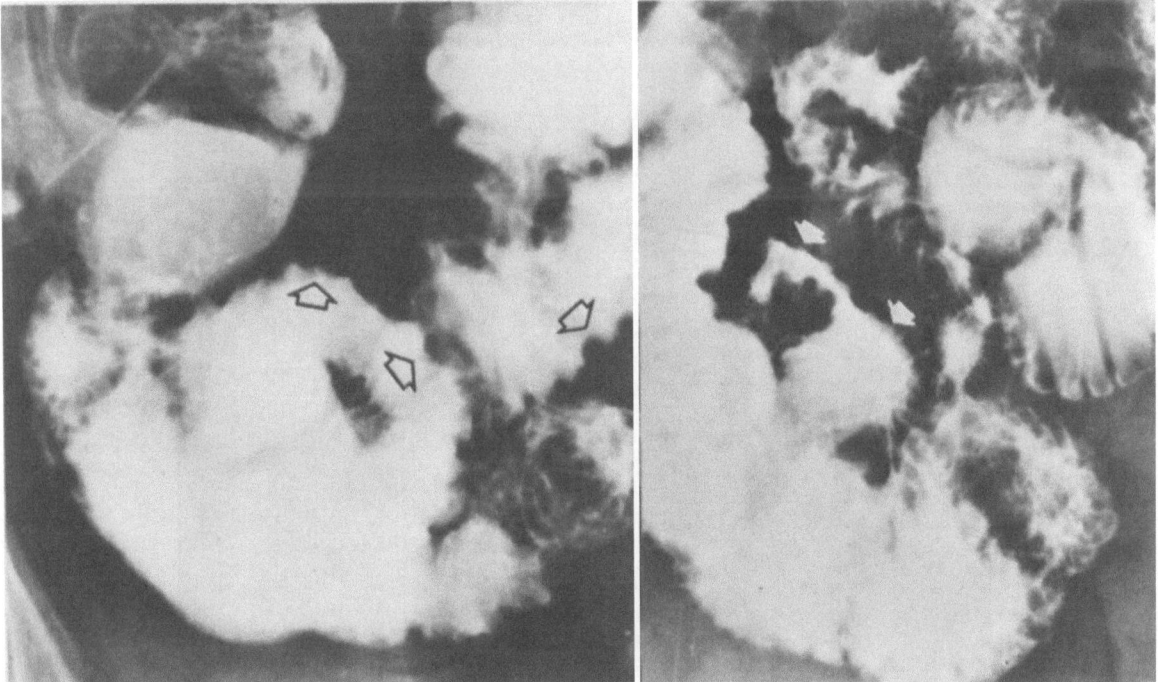

Fig. 9.5
Slight abnormalities in the more proximal part of the ileum in a patient with aphthous stomatitis due to Crohn's disease.

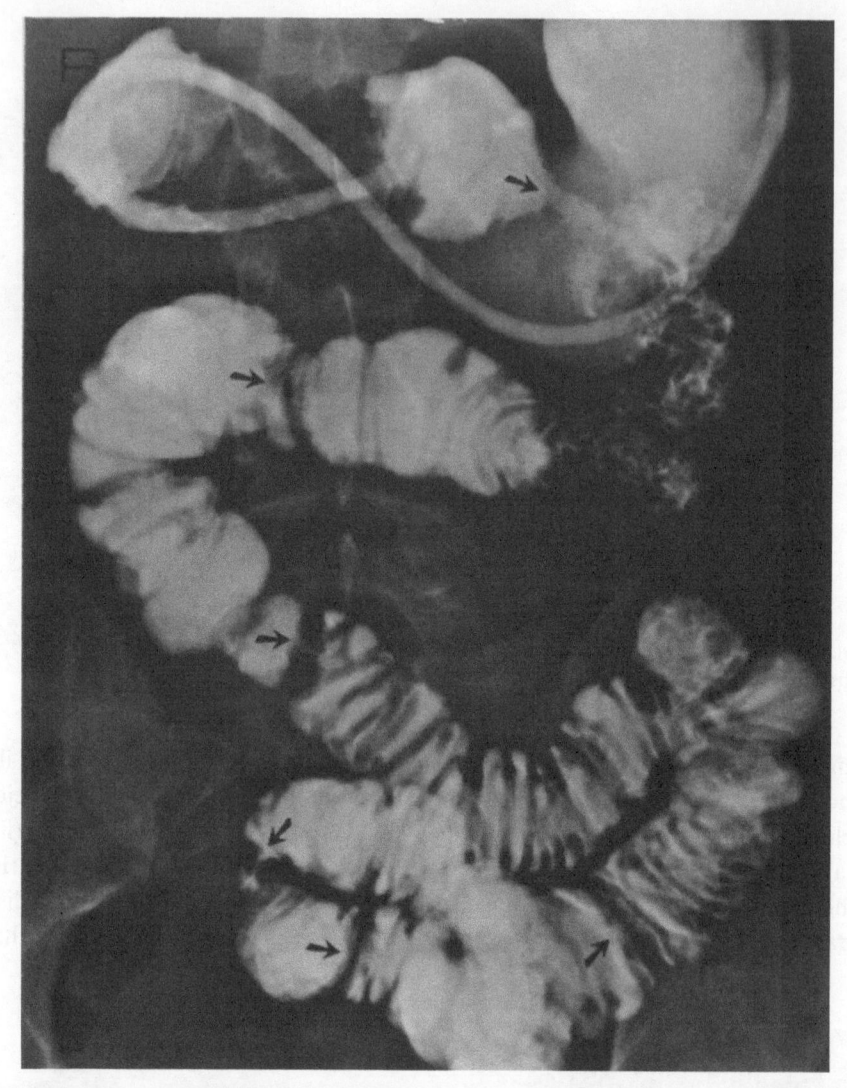

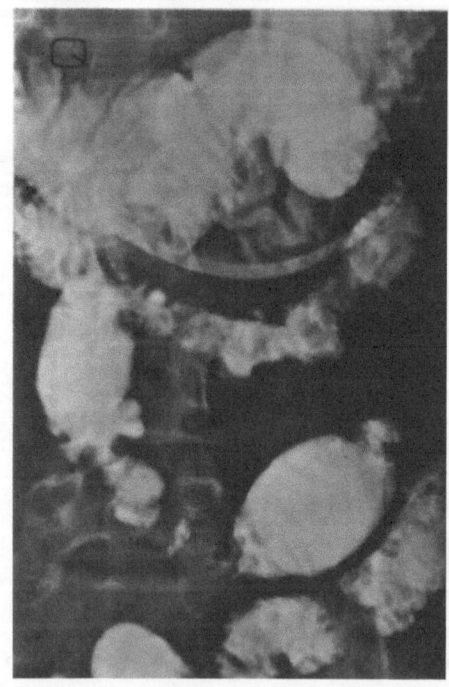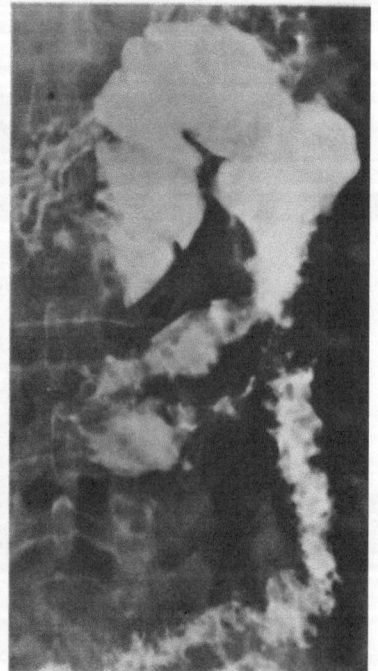

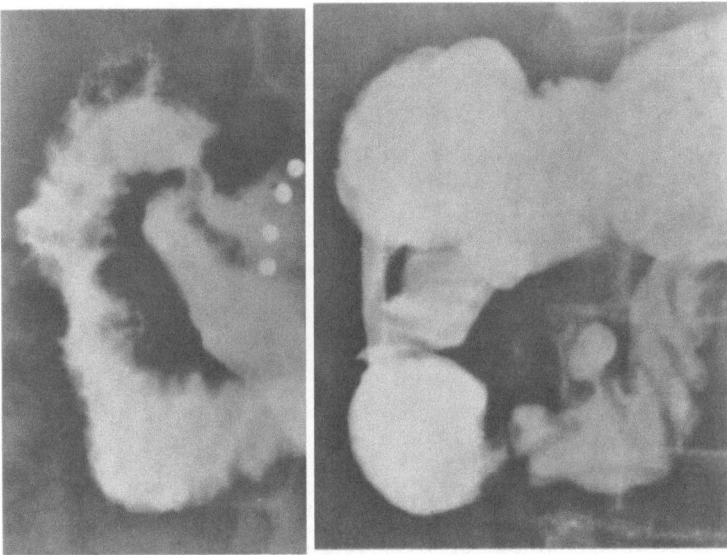

Fig. 9.7
Two patients with Crohn's disease of the duodenum.

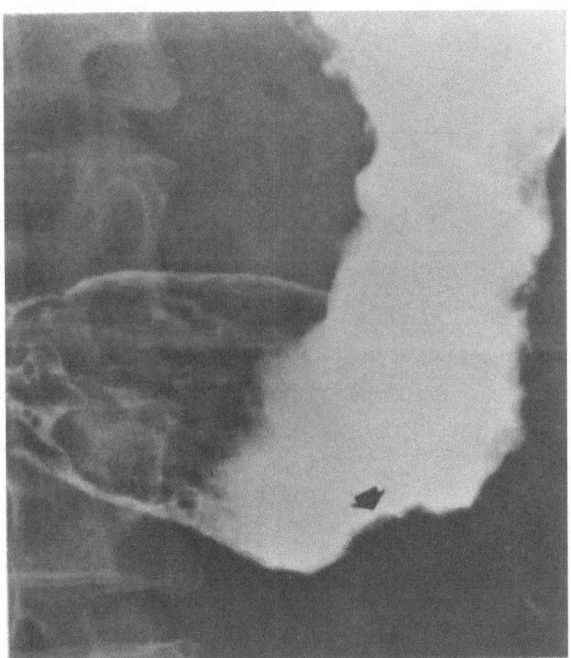

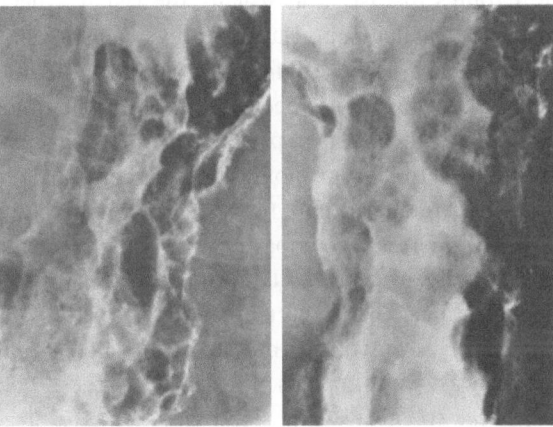

Fig. 9.8
Crohn's disease of the stomach. The mucosal pattern in the stomach somewhat resembles that of a lymphoreticular malignancy, a hypertrophic gastritis or Zollinger-Ellison disease except that the thick folds are often interrupted in the transverse direction so that a highly irregular network is observed.

Fig. 9.6
Two patients with Crohn's disease of the jejunum. Longitudinal ulcer (→) and multiple more or less constricting skip lesions.

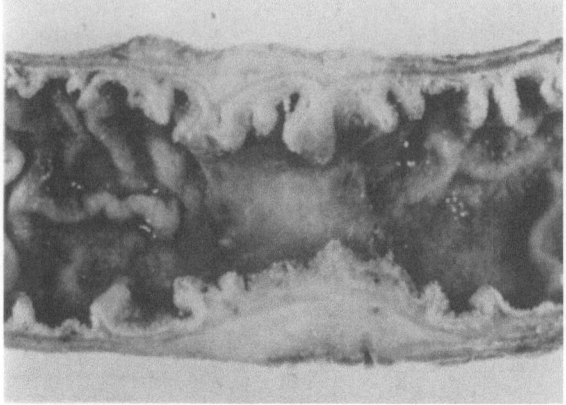

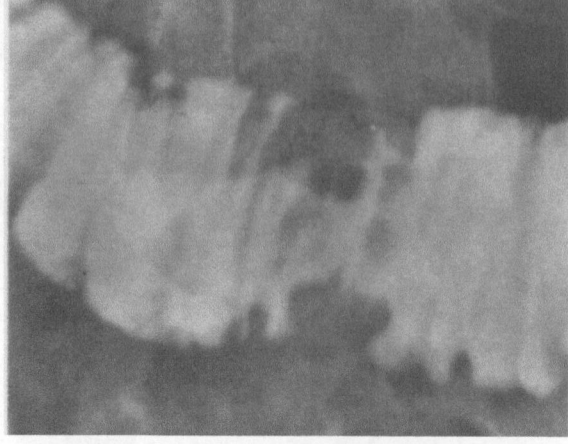

in that of the mouth. Careful inquiry would reveal that certainly one out of every 10 patients has a history of aphthae. Finally of every 10 patients with a Crohn's lesion in the small intestine, there is approximately one with one or more 'skip' lesions proximal to the primary lesion; skip lesions are clearly circumscribed sites in the middle of a fairly normal mucosa (fig. 9.9). An intestinal loop affected by Crohn's disease, thus usually the last few decimeters of the ileum, appears red and swollen during the acute phase of the infection. Although the diameter of the lumen has decreased slightly, the outer diameter of the diseased part of the intestine is still larger due to the pronounced thickening of the wall. This is due in part to the fact that Crohn's disease is often accompanied by a pronounced hypertrophy of the muscular layers in the wall of the intestine. This hypertrophy causes prolonged spasms in the involved intestinal segment so that the contrast fluid appears thread-like on the x-ray: this is the so-called string sign (fig. 9.10). An intraluminal increase in pressure in these loops may lead to herniation of the intact mucosal tissue right through the intestinal wall. Fluoroscopic examination shows that each of these so-called 'false diverticula' alternates in size (fig. 9.11). False diverticula are lined with mucosal tissue only and consequently they are extremely thin-walled. They are situated on the mesenteric side of the intestine, and have to be differentiated from still another type of diverticula, the so-called pseudo-diverticula (fig. 9.12). Pseudo-diverticula are usually situated on the antimesenteric side of the instestine and the wall of these diverticula, indeed, contains all layers of the intestinal wall. They are formed by contractions or

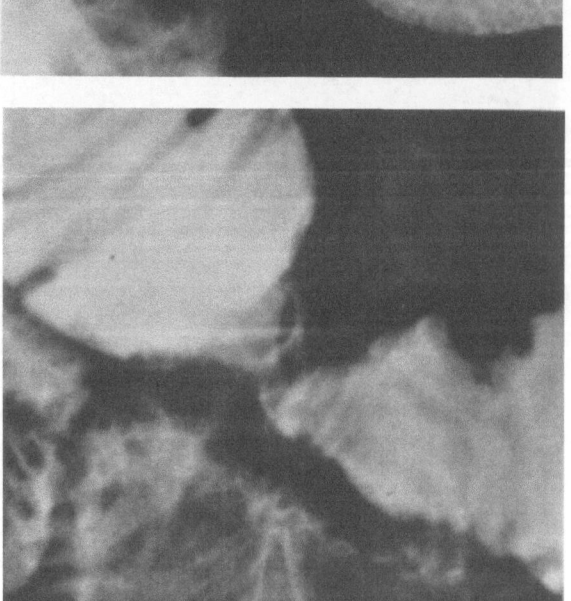

Fig. 9.9
vw. Skip lesions in Crohn's disease; fairly normal mucosa on either side of the lesion.

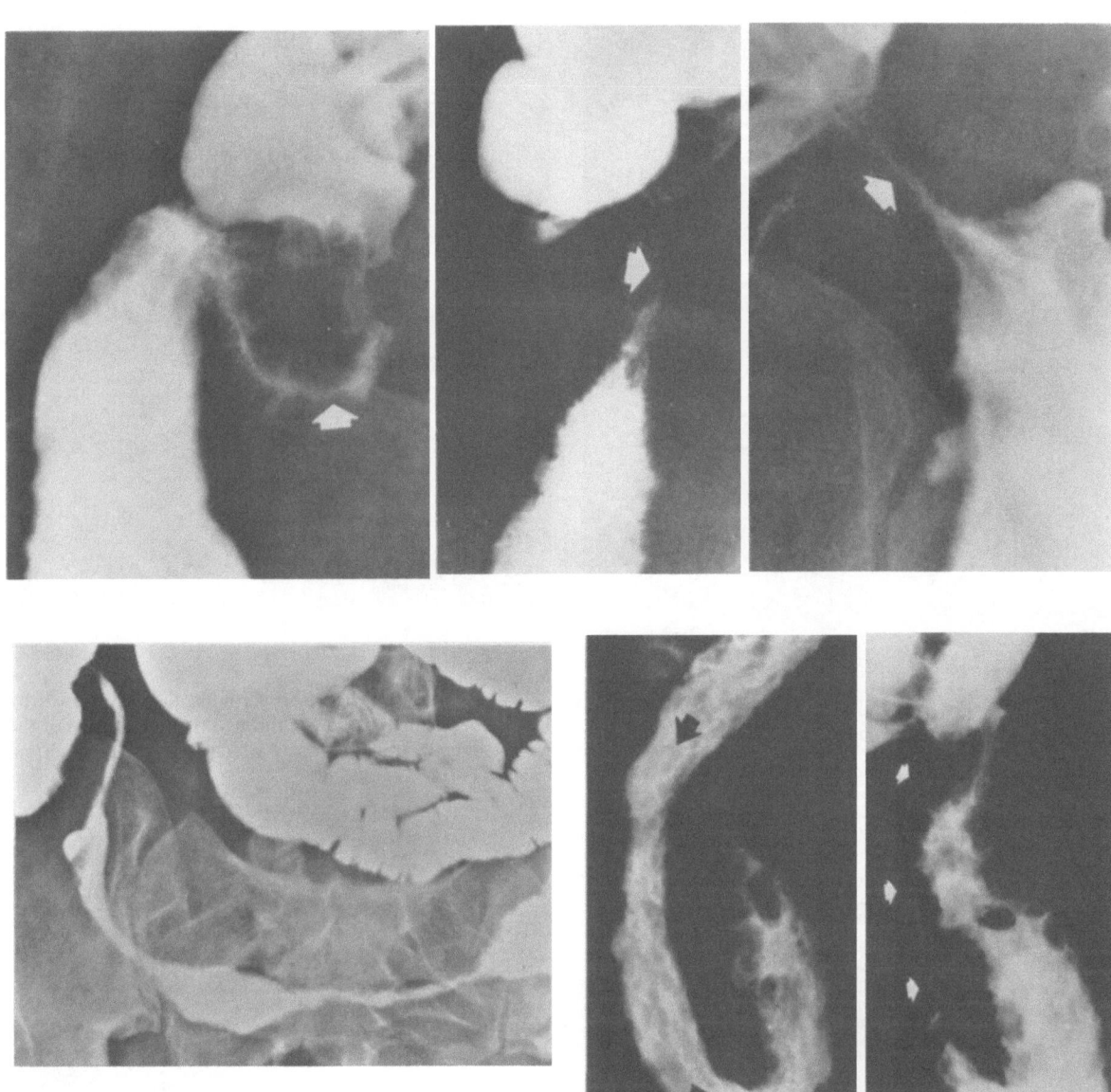

Fig. 9.10
Several examples of the so-called string sign in Crohn's disease caused by spasms due to a marked hypertrophy of the muscular layers. There is no indication of either a stenosis or a prestenotic dilatation.

fibrotic rings originating in the intact intestinal wall opposite the site of an ulceration at the mesentery attachment which has healed with fibrous degeneration and shriveling. In contrast to the former type of diverticula which are spherical with a narrow and sometimes long neck, the second type usually appear to be much larger, vary in shape and join the wall of the intestine with a more or less broad base. Fig. 9.13 illustrates that this type of shriveling cannot be differentiated from that seen in the colon. Sometimes it is quite obvious that there is little or no fibrosis; the sacculations then change so completely that it would be better to call them pseudo-pseudo-diverticula (fig. 9.14).

Another factor which can cause thickening of the intestinal wall in Crohn's disease is that the mesentery is usually thickened as a result of edema and an increase in the fat tissue which encircles the intestine somewhat like claws (fig. 9.15). The lymph nodes in the mesentery and the retroperitoneal area are often obviously enlarged, but sometimes they also show no change at all.

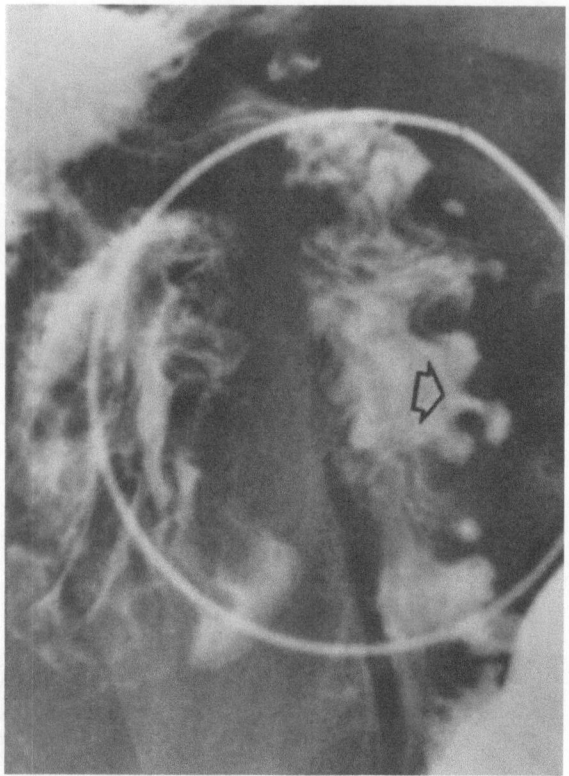

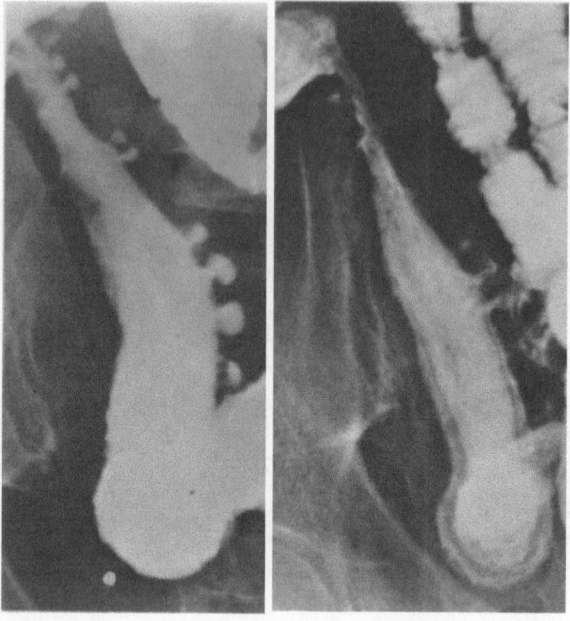

Fig. 9.11
So-called false diverticula in Crohn's disease caused by herniation of the mucosa out through the other layers of the wall. Compare true diverticula which originate in a normal mucosa (→).

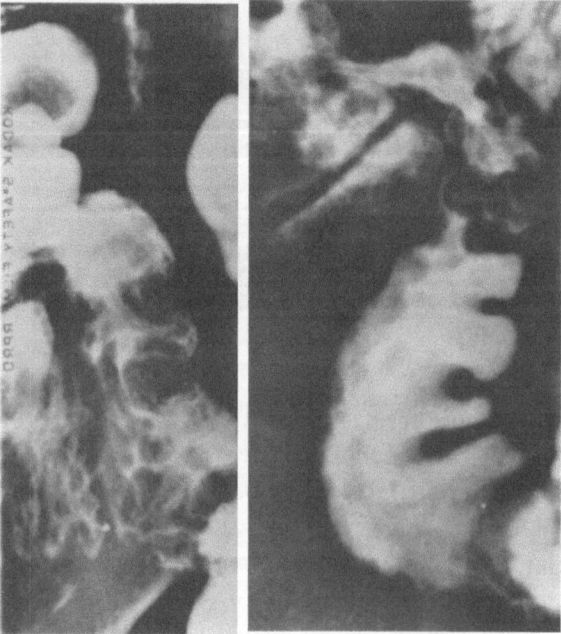

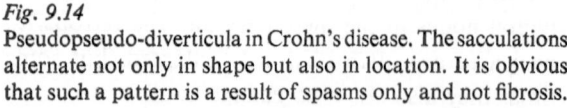

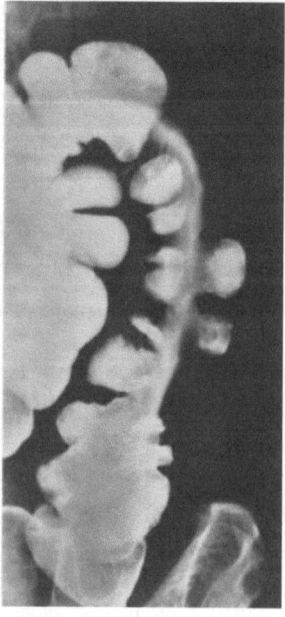

Fig. 9.14
Pseudopseudo-diverticula in Crohn's disease. The sacculations alternate not only in shape but also in location. It is obvious that such a pattern is a result of spasms only and not fibrosis.

Fig. 9.13
Pseudo-diverticula in the colon in Crohn's disease cause the same pattern as those in the small in intestine.

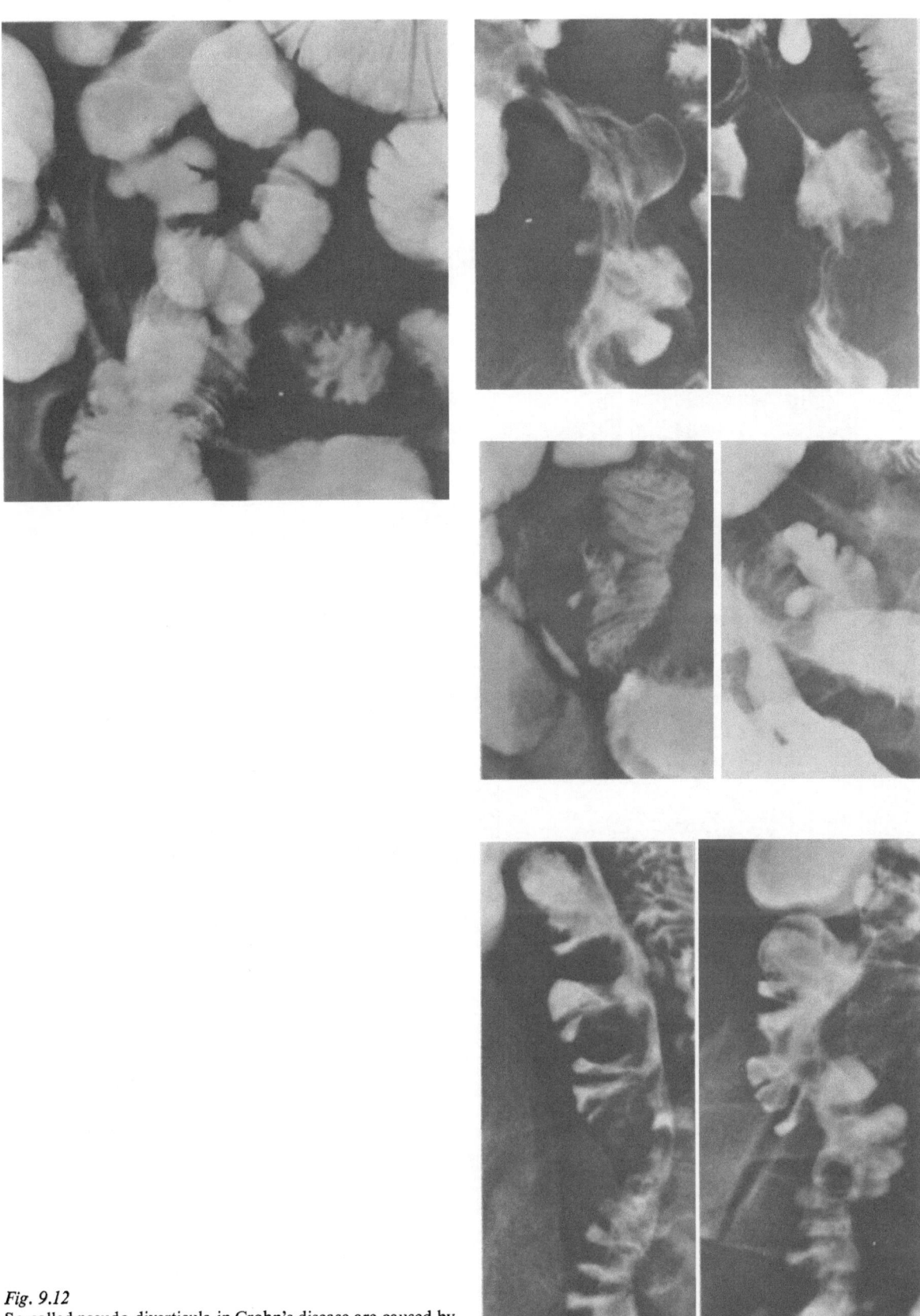

Fig. 9.12
So-called pseudo-diverticula in Crohn's disease are caused by
fibrous constrictions and contractions on the healthy side of
the intestinal wall opposite a longitudinal ulcer.

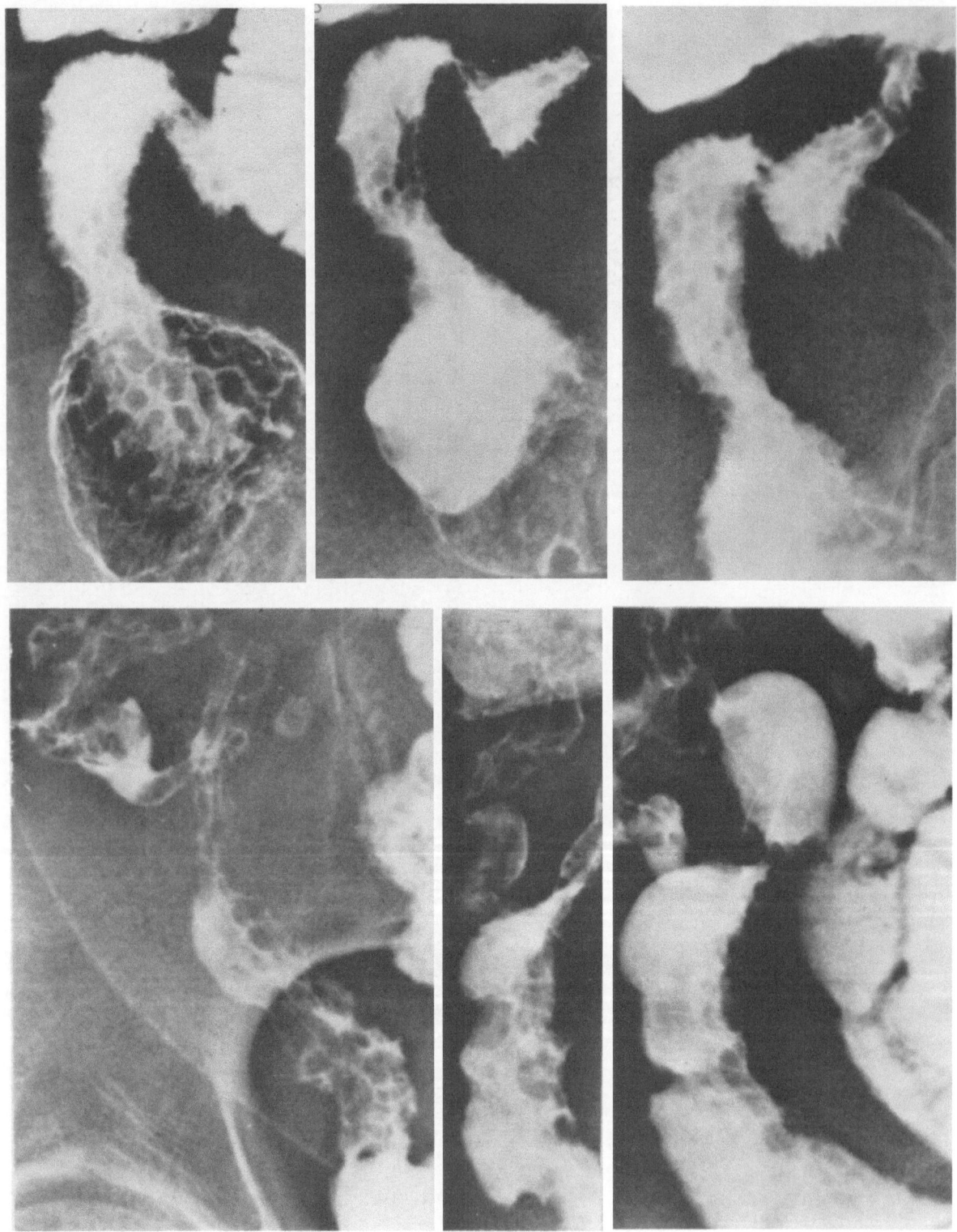

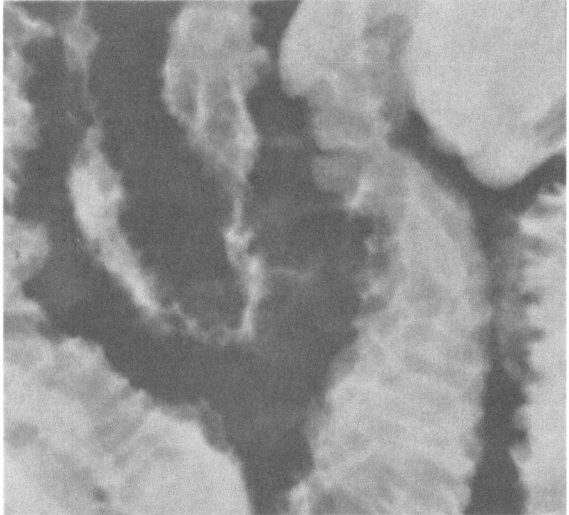

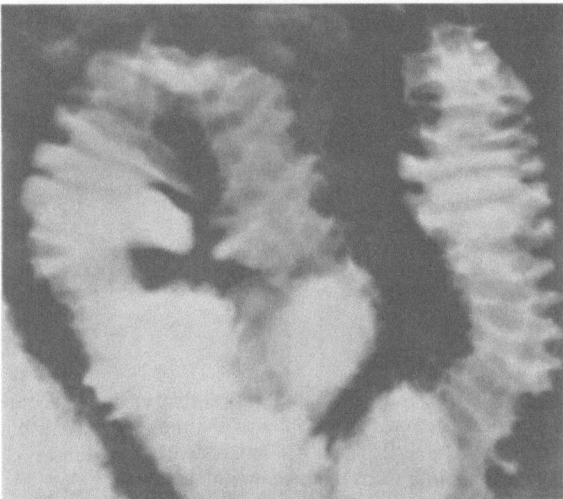

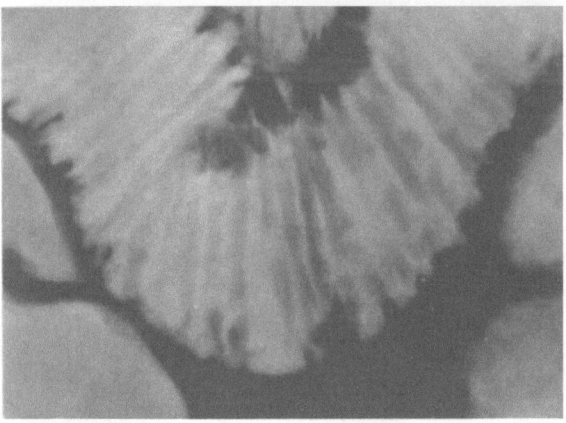

Fig. 9.17
Several examples of the so-called cobblestone pattern in Crohn's disease. The mucosa between the fissure-like ulcerations, which penetrate deep into the intestinal wall, is swollen like a cushion. Because the mucosal folds are more numerous in the jejunum, the cobblestone relief is more pronounced there than in the ileum.

These abnormalities are actually never visualized on the x-rays and in any case cannot be recognized as such.

In Crohn's disease the intestinal mucosa is usually swollen and cushion-like, mainly as a result of a lymphedema, an inflammatory infiltrate and lymphoid hyperplasia of the submucosa (fig. 9.16). Between these cushions or 'cobblestones' (fig. 9.17), which must be seen as islands of relatively intact mucosal tissue, are fissures or ulcers which penetrate deep into all layers of the intestinal wall. Abscesses form within the depths of these fissures which perforate quite easily forming fistulas to adjacent ileal loops, the sigmoid or the apex of the bladder (fig. 9.18). Fistulization is not only enhanced by the fusion of adjacent inflamed ileal loops. but probably also by minute intestinal infarctions resulting from the frequently concomitant endarteritis.

The ulcerations in the mucosa are found mainly on the mesenteric side of the intestine; they extend along the length of the intestine as well as perpendicular to it, thus sometimes causing a railroad track pattern. Near the ulcers there is often pus as well as an enhanced secretion due to hyperplasia of the mucus-secreting glands so that it can be difficult to obtain a sufficiently sharp x-ray of these ulcerations (fig. 9.19). Due to the richer mucosal folding the formation of cobblestones and deep linear ulcers is greater in the proximal part of the small intestine than in the distal segments – independent of the direction of the spread of the disease.

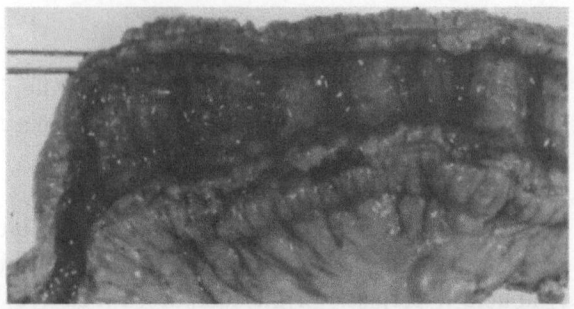

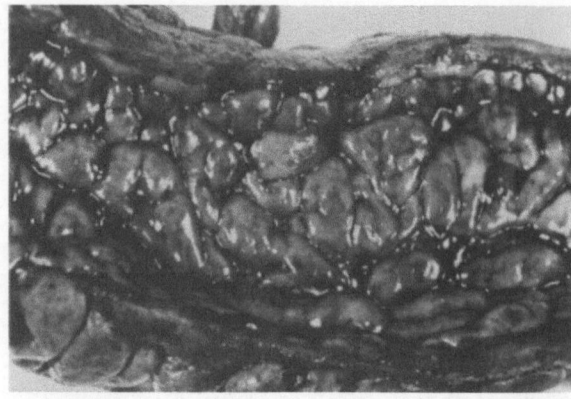

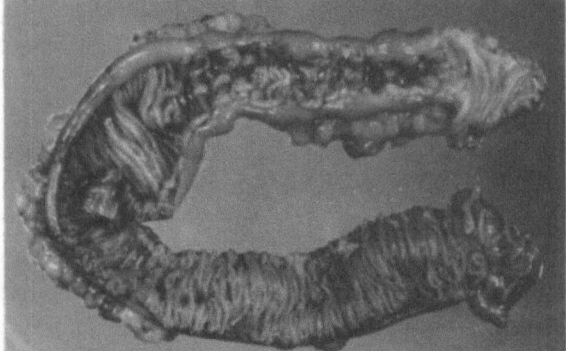

Fig. 9.16
Macroscopic examples of swollen mucosal folds and the cobblestone pattern in Crohn's disease.

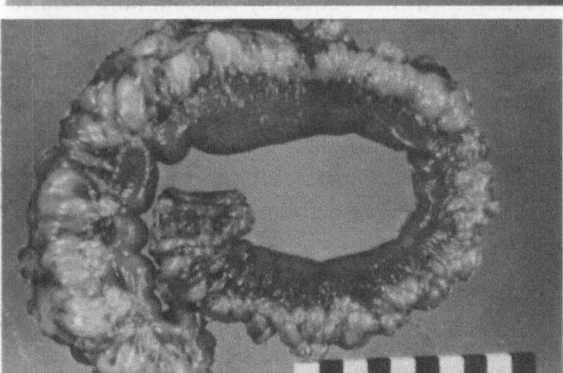

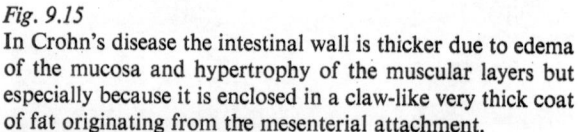

Fig. 9.15
In Crohn's disease the intestinal wall is thicker due to edema of the mucosa and hypertrophy of the muscular layers but especially because it is enclosed in a claw-like very thick coat of fat originating from the mesenterial attachment.

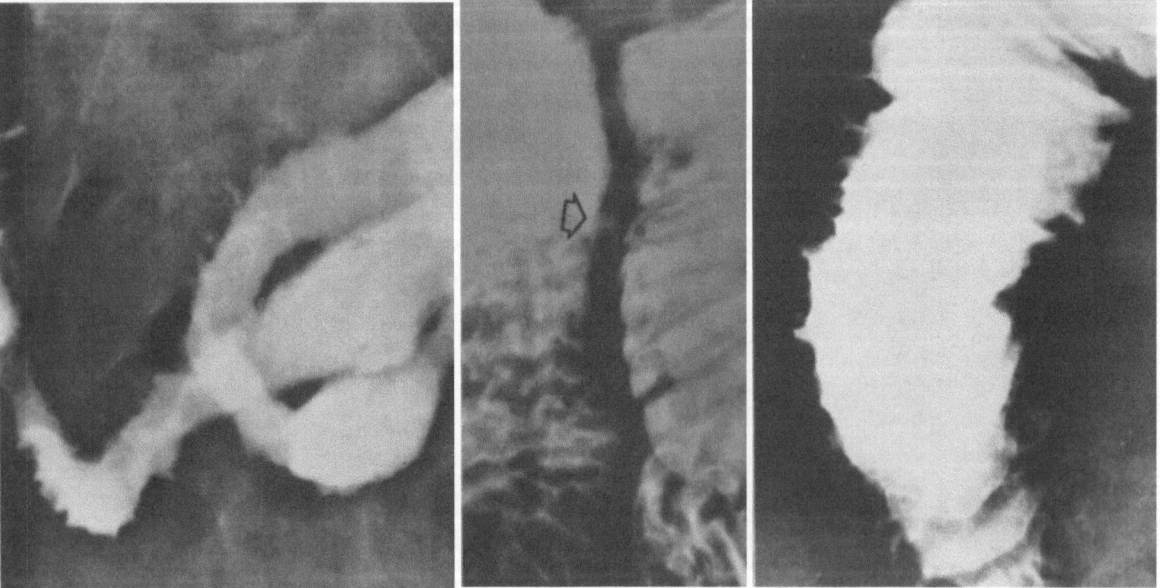

Fig. 9.18
x. Deep ulcerations in the intestinal wall in Crohn's disease, some clearly mushroom-shaped.

In general it is assumed that a pure mucosal swelling as a result of a submucosal lymphedema would be the earliest demonstrable symptom of an incipient Crohn's disease (fig. 9.20A). The formation of cobblestones and fissures would not develop until later; ulcerations in the fissures would then occur because the circulation is highly disturbed as a result of the edema. This hypothesis is based on the observation that in the event of a recurrence after an ileocecal resection, edema of the mucosa is observed first (fig. 9.20BCD). There is a greater chance of finding the earliest symptom of Crohn abnormalities in these patients than in patients who are being examined for the first time for as yet unexplained abdominal complaints. After all surgical patients come back regularly for a check-up even if they have no complaints. The findings of the pathologist and early roentgenological examination of patients with a family history have shown, however, that this concept is not always correct.

Furthermore we have also noted that the ulcerations can be limited in size and very superficial (fig. 9.21vw) and also sometimes occur in the center

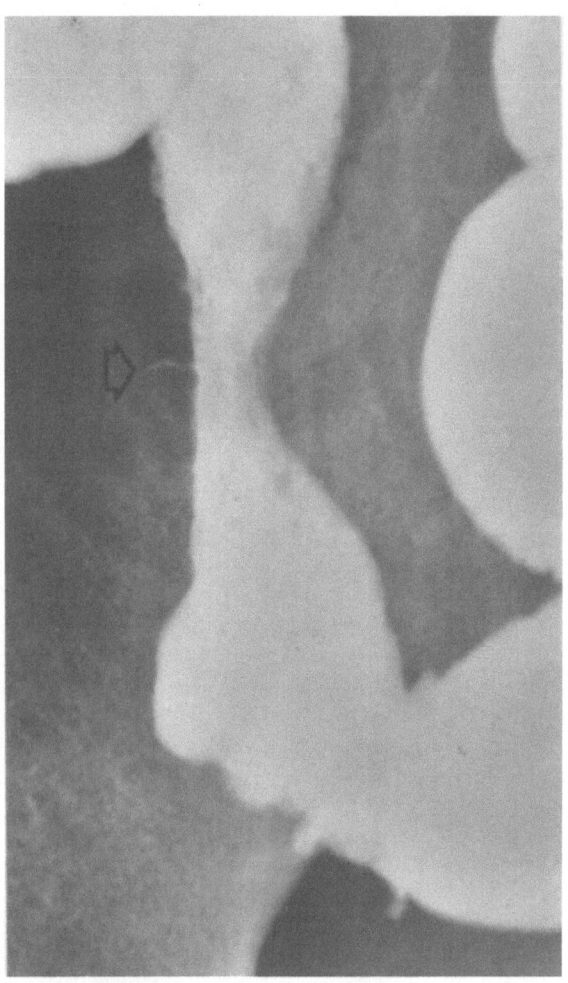

Fig. 9.18
Y. Probably the beginning of a fistulous tract.

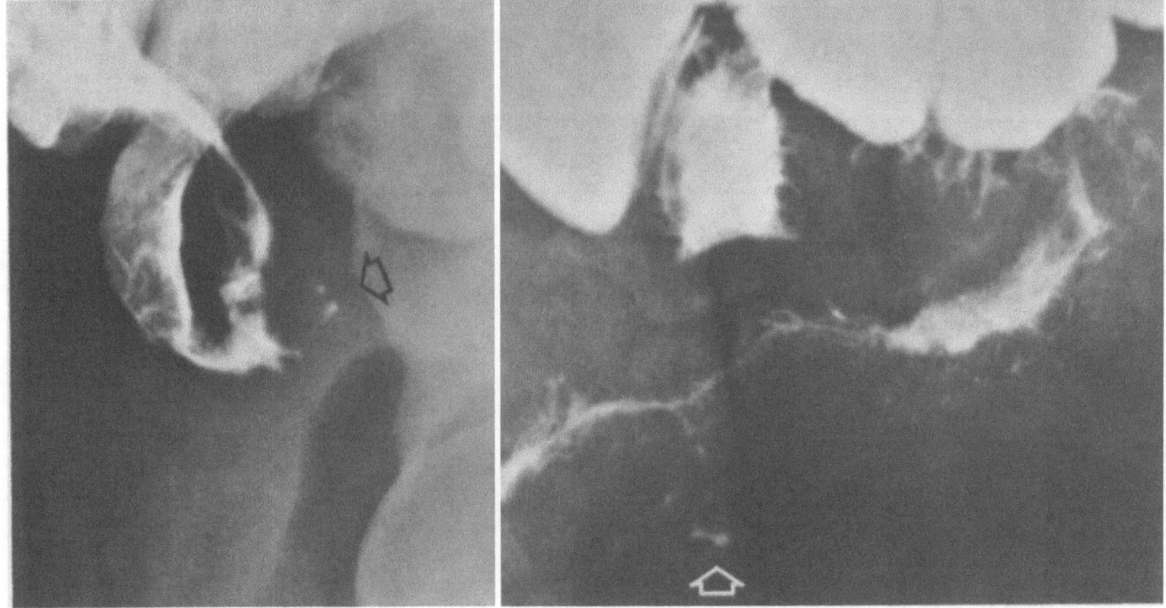

Fig. 9.18
z. Fistulization to the bladder.

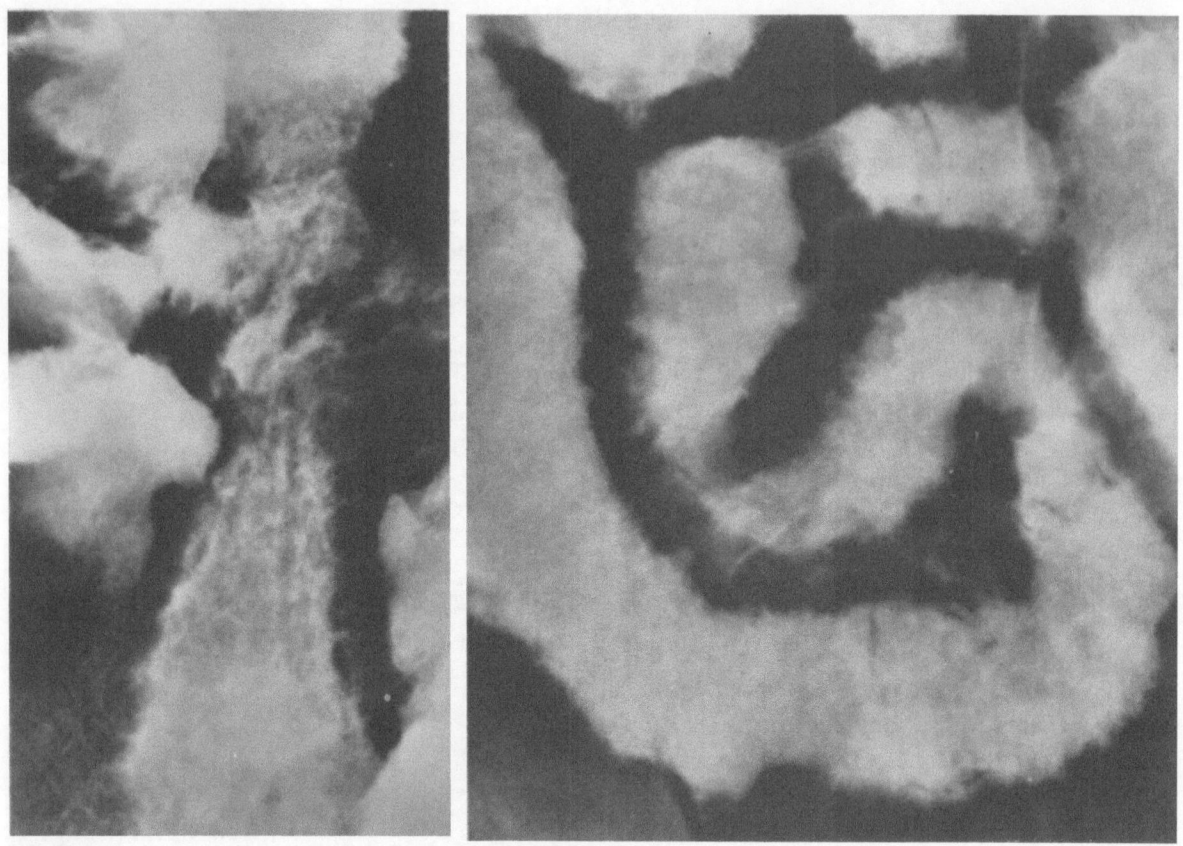

Fig. 9.19
Vague representation of the intestinal wall as a result of the purulent secretion covering the mucosa.

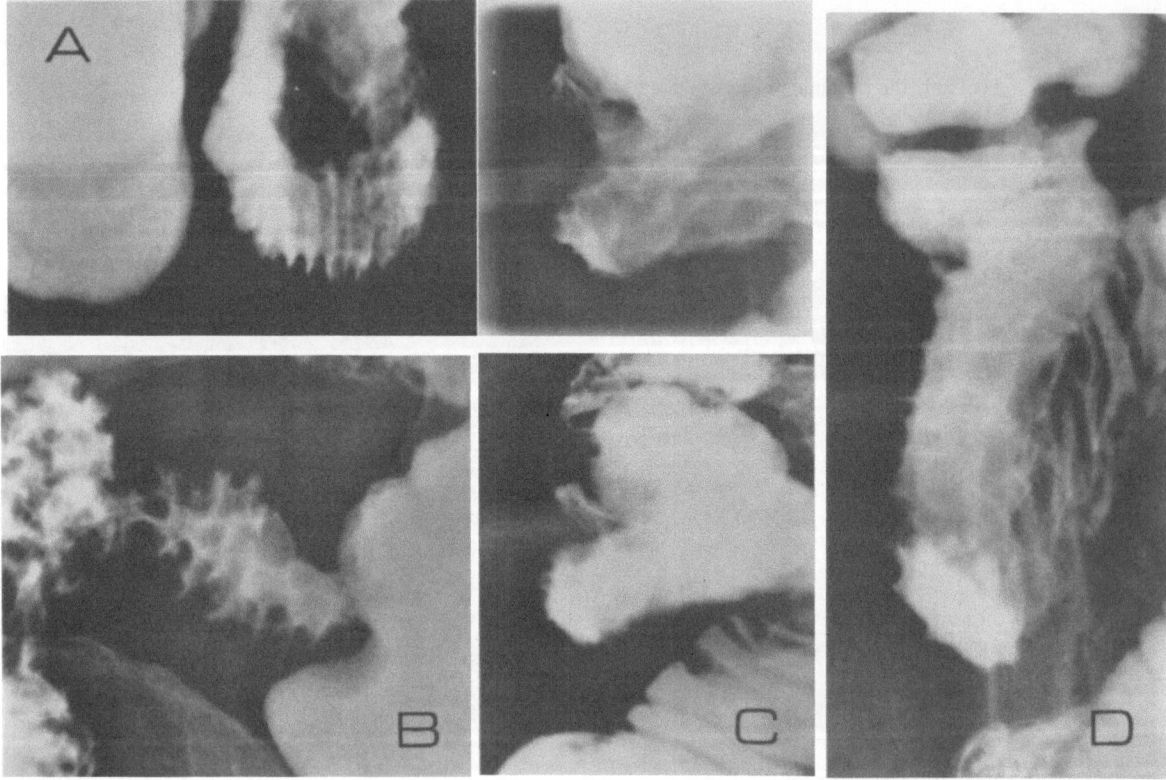

Fig. 9.20
A. Local lymphedema of the intestinal wall, in most cases the earliest demonstrable sign of a beginning Crohn's disease.

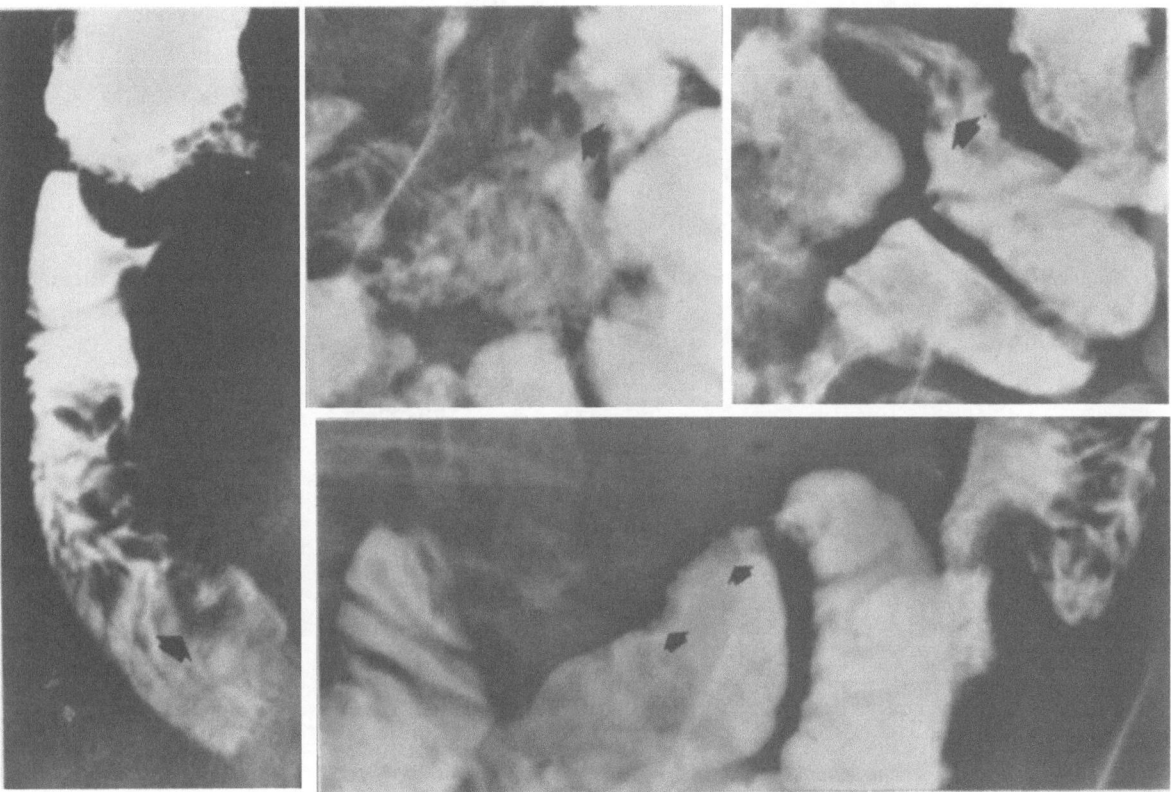

Fig. 9.22
Four cases of granulomas with a central ulcer crater in
Crohn's disease. The mucosa in such an area can show highly
divergent abnormalities, but sometimes also none at all.

of granulomas in a mucous membrane which shows
no signs of submucosal edema (fig. 9.22). This
appears to be true in the distal ileum in particular,
possibly because the disease occurs there more
frequently and because diagnosis of such subtle
abnormalities is somewhat easier in this segment
than in the jejunum where the folds are so much
more numerous. Such a loop sometimes feels
completely normal when examined during surgery
or at autopsy, so that negative findings of this type
should not be accorded too much significance. If
granulomas or cobblestones are large, they may
occasionally even be visible in an air-filled loop on
a survey exposure of the abdomen (fig. 9.23).

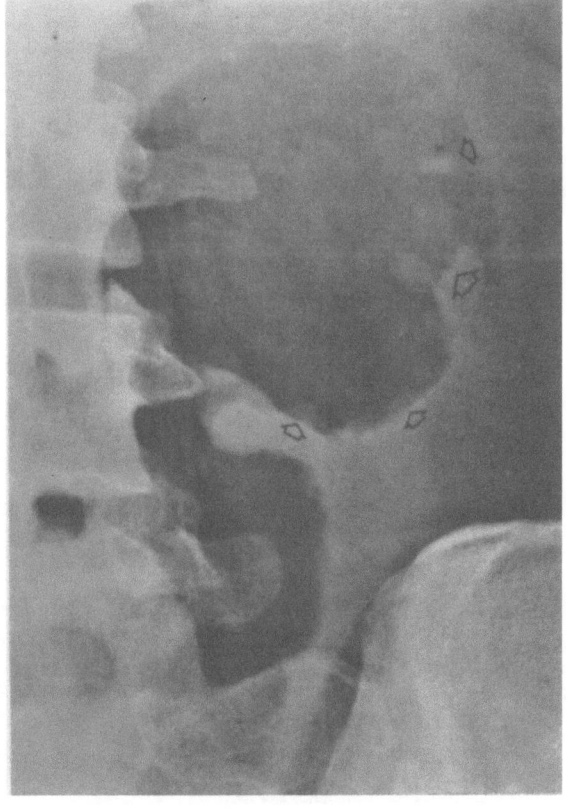

Fig. 9.23
Under favorable conditions solitary granulomas or cobblestones in Crohn's disease are sometimes visible on a survey
film of the abdomen.

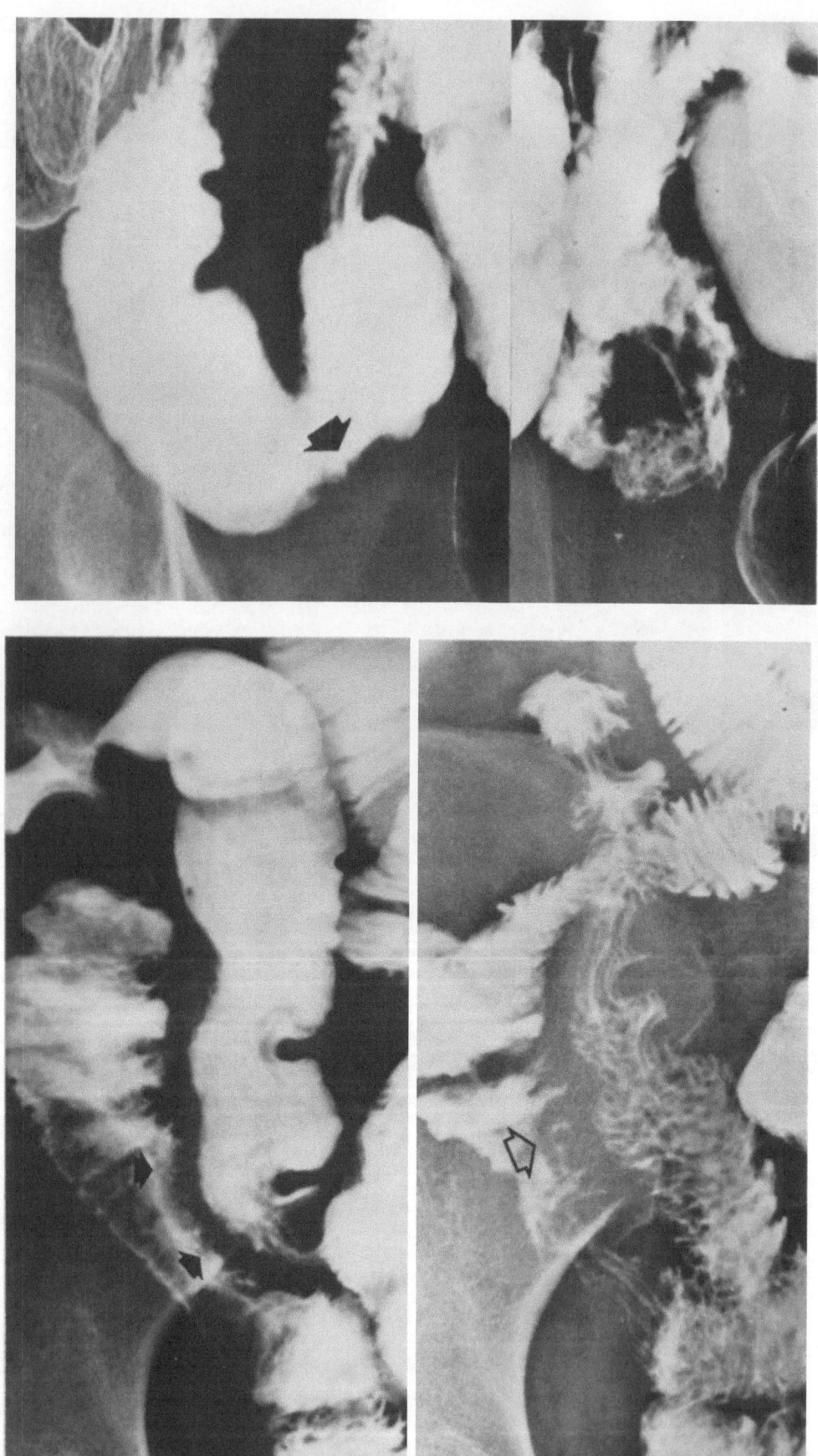

Fig. 9.21v

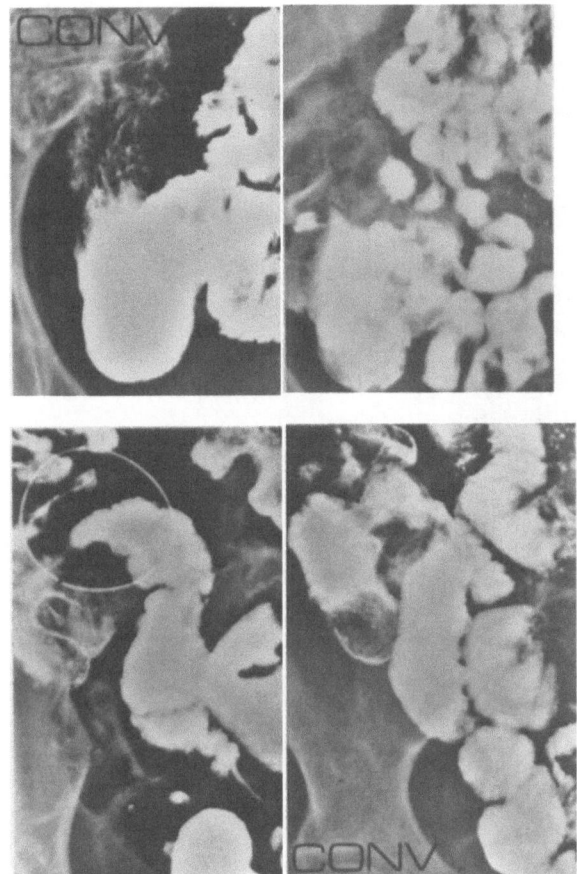

*Fig. 9.21*w

Fig. 9.21
v. Slight abnormalities of the mucosa without signs of edema in two patients;
w. several years later an extensive Crohn's disease was demonstrated. In both cases, the conventional examination showed no abnormalities.

Histologically this type of Crohn's disease is characterized by a chronic inflammatory infiltrate in all layers of the intestinal wall. However, the most pronounced abnormalities in Crohn's disease are found in the submucosa where lymphedema and hyperplasia of the lymphoid tissue are seen. Another characteristic is sarcoid formation manifested as granulomas with Langhan's giant cells which are also found to a lesser extent in Boeck's disease but are more common in tuberculosis. In spite of extensive examination the pathologist is not always able to locate these granulomas with giant cells so that the transmural character of the infection can sometimes be the decisive factor in establishing the diagnosis. In tuberculosis of course the acid-fast rods can be demontrated and the submucosa should be thinner and not thickened by edema.

The resemblance between the patho-anatomical pattern of Crohn's disease and those of Boeck's disease and tuberculosis has not solved the mystery surrounding the etiology of the former.

Moreover, Crohn's disease resembles tuberculosis in that the radiological abnormalities cannot be differentiated from one another and the skin reaction to purified tuberculin is positive in both cases. Crohn's disease resembles Boeck's disease in that an erythema nodosum, iritis or uveitis as well as vague complaints in the joints may appear in the histories of both.

Partly because of the identical clinical course of Crohn's disease and rheumatoid arthritis as well as the therapeutic reaction to corticosteroids and immunosuppressive drugs, it is generally assumed nowadays that the origin of Crohn's disease is immunobiological.

Although a history of recurrent skin and joint complaints in addition to aphthae in the oral cavity and anal fistulas, fissures or abscesses can be important indications of Crohn's disease, the establishment of this diagnosis at an early stage is often very difficult.

The most prominent complaints (abdominal pain, diarrhea, loss of weight and recurrent high temperatures) are so nonspecific that it can be 6 months to a year before the diagnosis is definitely established by means of a rectal biopsy or roentgenological examination. In the more advanced stages of Crohn's disease palpation will reveal a resistance in the abdomen – usually in the lower right quadrant – and fistulas may also be found. Most of the internal fistulas develop between the ileum on the one hand and another ileal loop, the sigmoid or the bladder and vagina on the other. In addition to this fistulization, rectovaginal fistulas and, after surgery, fistulas to the abdominal wall or the surgical scar in particular also occur. In young females frequent painful micturition with pneumaturia can even be the first complaint!

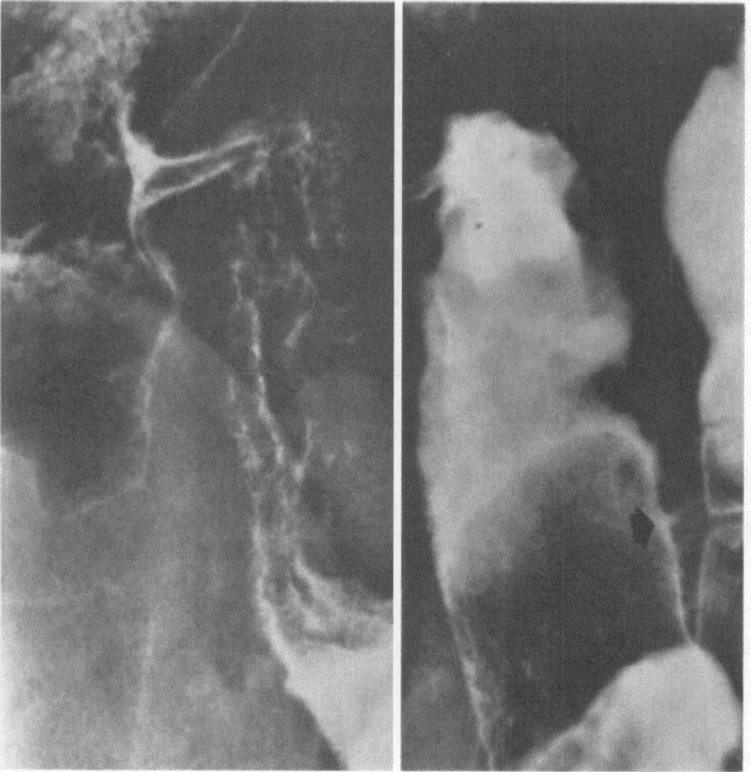

Fig. 9.24
Ulcerative colitis with superficial reflux ileitis in the distal ileum. Rather shriveled cecum and wide open Bauhin's valve.

Clinical differentiation from an ulcerative colitis can also be a problem, especially when the radiological abnormalities closely resemble those of the latter. In ulcerative colitis, diarrhea is usually more frequent and is often accompanied by loss of blood and mucus. Colics and a palpable resistance are not encountered in ulcerative colitis nor are there fistulas, fissures and abscesses around the anus.

It is, however, fortunate that differentiation of a reflux ileitis in ulcerative colitis localized in the cecum from a Crohn's disease is usually obvious on the roentgenograms. In ulcerative colitis, Bauhin's valve is as a rule wide open and the cecum is often shriveled. The distal ileum is moderately dilated and the wall appears smooth over 15–20 cm since ileitis in ulcerative colitis is so superficial that it usually cannot be visualized roentgenologically (fig. 9.24). In Crohn's disease Bauhin's valve is in fact often somewhat constricted and in many cases there is no shriveling of the cecum (fig. 9.25).

Fig. 9.25   →
Five cases of Crohn's disease involving Bauhin's valve and the ileocecal region. More pronounced mucosal abnormalities in the distal ileum and frequently an obvious constriction in the region of Bauhin's valve. Shriveling of the cecum depends upon the stage and the spread of the disease.

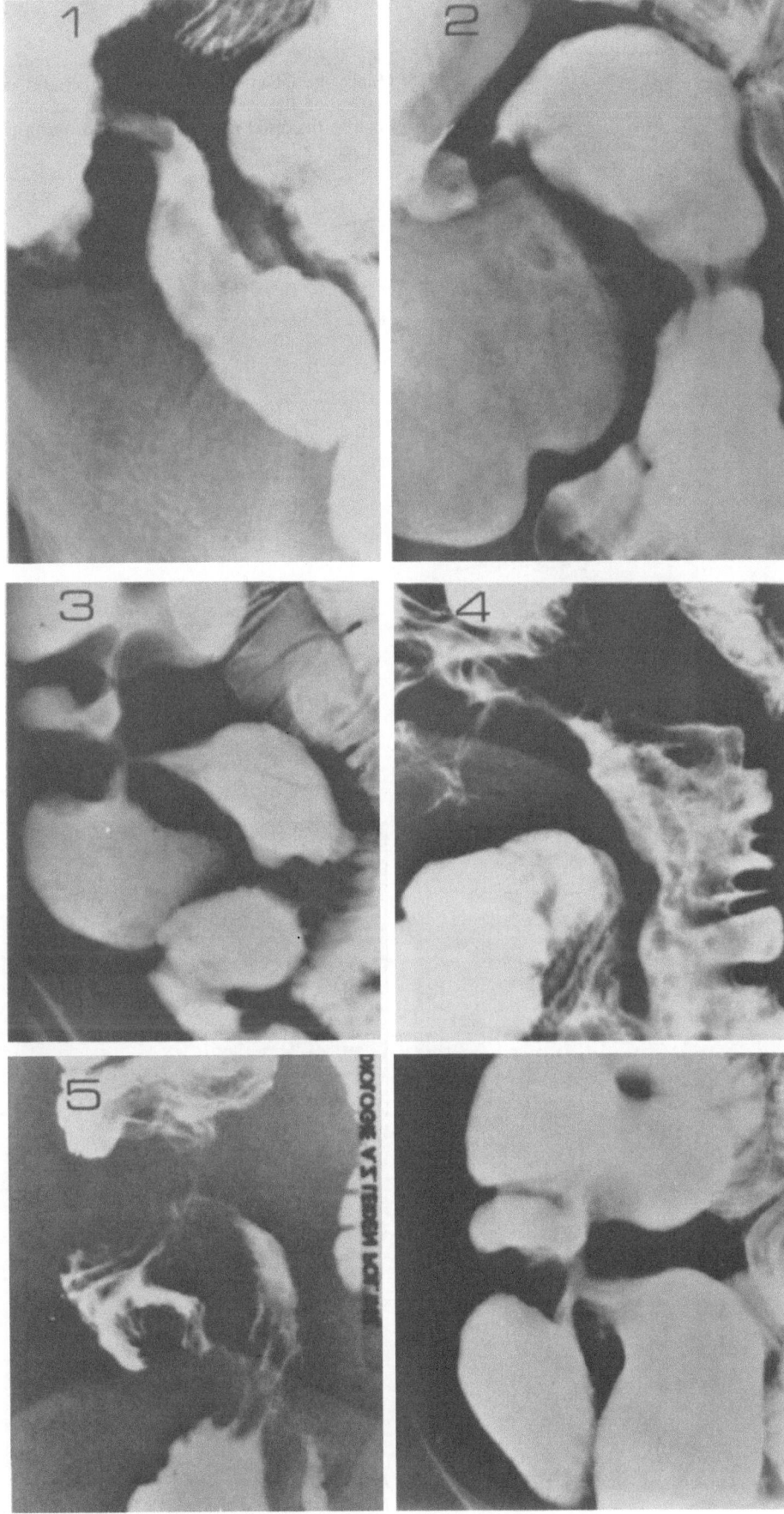

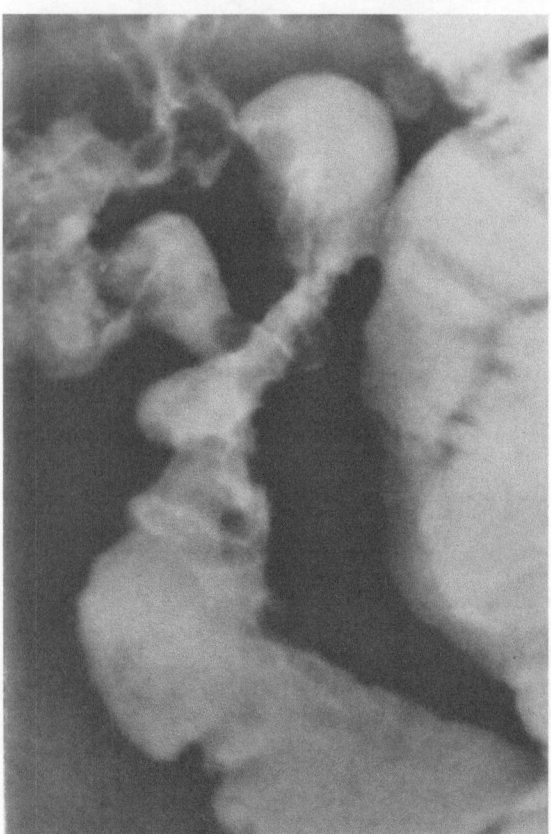

Fig. 9.26
Since the inflammatory process penetrates deeper into all layers of the wall in Crohn's disease than in ulcerative colitis, the distal ileum is often narrower instead of dilated.

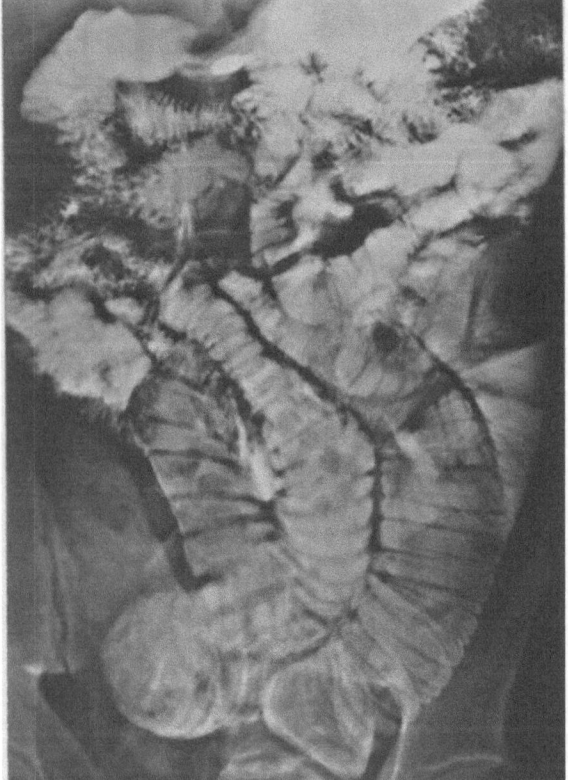

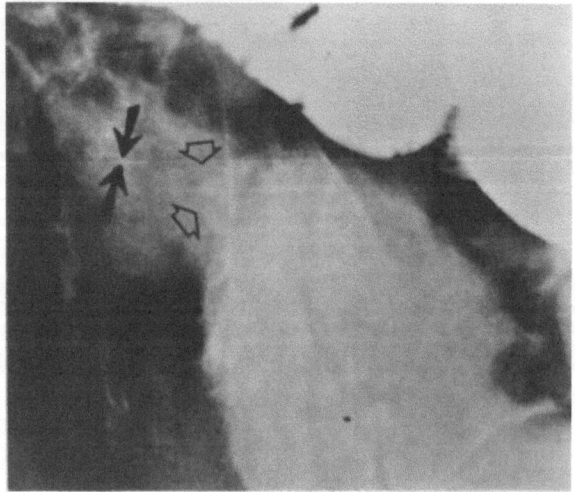

Fig. 9.27
Marked shriveling of Bauhin's valve can cause an ileus.

In a classical case the irregularly defined mucosal abnormalities which bulge out into the lumen cause the distal ileum to also appear narrower on the x-ray instead of dilated (fig. 9.26). Pronounced shriveling of Bauhin's valve can in fact cause a stenosis which may give rise to an ileus (fig. 9.27).

In contrast differentiation between a single occurrence of ulcerative colitis with reflux ileitis and a cured Crohn's disease involving the colon and the distal ileum is often exceedingly difficult. This is particularly true if:

1. The patient's history is not really typical or can no longer be determined with accuracy.
2. The entire colon has atrophied and the distal ileum is not longer than about 20 cm.
3. Bauhin's valve is wide open and the cecum has obviously shriveled (fig. 9.28).

A totally atrophied distal ileum and an open Bauhin's valve are also encountered in patients who use laxatives chronically. However, in these cases there is an atrophy of the mucosa and the muscular layers instead of a superficial inflammation of the intestinal wall and secondary fibrosis so that the cecum is dilated rather than shriveled. Furthermore in contrast to an ulcerative colitis, these abnormalities are more pronounced in the ileocecal region than in the descending colon and the rectosigmoid (fig. 9.29). Rectoscopic examination of these patients, almost always females, reveals the typical so-called pseudo-melanosis aspect.

In exceptional cases Crohn's disease may appear as an 'acute abdomen' without muscular defense. An inflamed appendix may also be the only localization of the – at that moment – usually unrecognized Crohn's disease. If an appendicular abscess with or without fistulization should develop later, then Crohn's disease should still be considered.

Roentgenologically it is difficult or impossible to differentiate Crohn's disease not only from tuberculosis (fig. 9.30) but also from ischemic abnormalities and eosinophilic gastroenteritis. Both of these diseases may be characterized only by a swollen fold relief in the early stage and by more irregular changes in the wall as well as ulcerations later on. The totally different history, however, indicates the diagnosis in most cases; in addition there is always marked eosinophilia in the blood in cases of eosinophilic infiltration.

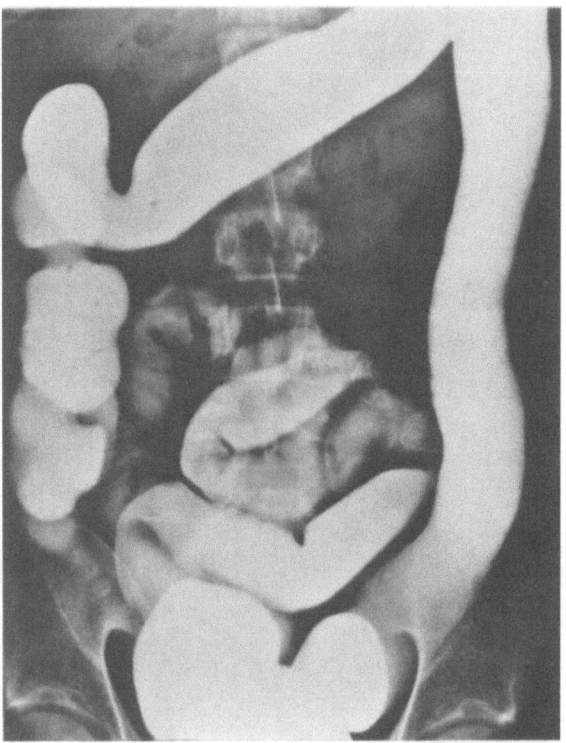

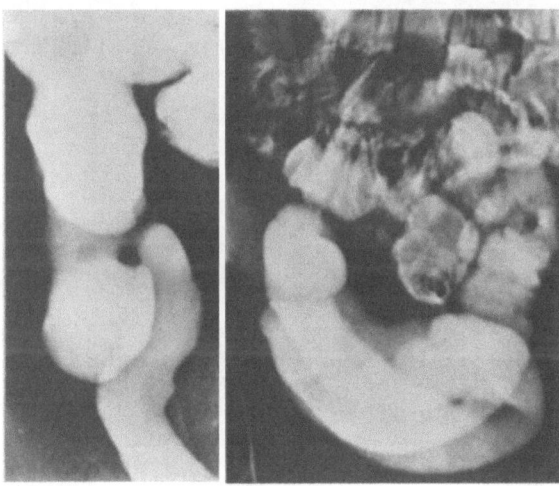

Fig. 9.28
Remission of Crohn's disease of the colon and the last 50–60 centimeters of the ileum. Here the cecum has shriveled and Bauhin's valve is wide open. The only complaint was a gradually increasing diarrhea of 7 years duration.

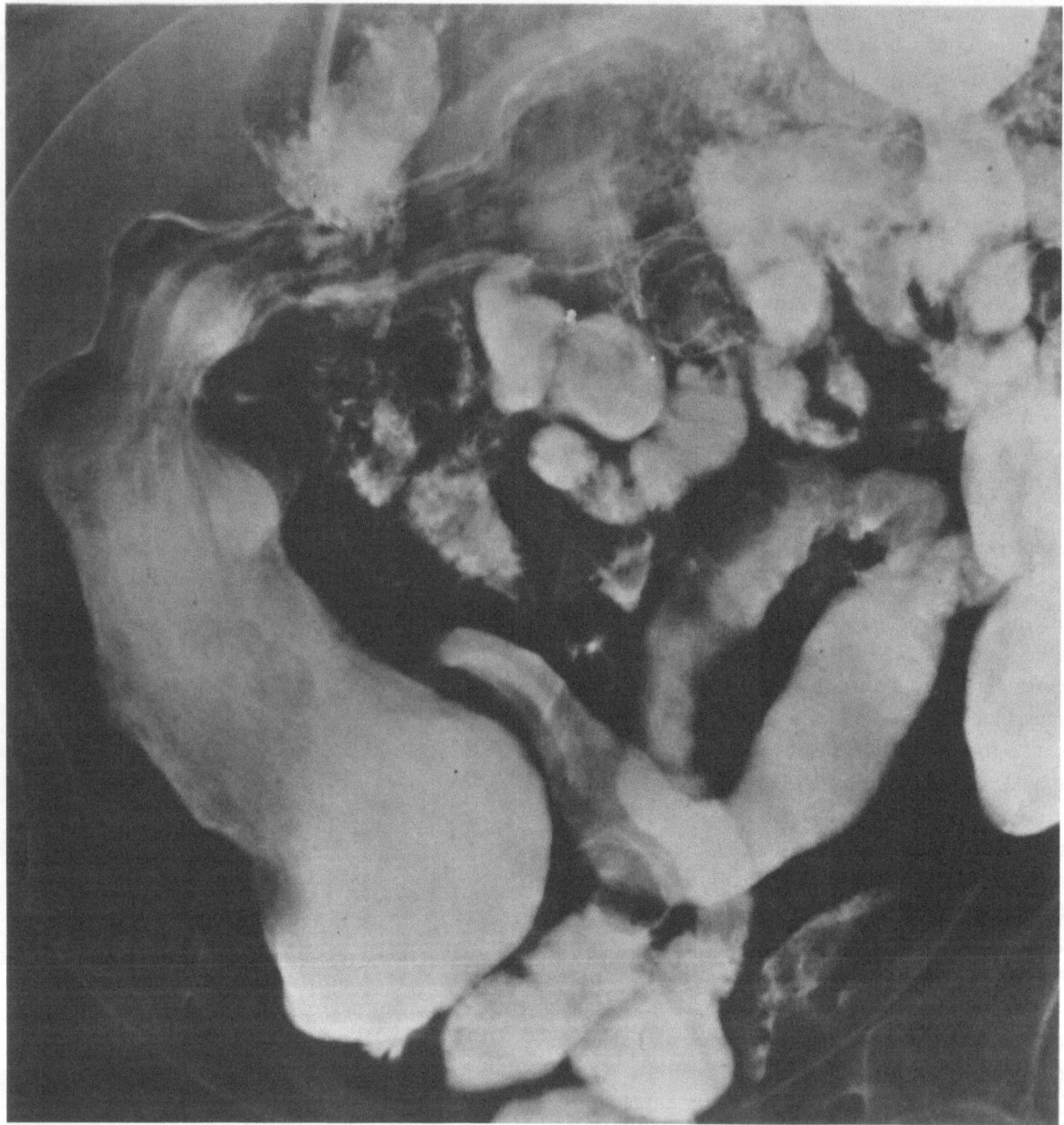

Fig. 9.29
Atrophy of the mucosa in the colon and the distal ileum as a result of the chronic use of laxatives. In such cases the cecum is often dilated instead of narrower.

As we have already seen, ulcerations in Crohn's disease heal with pronounced fibrosis and later also shriveling (fig. 9.31). As a result of the stenoses which may then develop (fig. 9.32), the abdominal pain can become colic-like and borborygmus may become pronounced. In exceptional cases the disease can have such a mild course during the active phase that these symptoms, suggesting ob-struction, may even be the patient's first complaint.

Especially if the inflammatory process was fairly superficial, the tendency to form strictures will be less, and fibrous plaques will be seen at the sites of the destroyed mucosa. The mucosal folds which have remained intact are visible in between the plaques as round, oval or elongated ridges (fig. 9.33).

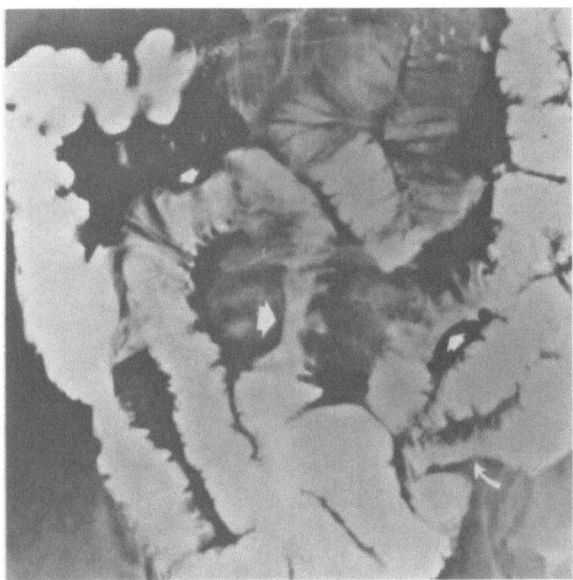

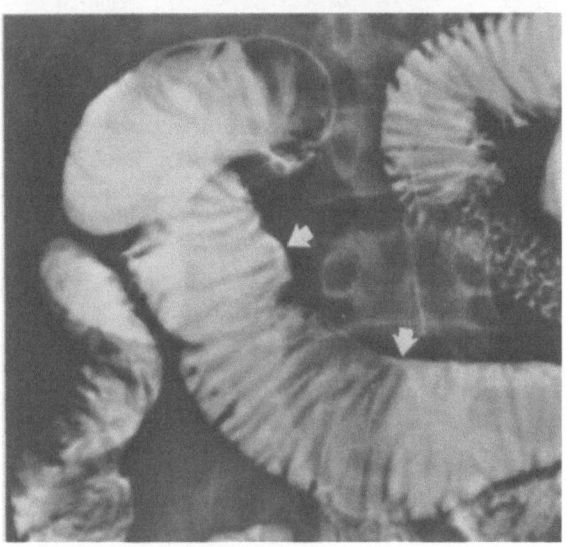

Fig. 9.30
Shriveling processes due to tuberculosis with pseudo-diverticula which cannot be differentiated from those seen in Crohn's disease. In ischemia, the abnormalities generally merge together.

Fig. 9.31
Ulcerations due to Crohn's disease which have healed with fibrotic shriveling. On one side of the intestine the mucosal pattern has disappeared completely.

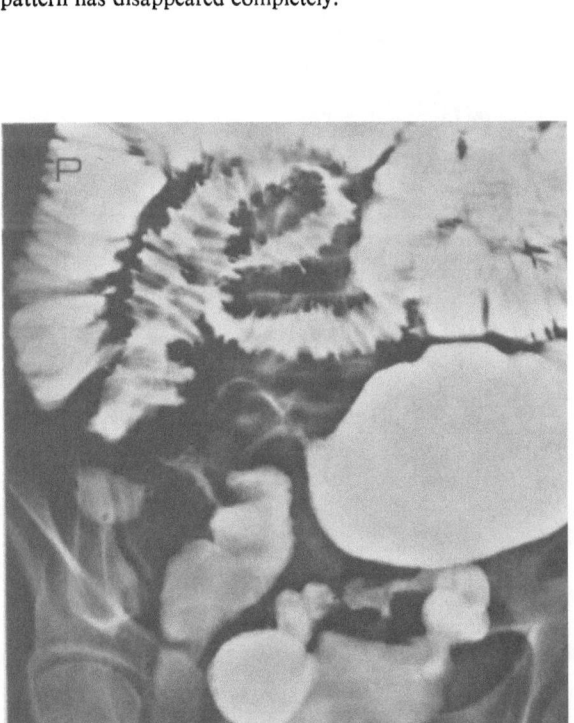

Fig. 9.32
PQ. Two patients with Crohn's disease show multiple stenoses as a result of ulcers which have healed with fibrosis. In patient Q the abnormalities could only be seen on the spot films taken under compression! (see also page 196).

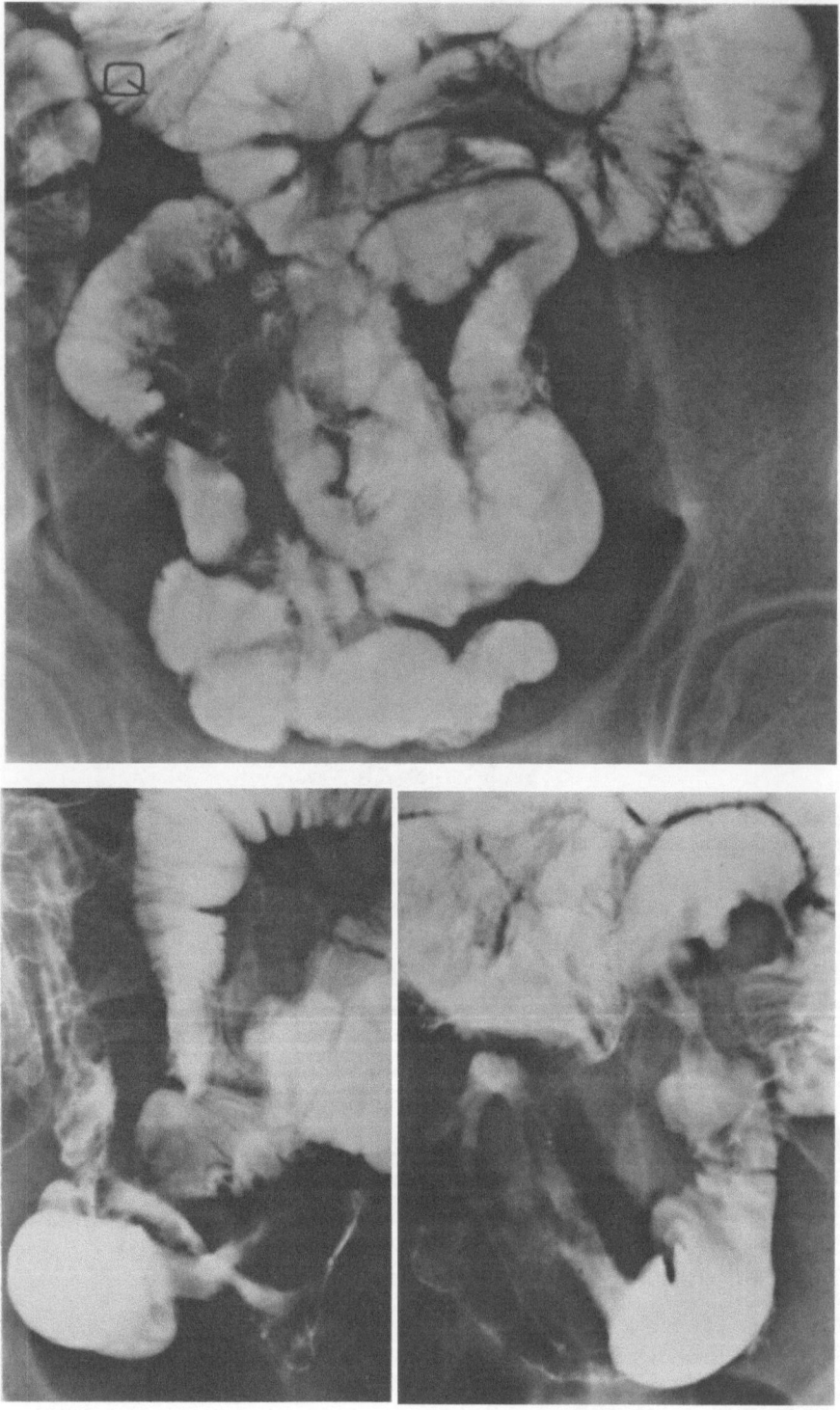

*Fig. 9.32*Q

PQ. Two patients with Crohn's disease show multiple stenoses as a result of ulcers which have
      healed with fibrosis. In patient Q the abnormalities could only be seen on the spot films taken
      under compression!

Fig. 9.33

Spot films of four patients with fibrotic plaques which have developed as a result of local destruction of the mucosa. The
remaining intact mucosal folds can be seen as round, oval or elongated rather broad clarifications.

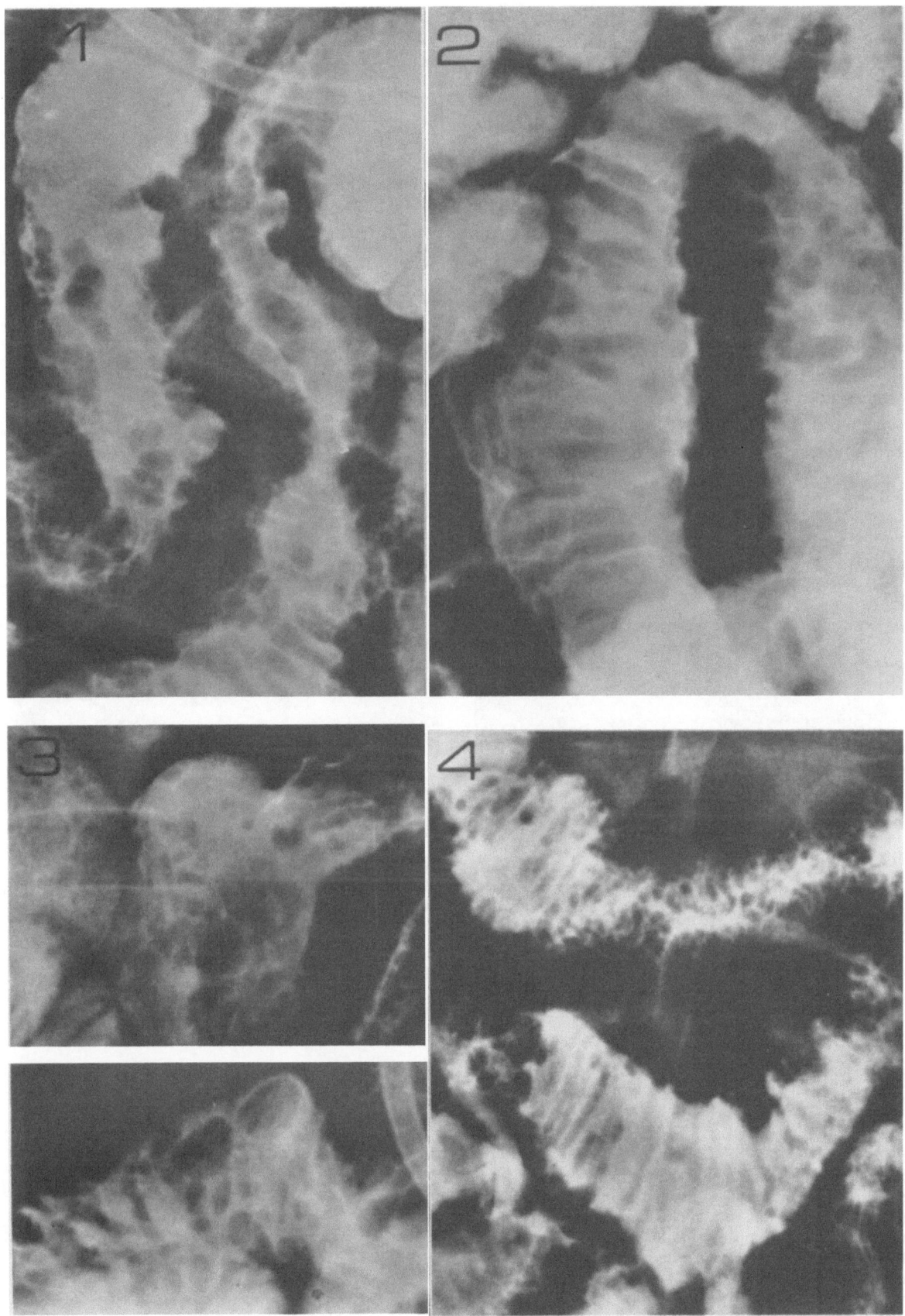

The differentiation between skip lesions which have become fibrotic and other ulcers in the small bowel which have healed with shriveling and formed stenoses can cause difficulties.

However, the history of a patient with celiac disease or ulcers due to ischemia differs completely from that of a patient with Crohn's disease.

Particularly when the stenosis is located in the distal ileum, the differentiation between post-ischemia and a cured Crohn's disease can be impossible. In both diseases, an asymmetric shriveling produces the same 'shell sign' (figs. 9.34, 9.35).

Also a very marked atrophy of the mucosa in the ileocecal region, sometimes fairly irregular in nature with strictures of various sizes, can be due to an ischemia of the intestinal wall (fig. 9.36) and therefore mimic a Crohn's disease (compare fig. 9.28).

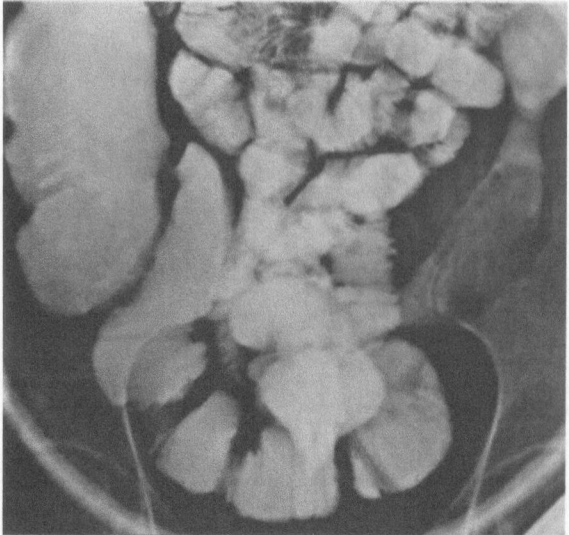

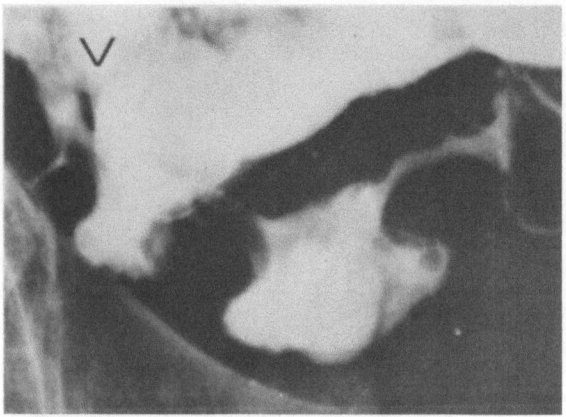

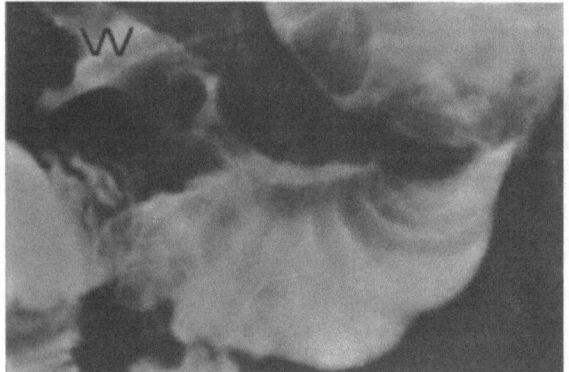

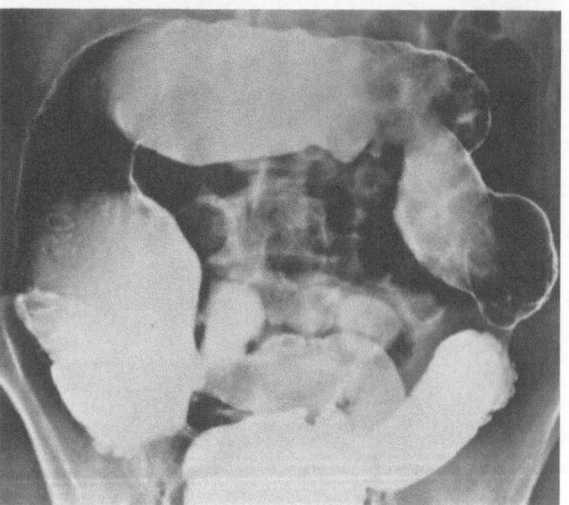

Fig. 9.36
Two cases of so-called ischemic colitis. In one of the patients, the strictures were constantly visible in the distal ileum (→).

Fig. 9.35
Asymmetric shriveling of ulcerations in the intestinal wall causes the mucosal folds to assume a radial course directed toward the ulcer; this pattern closely resembles the emblem of the Shell Oil Company (the Shell sign). Differentiation between old ulcers in Crohn's disease, ischemia and tuberculosis is impossible.
v. Ischemia.
w. Crohn's disease after 14 years of remission.

Fig. 9.34
Emblem of the Shell Oil Company

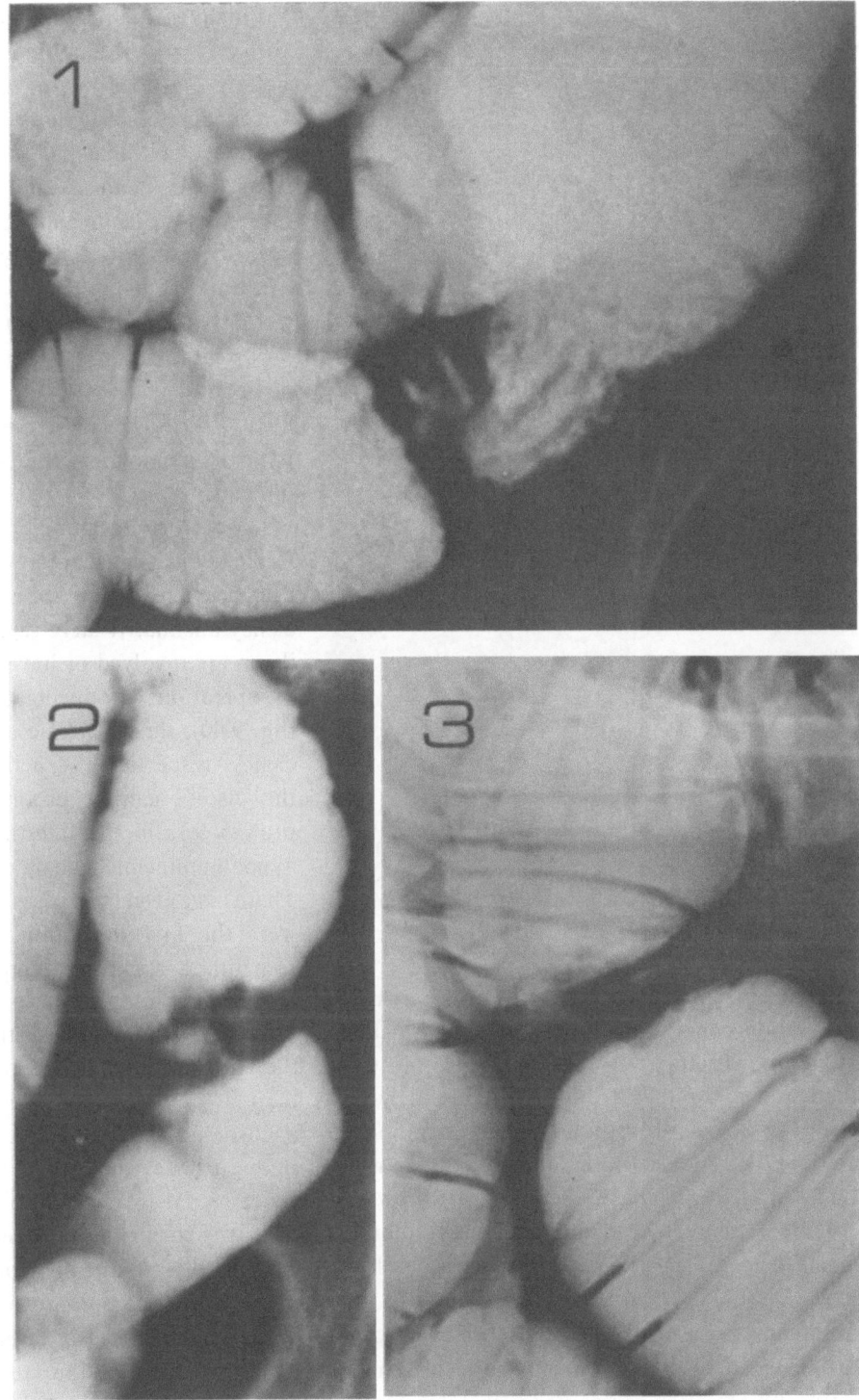

Fig. 9.37
Three patients with short constricting ulcerations of aspecific origin in the small intestine. For patients 1 and 3, ingestion of enteric-coated KCl tablets could be established from the history.

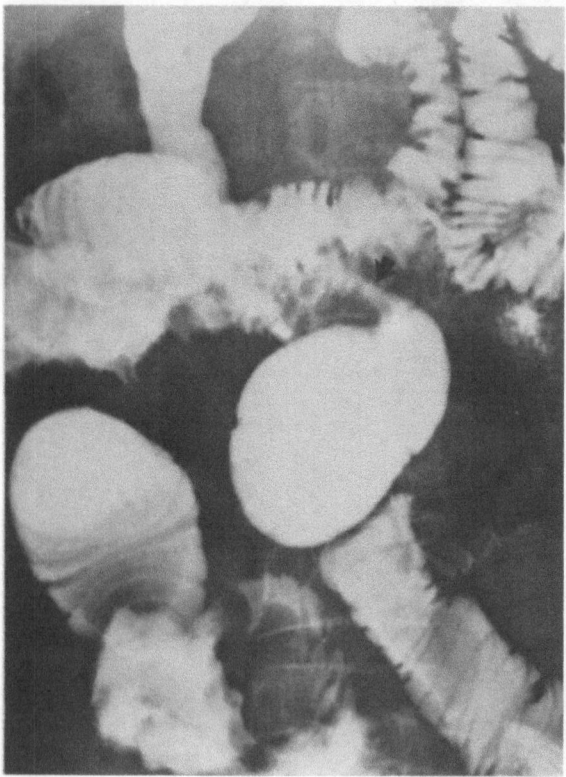

Fig. 9.38
Stenosis (→) in the small intestine as a result of lympho-sarcoma resembles a skip lesion. However, erratically en-larged spaces between the intestinal loops, compression phenomena and areas of extensive mucosal destruction can also be seen.

Therefore it remains imperative to obtain relevant information concerning the history of the patient.

Crohn's strictures in the jejunum must be differentiated carefully from those caused by cor-rosion or localized vasculitis after ingestion of enteric-coated tablets containing potassium or other drugs. In such cases the ulcers are, however, very short, generally circular and the rest of the jejunal mucosal relief appears to be completely intact (fig. 9.37). When there is a stricture of lym-phosarcoma considerable diagnostic evidence is also provided by the accompanying signs. In this disease, we are often confronted with extensive and disordered mucosal destruction. Furthermore there are several clearly defined areas in which the loops of the intestine are separated from one another and multiple compression phenomena can be observed, as a result of advanced thickening of the wall as well as clustering of the mesenteric lymphnodes (figs. 9.38 and 8.20).

Finally strictures of a spastic origin in a jejunum with an atrophied and more or less smooth mucosal pattern may occur in celiac disease (fig. 9.39). Ulcers due to celiac disease are only encountered in the most proximal part of the small intestine and never in the ileum. Although a carcinoid is usually located in the ileum and, because of the concomitant excessive fibrosis, is easily identified by the stric-tures and sudden changes in the course of the in-testine (so-called 'kinking'), these lesions sometimes occur as scattered strictures which cannot be distinguished from skip lesions or tumors (fig. 8.40L). If, however, we are well-informed as to the patient's complaints, diagnosis should not prove difficult.

Laboratory examination of a patient with Crohn's disease usually reveals a markedly elevated erythrocyte sedimentation rate with an iron defi-ciency anemia. If large segments of the jejunum or ileum are involved or have been resected in a series of operations producing a so-called short bowel (fig. 9.40), then a folinic acid or vitamin B_{12} defi-ciency, respectively, can develop. Exacerbation of the disease can be accompanied by pronounced protein loss in the intestine and as a result of a hypoalbuminemia, edema of the ankles will be seen. There have even been cases in which these symptoms were the first indications of Crohn's disease or sometimes, a chronic lymphoreticular malignancy in the small intestine.

The liver function is disturbed in one-quarter of the patients but renal biopsies reveal that in more than 50% of the patients there is fatty infiltration or a fibrotic and lymphocytic inflammatory reaction. If one realizes that all toxins of the inflammatory process pass through the liver via the portal vein, then it is surprising that healthy livers can exist in Crohn's disease and that only a small percentage of the patients acquire liver cirrhosis.

In about one out of every 25 patients, hydro-nephrosis will develop later as a result of fibrosis in the retroperitoneal region or the pelvis minor.

That one out of every 12 patients with Crohn's disease ultimately dies as a result, either direct or indirect, of this disease must be attributed not only to the above-mentioned complications but also to the increased risk of malignancy. As in ulcerative colitis there is a greater chance that an adeno-carcinoma will develop if a patient has had Crohn's

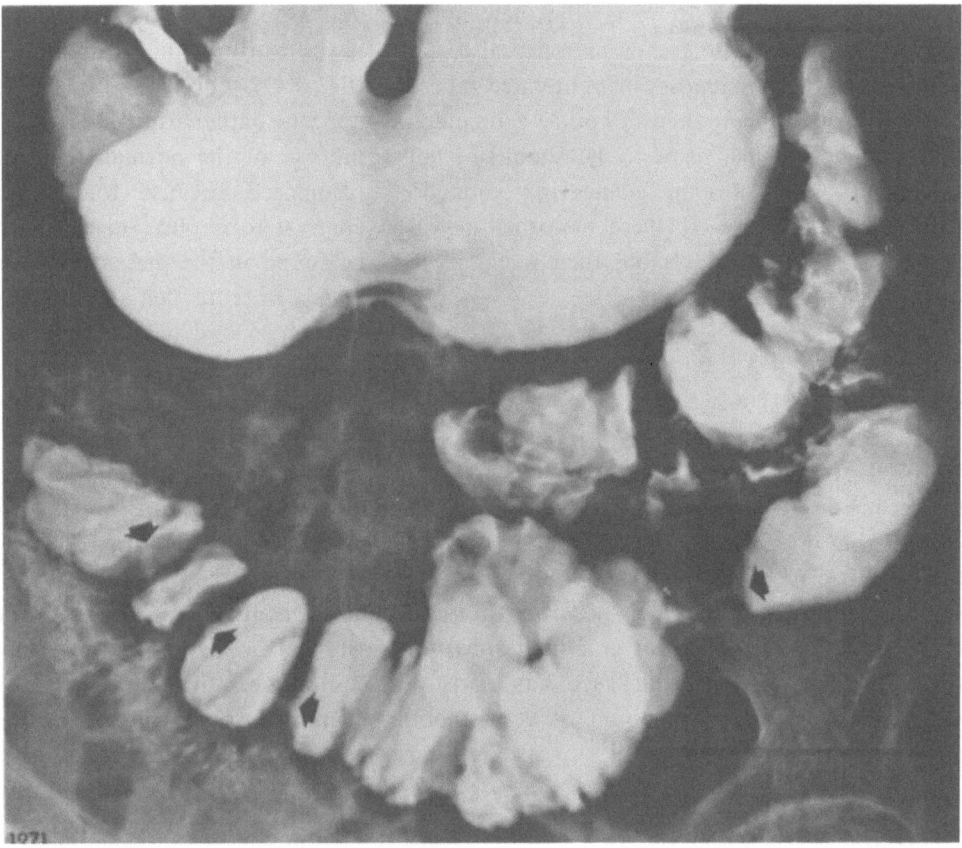

Fig. 9.39
Stenotic areas in the jejunum of a patient with celiac disease. During surgery it was found that the constrictions were located at ulcer sites and were partly due to spasms. Angiographic examination showed that the blood vessels in the small intestine were very fragile.

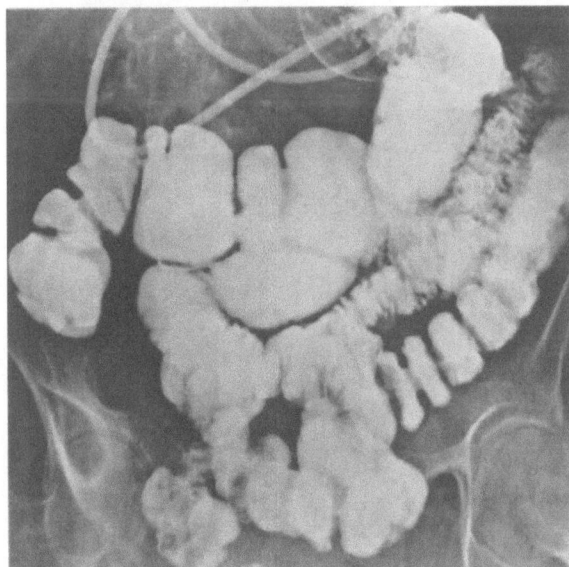

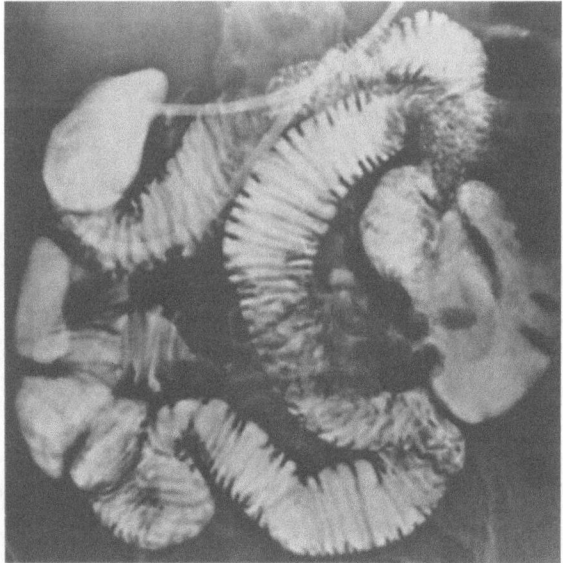

Fig. 9.40
Two examples of a so-called 'short bowel': after multiple resections the small intestine is at the most 1 meter long.

Left: 23-year-old patient. Right: recurring stenosis ±10 cm long in the region of the anastomosis with the remaining segment of the colon.

disease for more than 15 years. If a new patient with a fairly short history shows a mucosal pattern with either multiple stenoses or obliterated mucosa suggestive of a tumor, then of course a reticulosis or a lymphosarcoma, respectively, should be considered first and not a malignancy in conjunction with Crohn's disease. If these abnormalities are found in the ileocecal region, then a carcinoma of the cecum is also possible.

3. Reflux ileitis

In 10–20% of the cases of ulcerative colitis involving the cecum, a so-called reflux ileitis of the most distal 10 or 20 cm of the ileum will occur. In most cases this ileitis can be distinguished quite easily in several respects from the ileitis in Crohn's disease. It is neither hypertrophic nor granulomatous; furthermore the wall is not thickened but is instead very thin. The mucous membrane is very smooth and there are only very small superficial ulcers

and abscesses in the crypts of Lieberkühn which never lead to the formation of fistulous tracts (fig. 9.41). On the x-ray an ileum without folds appears rather tube-like. The transition to the mucosa of the normal ileum can in fact only be recognized because folds are again visible. In contrast to Crohn's disease, no abnormalities can be found in the mesentery or the regional lymph nodes. In reflux ileitis Bauhin's valve is quite often wide open and lies perpendicular to the diseased cecum. Every time the patient pushes as if to move his bowels, there is marked reflux of the colon contents into the distal ileum causing clarifications on the contrast column. Sometimes these dingy looking clarifications are incorrectly attributed to mucus and secretion products due to the ileitis, which therefore appears to be more serious than it in fact is. It is necessary to force the colon contents out of the ileum by increasing the amount of contrast medium administered; in this manner the ileum is flushed clean so that the abnormalities can be seen in their true proportions (fig. 9.42).

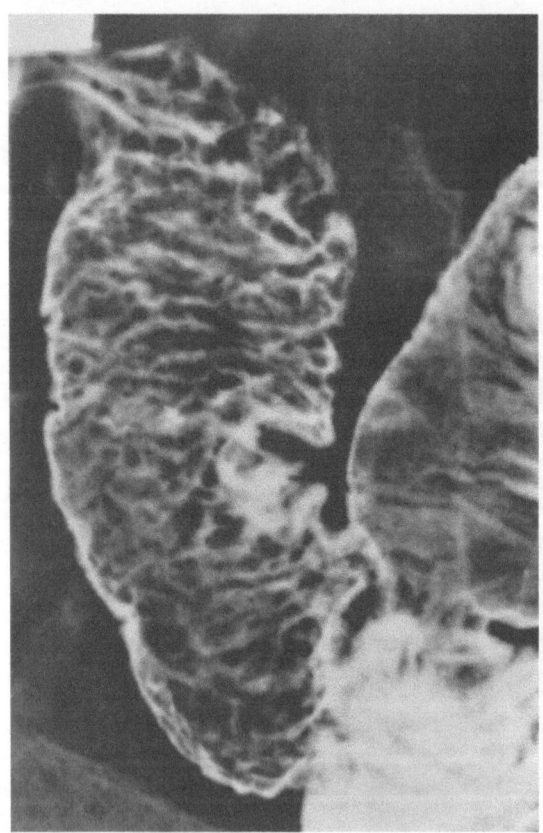
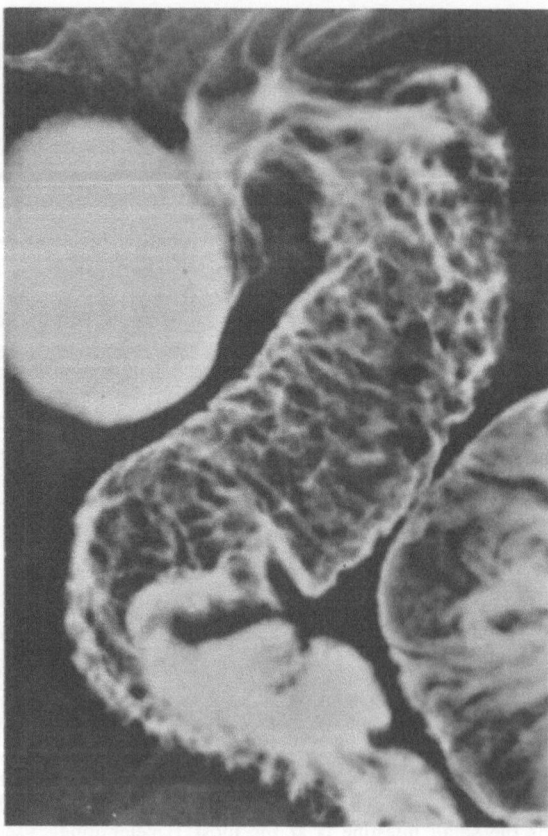

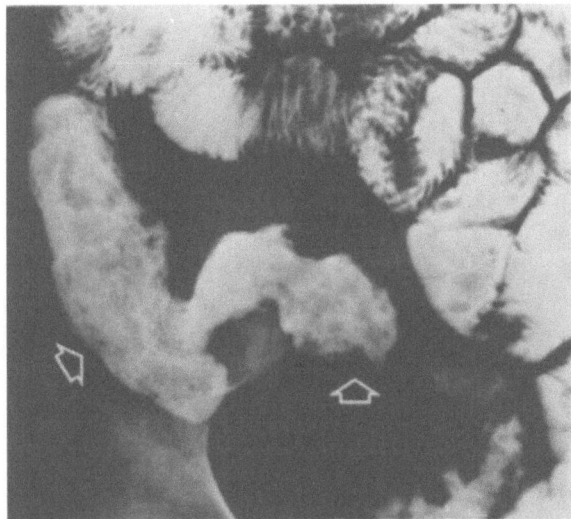

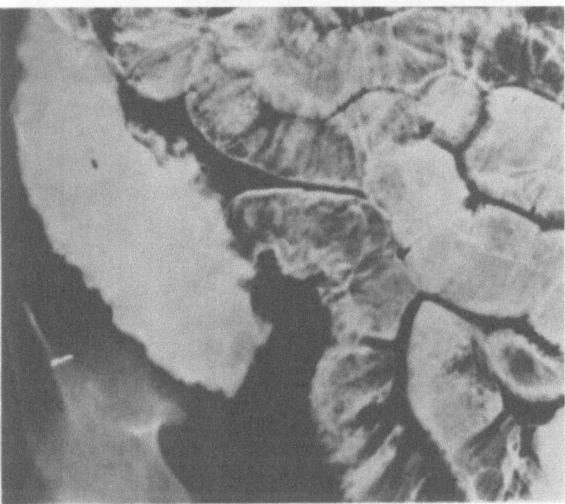

Fig. 9.42
A reflux ileitis sometimes appears worse than it in fact is, or is incorrectly presumed, if the distal ileum remains contaminated when the intestine is flushed clean.

←

Fig. 9.41
Granular appearance of mucosal surface and very superficial, transversely directed ulcerative grooves in the distal ileum as a result of reflux ileitis in ulcerative colitis. A transverse course of ulcerations in the distal ileum is probably a result of a rather superficial edematous swelling of the mucosa. In Crohn's disease the edema is much more pronounced which necessarily leads to a predominantly longitudinal folding of the inner surface of those parts of the bowel which are only scarcely provided with mucosal folds.

4. Yersinia EC infections

Already in 1945, Golden described a disease of the small intestine which he differentiated from the regional ileitis found in Crohn's disease. His patients were females 10–30 years of age who complained of pain in the lower right quadrant highly similar to that encountered in acute appendicitis. The painful terminal ileum was palpable in some cases. Radiological examination showed mucosal changes in the terminal centimeters of the ileum. Round filling defects suggestive of polyps were seen, and in some cases the mucosal folds were broadened. In those cases in which an appendectomy was performed, the appendix proved to be normal but the distal ileum was thickened and there were swollen mesenteric lymph nodes. In the course of a follow-up study over a period of 10 years Crohn's disease could not be demonstrated in any of these patients. In other cases, the symptoms were suggestive of Crohn's disease and the patients were referred to the internist or the gastroenterologist. In such cases, there was usually a brief history of cramp-like pain in the lower abdomen, sometimes associated with diarrhea and pyrexia.

Between 1950 and 1962 analogous patients were described by Prevot and others. They were all unable to identify the cause of this infection and believed that the mucosal abnormalities found resulted from hyperplasia of the lymphoid tissue.

In recent literature there is an increasing tendency to consider yersinia enterocolitica as the causative agent in these infections of the terminal loop of ileum. In veterinary medicine this bacterium has long been known as the gram-negative Pasteurella X, which causes lethal infectious diseases. Serological tests for the presence of yersinia EC proved to be positive in a number of cases in the abovementioned groups of patients.

The titers become elevated during the acute phase of this infection, which usually lasts only several weeks, and then gradually during recovery return to normal values.

The clinical manifestations of this disease do not always resemble those of a common gastroenteritis or appendicitis; in rare cases they can mimic a systemic sepsis or they can be accompanied by an erythema nodosum or a polyarthritis. The cardinal symptoms are a brief history of cramp-like pain in

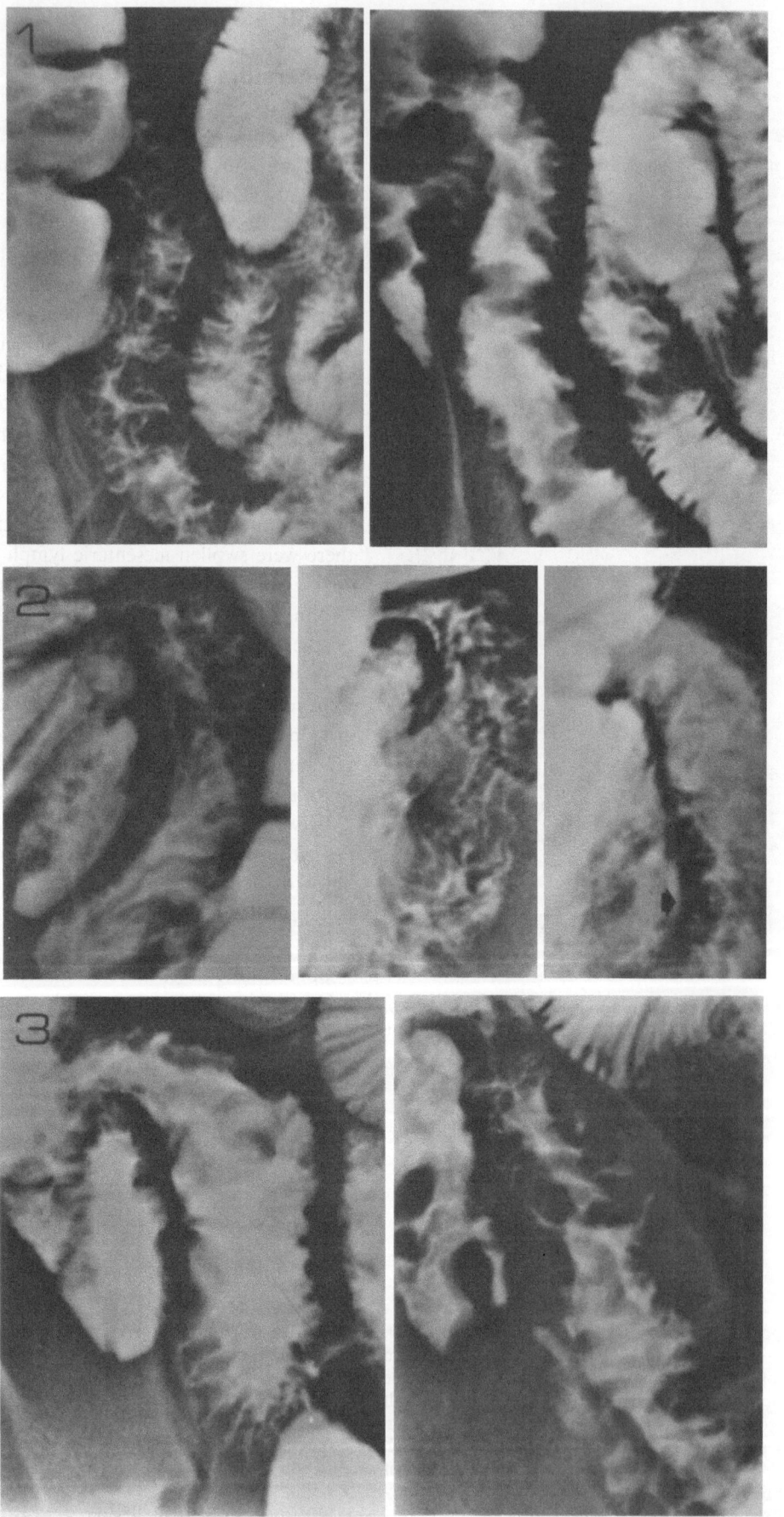

Fig. 9.43

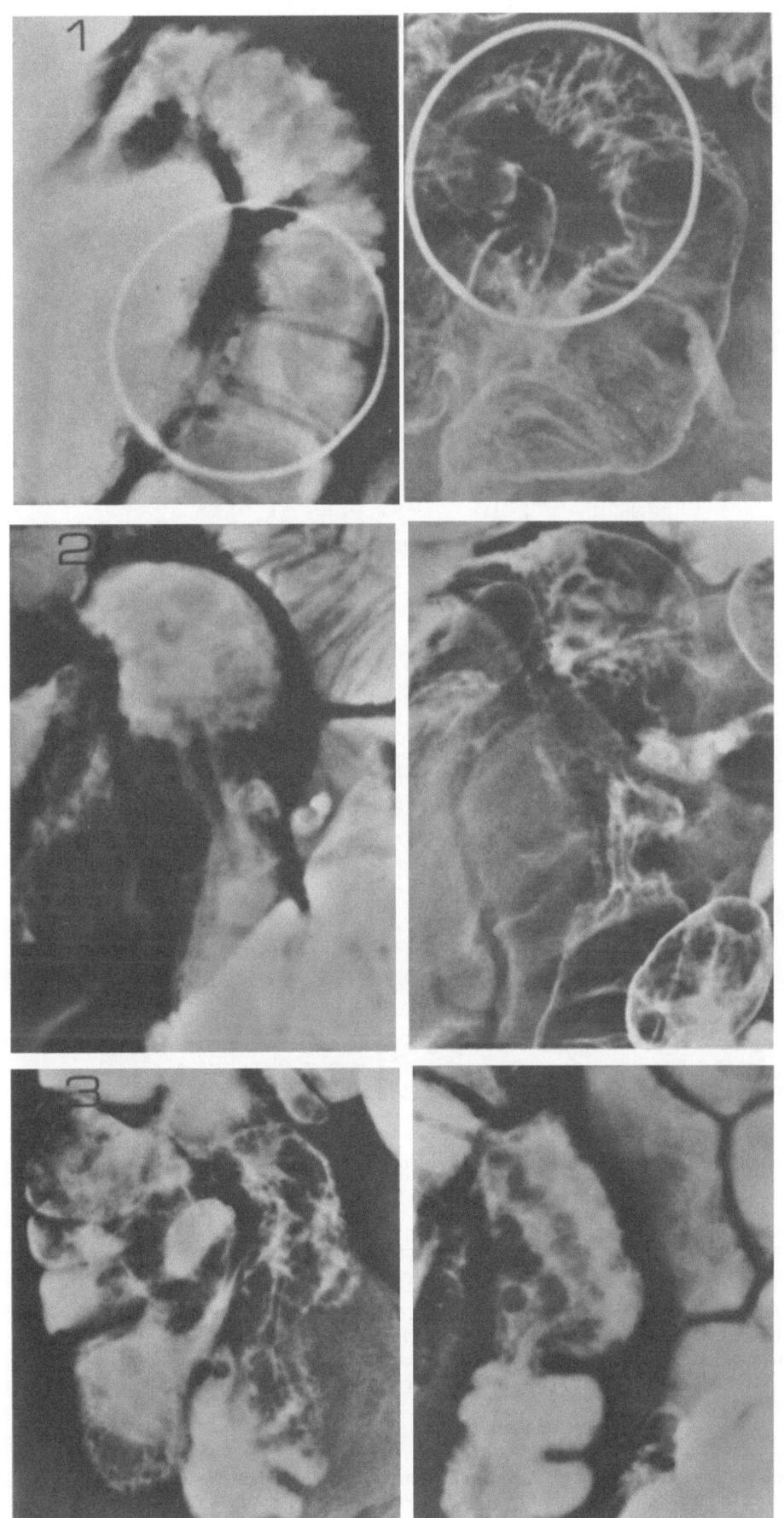

Fig. 9.44

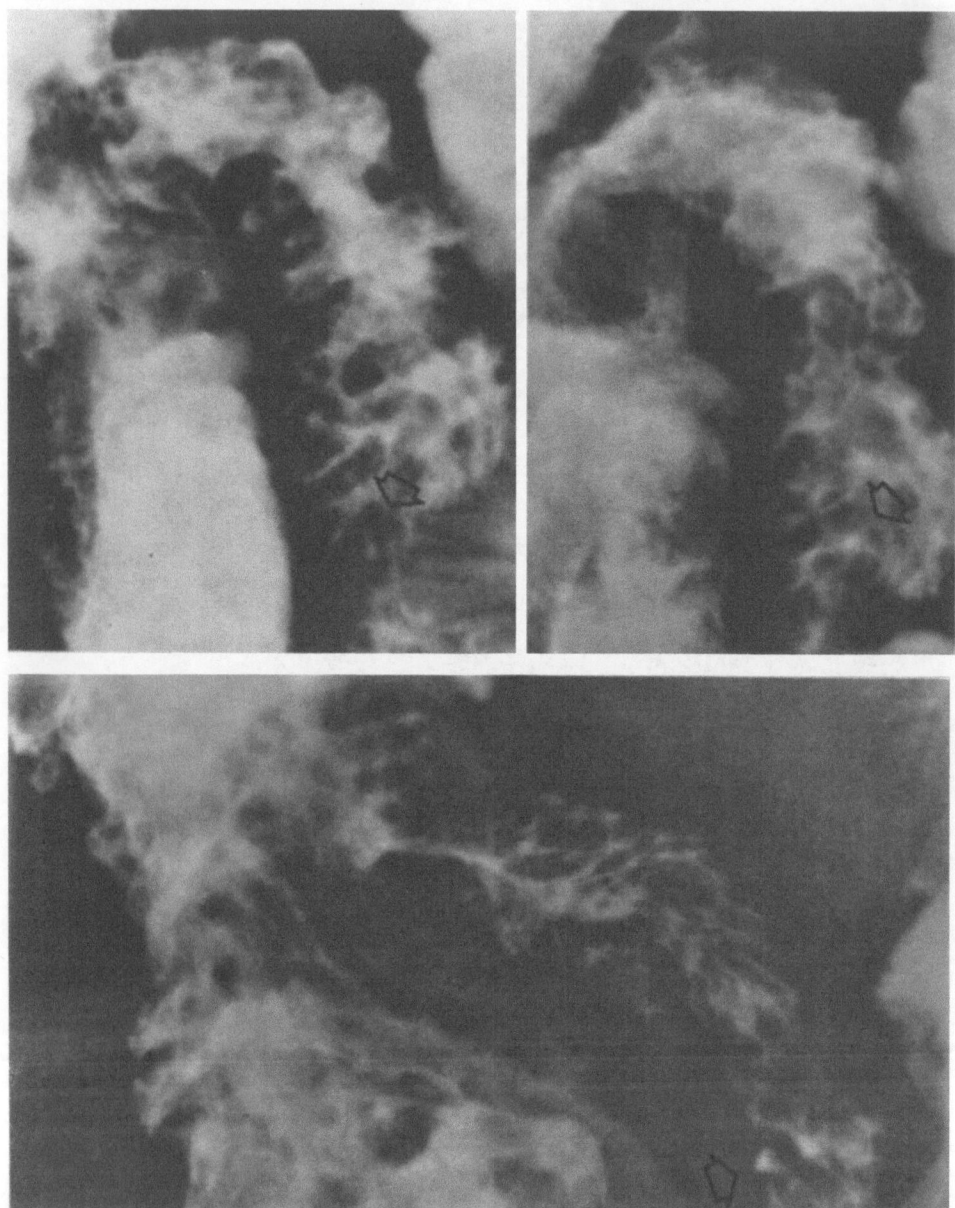

Fig. 9.45
Yersinia EC infection in the distal ileum; pattern is suggestive of aphthous ulcers (→).

←

Fig. 9.43
Three patients with yersinia ÉC-infection in the small intestine. In a 10–20 cm segment of the
distal ileum there are more or less round filling defects, which resemble lymph follicles or
inflammatory granulomas, as well as greatly broadened mucosal folds which follow an undulating course. Some filling defects contain a barium deposit (→) which is suggestive of a
central ulcer crater (see p. 204).

Fig. 9.44
The same patients as those seen in fig. 9.43, 2–3 months later. The abnormalities have clearly
diminished in all cases; they have not spread as would be expected in for example Crohn's
disease (see p. 205).

the lower abdomen, diarrhea and pyrexia. Because there are often more or less acute exacerbations, the possibility of a Crohn's disease is considered and as a rule a radiological examination is then carried out. When the symptoms are suggestive of acute appendicitis the situation is, however, more difficult. When it seems likely that surgery will be necessary in the near future, a radiological examination of the small intestine is in fact not recommended. In such cases, the patient can be spared the inconvenience of an operation by performing the serological and bacteriological tests first. The radiological changes observed only last for several weeks or 2–3 months at the most (fig. 9.44) and are limited to the terminal 20 cm of the ileum. In this area, we can see filling defects, sometimes reminiscent of cobblestones, which are probably due to hyperplasia of lymphoid tissue or granulomas with centrally located ulcers (fig. 9.45). The mucosal folds follow a very tortuous course, are increased in number and unmistakably broadened. The separation between the distal ileum and the adjacent cecal loops can be increased (fig. 9.43). The broad folds and the increased distance between the intestinal loops are the result of inflammatory edema of the mucosal folds and the intestinal wall, respectively.

These radiological findings are slightly different from those encountered in the initial stages of Crohn's disease. In the latter, the number of mucosal folds does not increase and the filling defects causing the typical cobblestones appearance are more pronounced and more oval in shape. In more advanced cases of Crohn's disease, the margins of the intestine are vaguely defined due to the numerous ulcerations which may be present. In comparison with the normal terminal loop of the ileum, the abundance of mucosal folds is the most striking feature and has proved to be a valid criterium for diagnosis of yersinia EC infection.

The radiological features of nodular lymphoid hyperplasia, as observed especially in children and not to be regarded as pathological, are readily distinguishable from the radiological findings in yersinia EC infections. In lymphoid hyperplasia, the filling defects are regularly arranged and rarely exceed a diameter of 1–3 mm.

5. Eosinophilic gastroenteritis

This recurrent disease, which is also often self-limiting, develops in patients with an allergic diathesis and should not be considered a true inflammatory process. Histologically it is characterized by extensive eosinophilic infiltration throughout all layers of the intestinal wall, particularly the mucosa and the lamina propria of the submucosa. The main localizations are the jejunum and the pars antralis of the stomach as well as, although less common, the duodenum and the proximal ileum. In addition to abdominal pain and malabsorption accompanied by diarrhea, there can also be such a marked loss of protein in the digestive tract that edema of the ankles also occurs. In addition to a hypoproteinemia there will also be a blood eosinophilia which may even reach values of 80 per cent. On the x-rays the infiltrates which bulge out into the intestinal lumen appear as polypous growths of various sizes; the mucosal folds show pronounced thickening and follow a tortuous course. The lumen of the involved intestinal loops is usually decreased; if the eosinophilic infiltration has damaged the muscular layers, the lumen may also be dilated locally. Because of the thickened intestinal walls and the edematous swelling of the mesentery, the distance between adjacent intestinal loops is obviously increased on the x-ray (fig. 9.46). Ulcerations and fistulas are not seen as a rule but if they do occur then a lymphosarcoma can be difficult to distinguish from an eosinophilic gastroenteritis (fig. 9.47). Differentiation from a Crohn's disease localized in the proximal intestine as well as a mild case of Whipple's disease can also cause problems. In Whipple's disease, however, the jejunal loops are dilated rather than narrowed and there is no increase in the separation between intestinal loops.

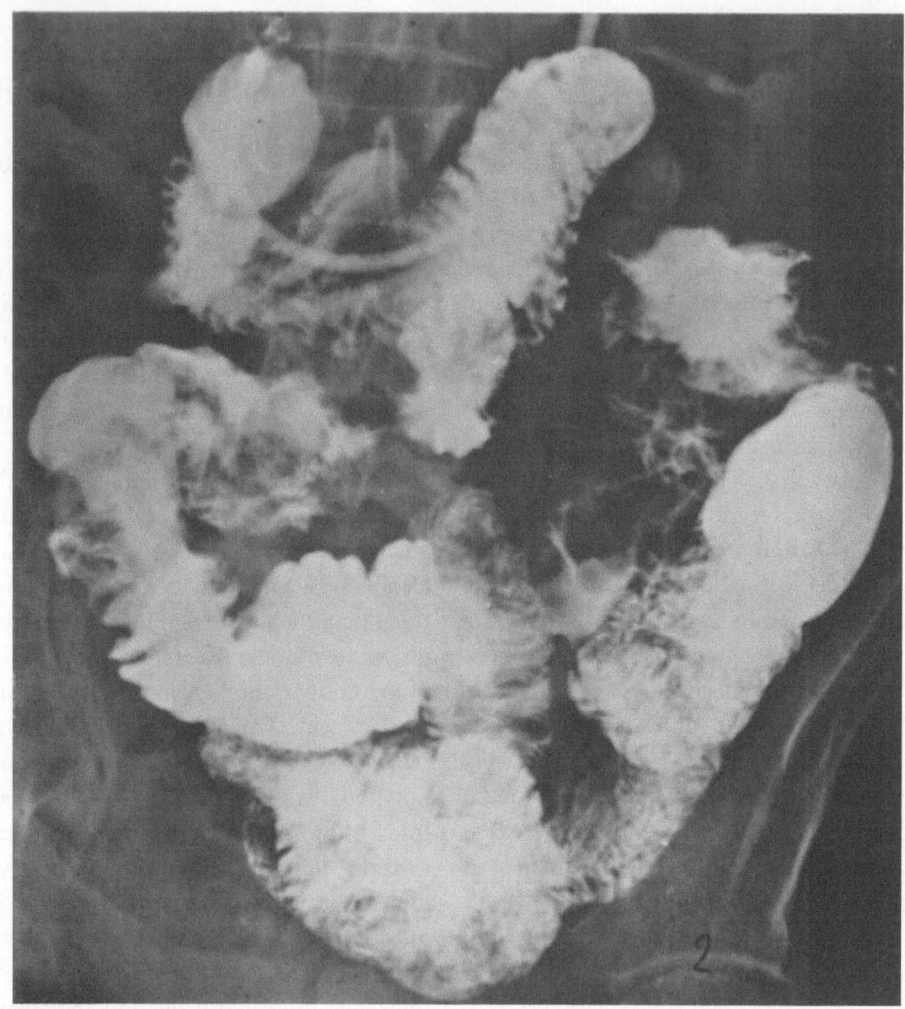

Fig. 9.46
Eosinophilic gastroenteritis, in this case with large infiltrates and extensive destruction so that differentiation from a lymphosarcoma (fig. 9.47) on the base of radiological criteria is not possible.

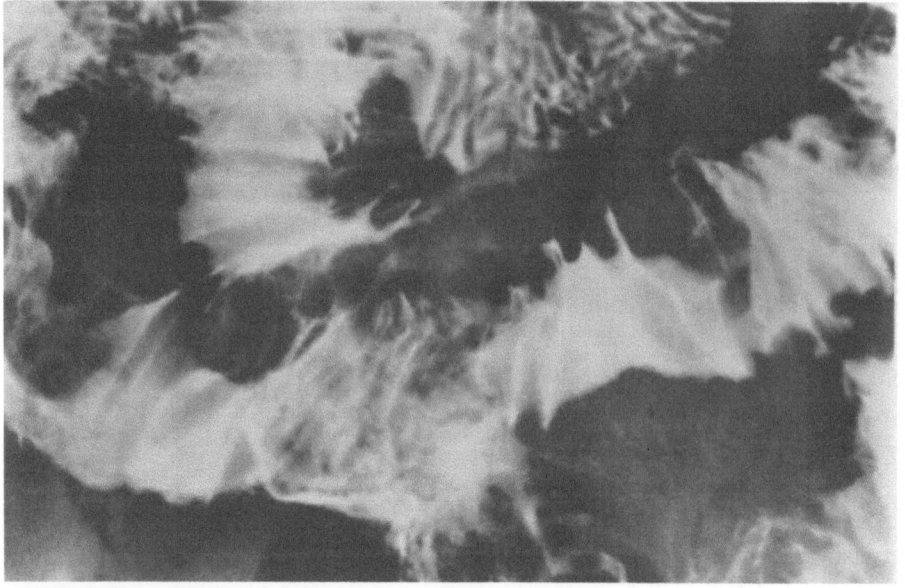

Fig. 9.47
Lymphosarcoma which cannot be differentiated from the highly destructive eosinophilic gastroenteritis in fig. 9.46.

6. Radiation enteritis

In the fight to increase the chances of survival for patients with malignant tumors by using radiotherapy, one must always be aware of the possibility of permanent damage to adjacent tissues.

Irradiation of tumors in the abdomen implies damage to the digestive tract in particular. In 1931 Desjardin showed that in the digestive tract of animals the small intestine is the most sensitive to roentgen rays. If the small intestine were less mobile, then abnormalities could be expected in the small bowel of all patients treated with a therapeutic dosage of radiation. The vulnerability increases from the duodenum towards the ileum; the sensitivity of the transverse colon, sigmoid, rectum and stomach is, however, less pronounced. Roswitt and his associates believe that the maximum therapeutic dosage is determined by the vulnerability of the small intestine and the kidneys.

The ileum is damaged by irradiation much more frequently than the jejunum since the ileum is more or less fixed in the pelvis minor and is therefore much less mobile than the jejunum. If adhesion has also occurred, then radiotherapy of the genital organs can sometimes cause an acute radiation enteritis of the ileum. Reports of radiation enteritis are fairly scarce in the journals of radiology. In part this can certainly be attributed to the fact that the mucosal patterns obtained during the conventional follow-through examination in such cases usually cannot be evaluated. We now know that these vague patterns are often caused by an increase in the motility and mucus secretion in the irradiated field; as a result there is a pronounced tendency toward flocculation of the barium suspension in this region.

A radiological examination of the small intestine before irradiation of organs in the abdomen is certainly worthwhile. In this manner adhesion and fusion of ileal loops in the pelvis minor can be discovered and irradiation can then be performed with the patient in the position of Trendelenburg. If the bladder is full and rectal air insufflation is used, the ileal loops can be forced back into the abdominal cavity insofar as possible, thus considerably reducing the chance of radiation enteritis.

The histological changes characterizing radiation enteritis consist mainly of ulcerations and signs of sclerosis, either isolated, multiple or in combination (Warren & Friedman, 1942). Both the ulcerations and the fibrosis can lead to the formation of strictures. The ulcerations can be deep-seated but may also develop as only superficial erosions. In addition there can be numerous changes which generally occur secondary to an inflammatory process such as perforations, fistulas and adhesions. There is almost always a more or less extensive necrosis; in extreme cases, an entire intestinal loop may be gangrenous.

In the early stages, the changes consist of edema and fibrinous exudation. As a result of the deposit of albumin, there is a hyalinization of the collagenous tissue, in particular the connective tissue of the mucosa and the submucosa as well as the walls of the vessels in the intestinal wall and the mesentery. The walls of both the intestine and the vessels become thicker, initially as a result of the edema and hyalinization but later also because of the eventual hypertrophy of the muscular tissue. Although the mucosa sometimes appears completely normal without any signs of ulceration, it is in these cases in fact atrophied and fixed to the submucosa. Not only arteries but also veins are involved; histologically they are characteristic of an endarteritis obliterans with endothelial proliferation, medionecrosis and thrombosis. Moreover, there can also be hyaline degeneration in the walls of the lymph vessels as well as a thickening of the endothelial layer; these lymphatic channels are also often ectatically dilated. Bosniak et al. (1969) clearly demonstrated these changes in the vessel in an experiment with rabbits. They irradiated a 3 cm exposed segment of the small intestine prepared surgically and then evaluated the circulation immediately after irradiation (1500 and 3000r) and periodically for 5 weeks using angiography. They observed the following:

1. Striking vascular spasms 2 days after irradiation: reacted favourably to antispasmodics.
2. Five days after irradiation: a deep hemorrhagic ulcer in the irradiated field.
3. Two weeks after irradiation: vascular constriction which could no longer be relieved with papaverine and therefore was caused by an organic change. In this stage there was a chronic inflammation in the intestinal wall.

Macroscopically an intestine which has been damaged by a radiation overdose (5000–6000r) usually shows edematous swelling along a fairly large segment and appears indurated. The intestine is coated with an opaque serous membrane which is highly telangiectatic, particularly where the intestine is attached to the mesentery.

The intestinal abnormalities resulting from irradiation are due largely to damaged blood vessels in the intestinal wall or the mesentery. The occurrence of vasculitis with thrombosis and perivascular fibrosis disturbs the circulation in the wall of the loops in the irradiated field and sometimes in loops which are clearly beyond the field.

In their histological description, already, Warren and Friedman also noted abnormalities beyond the irradiated field.

The frequencies given in the literature for the occurrence of the clinical symptoms of radiation enteritis vary greatly. The values range from 0.6 to 17% for patients who have undergone abdominal irradiation (Aldridge, Colcock and Braatsch). Most authors indicate that the complaints develop within two years after radiotherapy (De Cosse et al., Graudins). Numerous exceptions are, however, known – complaints have even developed 30 years after irradiation. Neumeister and Pfeiffer found that intestinal adhesions as a result of surgery greatly increase the chance of lesions in the small intestine because of the decreased mobility. The 30 patients studied by Mason et al. included 24 surgical patients. The most severe abnormalities were localized in the immobile loops.

Since a specific dose causes abnormalities in the small intestine in one patient but not in another, it would seem that the sensitivity varies per individual. There have for instance even been cases with a fatal outcome after only a few days of irradiation

with a minimum dosage – the so-called x-ray intoxication (Todd). In 1973 Pekka Nummi described two patients with severe diarrhea and a diffuse ulceration in the jejunum and the ileum after irradiation with 1500 rads.

The symptoms of a radiation enteritis can be separated into an acute and a chronic syndrome. The acute symptoms usually include a severe pain in the abdomen, nausea, vomiting and bloody diarrhea. Examination reveals a distended abdomen with a palpable tumor-like mass which is often mistaken for a recurrent tumor. Acute therapeutic measures, such as direct decompression using a Miller-Abbot tube, are often necessary since the course of the disease may otherwise become catastrophic within a short period. This is, however, often not sufficient and then a laparotomy is necessary. Unfortunately the postoperative course is often severely complicated by a peritonitis which usually results in death (Roswitt and Malsky).

In most cases, however, the patients have a chronic radiation enteritis which can develop one to twelve years after radiotherapy (Chau and Fletcher). The complaints are intermittent attacks of colic, obstipation, anorexia, vomiting, diarrhea, fatigue and loss of weight, sometimes even cachexia (nutritional cripple).

Out of a group of 3000 patients who underwent radiotherapy, Duncan and Leonard saw 6 with a malabsorption syndrome which consisted of diarrhea, alternating in some cases with obstipation, megaloblastic anemia and osteomalacia. Before their publication (1965), only 5 cases of radiation enteritis had been reported. The malabsorption is due to destruction of the mucosal epithelium so that resorption in the intestine is disturbed. We have also found that radiological abnormalities as a result of irradiation of the small intestine can sometimes already be observed within several weeks, even if the patient has few or no complaints; this agrees completely with the experiments of Bosniak et al.

The wall of an intestine damaged by an overdose of roentgen rays shows hyperemia and edema.

The edema is localized mainly in the submucosa; this is seen on the x-rays as a clear broadening of the mucosal folds with very thin fairly pointed spaces in between (spikes). As a result of the thicker intestinal wall, the distance between adjacent in-

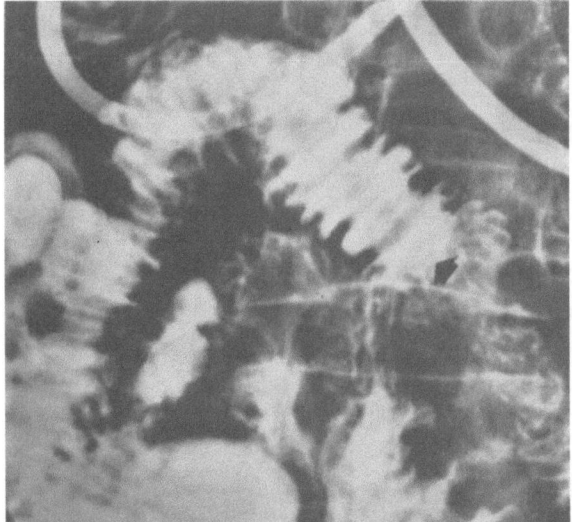

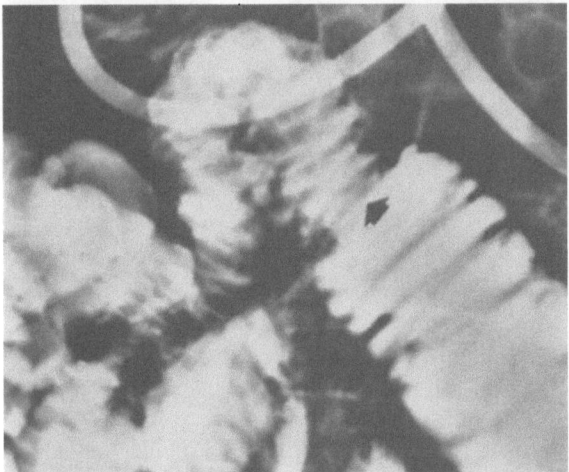

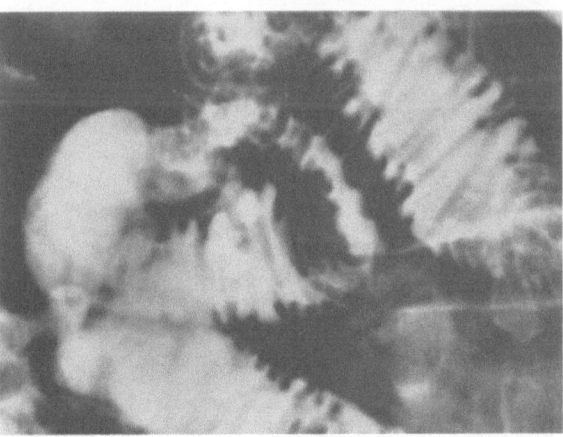

Fig. 9.48
Radiation enteritis with edematous mucosa. Between the highly swollen mucosal folds are narrow spaces filled with barium which resemble a coarsely toothed saw. The transition to the normal intestinal segments is very abrupt (→).

testinal loops is also obviously increased (fig. 9.48). These abnormalities are probably due to a local anoxia of the intestinal wall and are highly similar to those seen in cases of hypermotility (fig. 8.59). The edema probably develops only when the anoxia is rather prolonged or irreversible. As in ischemia, a fibrinous coating develops on the outside of the intestinal loops which causes multiple adhesions with adjacent loops (fig. 9.49). Moreover, ulcerations and necrosis can develop which may lead to bleeding, perforation and fistulas to nearby organs, usually therefore the bladder, sigmoid or rectum. Because of the rigidity and the absence of peristaltic movements, the average diameter of the intestinal lumen can be somewhat greater; the relief of the thickened folds is regular at first but often becomes more disorderly in a later stage.

After a period of months, sometimes even years, the scars or fibrotic tissue can lead to obstruction (fig. 9.50). If these local shriveling processes are localized in the mesentery, then 'kinking' is observed just as in the event of a carcinoid lesion. In later stages of a radiation enteritis the space between the intestinal loops remains enlarged, partly as a result of the thicker intestinal wall and also because shriveling causes the mesentery to become shorter. In this stage, however, the thickening of the intestinal wall is not due to edema in the submucosa but usually to a fibrosis involving all layers.

If the roentgen damage to the small intestine is limited and there are neither ulcerations nor necrosis, the fibrous shriveling will not be extensive and will be more diffuse in nature.

In that case stenoses will not develop in the small intestine; instead atrophy of the mucosa will be the predominant feature. As in a colon or stomach damaged by roentgen rays, we will only see a smooth mucosal surface without many folds (fig. 9.51). In the mucosa the epithelium is the most sensitive to roentgen rays; the initial reaction of the more resistant muscularis propria to radiation is as a rule a pronounced hypertonicity. During the radiological examination therefore a marked 'intestinal hurry' is observed in the irradiated field and it is exceedingly difficult to achieve adequate filling of the irritated intestinal loops (fig. 9.52).

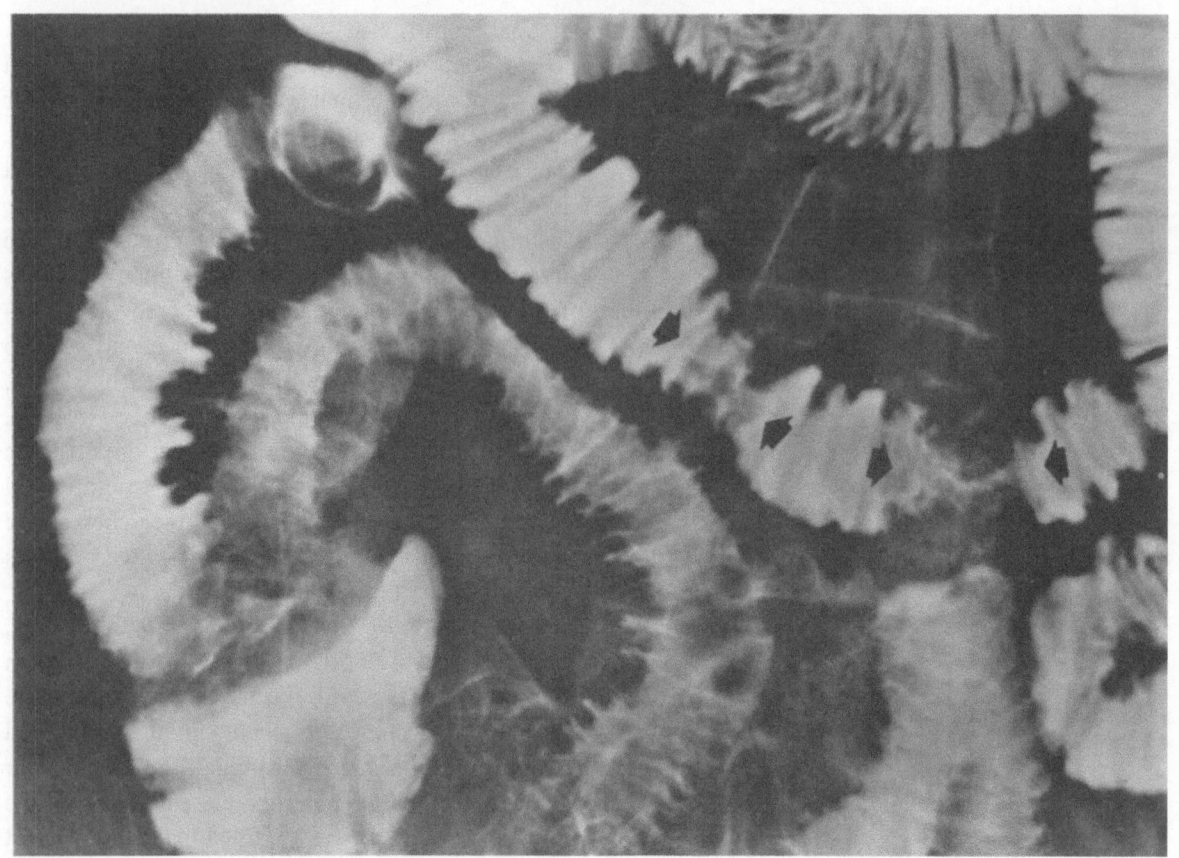

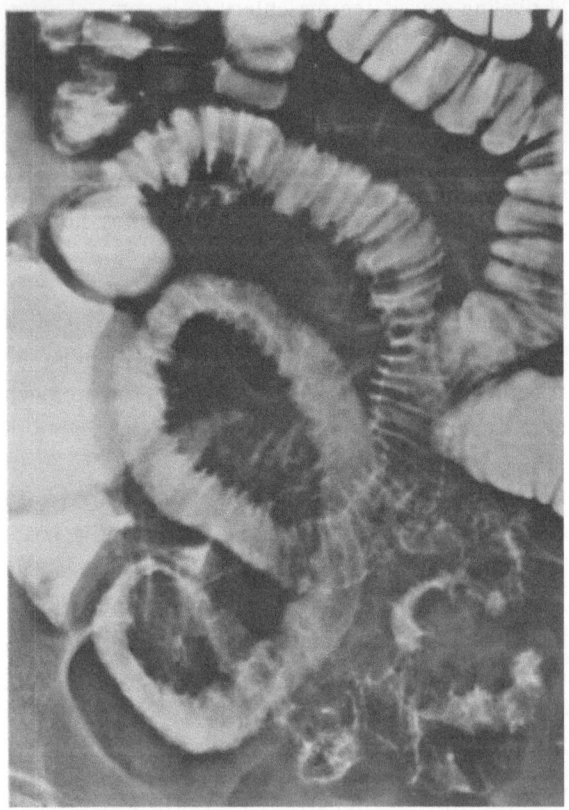

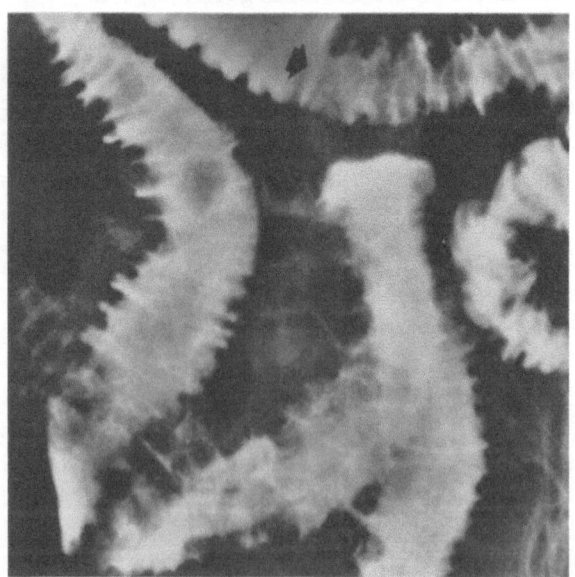

In terms of the various symptoms, the radiological abnormalities in radiation enteritis can be listed as follows:

1. spasms, recognized by the variation in the caliber of the intestinal lumen and the inability of the intestine to achieve total dilatation. The spasms are due to a moderate ischemia of the intestine and react favourably to antispasmodics.
2. thickening of the intestinal wall due to fibrosis or edema, mainly in the submucosa.
3. rigidity or stiffness of the intestinal wall, also due to edematous or fibrotic changes in the intestinal wall and recognized by the fact that the peristaltic movements have obviously decreased in number and particularly in intensity.

The edema as well as the fibrosis may develop only locally, depending mainly on where the blood or lymph vessels are (or were) occluded. If there is a pure edema of the mucosa, then the mucosal folds often have a cobblestone aspect and cause round or oval bulges in the margins of the contrast column. If there is an edema of the submucosa, the folds are also broadened but because the mucous membrane is completely intact, the regular arrangement is retained. In such cases the grooves between the folds which extend in parallel become exceedingly thin so that the so-called 'spiking' phenomenon (Mason and Clemett) is observed along the margins of the contrast column.

4. ulcerations can be deep, leading to stenoses and fistulas, but they can also be very superficial. In the latter case they are difficult to demonstrate radiologically. The regular arrangement of the mucosal folds is of course also retained when rigidity of the intestine is due only to a lymphedema which has developed as a result of a disturbance of the lymphatic flow in the center near the spinal column. In these cases, thickening of the intestinal wall is not as pronounced as in fig. 4.49 since there is no fibrosis at all (fig. 9.53).

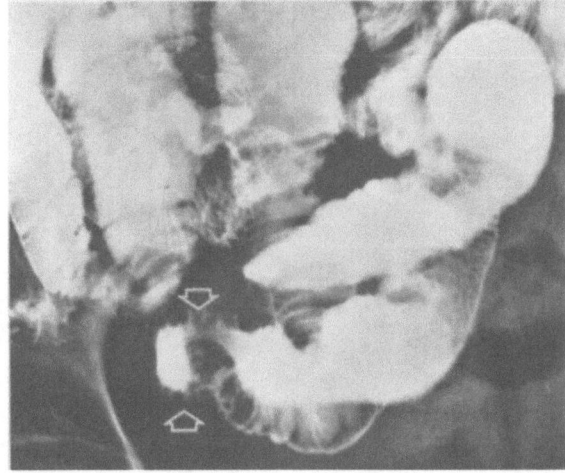

Fig. 9.50
Stenotic area in the intestine due to fibrosis in radiation enteritis.

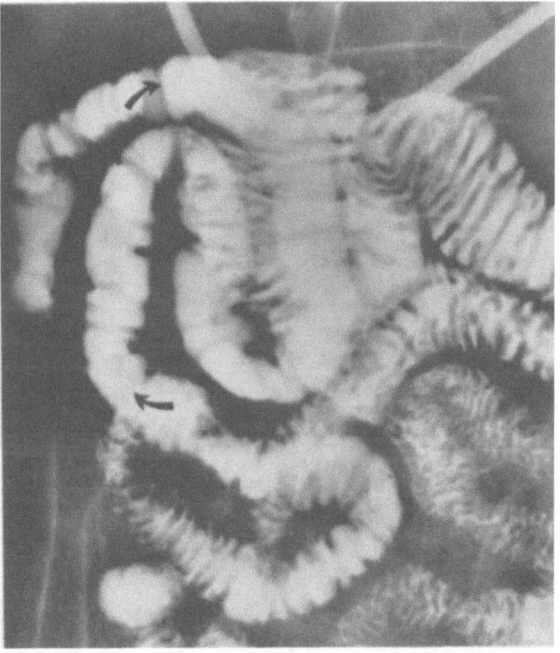

Fig. 9.51
Radiation enteritis with atrophy of the mucosal folds and a decrease in the caliber of the intestine, presumably as a result of fibrosis.

←

Fig. 9.49
Adhesion of intestinal loops in radiation enteritis; irregular mucosal surface and multiple small ulcerations. Thickened intestinal wall due mainly to fibrosis instead of edema. Areas resembling skip lesions indicated by arrows.

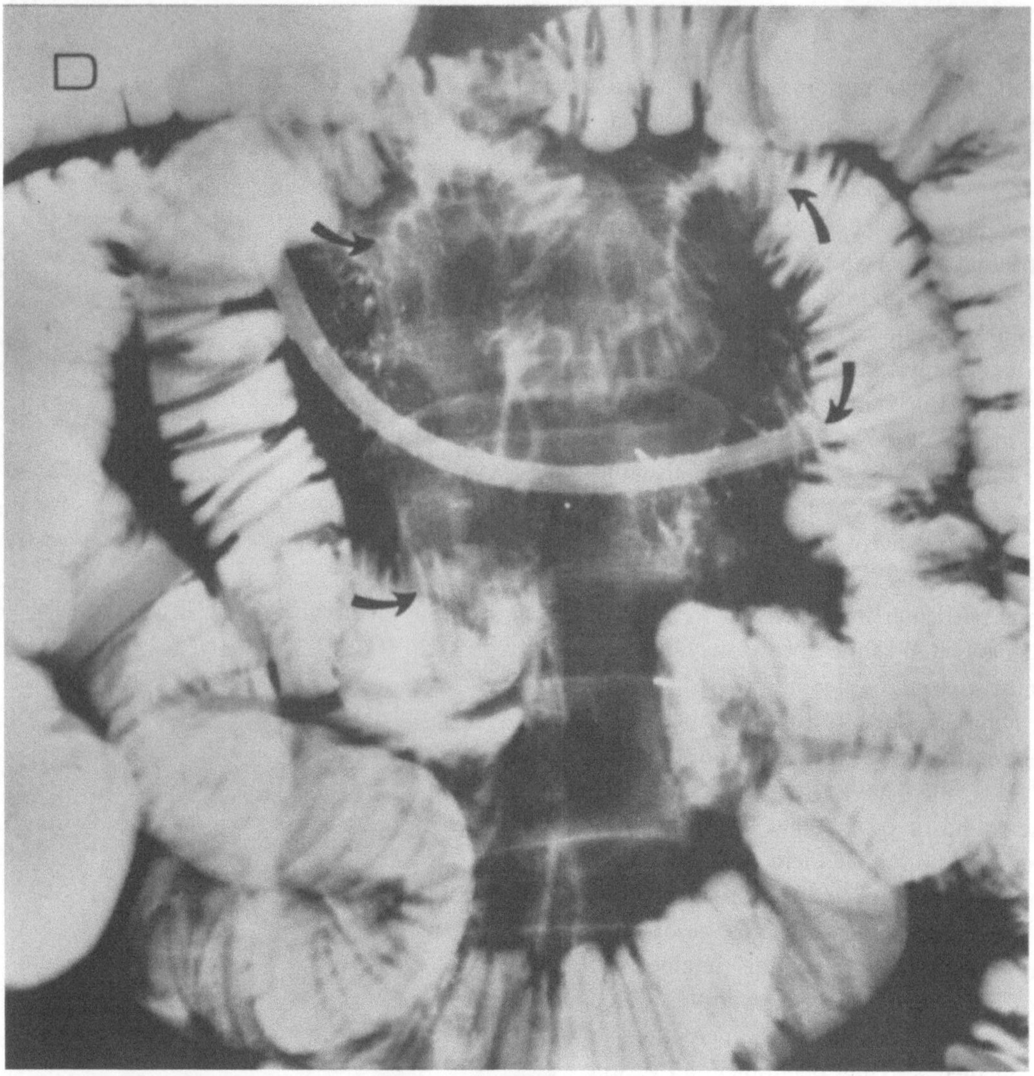

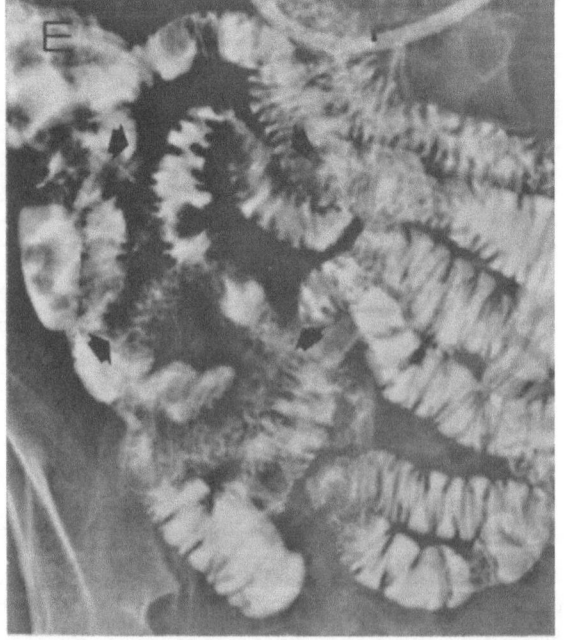

Fig. 9.52
Local intestinal hurry in an intestine with decreased caliber in radiation enteritis. The abnormalities are due to an ischemia and can therefore be found within (D) as well as beyond (E) the irradiated field.

5. Adhesion of the loops of the small intestine to other loops or surrounding organs is usually encountered in the pelvis minor. The loops can no longer be separated from one another or from the bladder or the cecum by means of compression. Peristaltic movements in a fused intestine can give a highly stretched mucosal pattern with a spiky aspect; this is called 'tacking down' in the literature.

6. Atrophy of the mucosa, recognized by the smooth wall; mucosal folds are more or less missing.

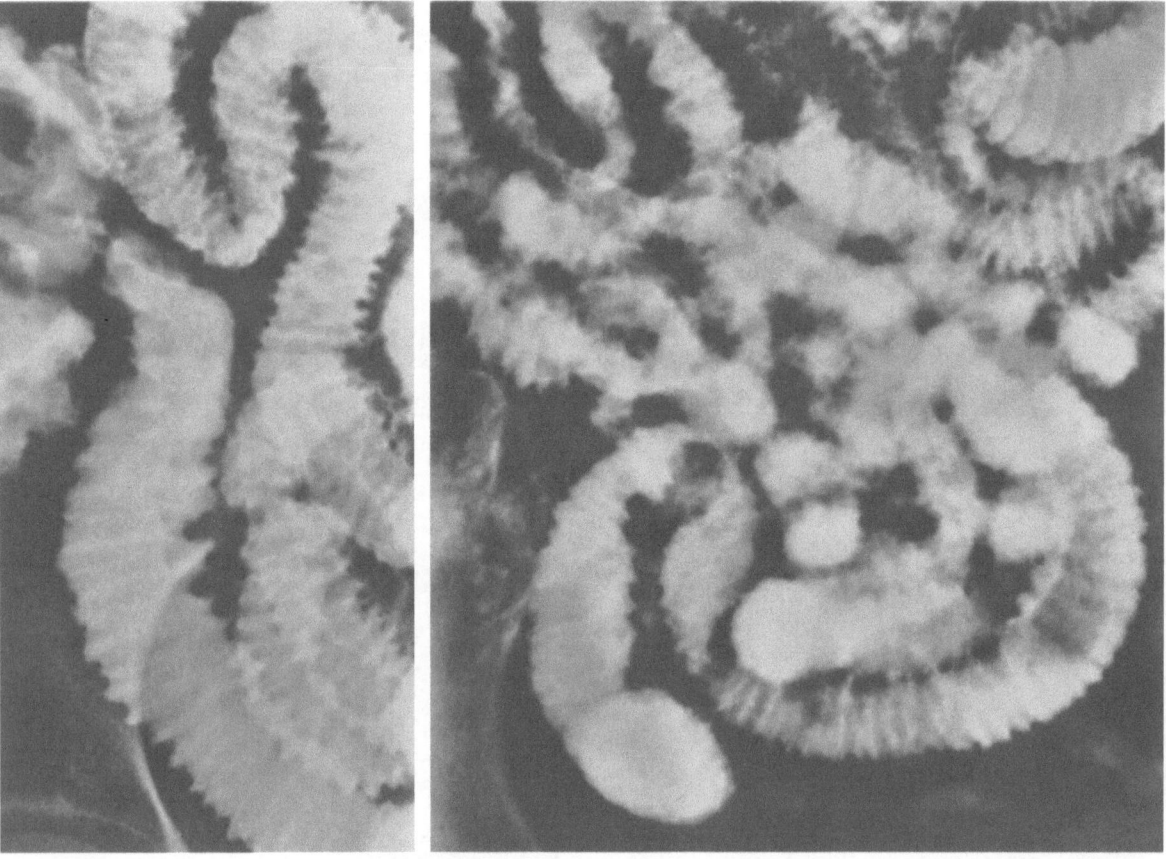

Fig. 9.53
Lymphedema of the entire small intestine as a result of a disturbed lymphatic flow in the center near the spinal column after irradiation. Due to the absence of fibrosis the intestinal wall here is not as thick as that in fig. 9.49 and the regular arrangement of the mucosa is retained.

7. Whipple's disease

This fairly rare disease which is sometimes hereditary is occasionally also called – incorrectly – lipodystrophy. Although more is known since Whipple's first description in 1907, this disease remains shrouded in mystery because of the unknown etiology.

The complaints of these patients, predominantly middle-aged males, include abdominal pain, steatorrhea, loss of weight, fatigue and recurrent shifting pain in the joints. Physical examination shows a generalized lymphadenopathy, enlarged liver and spleen and polyserositis. The skin is often pigmented as in Addison's disease. Hematological determinations reveal a low Hb and decreased protein and calcium concentrations; in addition the resorption of various food substances is clearly disturbed.

Post mortem studies and pathological examinations of laparotomia have shown that the lymph nodes and the lamina propria of the obviously thickened intestinal wall are filled with deposits of fat and fatty acids called 'lipogranulomas'. These deposits contain large foamy macrophages filled with a glycoprotein. Electron microscopy studies have established that during the active phase of the disease bacteria conglomerate in the macrophages but disappear after prolonged treatment with antibiotics.

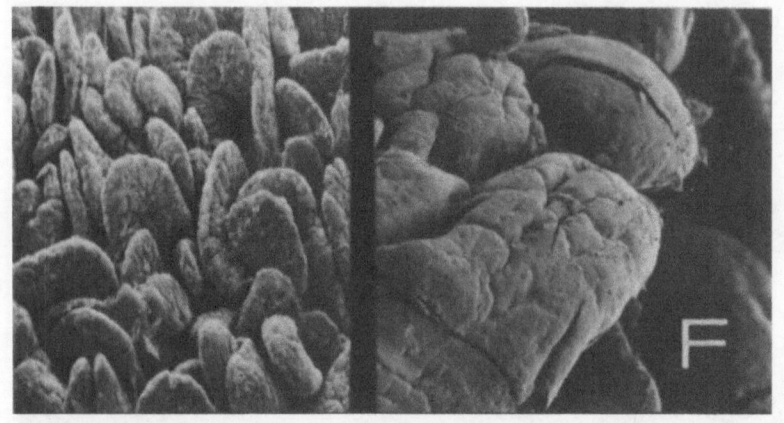

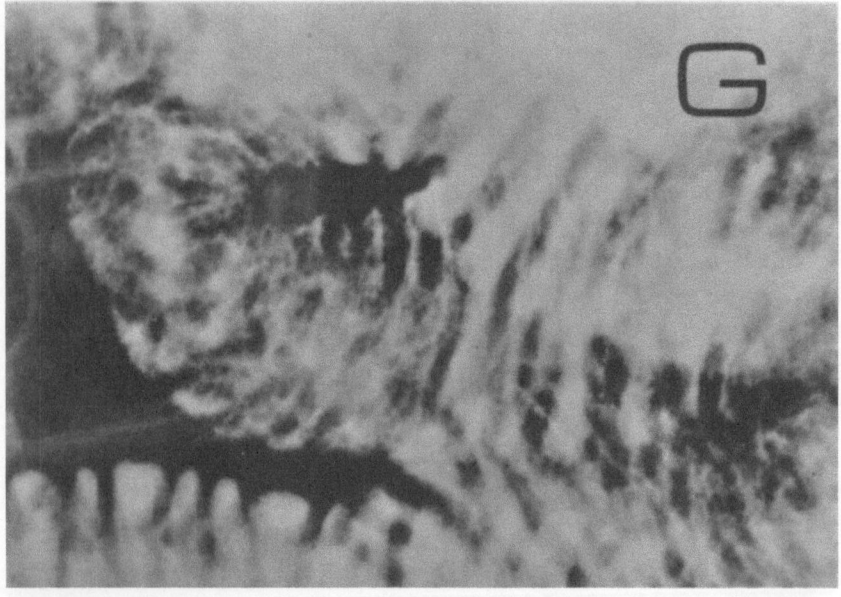

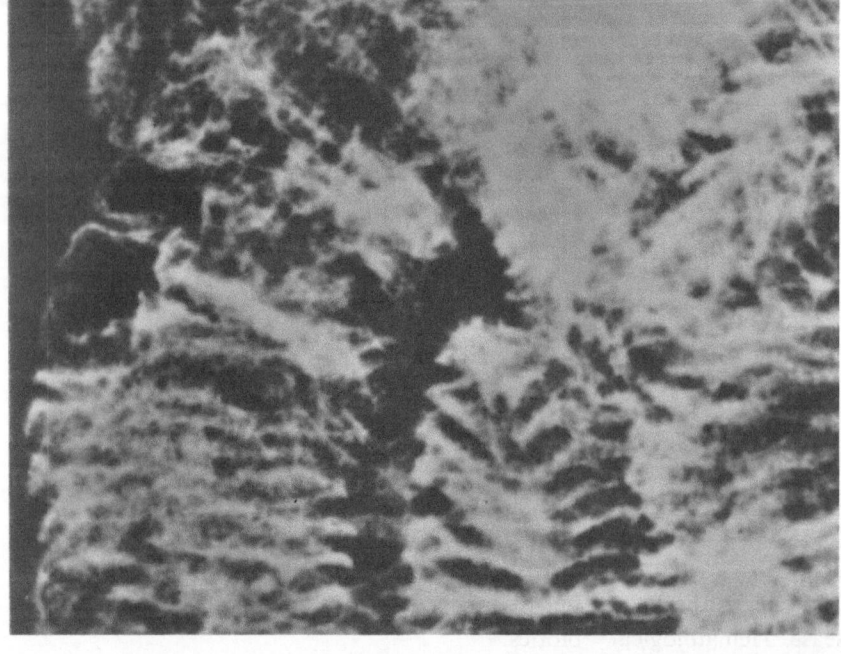

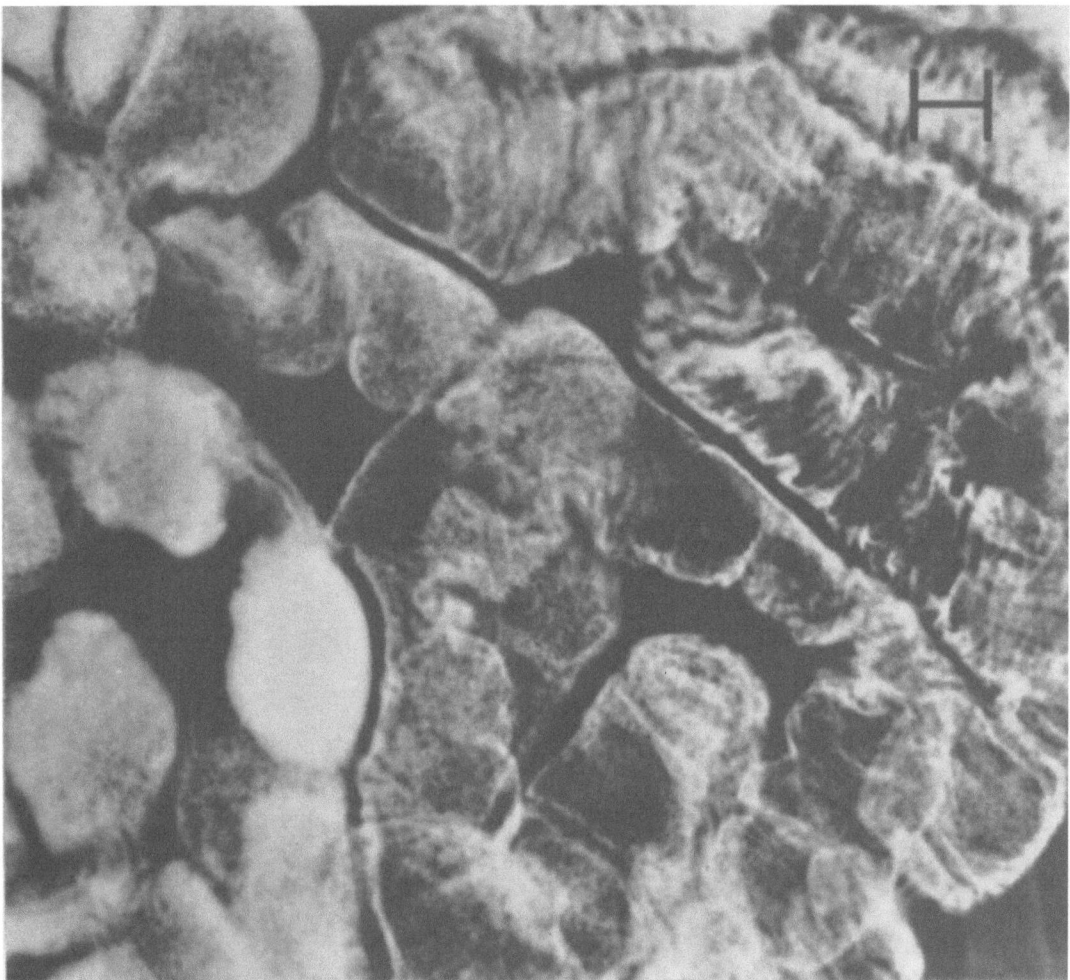

Fig. 9.54
In Whipple's disease the villi can be so swollen that they are ±0.5 mm in size; they then can be seen with the naked eye during endoscopic examination (F); on the roentgenograms (G) these villi are difficult to differentiate from foaming of the contrast fluid (H). The bubble-like villi, however, interrupt the contours of the intestinal wall.

By means of lymph node biopsies and biopsies of the jejunal mucosa obtained via duodenoscopy, it is now possible to establish the diagnosis and set up adequate treatment thus avoiding laparotomy. The villi on the thickened mucosal folds in the jejunum are so swollen due to lymphedema and accumulations of lipogranulomas that they sometimes are visible to the naked eye; they then appear on the x-rays as small nodules (fig. 9.54). The radiological abnormalities are further characterized by moderate dilatation of the jejunal loops and a slightly accelerated passage. There is a clear tendency toward flocculation or dilution of the contrast fluid so that the time available for making useful films is rather short. It appears that the marked coarsening of the mucosa in the jejunum, always mentioned in the literature and demonstrated on roentgenograms, can be attributed to a large extent to disintegration of the contrast fluid and, as far as we have been able to discover, is in fact less pronounced than is generally assumed. This is clearly demonstrated by comparing the x-rays of a conventional examination (fig. 9.55) with those obtained during an enteroclysis examination (fig. 9.56); these films were taken of the same patient two weeks apart. It is stated in the literature that the radiological abnormalities characteristic of celiac disease can closely resemble those of Whipple's disease but with the enteroclysis examination technique this is not true at all.

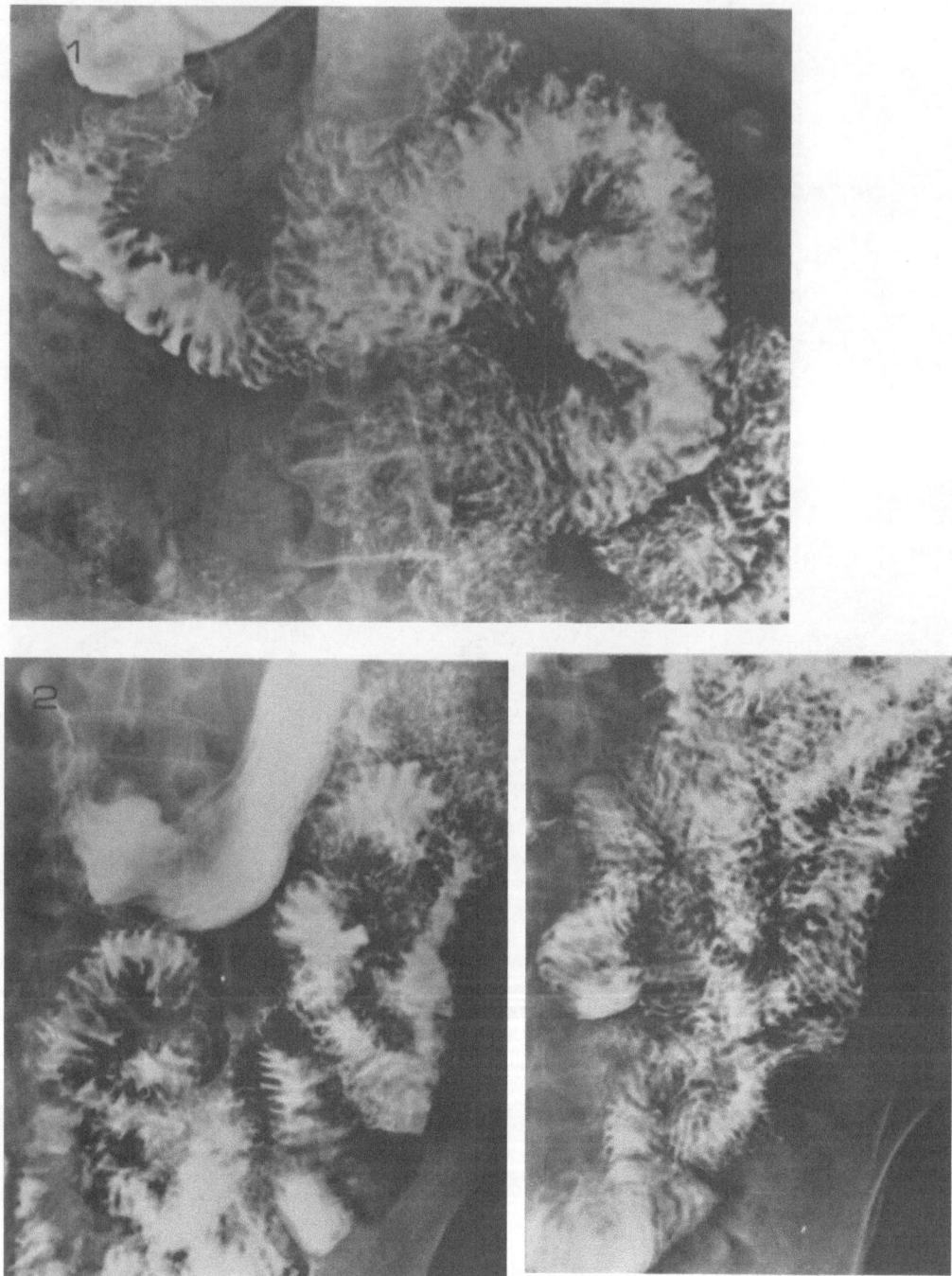

Fig. 9.55
Conventional transit examination of the small intestine of two patients with Whipple's disease. In both patients a coarse mucosal pattern, dilated jejunal loops and rapid flocculation of the barium suspension were observed.

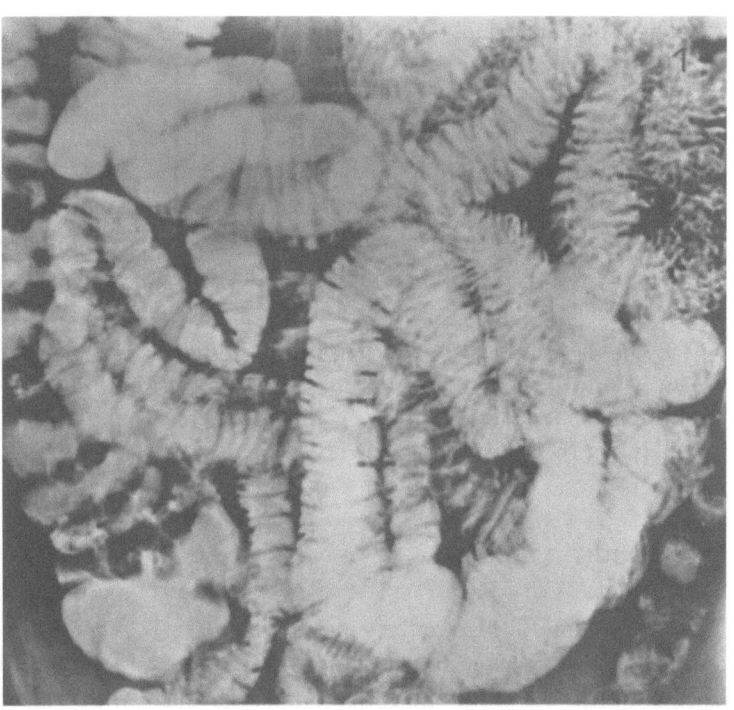

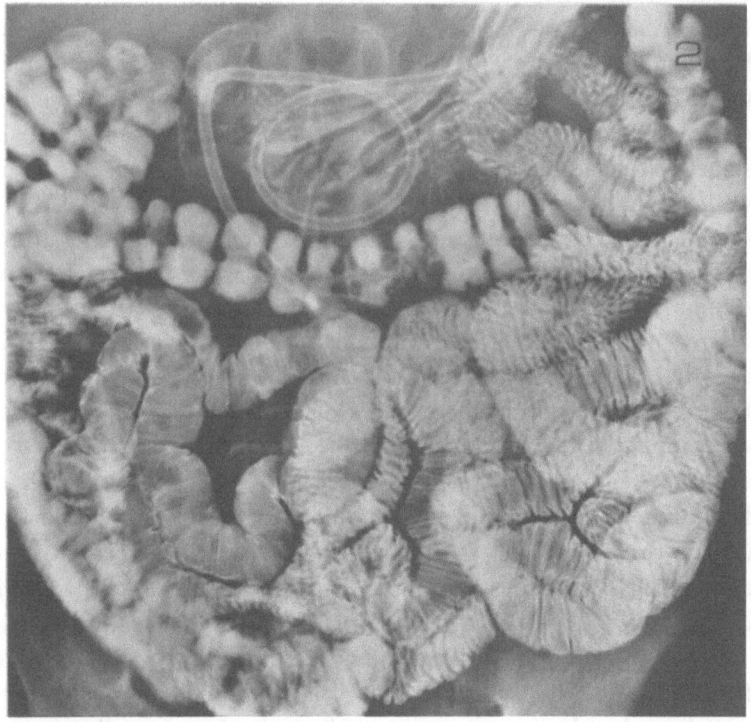

Fig. 9.56
The same patients as seen in fig. 9.55, examined by the enteroclysis method.
The mucosal folds now appear normal. Although patient (2) had been treated
for this disease during the interim period and patient (1) had not, we have
certainly not been able to establish on the basis of our experience that the
mucosal pattern will change significantly as a result of therapy.

Although the abnormalities in celiac disease are also localized mainly in the jejunum, the folds are atrophied rather than broadened; they sometimes are greatly reduced in number or even completely missing. Both the dilatation of the loops and the motility can be much more pronounced and may involve a much larger segment in celiac disease than in Whipple's disease. Strictly speaking the same moderate changes in the mucosal folds and the micronodular villous structure seen in Whipple's disease can also be demonstrated radiologically in lipoproteinemia; clinically, however, the differentiation between these two diseases is not difficult.

8. Aspecific ulcers

Not all circumscribed strictures in the small intestine can be attributed to skip lesions in Crohn's disease which heal with the formation of fibrous tissue and shriveling. In the ileum and in particular the jejunum, solitary or multiple stenoses are fairly common; they often contain a relatively small ulcer which usually is not visualized on the x-ray. In a large number of cases, the ulcer is annular and is located in the center of the stenotic segment. In other cases it is a normal crater-shaped ulcer which sometimes penetrates quite deep into the intestinal wall; the latter is markedly thickened at the ulcer site due to edema and fibrosis.

There is no agreement whatsoever as to what should be identified as an ulcus simplex or aspecific ulcer. Some believe that all ulcerations for which a causative agent cannot be demonstrated belong to this group; others, including ourselves, feel that this criterium depends too much on the diagnostic experience and capability of the diverse clinics, their laboratories and medical staff. According to Evert (1948), the aspecific ulcer is small and generally solitary, and is not accompanied by pathological changes elsewhere in the digestive tract.

From the above it will be obvious that the frequency of the aspecific ulcer in the small intestine as indicated in the literature will be of limited value. It is, however, striking that none of the values listed are very high so that it must in any case be a relatively rare phenomenon. It is interesting to note that the earliest mention of an aspecific ulcer in the small intestine dates from 1805 (Baillie) and in 1922 the American Richardson described the first jejunal ulcer of this type.

a. ETIOLOGY

Several causative agents for this type of ulcer may be an inflammatory process in the small intestine such as, for instance, a bacillary dysentery, injury of the mucosa by foreign bodies or the presence of ectopic mucosa from the stomach. Some believe that infections which are not enteral in origin can also cause an enteral ulcus simplex. Thus for example pneumococci were cultured from an ulcer in the small intestine of a patient with a pneumococcal infection in the upper respiratory tract; in another patient with furunculosis an ulcus simplex recurred with each exacerbation of the disease (Ebeling). Rosenow induced experimental ulcers with a specific species of streptococcus (Ebeling).

In the proximal part of the intestine ulcers can develop as a result of a Zollinger-Ellison syndrome, although in that case the cause is generally easily recognized. Strangely enough a marked increase and subsequent decrease in the frequency of the aspecific ulcer, also called the ulcus simplex, has been noted since 1964. This increase in frequency appears to be the result of treatment with enteric-coated KCl tablets, irrespective of the use of diuretics from the thiazide series (Lindenholmer). It is not known precisely how or why these tablets give rise to ulcers but presumably the locally enhanced KCl concentration causes vascular lesions and the ulcerations must be considered ischemic necroses. The possibility that the ulcers develop secondary to caustic injury of the mucosa which has healed with the formation of fibrous tissue can, however, not be ignored entirely. The stenoses are only $\frac{1}{2}$ to 1 cm long; they are smooth with an abrupt transition to the more or less funnel-shaped healthy intestine on either side.

Although experiments with rats, dogs and monkeys have proven that KCl causes ulcers in the small intestine, Jordan believes that there must also be other reasons for this increase in frequency since KCl had been in use many years before 1964 and the decrease in the frequency was signalized even before the use of enteric-coated KCl tablets was restricted. Although such drug-induced ulcerations satisfy the criterium of Evert and are considered an ulcus simplex by Sturges and Krone, Flendrig, Lubbers and Van Tongeren believe otherwise. Other medications which can induce ulcers in the small intestine are chlorpromazine, digitalis and adrenocortical hormones.

Quite often, however, the etiology of these solitary, but sometimes also multiple, ulcerations can no longer be determined.

The most common cause of ulcerations characterized by the formation of fibrotic rings and stenoses which lead to obstruction is probably a disturbance in the blood supply to the involved intestinal segment. Stenoses due to ischemia can be either solitary or multiple. They are generally 2–3 cm long, longer therefore than those caused by other factors.

The vascular anomaly may be the result of an embolus or a thrombosis, a vasculitis or a pronounced stenosis of the major branches of the celiac trunk and the superior mesenteric artery. The most common cause of vascular insufficiency is without a doubt arteriosclerosis. A congenital vascular anomaly or an insufficiency due to atrophy of the mucosa, as in celiac disease, is fairly rare.

A somewhat divergent point of view is postulated by Ravden and Litwin who suggest autodigestion after ischemia; Mecheles considers vascular spasms as the causative factor. The observations of Delavierre, Teicher and Morin support the theory that the origin is vascular in nature; they noted the microscopic changes of an endarteritis obliterans. Goehrs and his associates demonstrated the presence of multiple tiny emboli in the submucosa.

In rats acute ulcers can be induced by oral or parenteral administration of a dose of indomethacin equal to 5–80 times that given to man. Here, too, microscopic local changes in the vessels and thrombosis were observed. In man the ulcer will develop 3 months to 5 years after therapy is initiated. Often, however, no vascular anomalies can be found at all and if they are observed then it is difficult or impossible to determine whether they are primary or secondary.

b. PATHOLOGY

In about 2/3 of the cases the ulcus simplex develops in the ileum (Goehrs, Evert), usually within 80 cm of the duodenal flexure or within 60 cm of the ileocecal valve (Evert). Delavierre and Ebeling point out that a second ulcer can often be found in the stomach, duodenum, ileum or rectum. The aspecific ulcer is frequently multiple; it may even occur in groups of 2 or 3, sometimes even more (Holtzwessig). If several ulcers are found, then the various stages of healing can also be observed. According to some authors (Litwin, Dowdle), the ulcus simplex is usually located opposite the mesentery. Others (Watson, Evert) believe that this relationship, which implies a vascular lesion, is not clearly evident. Dockerty described a number of cases in which a thrombosis of the small mesenteric arteries could be demonstrated. Aspecific ulcerations are small and clearly circumscribed; they penetrate deep into the mucosa and the underlying layers, and there is little or no inflammatory reaction in the surrounding areas. If a stricture is evident, then fibrosis in the submucosa has advanced out of all proportion to the size of the ulcer. In such a case some edema of the submucosa may be seen on the proximal side of the ulcer.

Microscopically the ulcus simplex resembles the peptic ulcer in the stomach or duodenum. The ulcer floor which is smooth is covered with a thin layer of fibrin and leucocytes. The surrounding epithelium is not involved and the rim of the ulcer is sharply defined. The surface area of the damaged mucosa is greater than that of the underlying layers, thus the margins of the ulcer decrease stepwise with the depth. In the event of perforation the opening in the serosa is often as small as the head of a pin (Ebeling). The ulcer floor itself consists of granulation tissue with lymphocytic and plasmacellular infiltrates. The inflammatory reaction involves all layers and spreads beyond the ulcer. Beneath the granulation tissue is the collagenous connective tissue which will ultimately cause the stenosis.

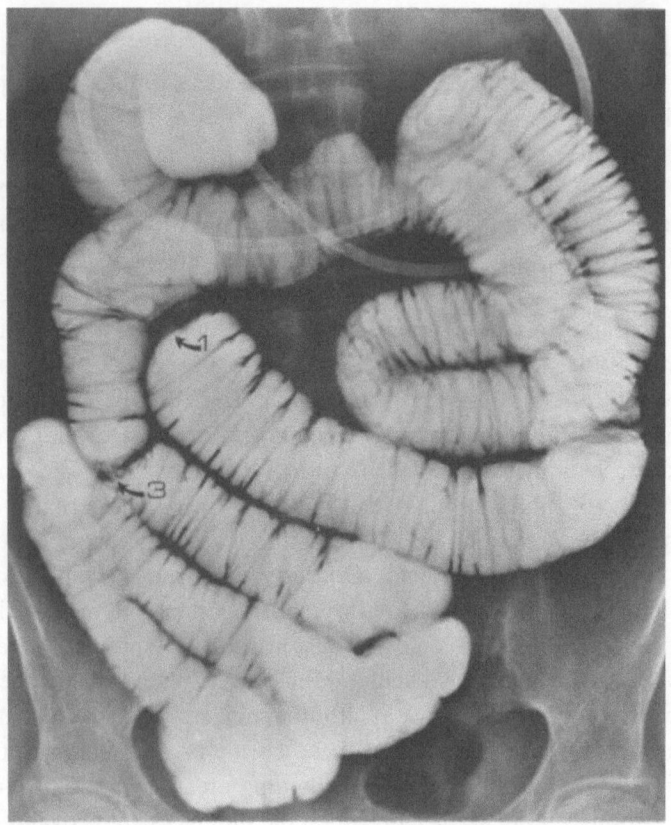

Fig. 9.57
Survey films of a patient who had complained of colic-like pain in the abdomen for years. Dilated intestinal loops with two short annular strictures (1 and 3). The spot films revealed, however, that there were in fact 3 stenoses which were only clearly visible when the loops were well-filled. The dilatation of the loops on the distal side of the third stenosis suggests that more constrictions probably exist further on: this was confirmed at surgery. None of the conventional examinations had ever revealed any abnormalities at all. This patient had been considered an unconfirmed Crohn's disease for 20 years and was scheduled for an ileocecal resection. It is obvious that Crohn's disease is not involved at all (see also p. 223).

c. SYMPTOMOLOGY

In contrast to the pathology, the symptomology of the ulcus simplex is not straightforward. In some cases the aspecific ulcer mimics a duodenal ulcer and in other cases, there are practically no complaints. The ulcer is found predominantly in patients between 30 and 50 years of age, although it has been reported in patients from 0 to 83 years of age (Ravdin). In males under 50 years of age the ulcers generally are localized in the terminal segment of the ileum. The ulcus simplex occurs in men more often than in women with a frequence of 2:1 (Dowdle) or 3:1 (Evert, Dockerty, Watson & Ebeling). The complaints can vary greatly and are unreliable for diagnosis; they are determined mainly by the localization of the lesion as well as the occurrence of complications such as strictures, bleeding and perforations. If the ulcer is in the ileum, there will be few or no complaints. If the ulcer lies in the

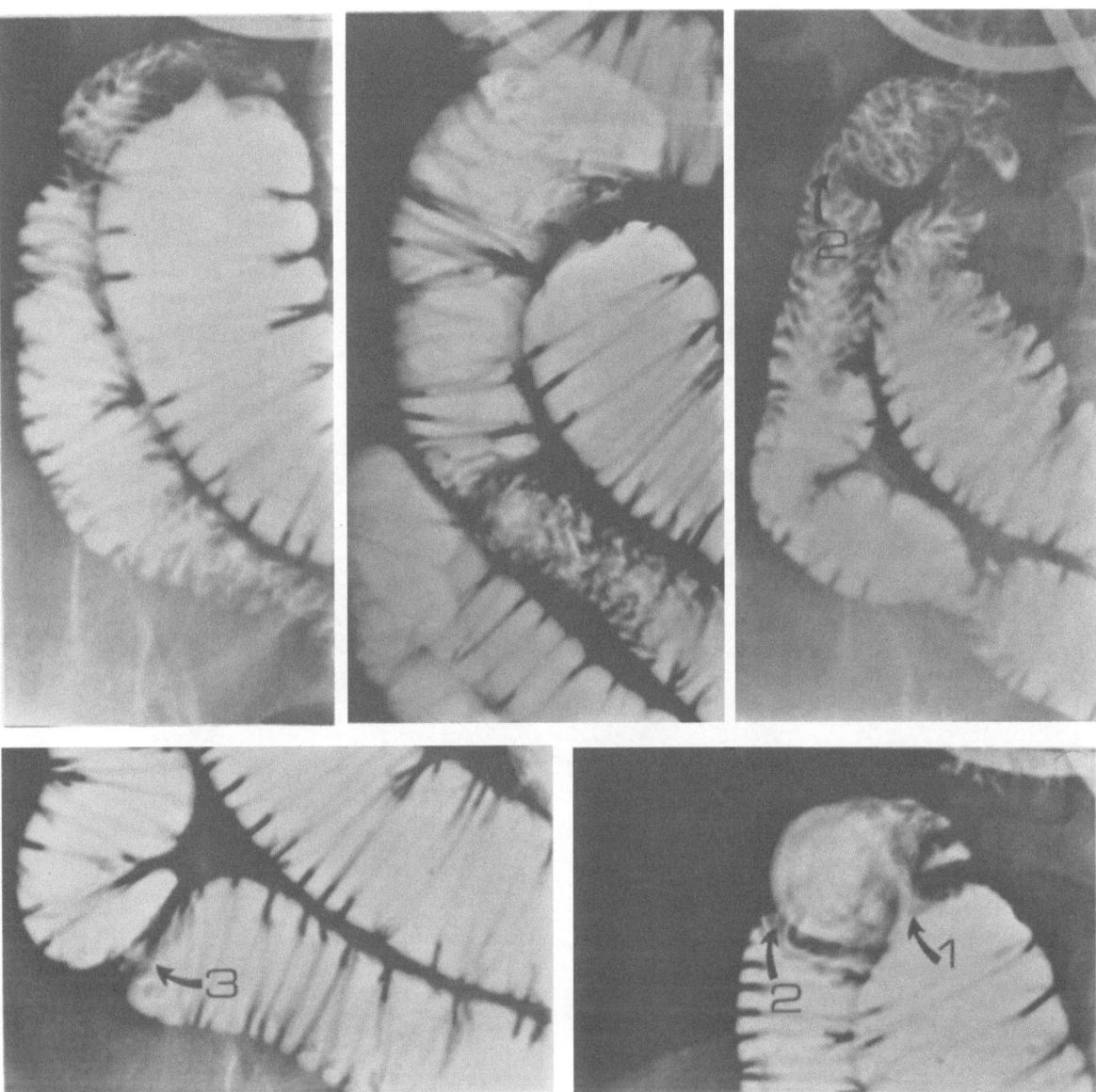

Fig. 9.57

jejunum the complaints will resemble those of a duodenal ulcer; this becomes more pronounced as the distance from Treitz's ligament decreases (Litwin). There is then a gnawing postprandial pain, often around the navel, which occurs later with respect to the meal than that of a duodenal ulcer.

In the past bleeding and perforation of these deep ulcers led to a high mortality of about 50%. The symptoms of these complications, especially the frequently occurring obstruction, should therefore also be considered very important. The patient complains of colic-like pains, sometimes accompanied by vomiting, diarrhea and eventually loss of weight. A partial obstruction need not always cause clinical phenomena; on the other hand sometimes even a swollen intestinal loop can be palpated (Sturges).

Occasionally there will be hemorrhage but usually the fecal benzidine reactions are positive (Evert) and anemia may develop. The symptoms of a perforation are similar to those of a perforating gastric ulcer, although the initial pain may be localized lower in the abdomen.

According to many authors (Ebeling, Goehrs, Ravdin), the duration of the complaints can vary greatly – from a few weeks to many years if perforation does not occur. A perforation incidentally

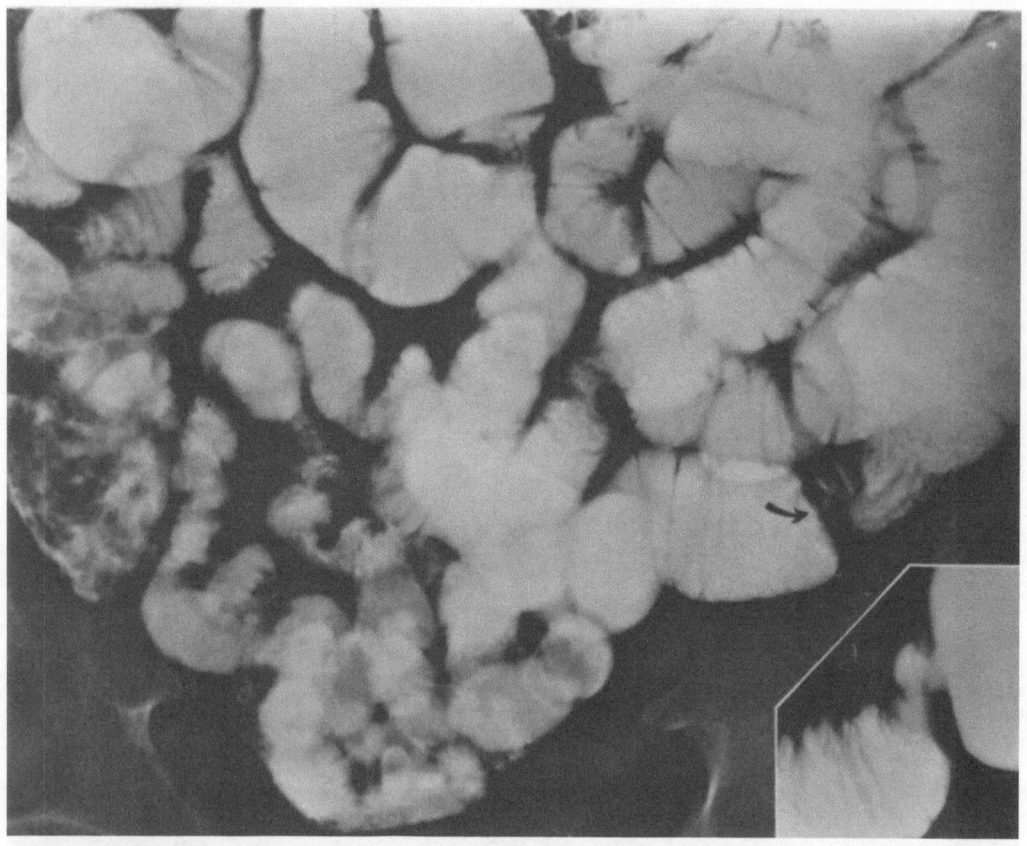

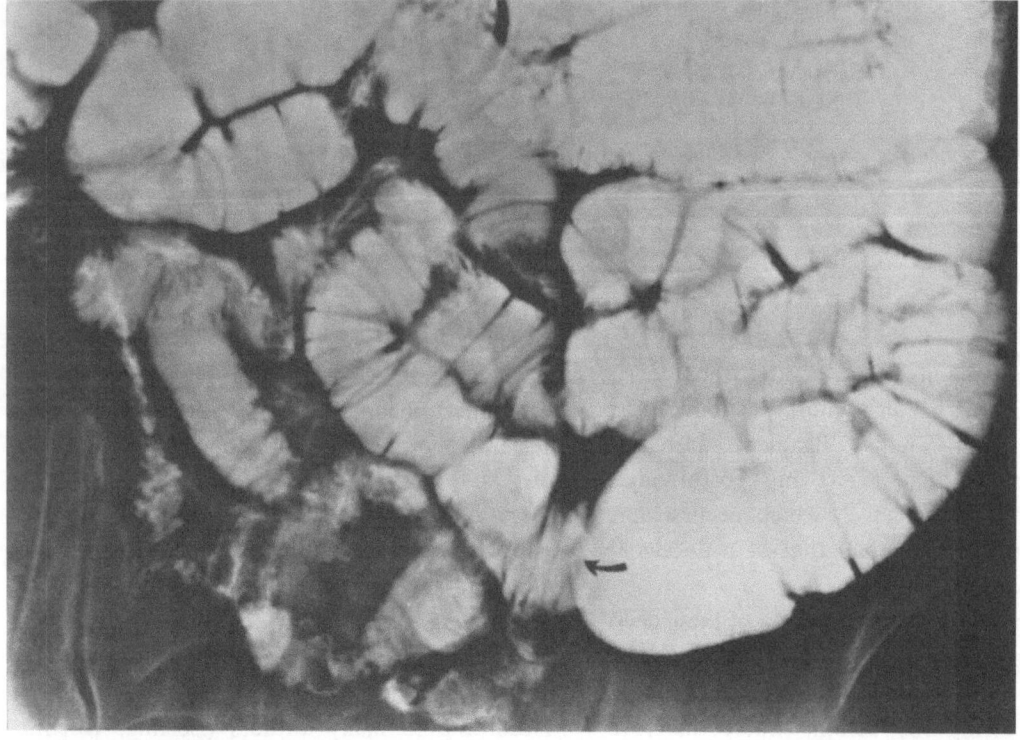

Fig. 9.58

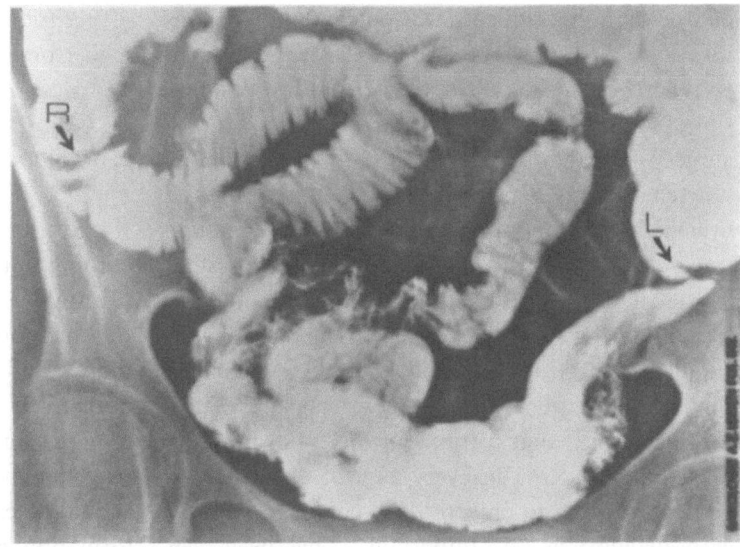

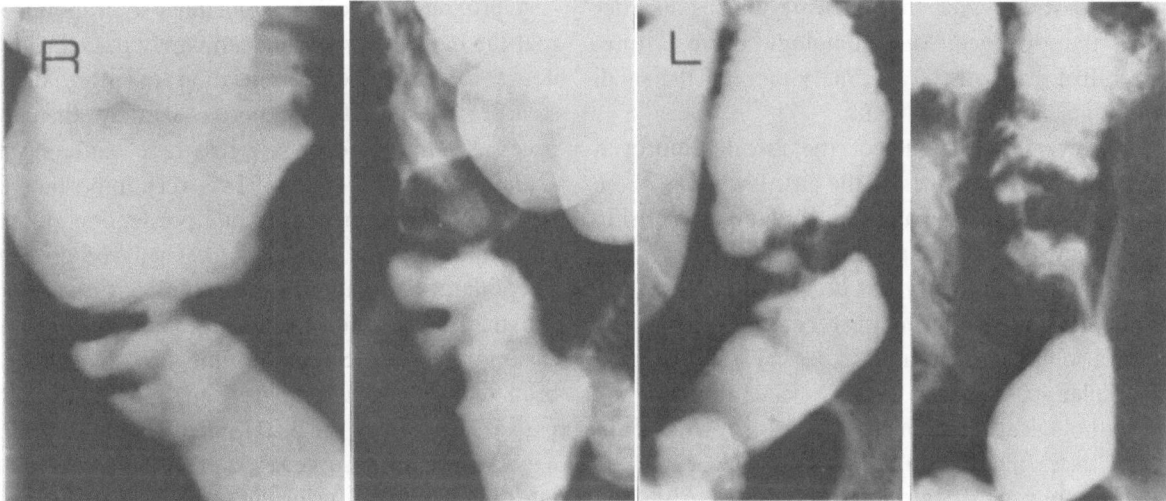

Fig. 9.59
Patient who complained of colic in the upper abdomen several times a week. The survey films showed a constant prestenotic dilatation on both sides. They appeared from the spot films to be due to short constricting aspecific ulcers. Strangely enough the intestinal mucosa on the distal side of the left-hand stenosis in particular is atrophied so that a primary vascular disease or damage due to corrosion involving a larger segment than normal is possible. There are neither radiological nor clinical indications of Crohn's disease. Because of a (too) low gastric acid concentration, the patient had taken pep-acid tablets over a prolonged period in the past.

←

Fig. 9.58
Solitary ulcer with pronounced prestenotic dilatation in the lower left quadrant in a patient who had complained of attacks of abdominal pain for many years although abnormalities had as yet never been demonstrated. Because of a prestenotic dilatation on one of the x-rays not shown here, it was assumed that there might be one more ulcer in the upper right quadrant; the surgeon, however, found 6!

can occur quite suddenly without any previous indications that such a possibility exists. According to reports in the literature, the perforation is sometimes so minute that it is not discovered during surgery (Litwin).

Even in 1927 Ravdin pointed out that in the event of obstruction or perforation in the digestive tract, it is essential to consider the small intestine as well, and if a gastric or duodenal ulcer cannot be located during surgery, then the jejunum and ileum should be inspected carefully. Sturges emphasizes that in connection with the increasing use of aggressive drugs, complications in the small intestine must be considered in every case of an acute abdomen. In order to prevent these complications, an early diagnosis is very important. It has been seen in the past, however, that the rarity of this disorder and the divergent symptomology make a preoperative diagnosis of a primary ulcer of the small intestine exceedingly difficult.

However, as a result of the greatly improved examination techniques of the past few years, these aspecific ulcers are being found with ever increasing frequency before the patient is on the operating table and the mortality has become quite low. It is sometimes noted during surgery that the stenosis may also have been caused in part by a pronounced muscular spasm.

Pathological anatomical studies show that in these cases there is an active ulcer and a marked hypertrophy of the prestenotic muscles. Although the patient's complaints, colic-like pain and eventually also vomiting after meals, clearly indicate an obstruction, experience has shown that this diagnosis has often not even been considered.

An ulcus simplex should be considered in the following cases:

1. complaints resembling those of a duodenal ulcer without roentgenological abnormalities in the stomach or duodenum.
2. gastrointestinal hemorrhage without abnormalities in the esophagus, stomach, duodenum or colon.
3. gastrointestinal bleeding or intermittent partial obstruction with attacks of colic-like abdominal pain or decreased peristalsis and dilatation of the intestinal loops.

4. peritonitis due to perforation although no perforated ulcer can be found.

d. RADIODIAGNOSIS

If a roentgenological examination is carried out according to the enteroclysis method, it is not difficult to establish the diagnosis (fig. 9.57—9.60). With this method the fluid is forced into the intestinal loops and striking prestenotic dilatations will develop. If this dilatation is overlooked during the examination and is discovered later during careful re-examination of the x-rays, a new examination should be carried out in order to obtain further information concerning the nature of the stenosis.

A proximal stenosis is sometimes so pronounced that the barium suspension can barely pass through it; as a result the identification of more distal stenoses is severely hampered. It may then be necessary to perform a retrograde enteroclysis examination via the colon. It is very important to remember that even if only one prestenotic dilatation can be seen, several strictures may be present. The dilatation may be visible only at the most proximal stenosis or the most constricting of the existing stenoses. Since the fluid flow has already been reduced by a more proximal stenosis it will pass easily through the distal stenoses. It is therefore necessary that the surgeon examine the entire small intestine carefully during the operation. If he does not do so, then there is considerable chance that one or more stenoses will be left and the patient's complaints will continue or recur within a sort period of time. A new roentgenological examination will then show a prestenotic dilatation at another location.

Aspecific stenoses and ulcerations in the jejunum or ileum are usually very short and can therefore be distinguished from those caused by tumors and those due to Crohn's disease. In the case of a tumor the margins are usually irregular and a space-occupying process can be seen; Crohn's disease usually involves much longer and irregularly defined segments and often similar ulcerations and stenoses are localized elsewhere.

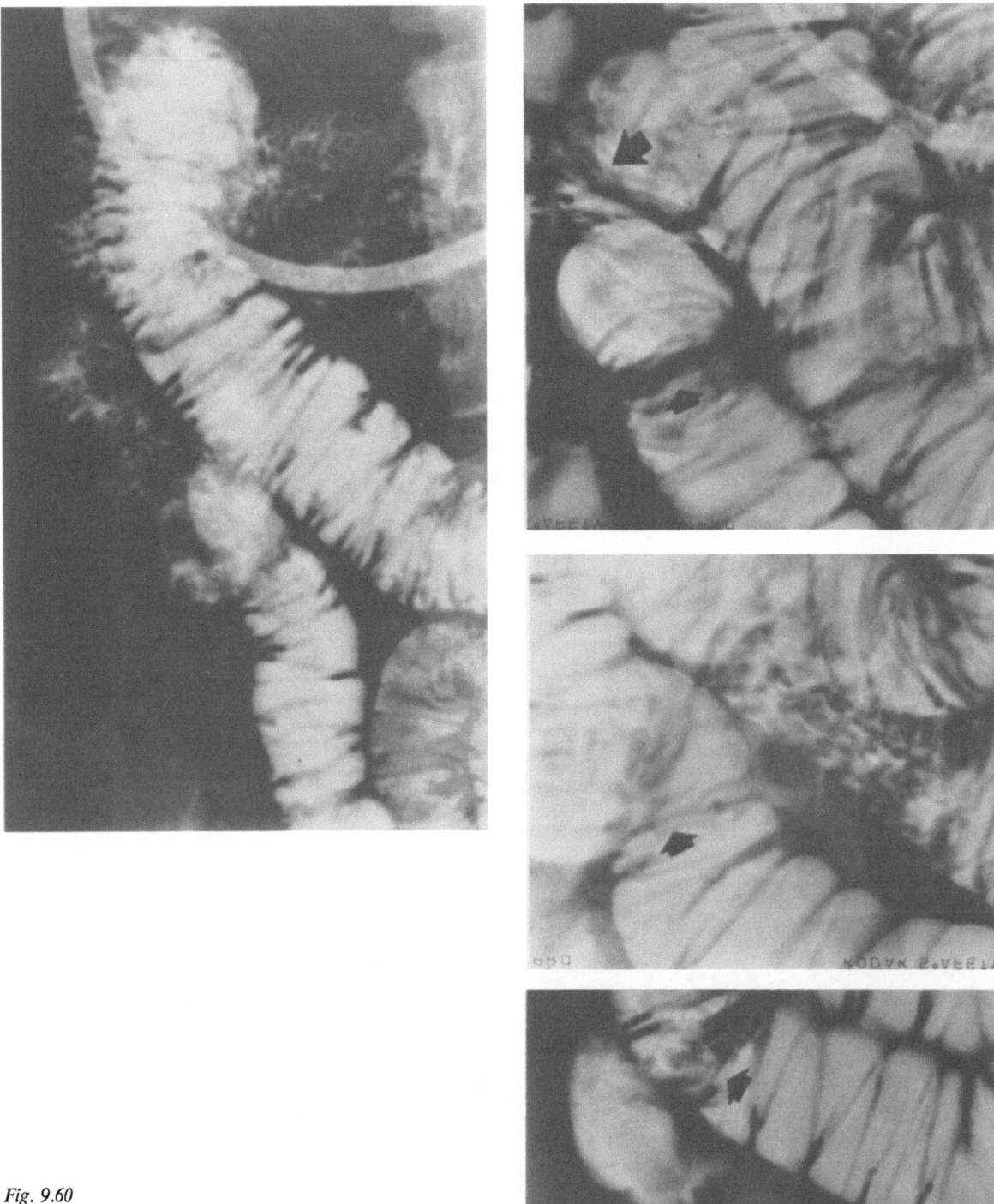

Fig. 9.60
Patient had suffered from colic-like attacks of pain in the abdomen during the past year. Seven years ago diuretics had been prescribed. In the upper right quadrant is one solitary stricture, and possibly there is a second one on the proximal side ±3 cm further on. The stricture was not observed during the examination itself so that no spot films of this region were made. Unfortunately subsequent developments are unknown.

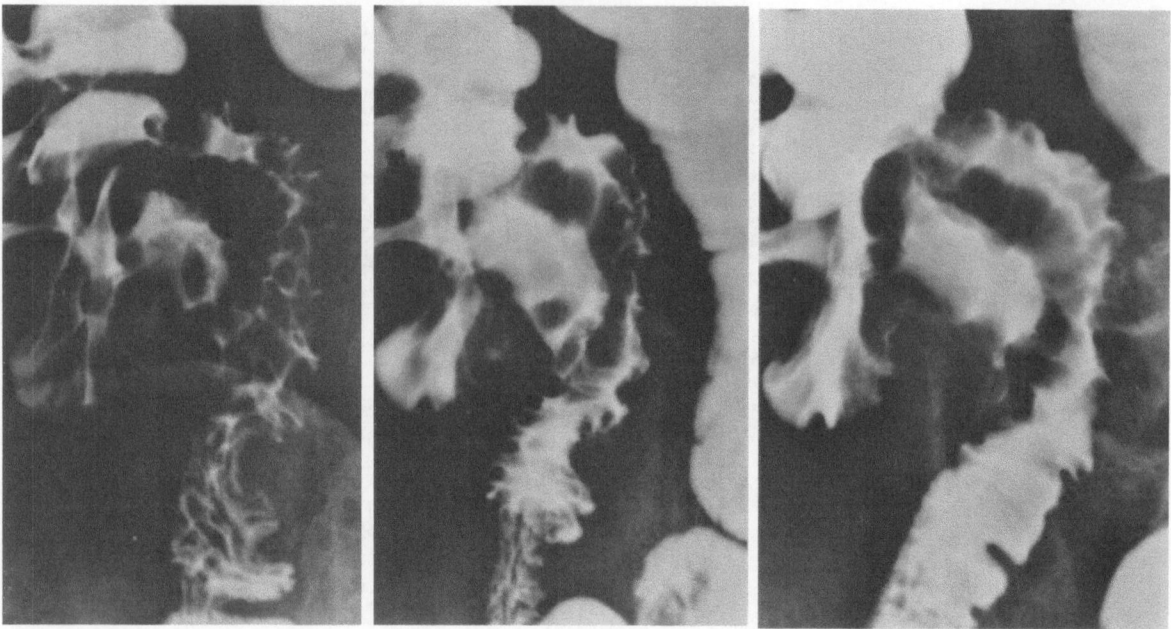

Fig. 9.61
Infiltrate of unknown origin in ileocecal region. Surgery revealed that the large oval accumulation of contrast medium was an ulcer crater. No indications of appendicitis or Crohn's disease.

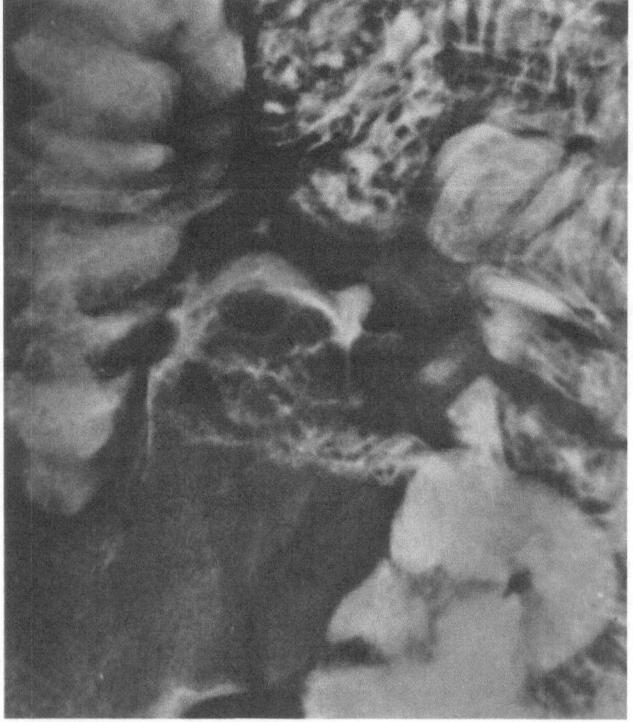

Fig. 9.62
Infiltrate in ileocecal region due to inflamed Meckel's diverticulum.
The correct diagnosis was not established radiologically.

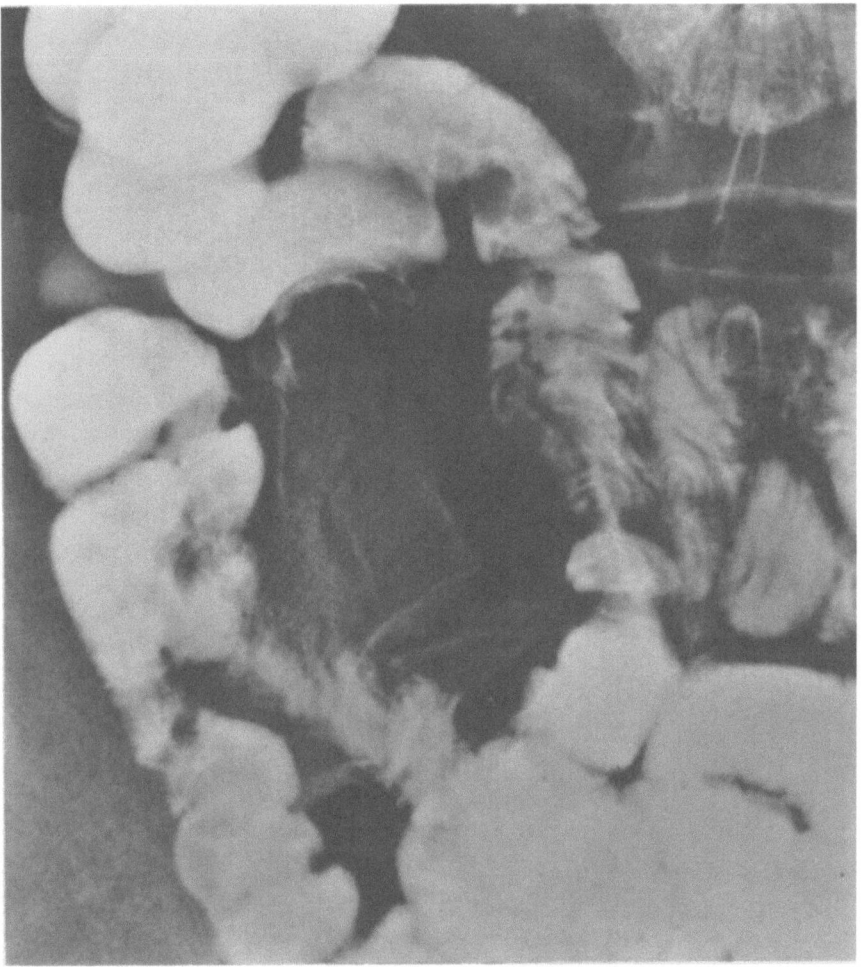

Fig. 9.63
Appendicular infiltrate which can be diagnosed with little difficulty.

9. Appendicular infiltrates

This term refers not only to the infiltrates which originate in the appendix but is also used in the broader sense to indicate all infiltration processes in the lower right quadrant which must be included in the differential diagnosis. After all inflammatory processes do develop in the lower right quadrant of the abdomen which cannot be explained (fig. 9.61). Obviously in such cases a process originating in the appendix or a Meckel's diverticulum should be considered first (fig. 9.62). Although these assumptions frequently turn out to be correct (figs. 9.63–9.64), it is not always true. In the course of several weeks, sometimes even months, the infiltration process heals with or without conservative or symptomatic therapy; often it disappears on its own without significant persistent abnormalities. The radiologically visible abnormalities are usually localized in the last 10 cm – 15 cm at the most – of the ileum and the medial wall of the cecum (fig. 9.65). If there is a definite space-occupying infiltrate, the abnormalities are more pronounced; the entire lower end of the cecum may then be involved and the deformation of the distal ileum can be so marked that the normal anatomy of this part of the intestine can no longer be identified. A misleading factor is that the inflammatory process can be localized elsewhere, for instance in the upper abdomen, if the appendix is directed upwards, and in the lateral flank if the cecum is mobile and is directed towards the median plane (fig. 9.66).

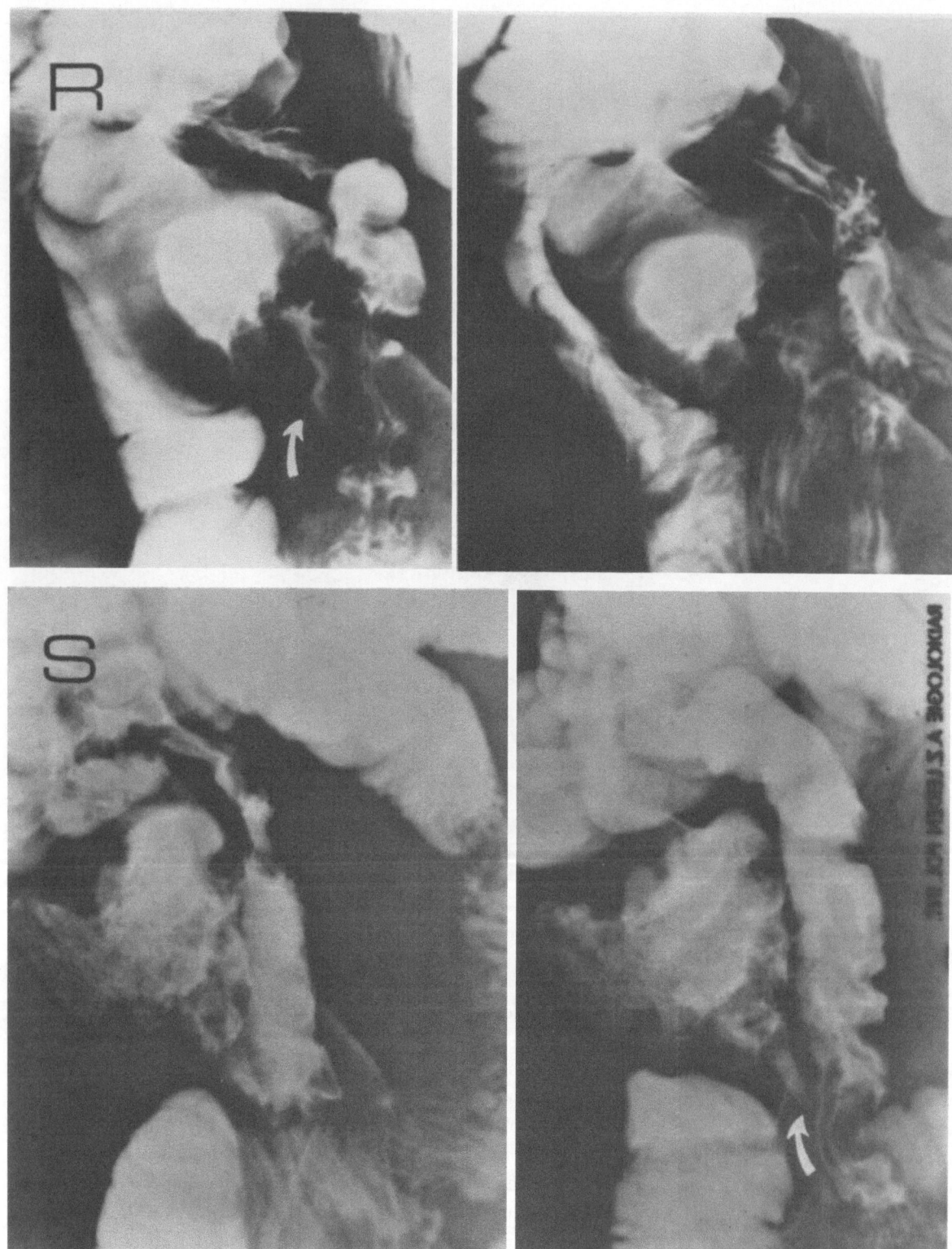

Fig. 9.64

R. Infiltrate in ileocecal region with a large deposit of contrast medium, similar to that seen in fig. 9.61, which presumably is a sacculation in the cecum with an ileal loop coiled around it. Short irregular filling of the appendix.

S. Two months later the infiltrate has disappeared and the filling of the appendix, although not longer, is more regular. Ileal loop is fused with lowest part of the cecum.

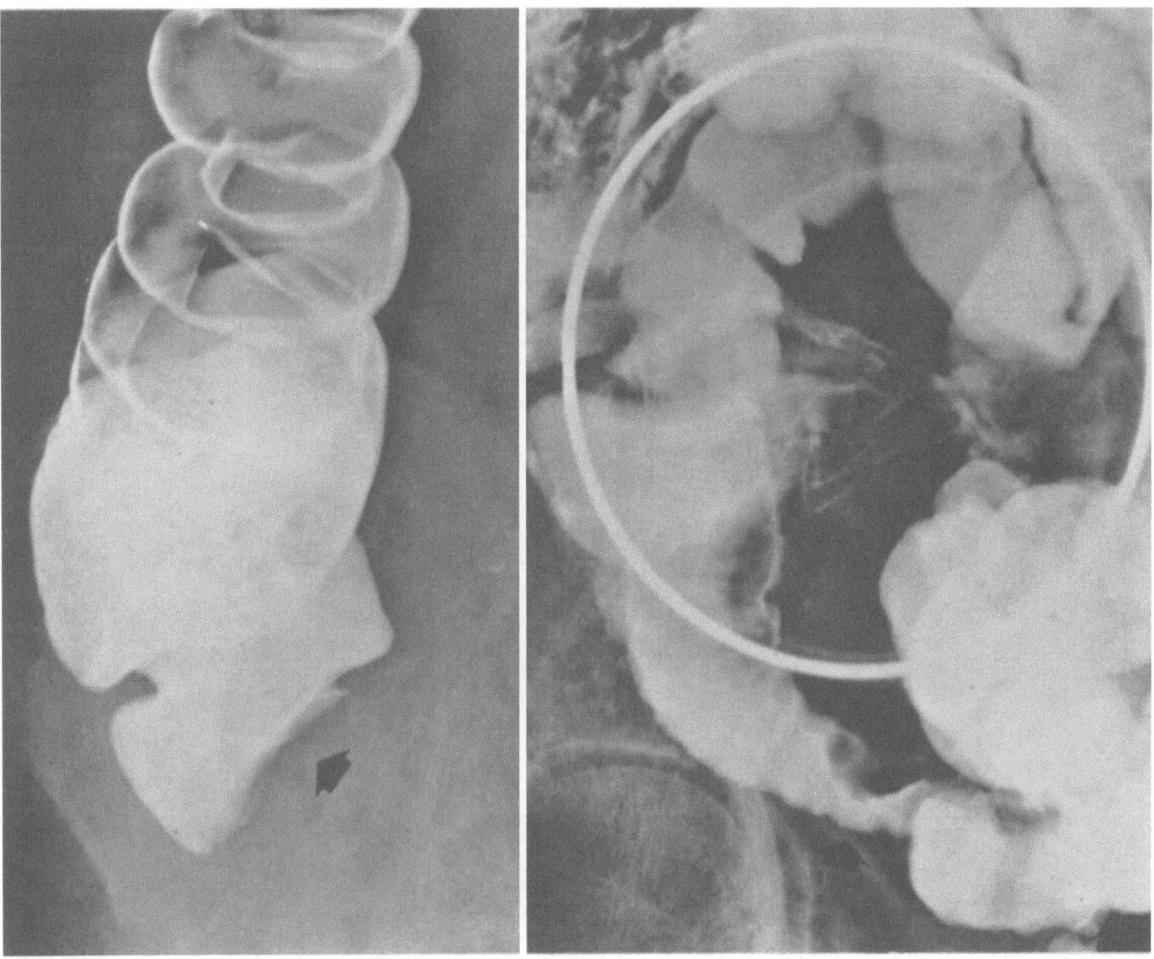

Fig. 9.65
Large appendicular infiltrate, obviously causing impressions on the medial side of the cecum and the ileal loops in the lower right quadrant, led to a moderate obstruction of the small intestine. Appendix is not filled. A tumor must also be included in the differential diagnosis.

Frequently an impression of the spread of the process can be obtained from the normal survey film of the abdomen, either because the gas in the intestinal lumen can be used to visualize the margins of that lumen or because a space-occupying soft tissue shadow contains no gas or appears abnormal (fig. 9.67R).

Of course the infiltration abnormalities can sometimes cause an ileus or perforation into a free abdominal cavity or Douglas' pouch (fig. 9.67s).

Infiltrations or abcesses as a result of an amebiasis are rare, at least in western European countries. However, if the patient is a so-called migrant worker from one of the Mediterranean countries or has had an abdominal infection during a stay in the tropics, this possibility should be considered (fig. 9.68). Another phenomenon which is observed almost exclusively in patients from Dutch harbor towns along the North Sea, where the herring catch is brought in and prepared for consumption, are the extensive infiltrates with fistulization caused by the herring worm (fig. 9.69). Today salting of the herring, which kills the worms is mandatory so that this delicacy can be consumed without fear of complications.

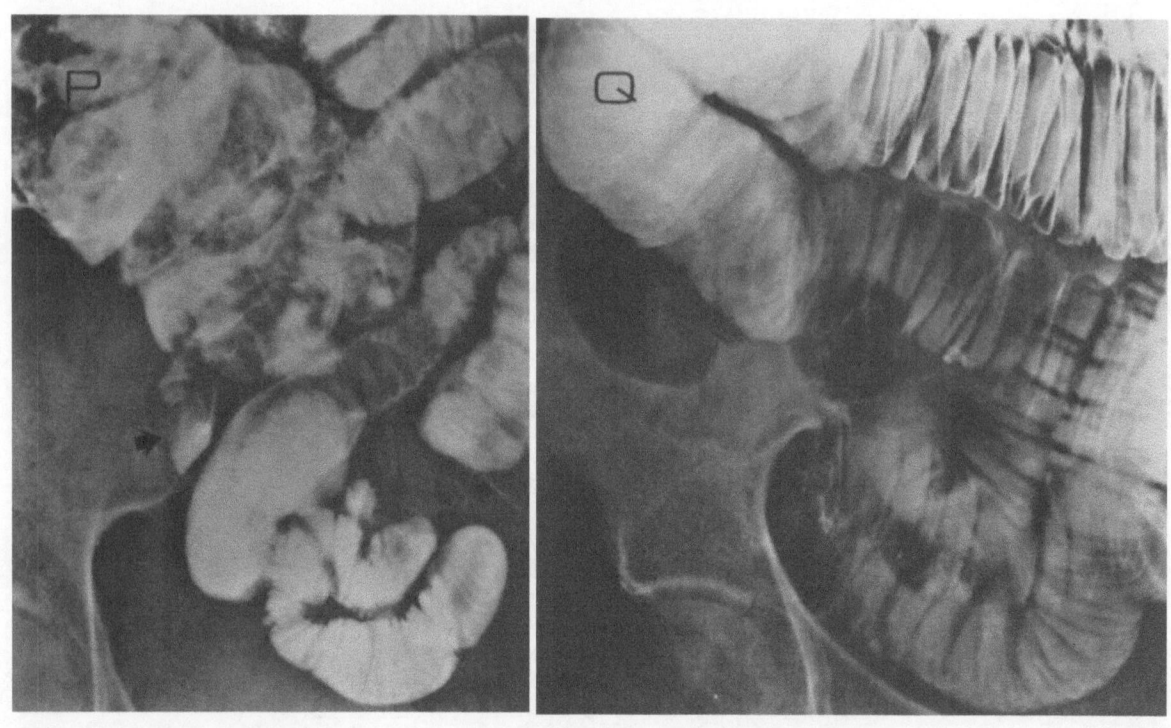

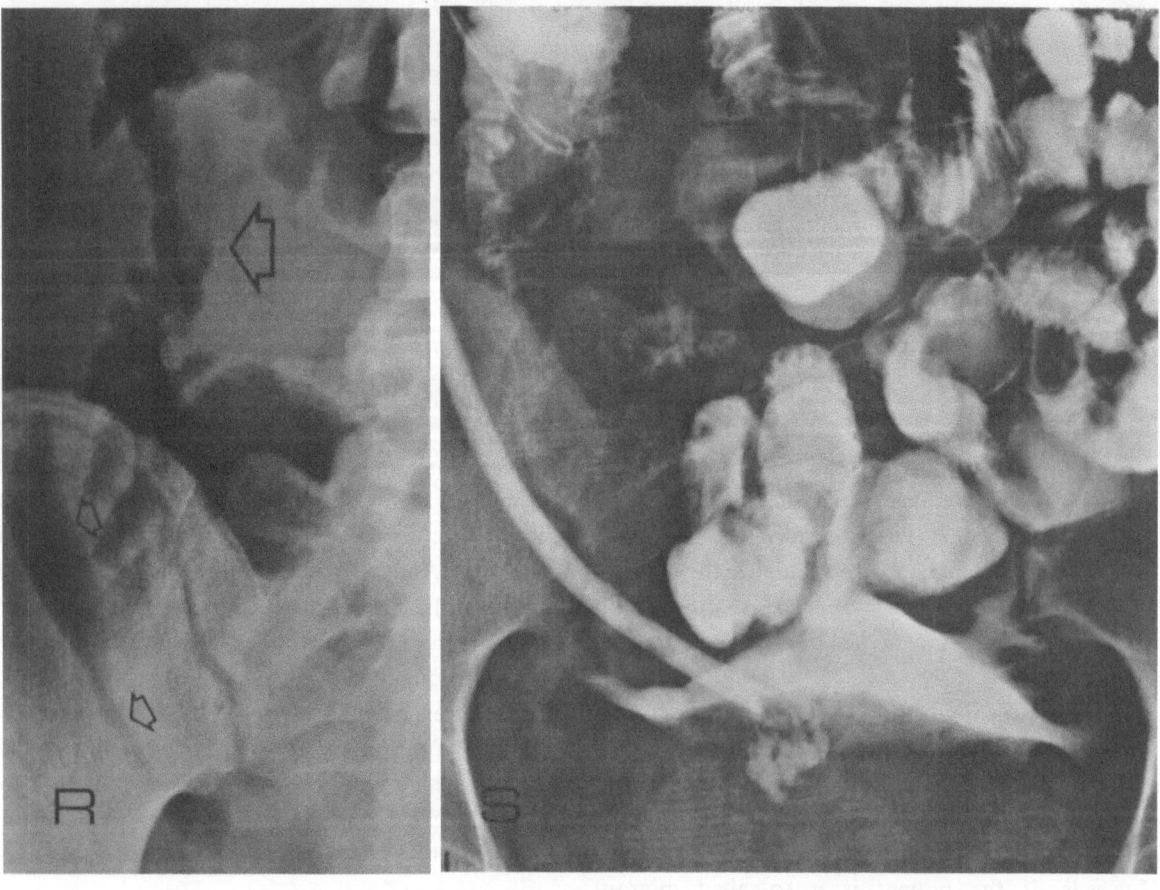

Fig. 9.66

P.   Clinical infiltrate on the lateral side of a high cecum with the lower end extending in the medial direction. No radiological indications of an infiltrate. Distal ileum partially visible (→); appendix is not filled.

Q.   Three months later: ileus as a result of an obstructing infiltrate in the lower right quadrant.
     Surgery: retrocecal appendicular infiltrate + abscess.

←——

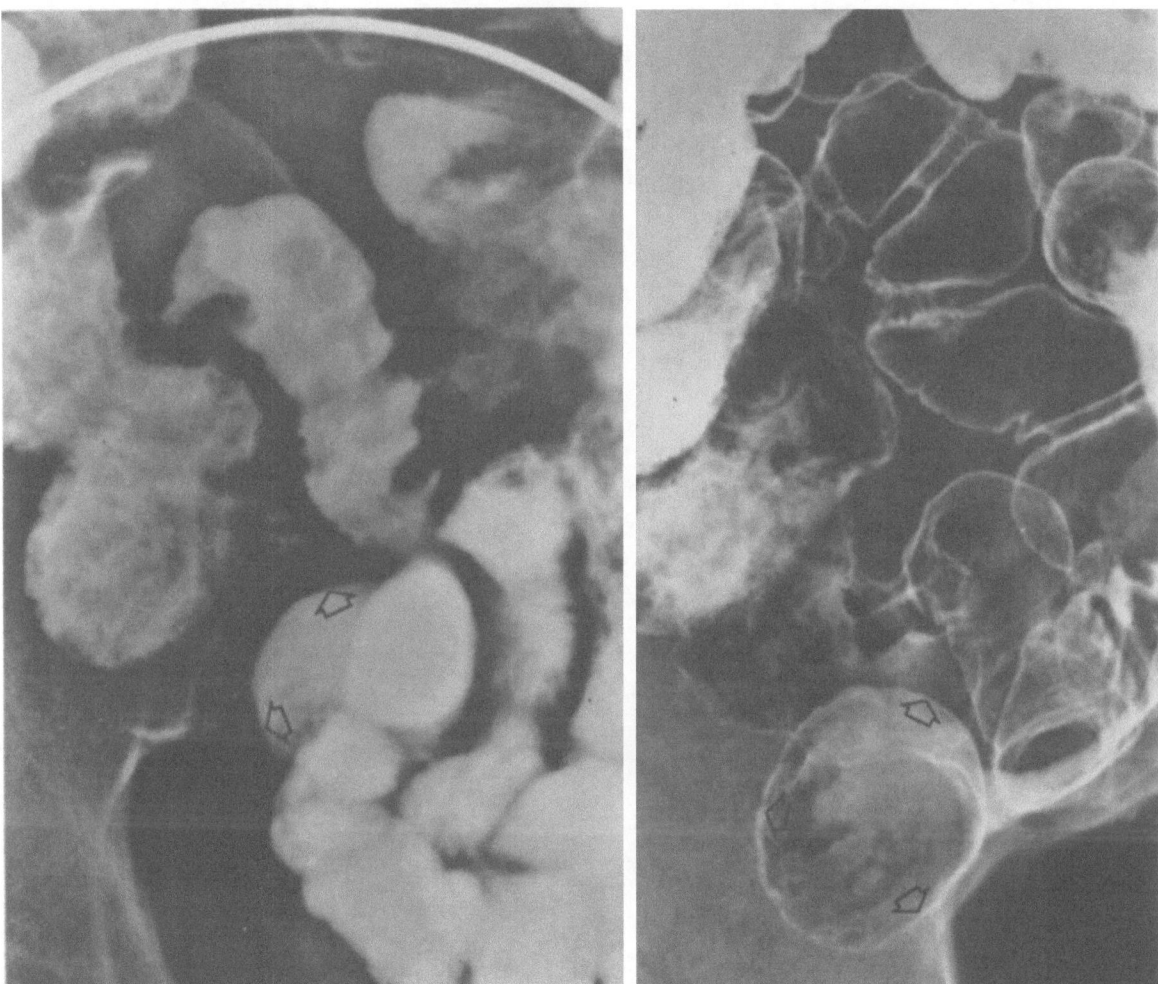

Fig. 9.68
Amebic abscess at lowest end of cecum.

——

←————

Fig. 9.67

R.   Pathological gas configurations in the ascending colon and lateral abdominal wall due to a high appendicular infiltrate with perforation to the retroperitoneal space.

S.   In the postoperative phase there was also perforation into Douglas' pouch.

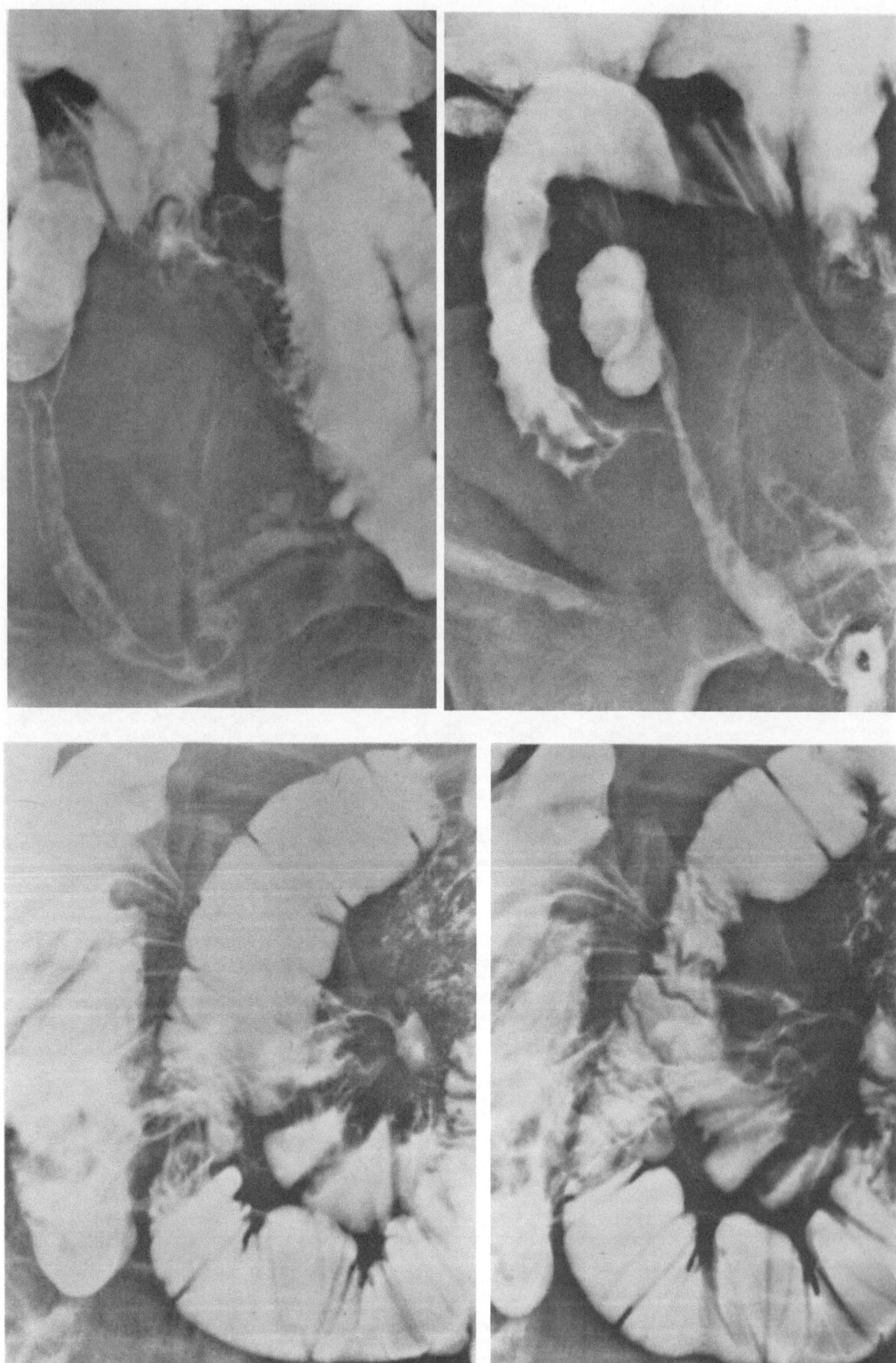

10. Zollinger-Ellison disease

In Zollinger-Ellison's disease solitary or multiple adenomas or slow-growth carcinomas involving the gastrin-secreting cells in the islands of Langhans in the pancreas cause the secretion of gastric acid to be markedly increased.

Since the mucous membrane in the various parts of the digestive tract cannot withstand this large quantity of gastric acid, the mucosal folds are obviously broadened in the jejunum as well as the stomach and the duodenum. This disease should therefore be considered a chemical enteritis; ulcers with secondary stenosis can be found in the jejunum and the distal half of the duodenum similar to those which develop as a result of the action of gastric acid on esophageal mucosa. Due to the low acidity in the duodenum the enzymes for the digestion of fats and proteins are inactivated and steatorrhea develops. In other cases there is only 'intestinal hurry' and a watery diarrhea. During the radiological examination, the unusually strong tendency toward flocculation of the contrast fluid is striking. In some cases the loops of the small intestine are highly dilated (figs. 9.70, 9.71). The cause of this dilatation is not very clear; it is questionable whether the increased fluid secretion to neutralize the excess acid and the increase in bulk resulting from disturbed digestion provide a complete explanation. Since the exceedingly small gastrin-secreting cell groups are usually multiple, and in addition metastases to the liver or other glands can be demonstrated during the examination in more than half of these cases, local excision is impossible and gastric resection is the only possible therapy.

11. Radiological manifestations of serum protein disorders

a. PROTEIN-LOSING ENTEROPATHY

Edema of the ankles and a hypoalbuminemia, with or without diarrhea, can sometimes be the first symptoms indicating a disease of the small intestine. Since hypoalbuminemia is often accompanied by an edematous swelling of the mucosal folds in the jejunum, it is important to be able to recognize this symptom (fig. 9.72).

Some protein loss through transudation of tissue fluid is a physiological phenomenon in the digestive tract; as a rule, however, these proteins are also resorbed. Loss of proteins from the digestive tract can be caused by a disturbed protein synthesis or pronounced leakage of proteins, due to various processes inside as well as outside the digestive tract, so that resorption is incomplete or the liver cannot handle the increased supply.

Protein loss can, when synthesis is unimpaired, also be congenital; then the discharge of lymph in the mesentry is disturbed because of hypoplasia of the lymphatic channels. Such a hypoplasia of the lymphatics is also accompanied by underdeveloped lymphatic channels in the extremities. In contrast the lymphatic channels in the intestinal mucosa are clearly dilated. On the roentgenogram it is noted that the mucosal folds are broadened, the intestinal loops are slightly dilated and the spaces between the loops are somewhat larger due to the thicker intestinal wall (see fig. 8.8). In most cases protein loss is, however, acquired as a result of various inflammatory processes in the small intestine, Whipple's disease or diverse tumors. Portal hypertension, disturbed liver function, cardiac insufficiency or disturbed kidney function can also lead to an elevated protein loss.

Fig. 9.69
Infiltration phenomena in the lower right quadrant due to herring worm disease. Multiple adhesions, fistulous tracts and stenotic intestinal loops. Differentiation from Crohn's disease is difficult; in this case, however, normal filling of the appendix indicates that it is not an appendicular infiltrate.

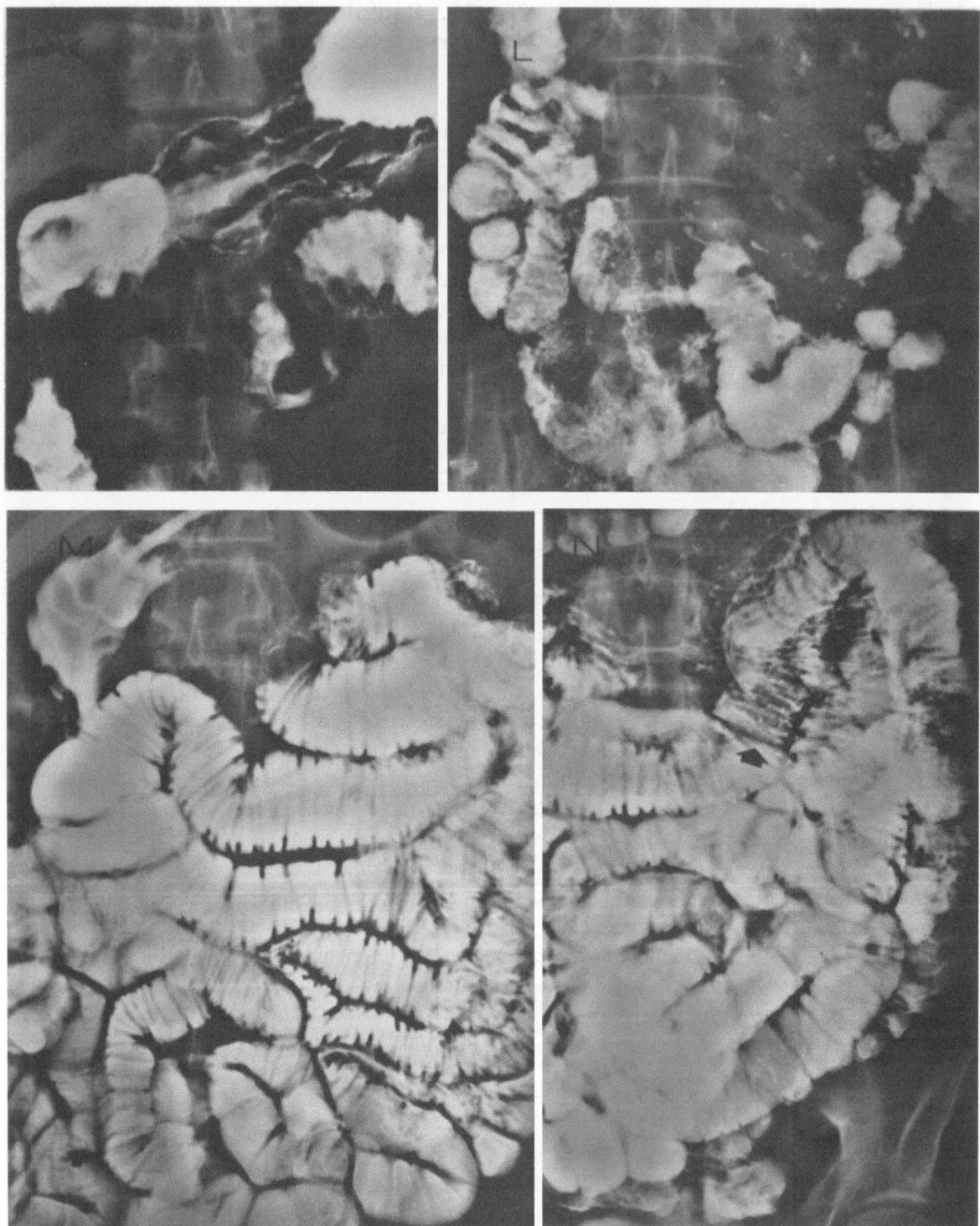

Fig. 9.70
Zollinger-Ellison disease.
K, L.   Conventional examination: coarse mucosal folds and highly disintegrated contrast fluid.
M, N.   Enteroclysis: moderately dilated intestinal loops both in the ileum and in the jejunum. Normal motility. Mucosal folds normal; only in the proximal duodenum are they obviously too coarse. In spite of the administration of large quantities of contrast fluid in order to withstand the damaging fluids as much as possible, flocculation developed immediately after termination of the infusion (N).

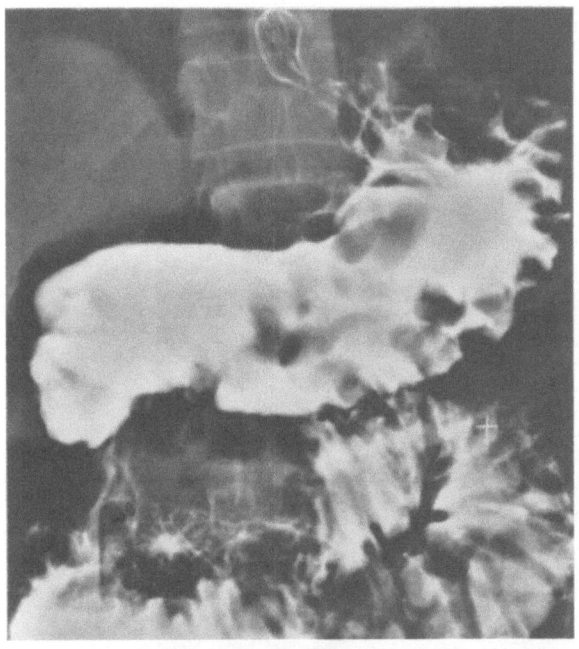

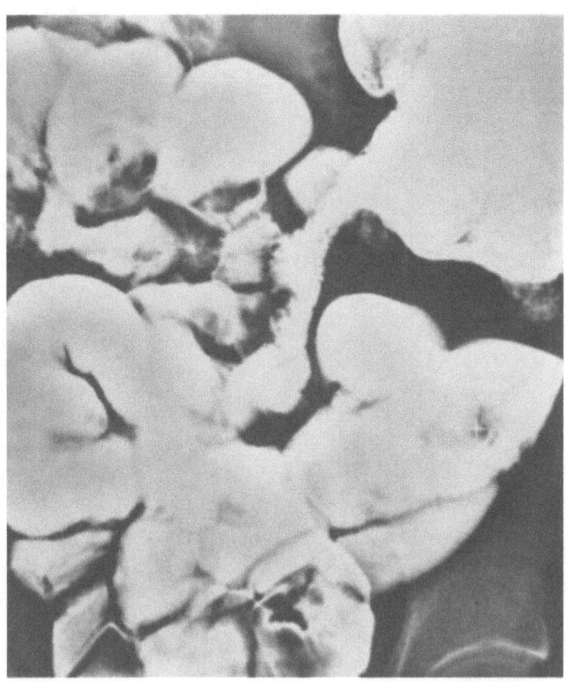

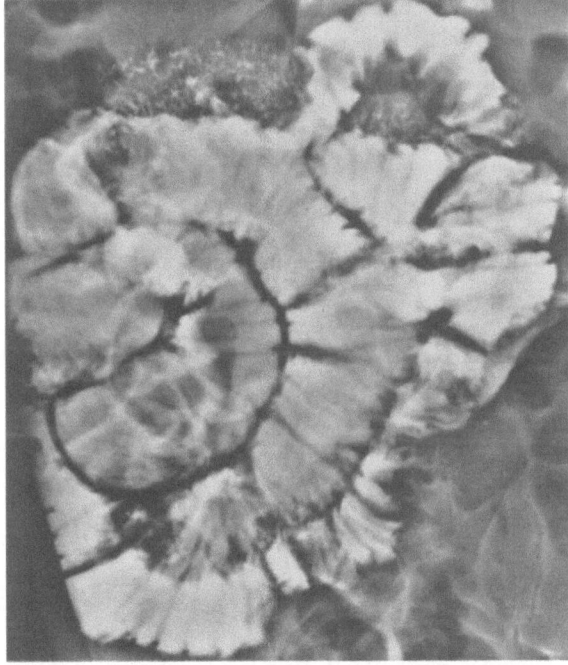

Fig. 9.71
Zollinger-Ellison disease. Very coarse mucosal folds in the stomach, duodenum and jejunum with pronounced dilatation of the loops in the jejunum and the ileum.

b. IMMUNOGLOBULIN DEFICIENCY

Much less common than albumin loss is a disturbed gamma globulin synthesis. Gamma globulins seem to play an important role in the immunologically determined humoral immunity against numerous, sometimes definitely malignant, diseases. Humeral immunity which must be distinguished from cellular immunity is connected with the so-called immunoglobulins, several types of which have now been identified, indicated as IgA, IgM, IgG, etc. A deficiency of these 3 types of gamma globulins can occur selectively or in combination as well as in various degrees giving rise to an agammaglobulinemia or a hypogammaglobulinemia. A disproportion of these immunoglobulins is called dysgammaglobulinemia.

An abnormally low level of immunoglobulins can be either congenital or acquired, the latter is probably more common. In agammaglobulinemia, hypogammaglobulinemia or dysgammaglobulinemia, the albumin level usually remains normal so that the total protein concentration is barely

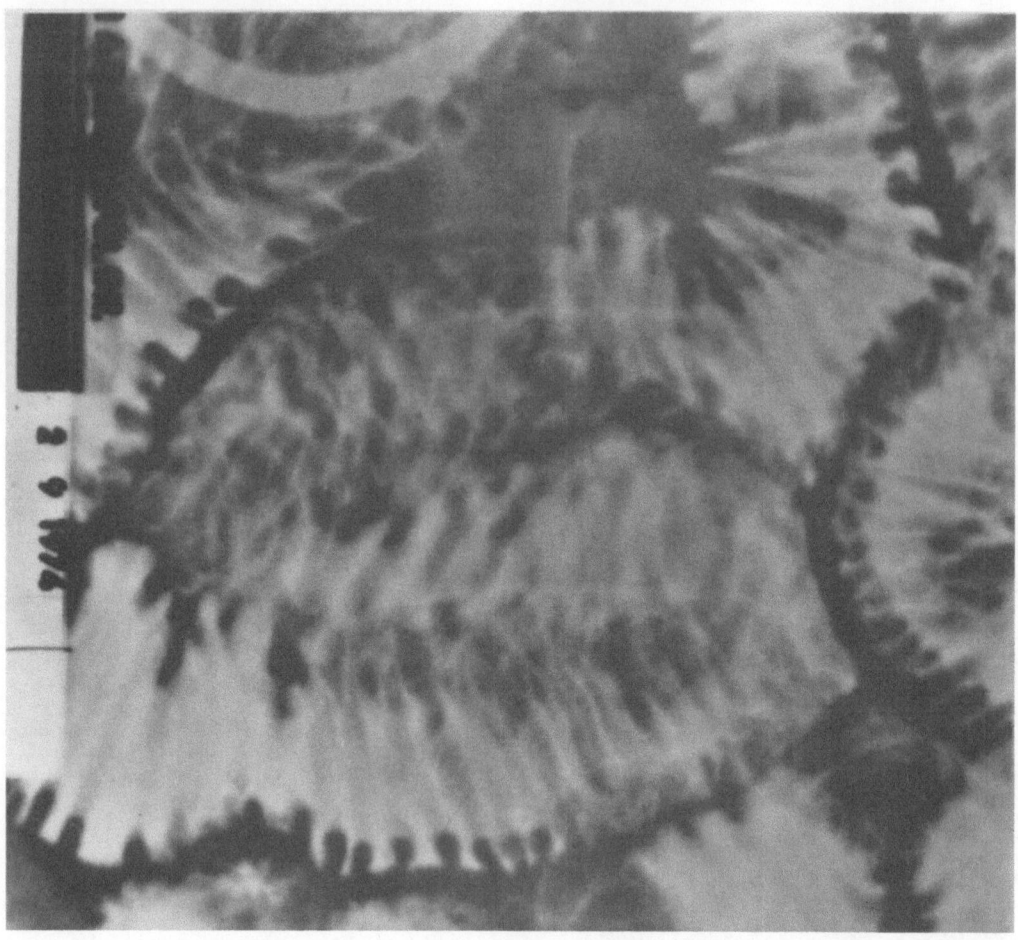

Fig. 9.72
Omega-shaped edematous swelling of the mucosal folds in a patient with protein loss in the small intestine as a result of an ulcerative colitis.

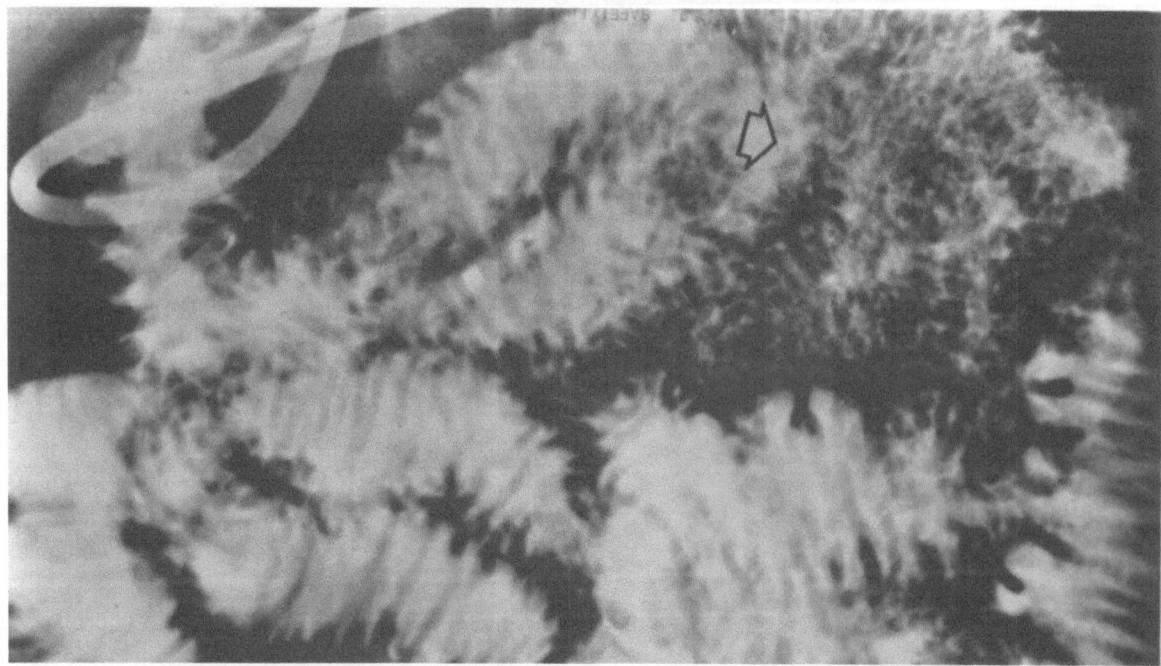

reduced and edema does not occur. However, patients with a disturbed gammaglobulin synthesis are highly susceptible to infectious diseases such as lambliasis which can lead to a reduced albumin concentration and swollen mucosal folds. Several diseases which involve a disturbance of the immunoglobulin pattern are celiac disease, pernicious anemia, atrophic gastritis, benign and malignant lymphoma (alpha chain disease), Waldenströms macroglobulinemia and primary amyloidosis.

It has been found that these diseases give a greater chance of malignancy, particularly in the digestive tract. The benign lymphoma is especially treacherous since it can suddenly turn into a malignant lymphoma after many years (fig. 9.76).

The clinical symptoms and laboratory findings for diseases accompanied by an immunoglobulin deficiency can vary widely. Several of the most common symptoms are:

1. Malabsorption, diarrhea and steatorrhea, due to secondary infections, achlorhydria, gluten-sensitivity and disturbed resorption as a result of changes in the intestinal wall.
2. Atrophied villi in the duodenum and proximal jejunum, sometimes accompanied by a gluten sensitivity.

3. Atrophied mucous membrane, sometimes in conjunction with an achlorhydria.
4. Either no plasma cells, or very many, in the lamina propria of the intestinal wall.
5. An agammaglobulinemia, hypogammaglobulinemia or dysgammaglobulinemia.
6. Increased susceptibility to intestinal infections.

Radiologically the following can be observed:

1. Greater tendency toward flocculation of the contrast fluid; this can be established by taking 1 or 2 residual exposures after the examination is completed.
2. Absence of mucosal folds on the side of greater curvature (atrophic gastritis) or in the duodenum and proximal jejunum (celiac disease).
3. Irritated mucosal patterns in the proximal jejunum (lambliasis) (fig. 9.73).
4. Very coarse more or less irregular mucosal folds and a thickening of the wall in a large segment of the small intestine, mainly the ileum (lymphoma) (fig. 9.74).
5. Lymphoid nodular hyperplasia; the mucosa is then covered with numerous 2–4 mm nodules caused by hyperplastic lymph follicles in the lamina propria (fig. 9.75).

←

Fig. 9.73
Irritability of the jejunum in a case of lambliasis. Rapid disintegration of the contrast fluid (→), probably due to hypersecretion.

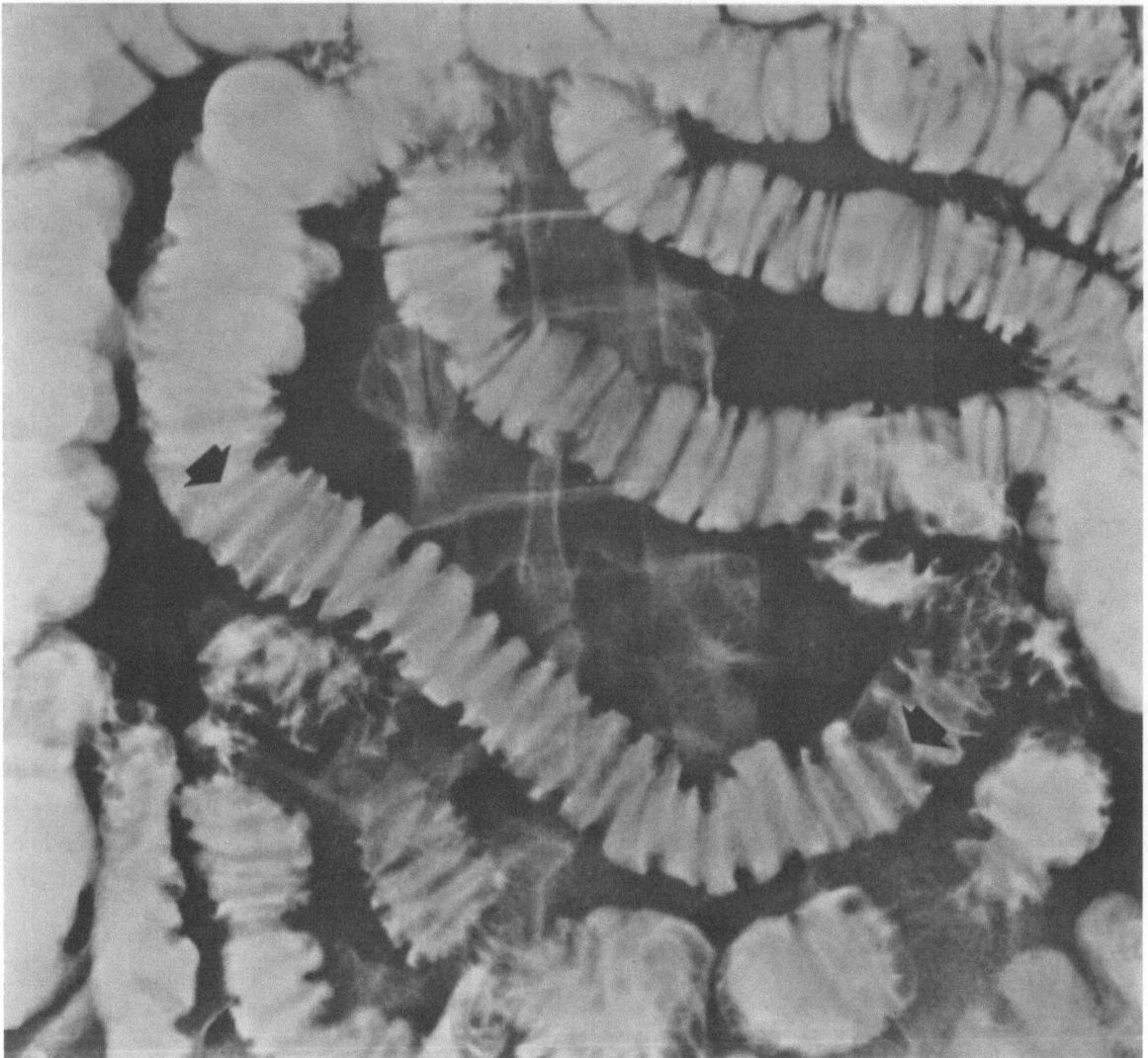

Fig. 9.74

v. Mucosal folds are obviously too coarse along several decimeters in the proximal ileum; this middle-aged patient had lost considerable weight in the last 6 months, and a malabsorption and a slowly increasing diarrhea had developed. For these abnormalities of the mucosa, the following must be considered:
1. superficial lymphoma
2. ischemia
3. Crohn's disease

w. Three months later a repeat examination revealed that the abnormalities had spread and increased slightly in severity. The mucosal surface has fairly irregular margins, possibly as a result of superficial ulcerations. On the basis of the course of the disease during this period and other examinations, ischemia and Crohn's disease can probably be excluded and a lymphoma must be seriously considered. Experience has shown that these abnormalities can suddenly, but also very gradually, develop into a malignant lymphoma. Follow-up of this patient was not possible since he refused further treatment. The biopsy revealed multiple deposits of plasma cells in the lamina propria.

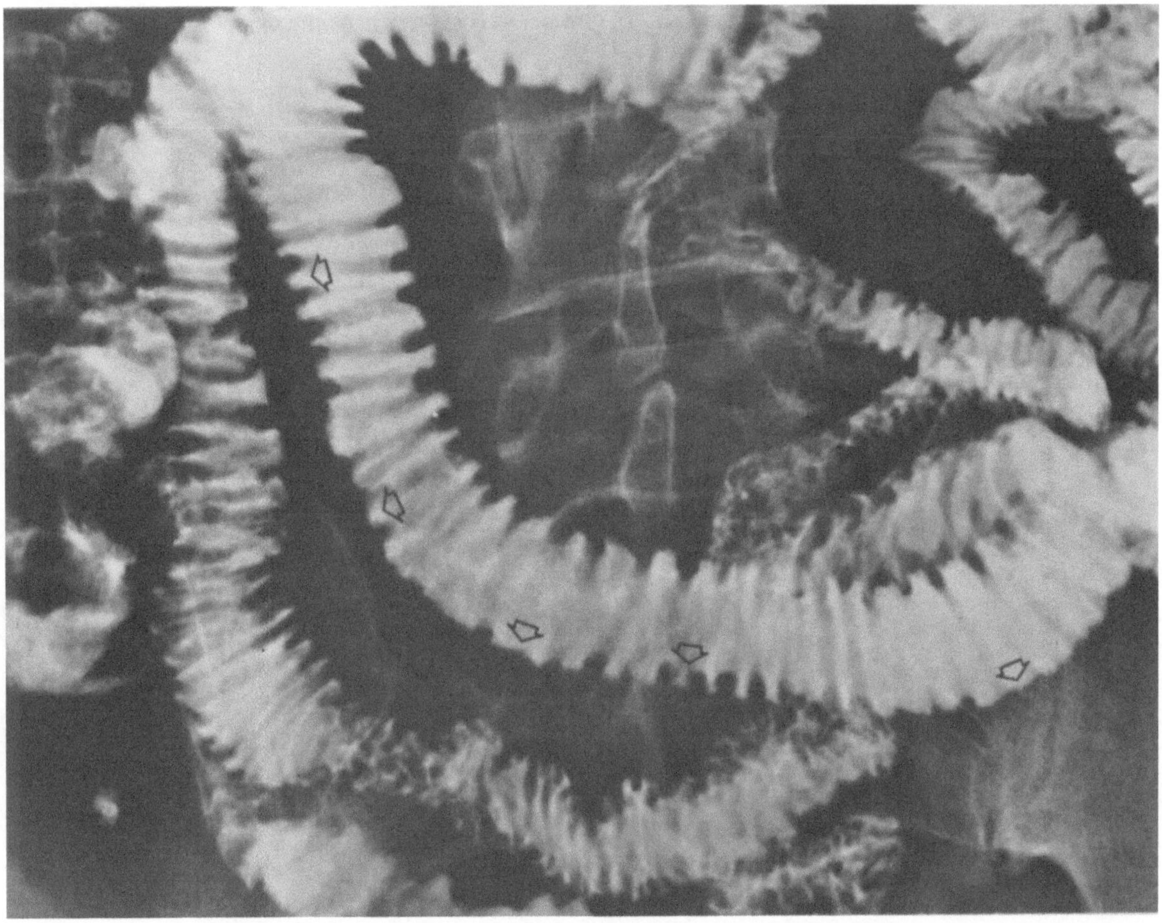

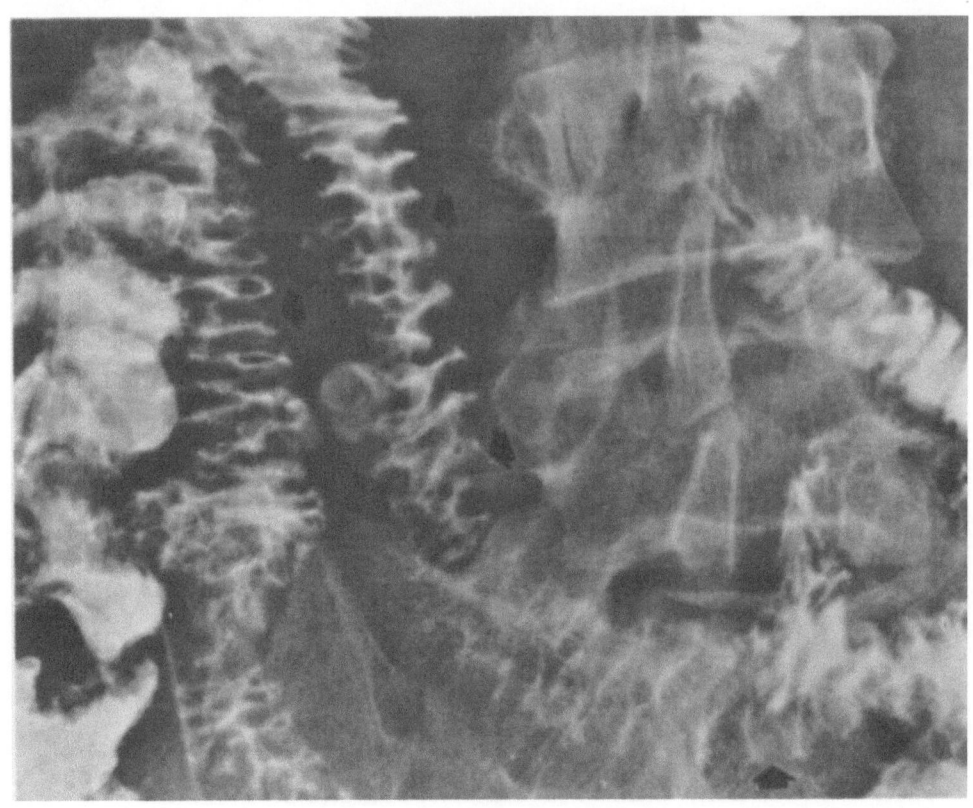

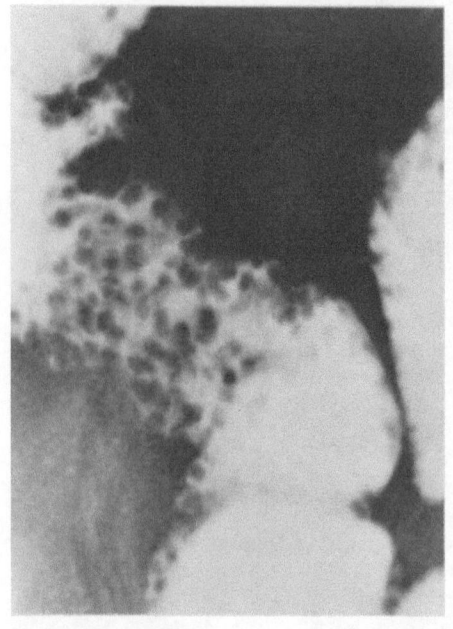

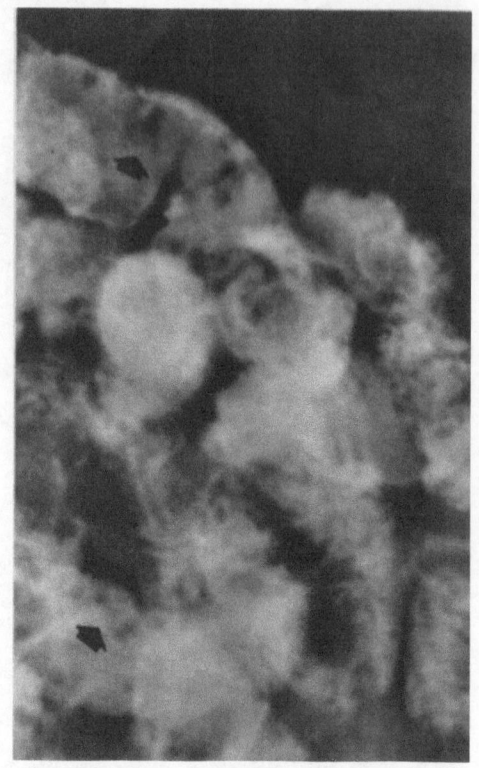

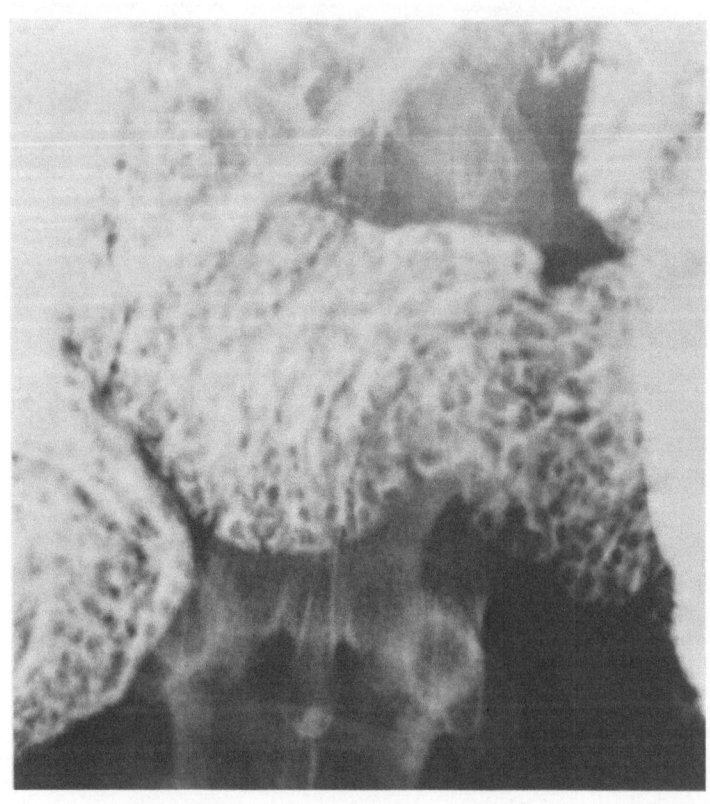

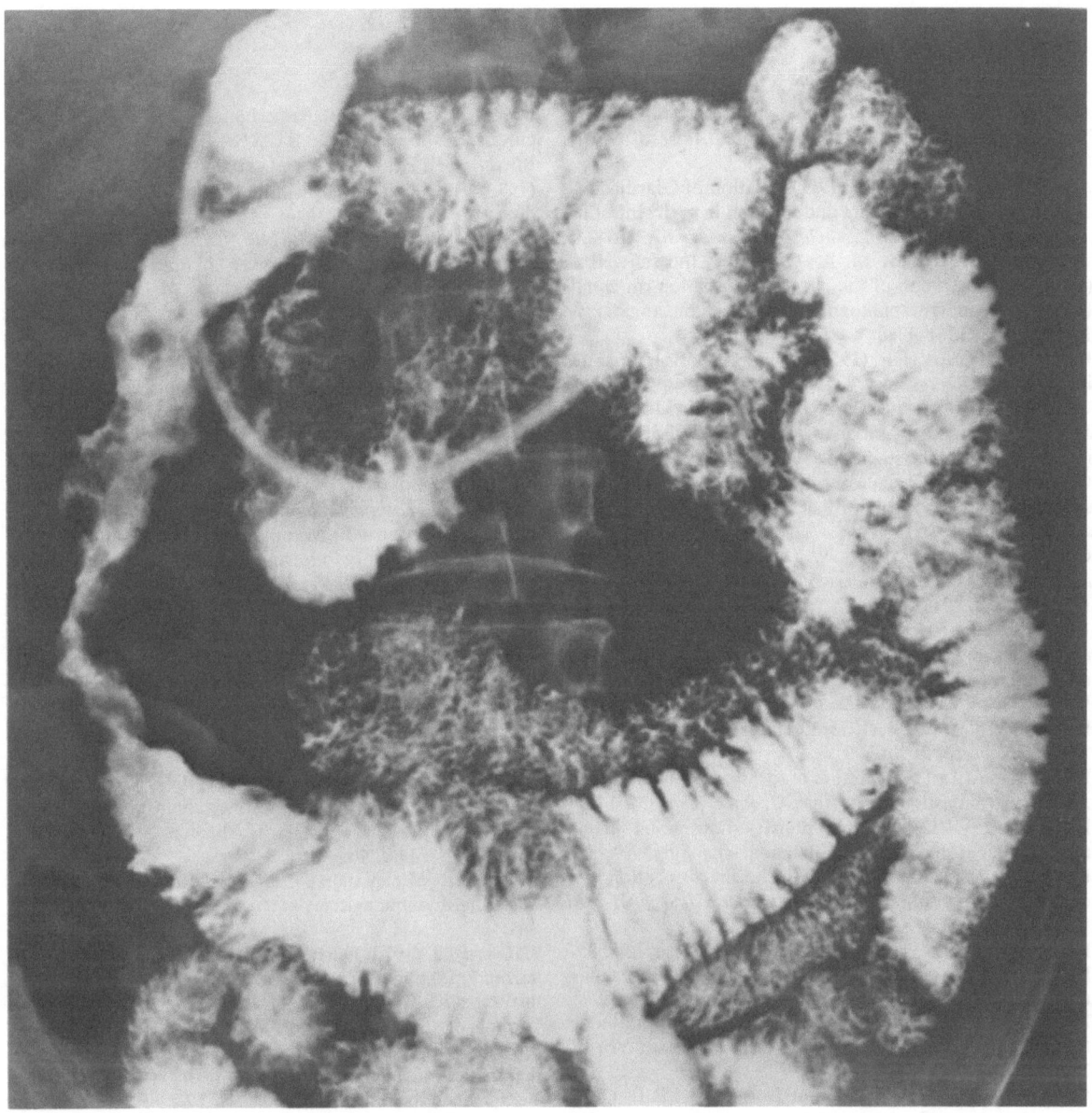

Fig. 9.76
Hypoglobulinaemia with an extensive lymphoid hyperplasia of the small intestine and a lymphosarcoma in the jejunum.

←

Fig. 9.75
Lymphoid nodular hyperplasia as seen in cases of immunoglobulin deficiency.

Bibliography chapter IX

ALDRIDGE A. H. (1942) Intestinal injuries resulting from irradiation treatment of uterine carcinoma. *Amer. J. Obstet. Gynec. 44*, 833–857.

AMENT M. E.; RUBIN C. E. (1972) Relation of Giardiasis to abnormal intestinal structure and function in gastrointestinal immunodeficiency syndromes. *Gastroenterology 62*, 216–226.

BOSNIAK M. A.; HARDY M. A.; QUINT J.; GHOSSEIN N. A. (1969) Demonstration of the effect of irradiation on canine bowel using in vivo photografic magnification angiografy. *Radiology 93*, 1361–1368.

BUCKER, J.; FEINDT H. R. (1951) Pseudopolyposis lymphatica ilei. *Fortschr. Röntgenstr. 74*, 59–65.

CHAU P. M.; FLETCHER G. H.; RUTLEDGE F. N.; DODD G. D. JR. (1962) Complications in high dose whole pelvis irradiation in female pelvic cancer. *Amer. J. Roentgenol. 87*, 22–40.

CLEMETT A. (1968) Lecture on 'Intestinal manifestations of systemic disease'. School of Medecine. University of California, march 1968.

COLCOCK B. P.; BRAATSCH J. W. (1968) *Surgery of the small intestine in the adult.* Saunders, Philadelphia, 161–165.

DE COSSE J. J.; RHODES R. S.; WENTZ W. B.; REAGAN J. W.; DWORKEN H. J.; HOLDEN W. D. (1969) The natural history and management of radiation induced injury of the gastrointestinal tract. *Ann. Surg. 170*, 369–384.

DELAVIERRE PH.; LEVASSEUR J.-C.; KRON B.; RUAULT P.; BASTIAN ET TRAN VAN B. (1973) Les ulcères primitifs du grêle. *Sem. Hôp. Paris 49*, 2052.

DESJARDINS A. U. (1931) Action of roentgen rays and radium on the gastrointestinal tract. *Amer. J. Roentgenol. 26*, 145.

DOWDLE E. (1942) Multiple primary nonspecific jejunal ulcers, with chronic duodenal dilatation. *Ann. Surg. 166*, 348.

DUNCAN W.; LEONARD J. (1965) The malabsorption syndrome following radiotherapy. *The quarterly Journal of Med.* Vol. XXXIV.

EBELING W. (1933) Primary jejunal ulcer. *Ann. Surg. 97*, 857.

EVERT J. A.; BLACK B. M.; DOCKERTY M. B. (1948) Primary nonspecific ulcers of the small intestine. *Surgery 23*, 185.

FRIEDMAN W. B. (1955) Pathogenesis of intestinal ulcus following irradiation. *A.M.A. Archives of Pathology* Vol. *59*, 2–4.

GOEHRS H. R.; MORLOCK C. G.; DOCKERTY M. B. (1957) Primary non-specific ulcers of the small intestine. *Proc. Mayo Clinic 32*, 351.

GRAUNDINS J. (1969) Über Strahlenspätschäden am Dünndarm. *Langenbecks Arch. Klin. Chir. 324*, 120–130.

GRYBOSKI J. D.; SELF T. W.; CLEMETT A.; et al. (1968) Selective immunoglobulin A deficiency and intestinal nodular lymphoid hyperplasia: Correction of diarrhea with antibiotics and plasma. *Pediatrics 42*, 833–837.

HODGSON J. R.; HOFFMAN H. N. II; HUIZENGA K. A. (1967) Roentgenologic features of lymphoid hyperplasia of the small intestine associated with dysgammaglobulinemia. *Radiology 88*, 883–888.

KHILNANI M. T.; KELLER R. J.; CUTTNER J. (1969) Macroglobulinemia and steatorrhea: roentgen and pathologic findings in the intestinal tract. *Radiol. Clin. N.A. 7*, 43–55.

KYLE J. (1972) *Crohn's Disease.* Heinemann, London.

LINDHOLMER B.; NIJMAN E.; RAF L. (1964) Nonspecific ulceration of the small bowel. *Acta chir. scand. 128*, 310.

LITWIN M. S.; CRANE C. (1960) Primary nonpeptic ulcer of the jejunum. *Ann. Surg. 151*, 594.

MARINA-FIOL C. (1962) Bemerkungen über die Ileitis follicularis. *Gastroenterologia*, Basel *98*, 19–29.

MARSHAK R. H.; HAZZI CH.; LINDNER A. E.; MAKLANSKY D. (1975) The small bowel in immunoglobulin deficiency syndromes.

MARSHAK R. H.; RUOFF M.; LINDNER A. E. (1968) Roentgen manifestations of giardiasis. *Amer. J. Roentgenol. 104*, 557–560.

MASON G. R.; DIETRICH P.; FRIEDLAND G. W.; HANKES G. E. (1970) The radiological findings in radiation induced enteritis and colitis. *Clin. Radiol. 21*, 232–247.

NEUMEISTER K.; PFEIFFER J. (1966) Klinische Analyse der Akuten Intestinalen Strahlenreaktionen bei Röntgen-Radium- und Telekobaltbestrahlungen. *Strahlentherapie 129*, 512–519.

NILEHN B.; SJOSTROM B. (1967) Studies on Yersinia enterocolitica. *Acta path. microbiol. scand. 71*, 612–628.

NUMMI P.; FRITMEN J.; MÄKÖNEN H. (1973) Radiationinduced small bowel injury following telecobalt therapy of bladder tumor. *Scand. J. Urol. Neprol. 7*, 30–32.

OSBORN ANNE G.; FRIEDLAND G. W. (1973) A radiological approach to the diagnosis of small bowel disease. *Clin. Radiol. 24*, 281–301.

PREVOT R. (1950) Röntgendiagnose der entzündlichen Darmerkrankungen. *Fortschr. Röntgenstr. 72*, 547–563.

RAVDIN I. S. (1927) Primary ulcer of the jejunum. *Ann. Surg. 85*, 873.

ROSWITT B.; MALSKY S. J.; REID C. B. (1972) Severe radiation injuries of stomach, small intestine, colon and rectum. Va Radist. Ther. Cent. – Va Hosp. Bronx, N.Y. – *Amer. J. Roentgenol. 144/3*, 460–475.

SHIMKIN P. M.; WALDMAN T. A.; KRUGMAN R. L. (1970) Intestinal Lymphangiectasia. *Amer. J. Roentgenol. 110*, 827–841.

SIELAFF H. J. (1970) Die radiologische Diagnostik der Dünndarmerkrankungen. *Therapiewoche 20*, 3207–3215.

SIMPKINS K. C. (1972) Some aspects of the radiology of Crohn's disease. *Brit. J. Surg.* Vol. *59*, No. *10*.

SJOSTROM B.; NILEHN B. (1968) Some aspects of the inflammation of the ileocoecal region with special reference to Yersinia enterocolitica. *Bull. Soc. int. Chir.* No. *5*.

STURGES H. F.; KRONE CH. L. (1973) Ulceration and structure of the jejunum in a patient on long-term Indomethacin therapy. *Amer. J. Gastroent. 59*, 162.

TEICHER I.; MUEULBAUER M. A.; ALLEN A. C. (1963) The clinical-pathological spectrum of primary ulcers of the small intestine. *Surg. Gynec. Obstet. 116*, 196.

TODD T. F. (1938) Rectal ulceration following irradiation treatment of carcinoma of cervix uteri. *Surg. Gynec. Obstet. 67*, 617–631.

WARREN J.; FRIEDMAN N. (1942) Pathology and pathologic diagnosis of radiation lesions in gastrointestinal tract. *Amer. J. Path. 18*, 499.

WATSON M. R.; HELWIG E. B. (1968) Primary nonspecific ulceration of the small bowel. *Arch. Surg. 87*, 600.

WIECHEN P. J. VAN (1974) Radiological changes in the distal part of the ileum in association with yersinia enterocolitica infections. *Radiol. clin. biol. 43*, 242–253.

See also the nrs. 38–91–143–145 and 190 of the bibliography of pages 164 and following.

X

TUMORS

1. General

Although the small intestine is approximately twice as long as the esophagus, stomach and colon together, tumors of the small bowel are relatively rare; they account for about 5% of all tumors of the digestive tract. The reason for this apparent immunity is a matter of conjecture; it is presumed that the lack of stasis in this part of the digestive tract is significant. In the absolute sense, however, tumors of the small intestine cannot be considered rare. They are found in about 20% of the autopsy material. In contrast to the colon and especially the esophagus and stomach, where malignant tumors are more common than benign ones, only 1/5th of all tumors in the small intestine are malignant.

In the past a tumor in the small intestine was seldom demonstrated preoperatively by means of radiological examination; in fact until recently this diagnosis was only established in about 1 out of every 5 cases. This poor score was due in part to the fact that benign tumors are usually asymptomatic, or at least until they reach a certain size when recurrent complaints of obstruction occur. In the jejunum, that part of the intestine where peristalsis is the most active, a (temporary) intussusception will sometimes develop. Malignant tumors, too, are not discovered until further growth of the tumor causes obvious stenotic phenomena. The patient then complains of colic-like pains in the abdomen which are usually localized around the navel. Intussusceptions are seldom or never seen in conjunction with malignant tumors since the latter never have a peduncle and growth tends to be extraluminal, sometimes with invasion of the surrounding tissue. Although these abdominal pains, often accompanied by diarrhea and sometimes also by a clinical malabsorption, are encountered in 2/3 of the patients with tumors, they are by no means a specific symptom for a tumor of the small intestine. The fact that there can also be periods without complaints is misleading. The same is true for bleeding in the digestive tract; this is encountered in one-half of the patients and it is often presumed, understandably, that the blood loss originates in the colon or the stomach. It should therefore first be established by means of physical and radiological examination that there are no abnormalities in these two parts of the digestive tract. Subsequently the possibility of a tumor in the small intestine must be considered and included in the differential diagnosis. Often, however, the correct diagnosis is not discovered until the patient is on the operating table, frequently after he has had complaints for at least a year; at this stage a palpable mass can be felt in 1/3 of the cases. From the preceding it will be clear that the tumors found in the small bowel during surgery are predominantly malignant, in contrast to the autopsy findings whereby most of the tumors of the small intestine appear to be benign. If a bleeding is diagnosed and localized, either clinically or angiographically, a laparotomy should follow. Negative findings based solely on external palpation of the intestinal loops are completely worthless; the lumen of the intestine must be inspected using multiple incisions. If there is even a moderate constriction of the intestinal lumen, the enteroclysis examination can be used to provoke a striking prestenotic dilatation.

Another advantage of the enteroclysis technique is that an obvious increase in the distance between the descending limb of the duodenum and the spinal column may already become evident during fluoroscopic monitoring of the position of the tube in the right lateral position (fig. 10.1). This can indicate a tumor of the pancreas, some other retroperitoneal tumorous growth or metastasis in a

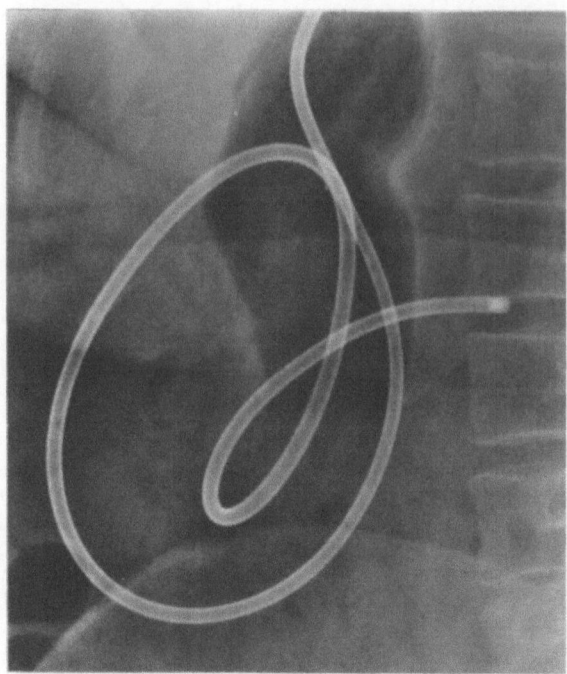

Fig. 10.1
Obvious broadening of the retroperitoneal space by metastases – in this case of a melanoma.

lymph node from a primary tumor elsewhere. Metastatic growth in particular may not involve the mass of intestinal loops at all so that the widening of the prevertebral space may be completely overlooked in the a.p. projection.

Although these factors have brought about a very real improvement in the diagnosis of tumors, the enteroclysis technique alone is not the only important aspect. In addition to the use of this method of examination, the precision with which the clinician scans each separate intestinal loop, using spot films, is essential, just as in the search for a Meckel's diverticulum.

It is obvious that once good roentgenograms which permit easy evaluation of the anatomy of the intestinal loops became possible, the need for further spot films became evident; after all spot films were of little use when the loops were inadequately filled. The enteroclysis technique also has stimulated many clinicians to make a greater personal effort, thus producing a sort of potential effect of all of these factors. The net result is that one out of every 100 patients who comes to our department for a roentgenological examination of the small intestine is found to have a tumor, either

benign, malignant or metastatic. Not all tumors cause obstruction phenomena. A precise examination of the mucosal pattern is therefore very valuable not only for inflammatory and vascular diseases but also for the detection of a malignant process. Thus an intramural process growing along the length of the intestine which, if peristalsis remains normal, only causes a somewhat coarsened mucosal pattern may be a benign or malignant lymphoma. At a somewhat later stage and especially more distal in the intestine, a lymphoma may only produce a smooth mucosa which appears atrophied, sometimes with ulcerative changes, and a barely thickened intestinal wall. Destruction or space-occupying processes, which we would like to see as evidence of tumor growth, may be missing entirely.

Of course an ileum without fold relief and an increase in the space between adjacent intestinal loops can also be caused by a primary amyloidosis or Crohn's disease. However, ulcerations rarely develop in amyloidosis and are frequently encountered in Crohn's disease. In Crohn's disease the broadening of the space between the loops can be due to either thickening of the intestinal wall itself or thickening of the layer of fat which surrounds the intestine. Usually in these cases the process is in an active stage. After remission of Crohn's disease or atrophy of the mucosa as a result of the chronic use of laxatives, the inner wall of the intestine is also smooth but there is no thickening of the wall. Finally in ischemia the segment without mucosal relief is usually not very long. Sudden rather erratic changes in the course of the intestinal loop can indicate fibrotic shriveling as a result of a nearby carcinoid and a local intussusception might suggest a polypous formation which is in itself not visible.

Displacement or compression of intestinal loops, sometimes only visible in the supine, prone or lateral position, can indicate benign or malignant tumor growth in the retroperitoneal space (fig. 10.2), the abdominal wall or the mesentery (fig. 10.3).

However, sometimes spread of a retroperitoneal tumor via the mesentery to or around the intestinal lumen can cause changes which give the impression that the tumor originates in the intestinal wall. Broadening of the mesentery then produces large empty spaces between the intestinal loops which

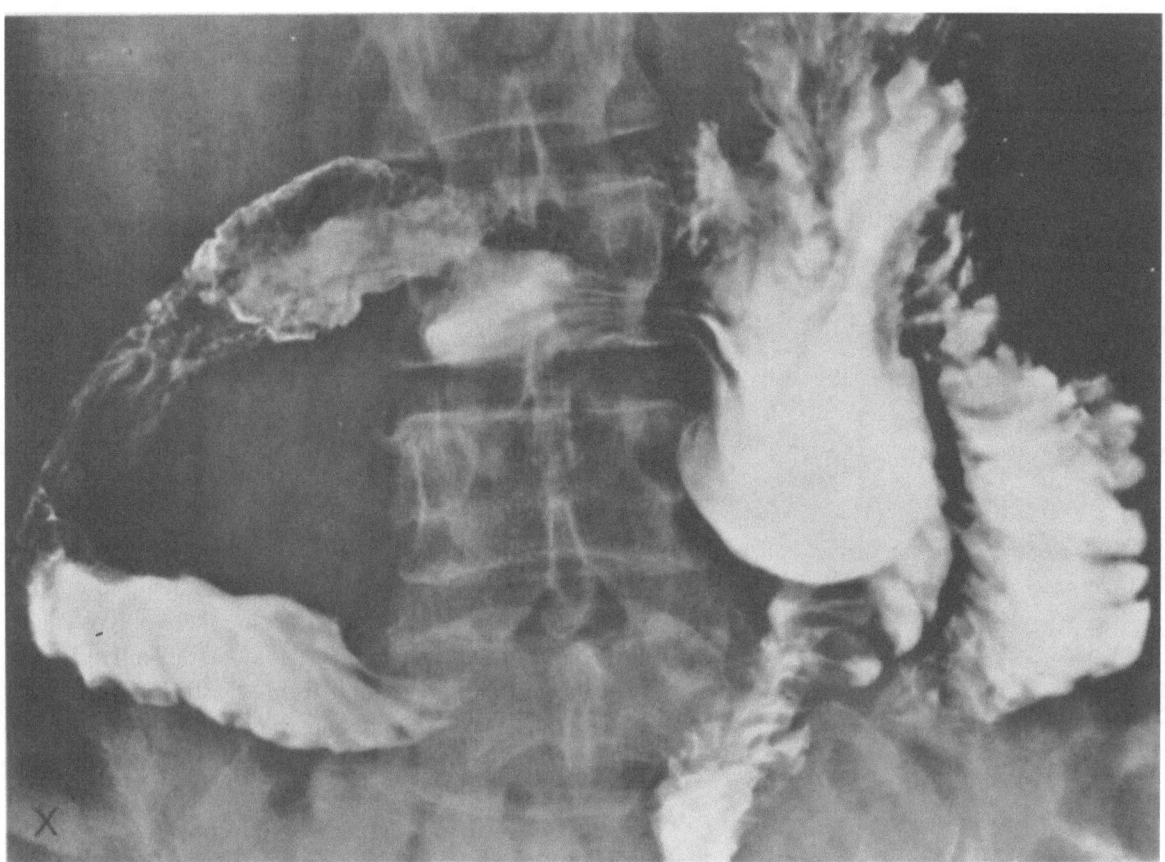

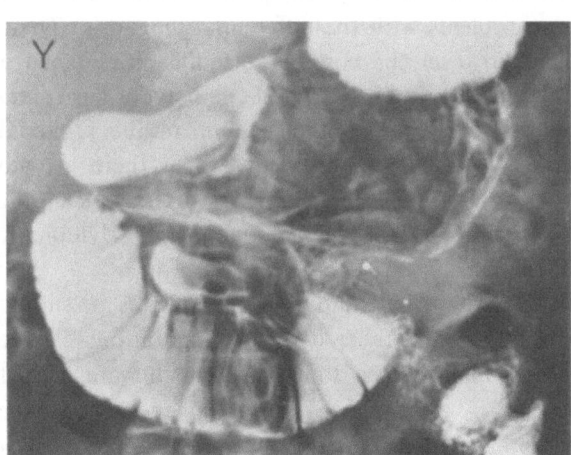

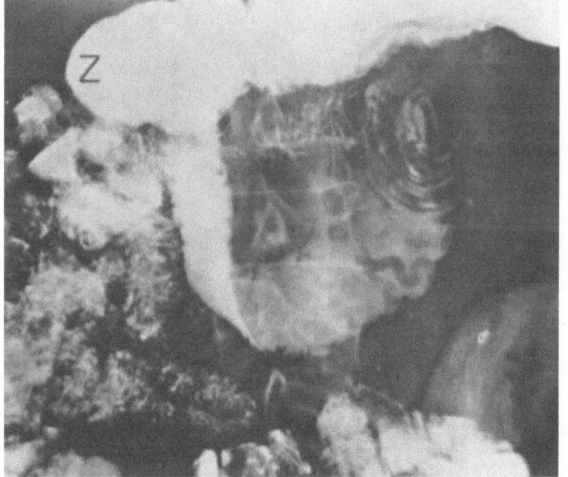

*Fig. 10.*2.

x. Retroperitoneal lymphoreticular malignancy with marked compression of a fairly long segment of the duodenum.

y. Compression at the duodenojejunal junction by a tumor of the pancreas tail.

z. Compression of the transverse limb of the duodenum by a large retroperitoneal leiomyosarcoma. There is also a developmental anomaly of the intestinal loops: the jejunum lies in the right half of the abdomen.

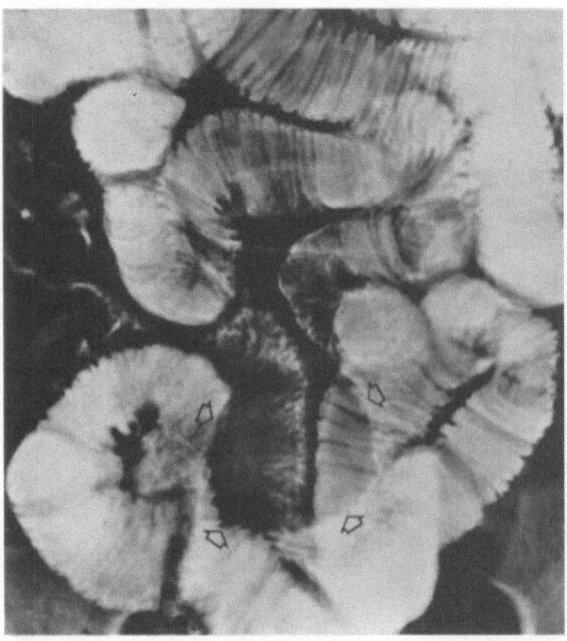

Fig. 10.3
Displacement of the intestinal loops by a mesenterial cyst.

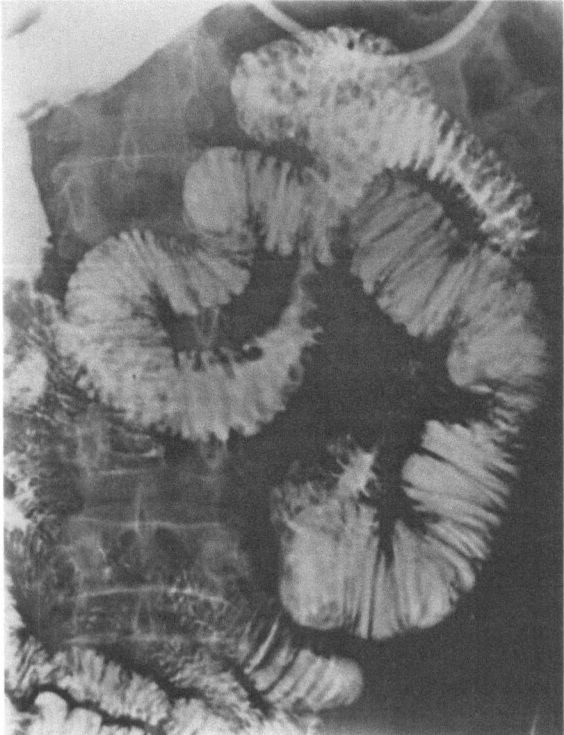

Fig. 10.4
Retroperitoneal liposarcoma which has spread via the mesentery to encircle the intestinal lumen so that, partly because of the empty spaces between the intestinal loops, a lymphosarcoma is suggested.

suggest a lymphosarcoma (fig. 10.4). Local dilatations of an intestinal loop without a subsequent stenosis can be the result of local injury to nerve tissue due to invasive tumor growth as in lymphosarcoma. Usually, however, in these cases there are also concomitant phenomena which reveal the diagnosis. Local stretching of the mucosal folds can be the result of an intramural leiomyoma which causes little or no bulging into the lumen or a duplication cyst. Compression can cause deceptively similar patterns (fig. 10.8); incorrect evaluation of this technique must therefore be avoided.

Polypoid masses in the intestinal lumen, often only discovered after a careful search of spot films, can be due to metastasis of tumors elsewhere, a (sometimes hereditary) systemic disease accompanied by polypous formations or lymphoreticular tumor growth. In the latter case these polyps can be very tiny and numerous so that it is difficult or impossible to differentiate it from a gastrointestinal polyposis or lymphoid hyperplasia. Lymphoid hyperplasia, also called lymphatic polyposis or pseudopolyposis lymphatica, accompanies diverse generally benign diseases such as infection with Giardia lamblia. If this hyperplasia of the follicles is restricted to the proximal jejunum or is seen only in the distal ileum of a young patient, there are usually no problems with the differential diagnosis. There can, however, be considerable difficulties when a more or less extensive lymphatic polyposis is found in the distal part of the jejunum or the proximal part of the ileum, especially when there are no signs of hyperplasia in the last decimeters of the ileum where the greatest quantity of lymphatic tissue is found.

Finally when evaluating the x-rays, it should always be remembered that configurations can be seen which suggest tumor growth but are in fact caused by a completely different phenomenon. One example is an inflammatory granuloma with a central ulcer crater which is deceptively similar to metastasis with central necrosis (fig. 10.5).

The polypoid formation in fig. 10.6B which is due to the invagination of the end of the afferent loop after a gastrectomy of the BII type resembles a bulge in the cecum caused by the invagination of the stump of the appendix after removal of this organ. Often it is only possible to fill this afferent loop with contrast medium after peristalsis has been eliminated by administering a hypotonic agent.

Configurations which suggest a tumor are not only caused by real structures of a completely different nature; they may also be due to misleading patterns which generally persist for only a short time. Sometimes these temporary misleading patterns are the result of inadequate filling of the intestine (fig. 10.7) or the use of compression by the clinician (fig. 10.8); sometimes there is auto-compression by adjacent tissue structures such as an intersecting vessel (fig. 10.9). A less common misleading pattern develops when in a specific projection a normally existing structure, often part of the skeleton, appears to enclose a space-occupying process (fig. 10.10).

The easiest way to classify tumors of the small bowel is as follows:

1. generalized gastrointestinal polyposis;
2. benign tumors;
3. semimalignant tumors;
4. malignant tumors;
5. metastasis.

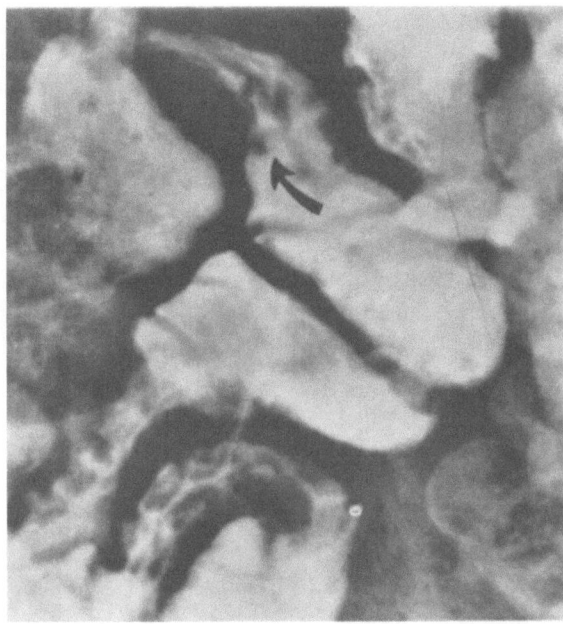

Fig. 10.5
Inflammatory granuloma with central ulcer crater in Crohn's disease.

2. Polyposis

A number of diseases occur in the digestive tract which are characterized by a widespread polyposis and a marked familial incidence. In two of these disorders, familial polyposis and Gardners syndrome, the small polyps are adenomas, which occur only in the colon and are very likely to become malignant. In two other forms of polyposis,

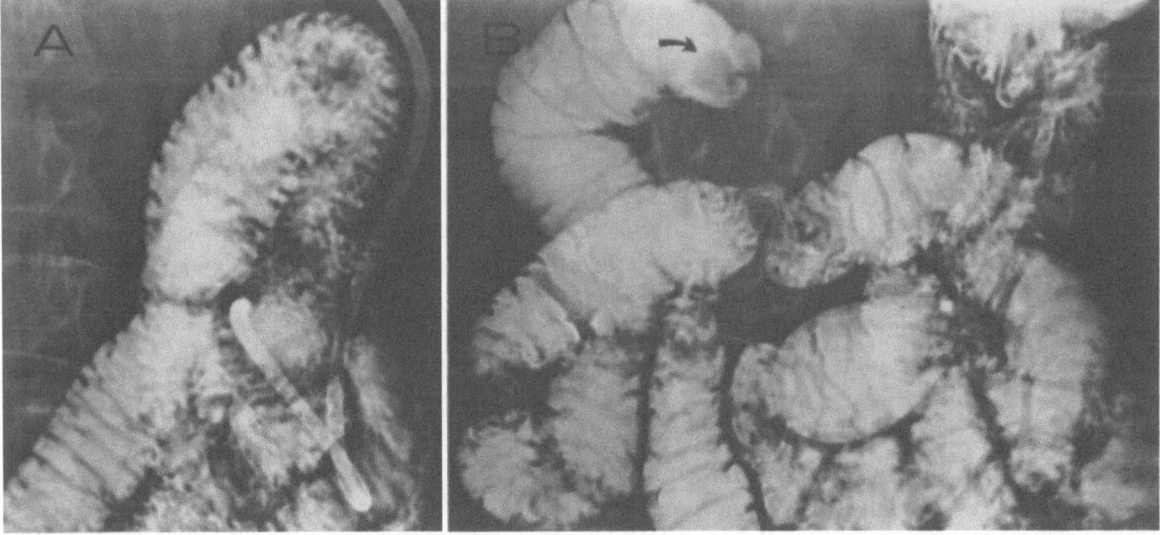

Fig. 10.6
Smoothly defined round bulge in the stump of an afferent loop after a BII resection due to invagination of the suture line. The afferent loop rarely fills spontaneously (A); however, in more than 50% of the cases filling is obtained after administration of a hypotonic agent (B).

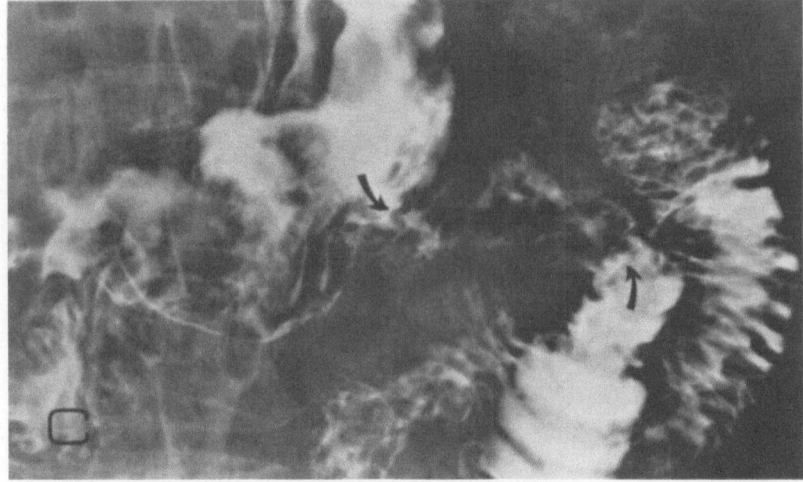

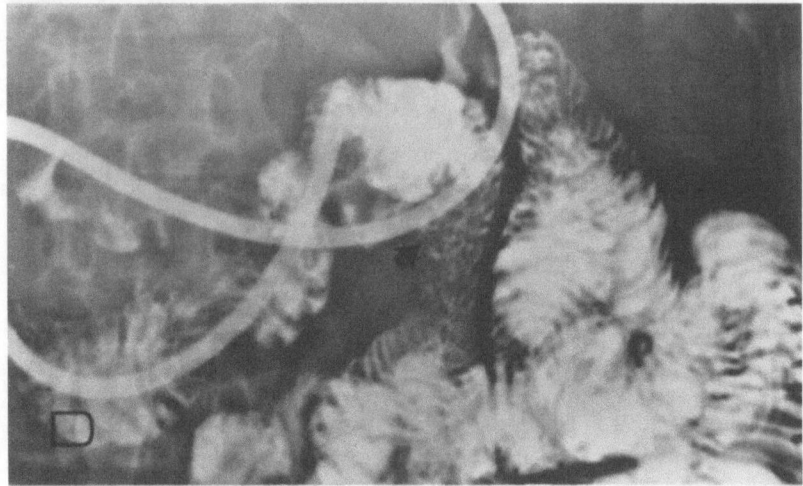

Fig. 10.7

C. Irregular mucosal pattern in the proximal part of the jejunum (→←) following gastric examination and due exclusively to inadequate filling of the intestine. Proximal and distal to the suspect region the mucosal relief was normal so that disintegration of the contrast fluid was out of the question.

D. In the course of an enteroclysis examination 1 week later, this part of the intestine was well-filled and no abnormalities could be seen.

the Peutz-Jeghers syndrome and the Cronkhite-Canada syndrome, the polyps are found not only in the colon but also in the small intestine (fig. 10.11). In these cases there is little or no tendency towards malignant degeneration. In the Peutz-Jeghers syndrome, the better known of the two, histological examination shows that the polyps are not adenomas but harmartomas originating from the muscularis mucosae. The diagnosis is easily recognized since this syndrome is also characterized by a pigmentation of the skin and the mucous membrane in and around the mouth and in some cases, also of the skin on the tensor side of several joints. This mucocutaneous pigmentation is due to a disturbed melanin storage and is somewhat suggestive of Addison's disease. The polyps can be so small that they are invisible or so large that they cause hemorrhage and attacks of pain as a result of recurrent intussusceptions. The polyps can be distributed diffusely or in

patches and are generally more numerous in the jejunum than in the ileum. The Cronkhite-Canada syndrome is much more rare; in addition to the hyperpigmentation, it can also be accompanied by alopecia, dystrophy of the nails and a very severe malabsorption. In this disease, which possibly should be considered a form of generalized juvenile polyposis, the polyps are inflammatory and epithelial in nature and often contain multiple cysts filled with mucin. The Cronkhite-Canada syndrome has a high mortality, is not hereditary and so far has only been found in adults over 40 years of age.

3. Benign tumors

As previously mentioned, although the benign tumors in the small intestine predominate over the

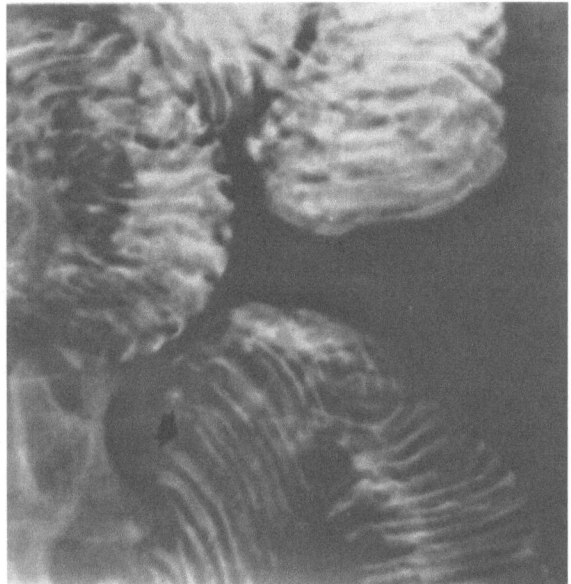

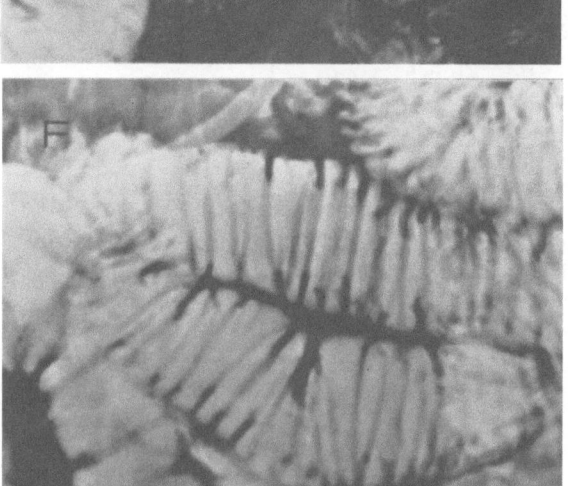

Fig. 10.8
Misleading pattern resembling leiomyoma due to local compression of the intestinal loops.

Fig. 10.9
Configuration resembling a round bulge in the intestinal loop (E) disappears when the intestine is well-filled.

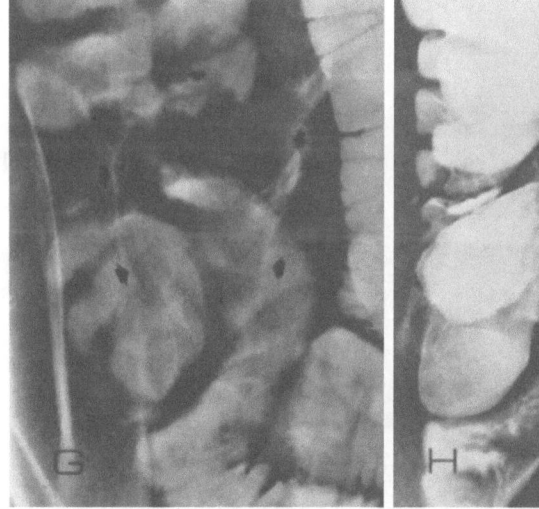

Fig. 10.10
This configuration, caused mainly by bone structures, somewhat resembles a space-occupying process in the region of Bauhin's valve (G). In a different projection the misleading pattern has completely disappeared (H).

malignant in number, they cause no obstruction – or at least not until quite late – and partly for this reason are only occasionally diagnosed. Even the fact that at least one-third of the benign tumors cause recurrent occult or gross bleeding via the rectum has not increased the frequency with which this diagnosis is established. In the case of teleangiectasia or hemangiomas, both occurring mainly in the jejunum, the bleeding can even be profuse but it still is seldom possible to discover the lesion during transit examination of the small intestine. Teleangiectasias are only dilatations of existing

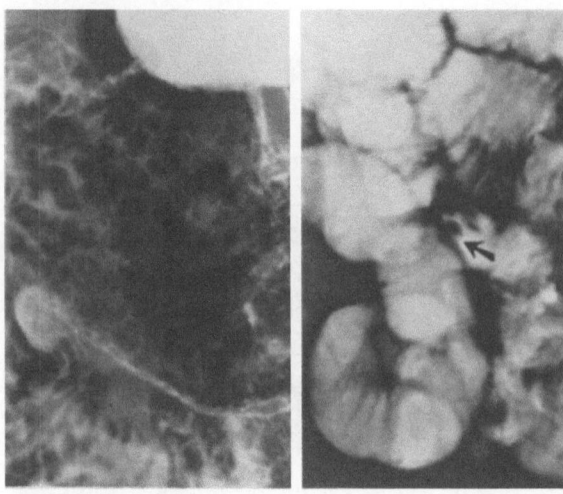

Fig. 10.11A
Polyps in the stomach and a few of equal size in the small intestine due to the Peutz-Jeghers syndrome. Polyps were also found in the rectum of this patient.

vascular structures and the hemangiomas, which originate in the submucosal vascular plexus, can be scattered and quite tiny. If the presence of calcified phleboliths does not indicate the nature of the disease, it is clear that an angiographic examination will be necessary to determine the diagnosis.

In addition to vascular tumors, we also find solitary adenomatous polyps, myomas, lipomas and fibromas with approximately equal frequency in the small bowel. Fibromas, like vascular tumors, often develop intramurally or extraluminally and are very rarely discovered by means of radiological examination.

Although leiomyomas lie within but mainly outside the intestinal wall, they are diagnosed more frequently than any of the other benign tumors of the small intestine because of their size. Leiomyomas can occur everywhere in the small intestine, but are most common in the jejunum. A central necrosis with ulcerations and hemorrhage can develop in leiomyomas even when there is no malignant degeneration. A characteristic of the larger intramural benign tumor is that the folds of the intact mucosa stretch across the growth. It should be mentioned, however, that external compression of the intestinal loops can produce a somewhat similar effect. The compression of intestinal loops resulting from the intraluminal or mesenterial spread of a lymphosarcoma can usually be recognized because of the concomitant stenoses and obliteration of the mucosa.

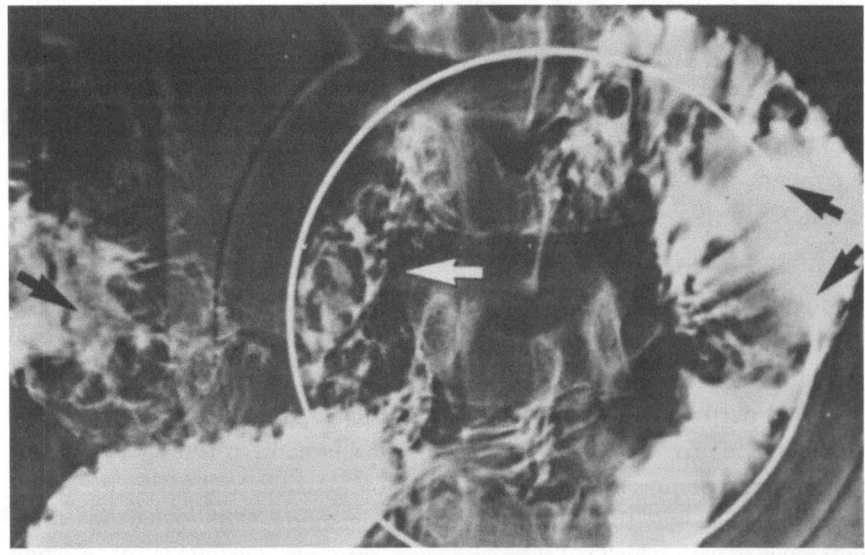

Fig. 10.11B
Polyps of different size in the duodenum due to a Peutz-Jeghers syndrome.

Lipomas can also be found throughout the small intestine but generally they are encountered in the most distal part of the ileum.

They are usually round or oval, but can sometimes be multipolypoid. In Bauhin's valve they cause sharply defined irregular masses in the contrast column which are quite prominent in the cecum. Because they spread mainly in the submucosa or intraluminally, which can lead to intussusceptions, lipomas sometimes cause recurring complaints of obstruction. One characteristic of

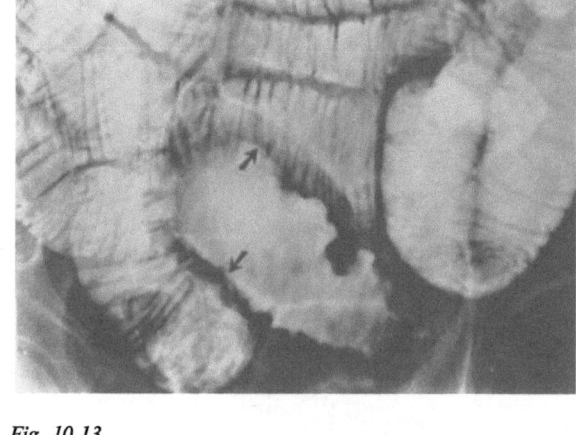

Fig. 10.13
Plaque-like carcinoids are rare; they are difficult to differentiate from a local intramural lymphosarcoma. The lumen of the intestine is dilated locally and the intestinal wall is thickened. There was metastasis in the liver.

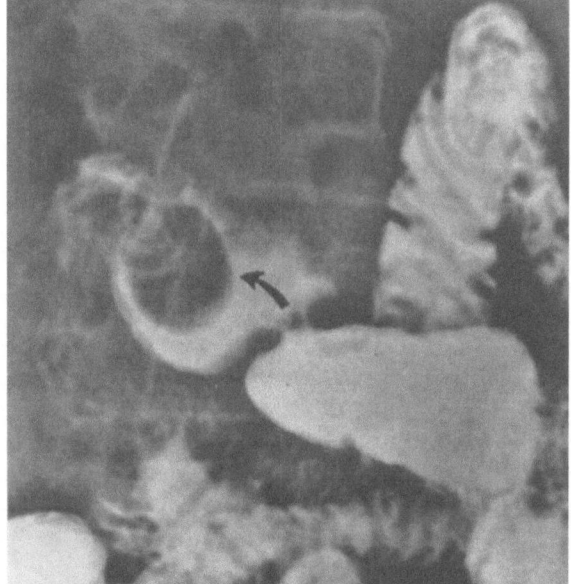

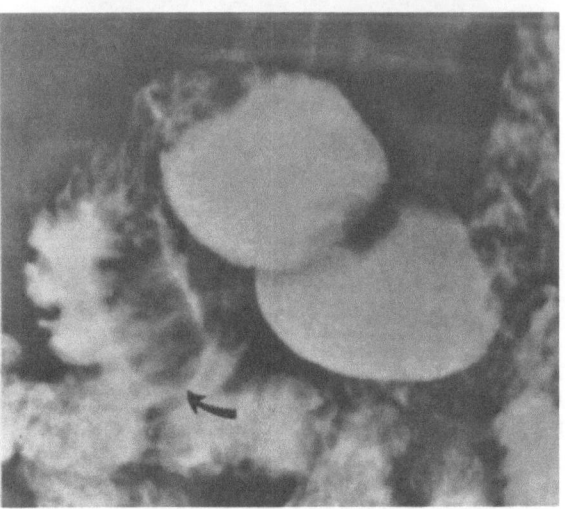

Fig. 10.12
A characteristic of lipomas is that they are easily deformed.

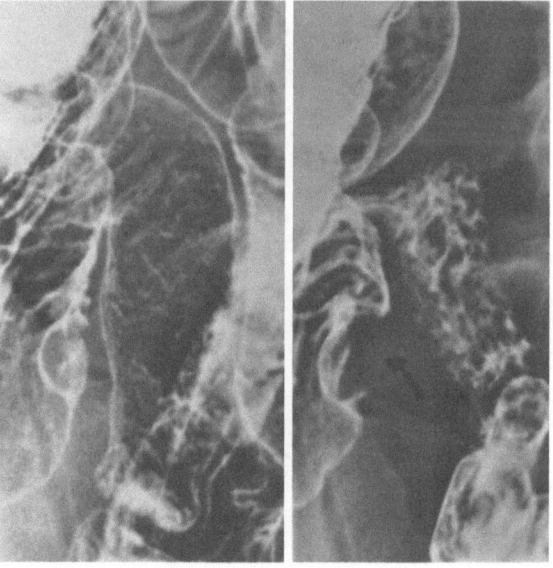

Fig. 10.14
Small carcinoid tumor at the base of the appendix which is almost impossible to distinguish from an invaginated stump after an appendectomy.

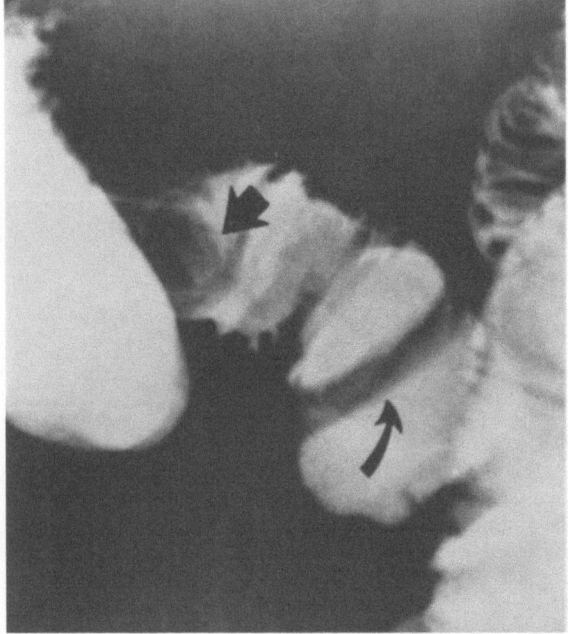

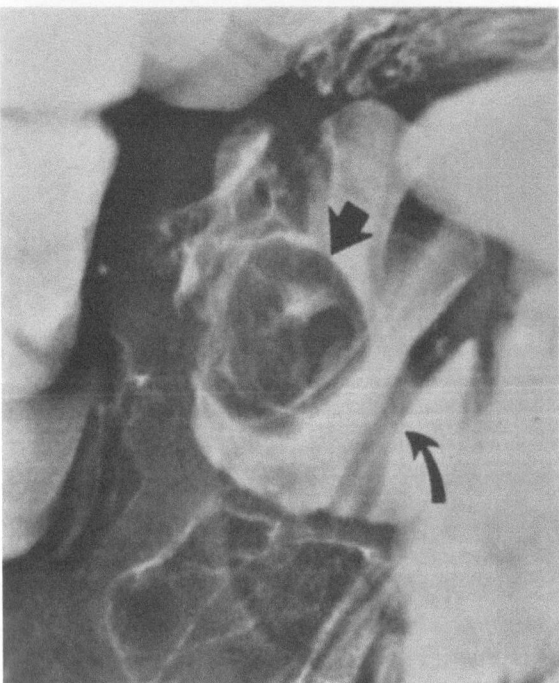

lipomas is their weak structure; as a result they are easily deformed (fig. 10.12) so that differentiation from air bubbles can be very difficult unless several films showing the abnormality are available.

4. Semimalignant tumors

Carcinoids are plaque (fig. 10.13) or nodule-like growths which originate in the serotonin-producing argentaffin cells in the floor of the crypts of Lieber-kühn in the intestinal mucosa. Carcinoids, solitary and multiple, can be encountered everywhere in the digestive tract but also occur elsewhere in the body such as the biliary ducts, the pancreas or the bronchial tree. The most common site is the appendix (fig. 10.14) but in almost one-third of the cases, they are found in the distal ileum (fig. 10.15). Carcinoids occur predominantly in younger patients; in general they grow very slowly and are therefore regarded as a low-grade malignancy. In

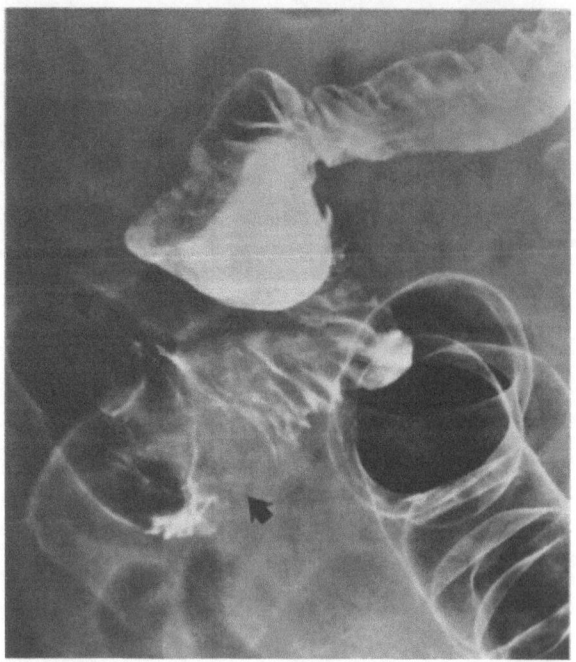

Fig. 10.15
Two cases of intramural carcinoids in the distal ileum (→). Extensive fibrosis in the intestinal wall and the mesentery causes constrictions of the intestinal lumen; when the intestine is well-filled, these constrictions are clearly visible as deep grooves (→).

Fig. 10.16
Extensive carcinoids with more or less smooth polycycloid margins in the cecum. Extensive metastases in the liver.

at least one-third of the cases there is also metastasis, almost always to the liver but sometimes also to other organs. Metastasis is most common when the carcinoid is localized in the ileum or colon (fig. 10.16) and is exceedingly rare when the primary site is the appendix.

The serotonin produced by the tumor is a protein-like hormone which enhances peristalsis and causes bronchospasms and diarrhea. Normally most of the serotonin produced is metabolized in the liver and only very minimal amounts enter the bloodstream. If larger quantities enter the liver or if the serotonin is produced in the liver by the metastases, then it also enters the right side of the heart and causes endothelial growths on the cardiac valves. A pulmonary stenosis, tricuspidal insufficiency and dilatation of the heart with a right-sided decompensation can result. The filtering action of the pulmonary circulation keeps the left side of the heart free of these complications. If there is metastasis in the liver, bradykinin is also produced. Like serotonin, bradykinin is a protein-like hormone which causes the 'flush syndrome' so characteristic of carcinoid. The flush syndrome lasts 5–10 minutes and is typified by a pronounced redness and hotness of the upper half of the body followed by tachycardia and vasodilatation and ending with cyanosis. Strain or fear, and sometimes consumption of alcohol or cheese, can provoke a flush reaction.

One-third of the patients who were found at autopsy to have had a carcinoid had no complaints. The diagnosis of carcinoid can be verified biochemically by the increased levels of the break down products of serotonin and bradykinin in blood and urine. Radiologically the easiest way to establish the diagnosis is an angiographic examination of the celiac trunk which reveals the highly vascularized metastases; the latter which are frequently present are always much larger than the primary lesions.

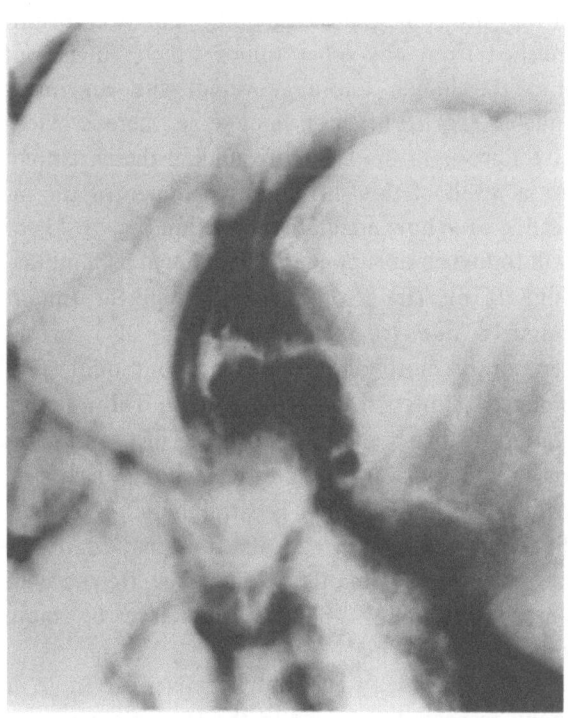

Fig. 10.17
Annular stricture due to small carcinoid tumor with marked shriveling. On the survey film an obvious prestenotic dilatation (→←) was noted which had to be located in the small intestine since the rectum and sigmoid were not yet filled with contrast medium.

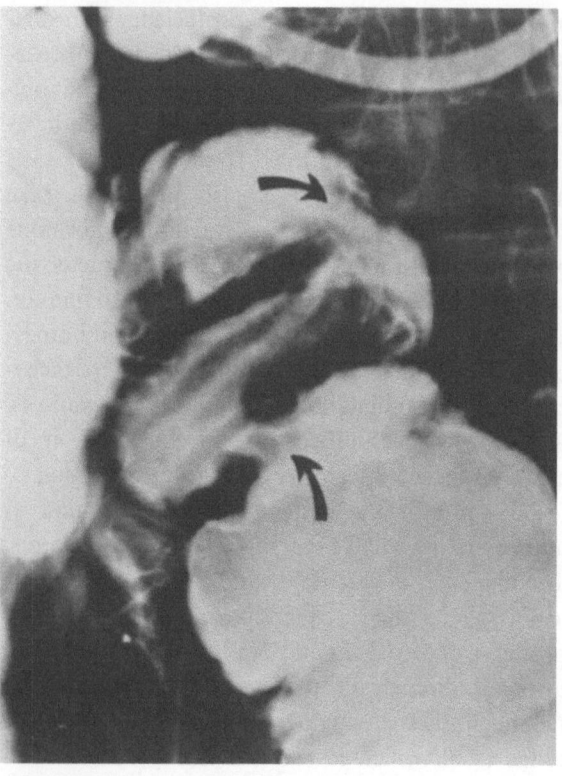

Fig. 10.18
Abrupt changes in the course of the intestine (kinking) due to local shriveling of the mesentery caused by a carcinoid.

In the intestine, carcinoids are often intramural and very small so that they cannot be demonstrated. If they are somewhat larger, they cannot be distinguished from any other tumor which bulges out into the lumen and is covered with an intact mucosa (fig. 10.15). In a later stage, there is extensive fibrosis in the area surrounding the carcinoid. As a result of this shriveling the lumen of the intestine can show annular constriction (fig. 10.17) or will follow an abrupt course designated as 'kinking' (fig. 10.18). The serotonin secreted by the tumor, possibly due to the compression, also causes temporary more or less localized but quite pronounced hyperperistalsis (fig. 10.19). The mucosal pattern is then somewhat feathered, just as in cases of mild anoxia in an intestine with a decreased caliber. When the tumor is extraluminal, a feather-like mucosal pattern can also be seen; as in the case of a leiomyoma the intestine lies stretched out across the tumor and may therefore be more dilated than normal.

A disease which somewhat resembles carcinoid in many respects but is not in the least malignant is endometriosis. This is the heterotopic localization of endometrium in females between 30 and 40 years of age, but sometimes older or younger.

Although occurring predominantly in organs and tissues in the pelvis minor and the sigmoid, localizations in the appendix, cecum and ileum are also occasionally seen. The disease is characterized by a dysmenorrhea and a pain which increases and decreases periodically because the ectopic tissue is totally involved in the menstrual cycle. In endometriosis, too, the tumor, which in this case is absolutely benign, is intramural. It is subserous and seldom grows through the mucosa in the direction of the lumen. Cyclic bleedings usually do not reach the lumen of the intestine so that there is no rectal bleeding. The mucosal pattern remains intact and is only lost when bleeding is so profuse that the stretched mucous membrane becomes necrotic. The recurrent bleedings lead to widespread fibrosis, annular obstructions, stenoses several centimeters long, angulation and kinking which radiologically cannot be distinguished from that due to carcinoid.

5. Malignant tumors

The most important primary malignant tumors in the small intestine are, in order of frequency, lymphoreticular tumors, adenocarcinomas and leiomyosarcomas. There are, however, numerous references in the literature which state that adenocarcinoma occurs more frequently than lymphosarcoma and reticulosarcoma together.

Leiomyosarcoma is usually discovered fairly late because it is a slow-growing tumor and, since it is extraluminal, does not cause obstruction in the early stages. At the time of diagnosis, the tumor is often already quite large and can be felt as a palpable mass. Even more than in leiomyoma, the radiological aspect is characterized by quite pronounced and more or less parallel intestinal mucosal folds (fig. 10.20) In the more advanced stages, invasion and destruction of the intestinal mucosa do occur so that this characteristic pattern disappears (fig. 10.21). Then there are also often clear signs of ulceration and central necrosis. Leiomyosarcomas are encountered everywhere in the small bowel although they seldom occur in the duodenum and retroperitoneal space (fig. 10.22).

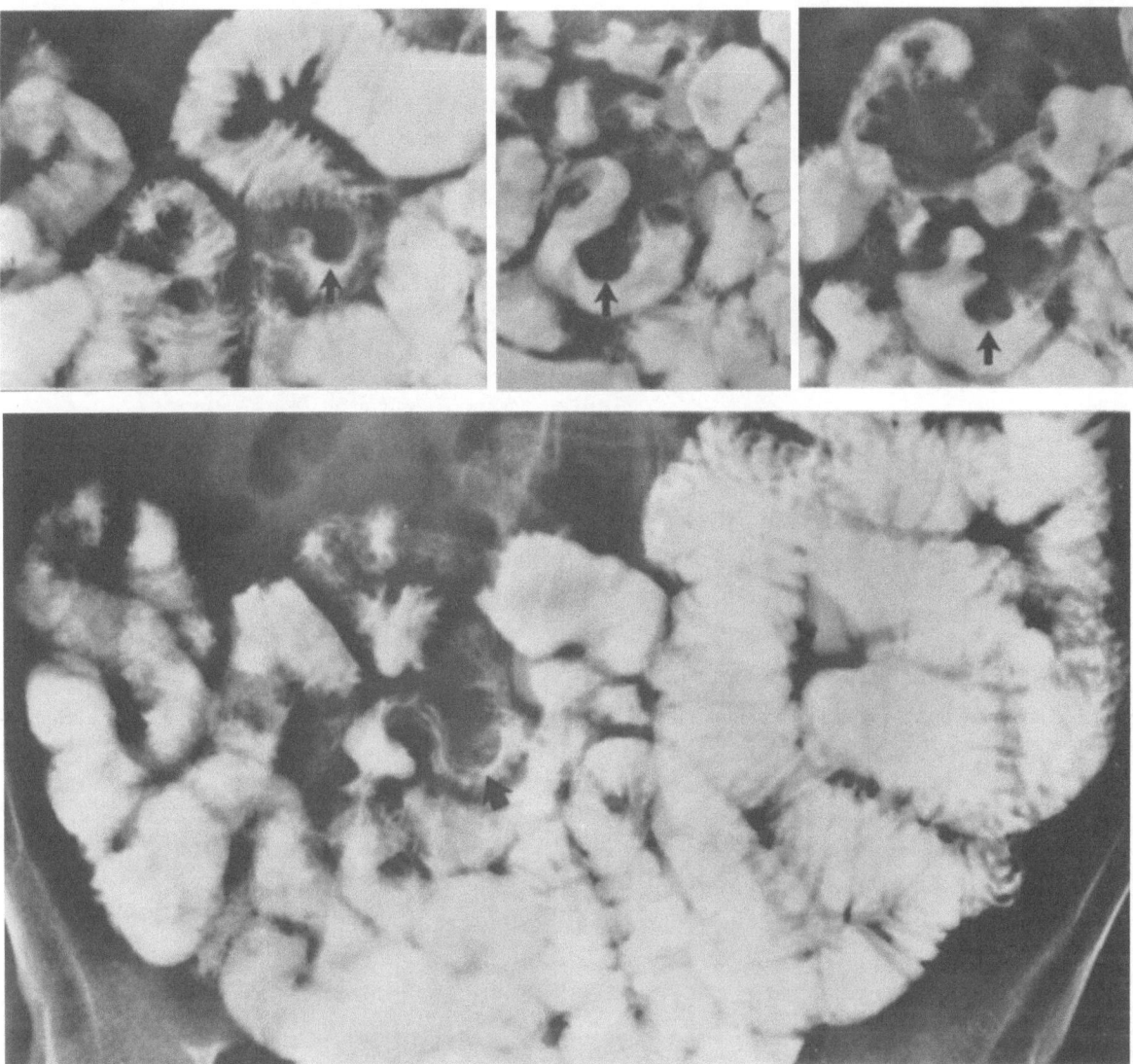

Fig. 10.19
Intestine with very local hypermotility and high tone (narrow lumen) due to serotonin produced by a carcinoid. The marble-sized space (→) seen next to the lumen must be the small tumor. There were metastases in the liver.

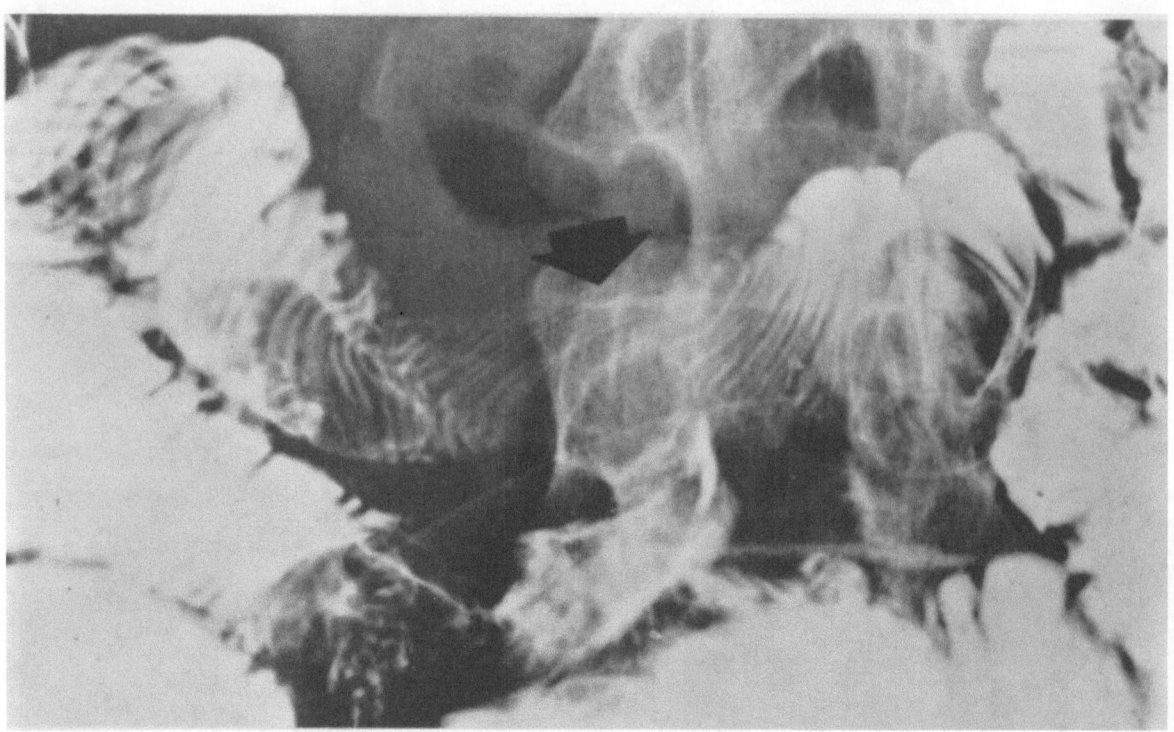

Fig. 10.20
Stretched and more or less parallel mucosal folds in a very long segment ($\pm$ 10 cm) of the small bowel caused by a leiomyosarcoma.

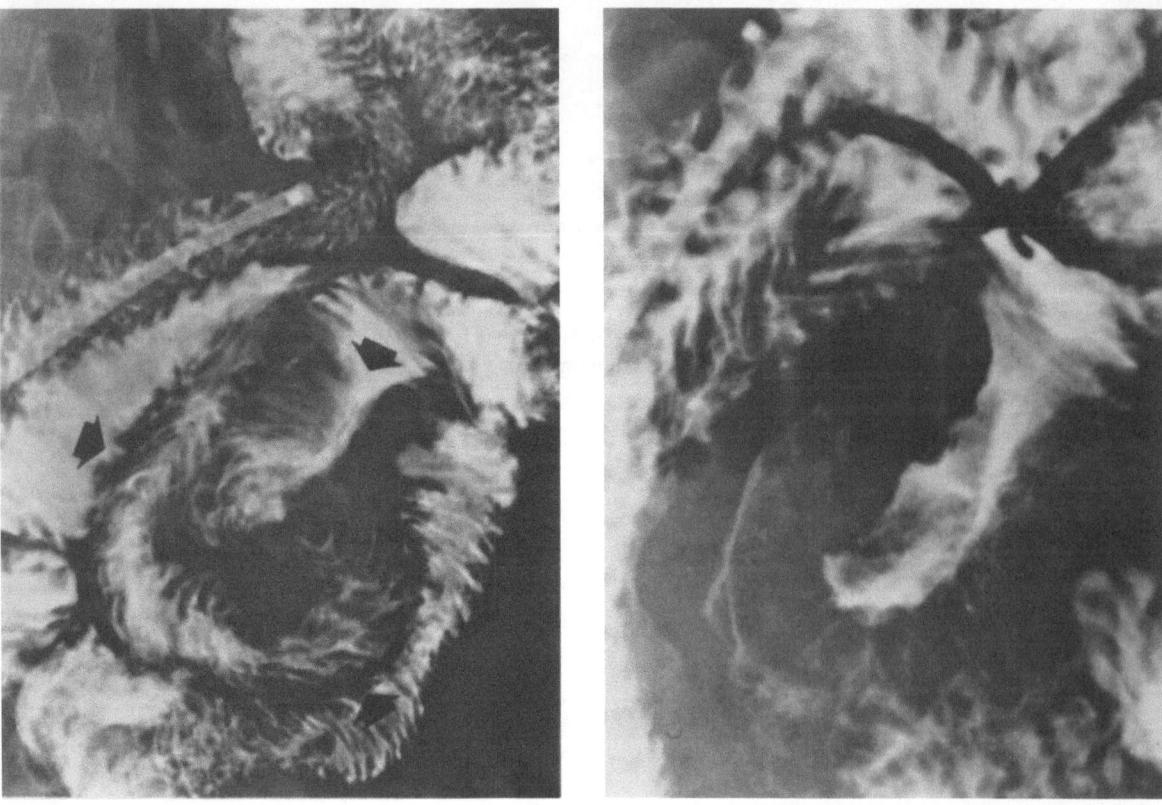

Fig. 10.21
Large leiomyosarcoma which can no longer be differentiated from any other extensive tumorous mass such as the liposarcoma in fig. 10.4 and the lymphosarcoma in fig. 10.28.

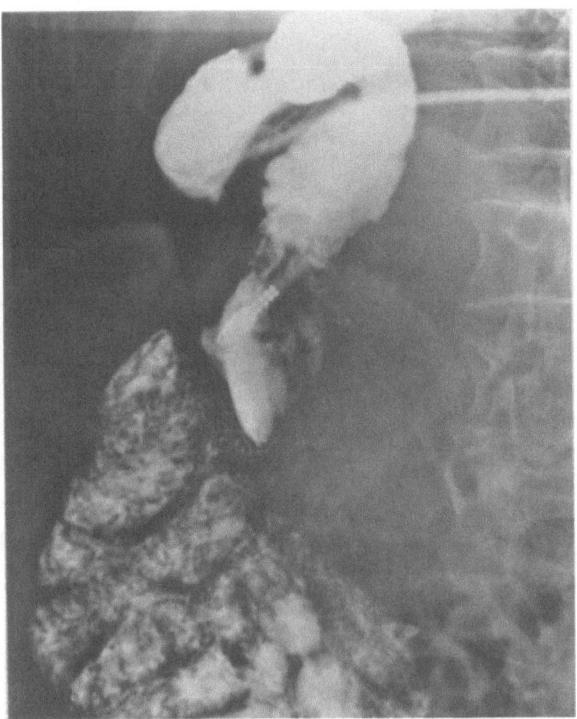

Fig. 10.22
Very large leiomyosarcoma growing in the retroperitoneal space, which probably did not originate in the duodenum. Very pronounced displacement of the mass of intestinal loops.

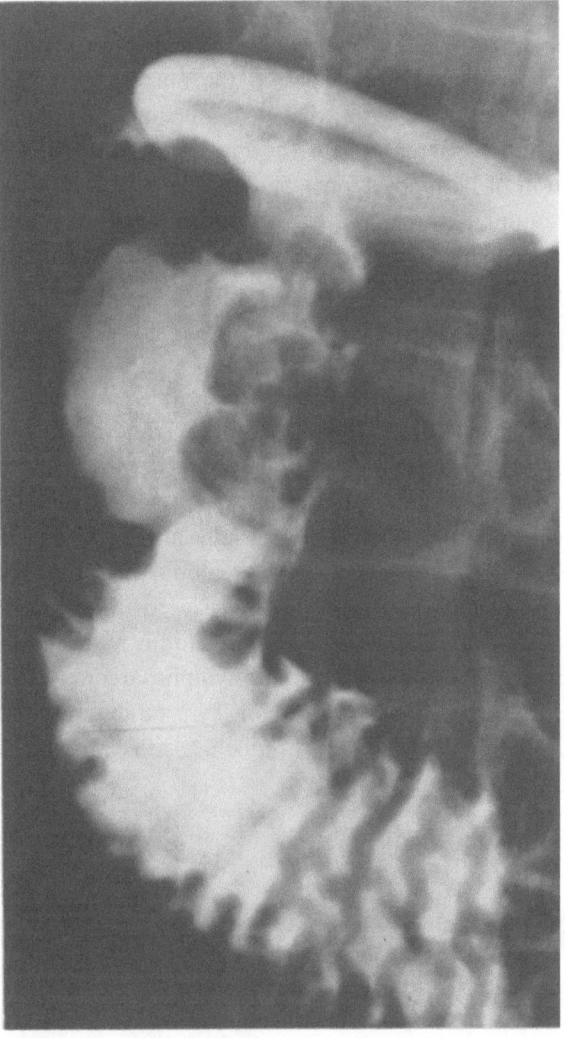

Fig. 10.23
Large ulcerous adenocarcinoma in the descending limb of the duodenum.

In spite of the fact that the diagnosis is usually not established until quite late, and only surgical intervention can be considered since these highly vascularized tumors barely react to chemotherapy and radiotherapy, the 5-year survival rate is almost 50%; the prognosis is therefore relatively favorable.

In adenocarcinomas, on the other hand, annular strictures develop very rapidly; as a result this disease is discovered much sooner.

Adenocarcinoma occurs more frequently in the proximal part of the small intestine, sometimes in the duodenum (fig. 10.23) and in particular near the duodenojejunal junction (fig. 10.24). A localization in the duodenum gives clinical symptoms which somewhat resemble those of a slightly atypical peptic ulcer; this is deceptive and does not lead to early diagnosis. In general adenocarcinoma appears as a short, irregularly defined constricting lesion (fig. 10.25). However, in the duodenum the tumor is sometimes multipolypoid in form, mucous-producing and not constricting. For these reasons it is also not discovered as quickly. Like leiomyosar-

coma, adenocarcinoma is more common in men than in women. The 5-year survival rate is about 20%; however, a tumor proximal to Treitz's ligament has a less favorable prognosis than one localized more distally. This difference in prognosis is partly due to the fact that a tumor in the distal intestine can be removed by means of a simple resection whereas a localization proximal to Treitz's ligament requires the more major 'Whipple' operation.

Lymphoreticular malignant growths are probably the most common in the small intestine, and not adenocarcinoma as stated in the literature. The

entire small intestine is rich in lymphoid tissue: it
is spread diffusely throughout the lamina propria
and is found in follicles in the mucosa and submucosa, mainly in the distal ileum. The distal
ileum is therefore also the most frequent localization of lymphosarcoma and reticulosarcoma; other
common sites are the duodenum, jejunum and
appendix. Solitary localizations are less common
(fig. 10.26). In most cases, however, the sites are
multiple and include several segments of the intestines.

Histologically reticulosarcomas differ little from
lymphosarcomas except that the lymphocytic infiltrates consist of less mature cells with larger
nuclei and there is more reticular tissue. Reticulum
cell sarcomas (fig. 10.27) usually grow faster than
lymphosarcomas and growth along the length of
the intestine is much less extensive in most cases;
it would seem that the tumor seldom reaches this
stage. If 5-year survival for lymphosarcoma after
surgical, radiotherapeutic or cytostatic treatment
is about 50%, that for reticulum cell sarcoma is
25%, at the most.

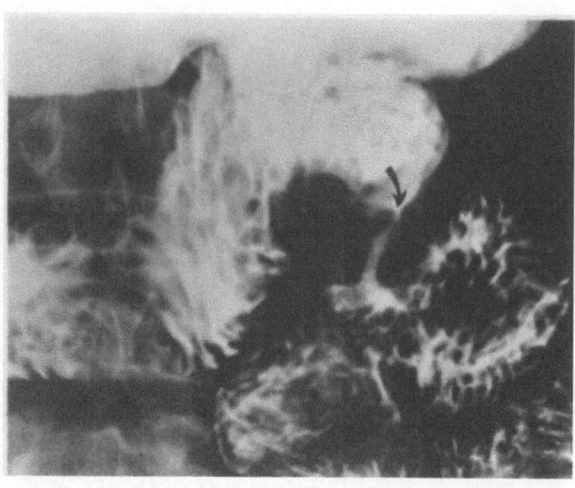

Fig. 10.24
Smooth stenosis, ± 3 cm long, in the duodenojejunal
junction due to an adenocarcinoma.

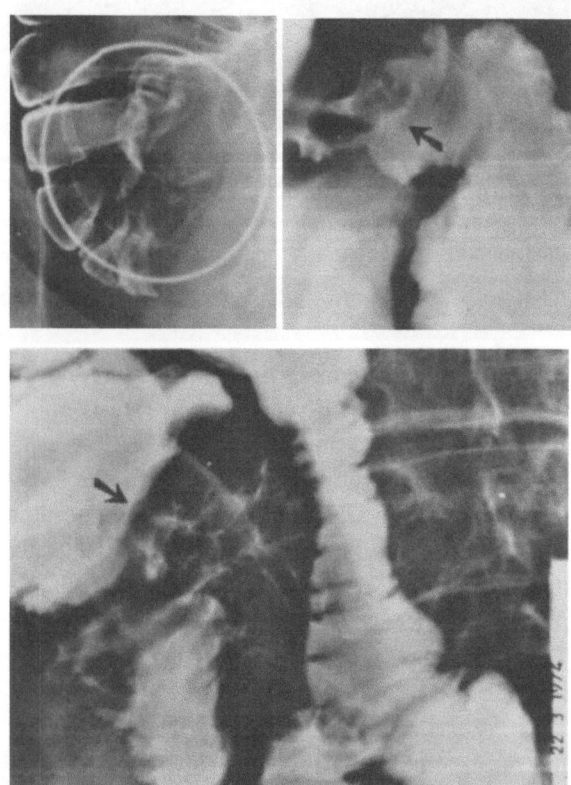

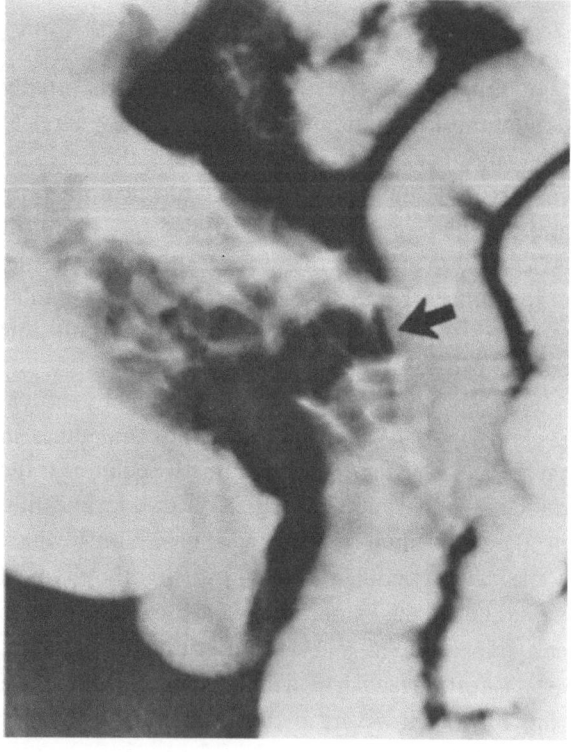

Fig. 10.25
Two cases of short strictures with irregular margins in the
ileum caused by adenocarcinoma.

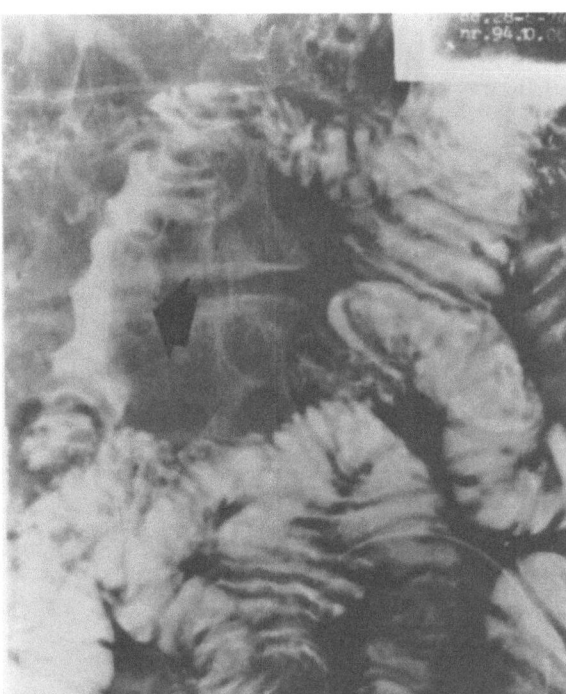

Fig. 10.26
A solitary lymphosarcoma is encountered less frequently; here it is presented as an extended stenosis in the jejunum.

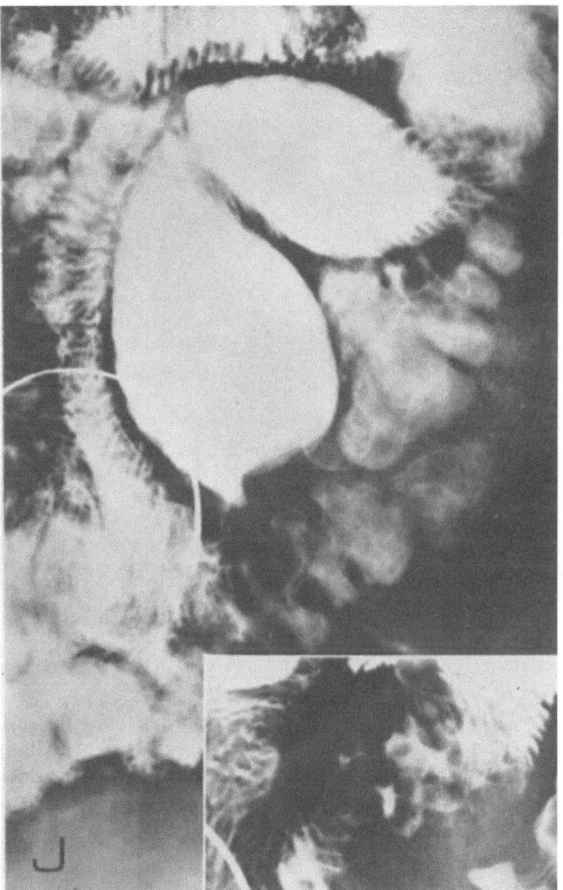

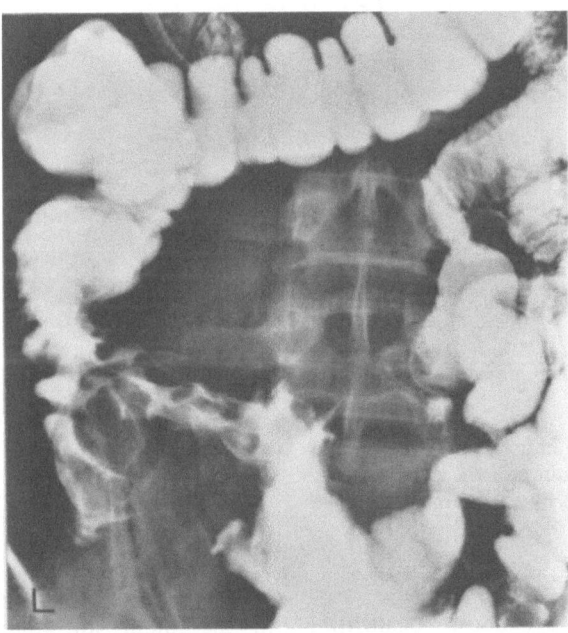

Fig. 10.27
Three cases of reticulum cell sarcoma.

J.   Short constricting tumor with irregular mucosal relief causing a striking prestenotic dilatation.

     Two years later metastases were found.

K.   see p. 262

L.   Very large and rapidly growing retroperitoneal reticulum cell sarcoma in a 23-year-old male which spread to the mesentery and did not cause obstruction until a late stage. Highly stretched folds with irregular course in the distal ileum. Initially the process was thought to be an appendicular infiltrate.

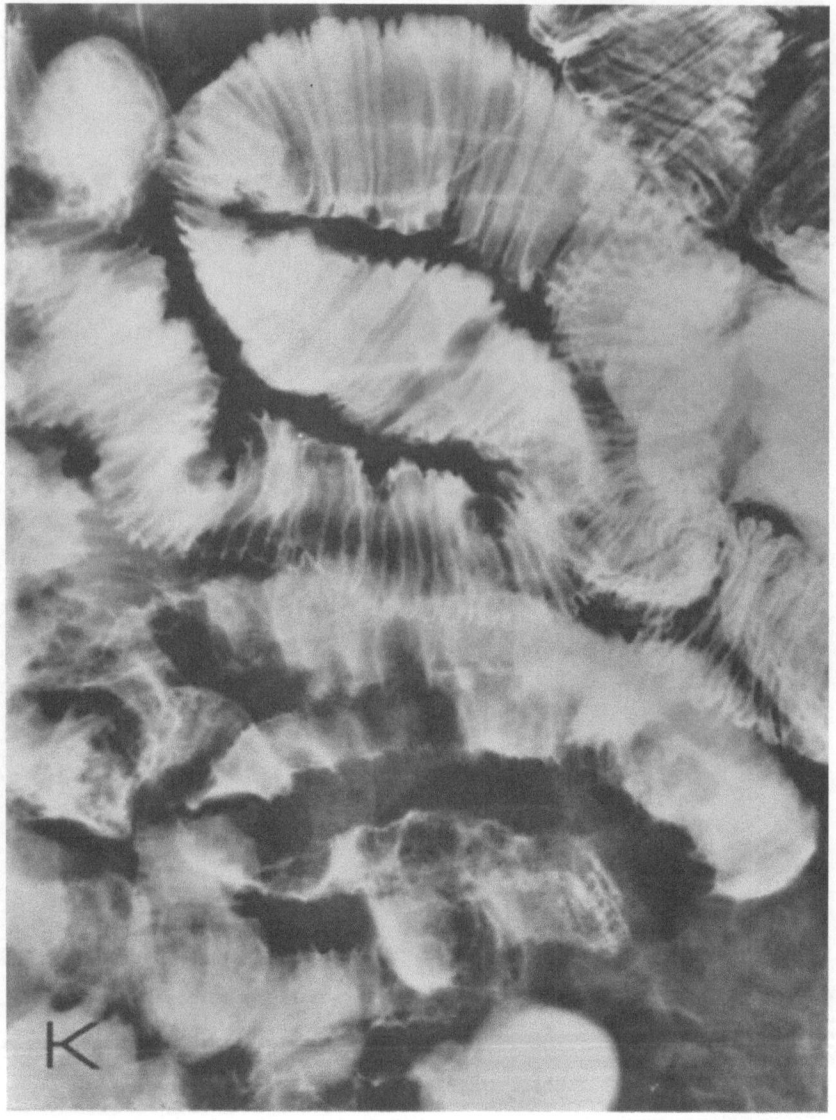

Fig. 10.27K
к.   Unusual reticulum cell sarcoma growing along the surface and involving a very   large
     segment of the small bowel causing the complete disappearance of the mucosal relief
     in some areas and folds which are infiltrated or thickened by edema in others. The
     intestinal wall is obviously thickened.

Tumors originating in the lymph follicles or the lamina propria are called primary lymphomas. The mesentery and the abdominal lymph nodes can also be involved but there are no or very few sites in other organs. A generalized lymphoreticular sarcoma or malignant lymphoma can be encountered in the liver, spleen or skeleton. In one-fourth of these cases, there are also localizations in the small bowel and then it is called secondary lymphoma. In small children certainly more than 50% show localizations in the small intestine.

A lymphoreticular process in the small intestine can manifest itself in many different ways clinically but especially radiologically. In primary or secondary lymphoma there may be multiple intramural lesions or polypoid defects bulging out into the lumen of the contrast column. The lesions can be so small that they are not much bigger than those seen in lymphoid hyperplasia; in other cases they can be quite large giving rise to intussusception or obstruction. The surface of the nodules may be ulcerous or show clear centralized necrosis as seen in a leiomyo(sarco)ma or a melanoma. Obviously perforations and fistulas may then also develop.

In the event of widespread growth of the tumors into the mesentery or outside the lumen of the intestine, multiple compression effects and large erratically shaped spaces between the intestinal loops will be seen on the x-rays (fig. 10.28).

In most cases there is only diffuse infiltrative growth into the lamina propria, mucosa or submucosa of the intestinal wall. The tumor can then spread extensively and even involve the full length of the small intestine without causing radiologically visible abnormalities (fig. 10.29). At the same time clinical symptoms may be absent entirely or may consist only of general complaints such as pain, malaise, anorexia, loss of weight and anemia, which are not at all specific. As a rule there are also multiple deficiencies as a result of malabsorption as well as protein loss and edema.

A lymphosarcoma often grows rather slowly and does not cause obstruction phenomena until fairly late, if at all.

The few complaints and the very subtle radiological abnormalities barely increase; in fact they may even decrease temporarily. However, there can be a sudden marked increase in the rate of growth such that a widespread tumorous mass develops within several months with pronounced widening of the spaces between the intestinal loops on the x-ray, extensive necrosis and destruction of the mucosal membrane (fig. 10.30).

It is possible that in the very slow initial phase the process is not yet malignant and that this first stage of growth should be called a 'benign lymphoma'. Because this first stage is so prolonged and there are so few clinical and radiological symptoms, the malignant lymphoma must be considered not only the most insidious tumor in the small intestine but also the most insidious disease of the entire pathology of the small intestine. Even the histological examination of mucosal biopsies has not changed this situation; if possible it has even increased the problems with respect to the differential diagnosis. Often no abnormalities at all are found; at the most the number of plasma cells or mature lymphocytes in the lamina propria of the intestinal wall has increased. In other cases the villi appear

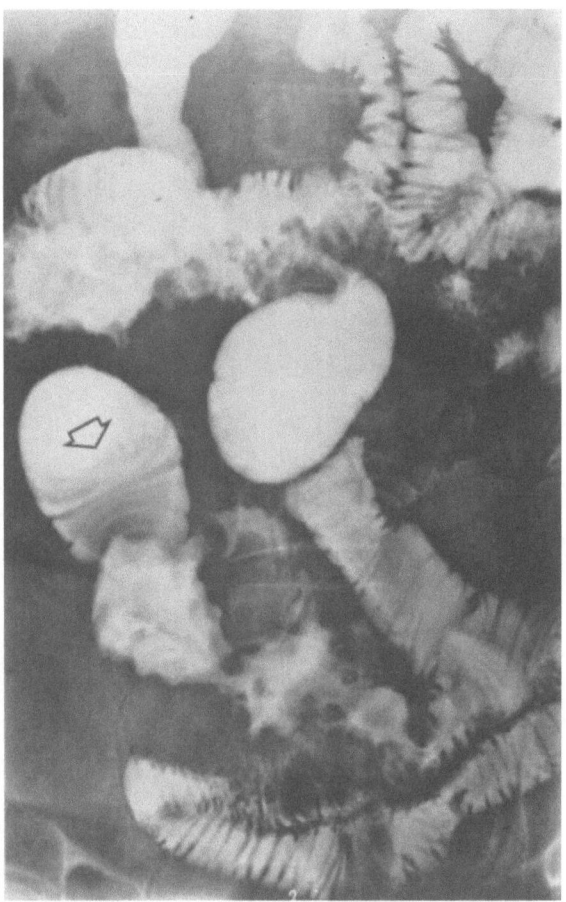

Fig. 10.28
Extensive lymphosarcoma with diverse localizations in the intestinal wall and the mesentery. Compression effects (→) and multiple empty spaces between the intestinal loops.

atrophied and in combination with the clinical considerations an initial diagnosis of celiac disease is then established. For a number of patients this is without a doubt correct, since there is an increased risk in celiac disease that a malignant lymphoma or some other tumor will develop in the digestive tract later (see chapter XII). If, however, it appears that the patients do not react favorably to a gluten-free diet, then the possibility of a malignant lymphoma must be considered seriously. This is also true if it is found that blood serum, urine or intestinal juices contain pathological immunoglobulins without the light IgA chains. These immunological disorders are characteristic of malignant lymphoma in young adults between 20 and 40 years of age who come from the countries around the Mediterranean Sea. Today in the Netherlands

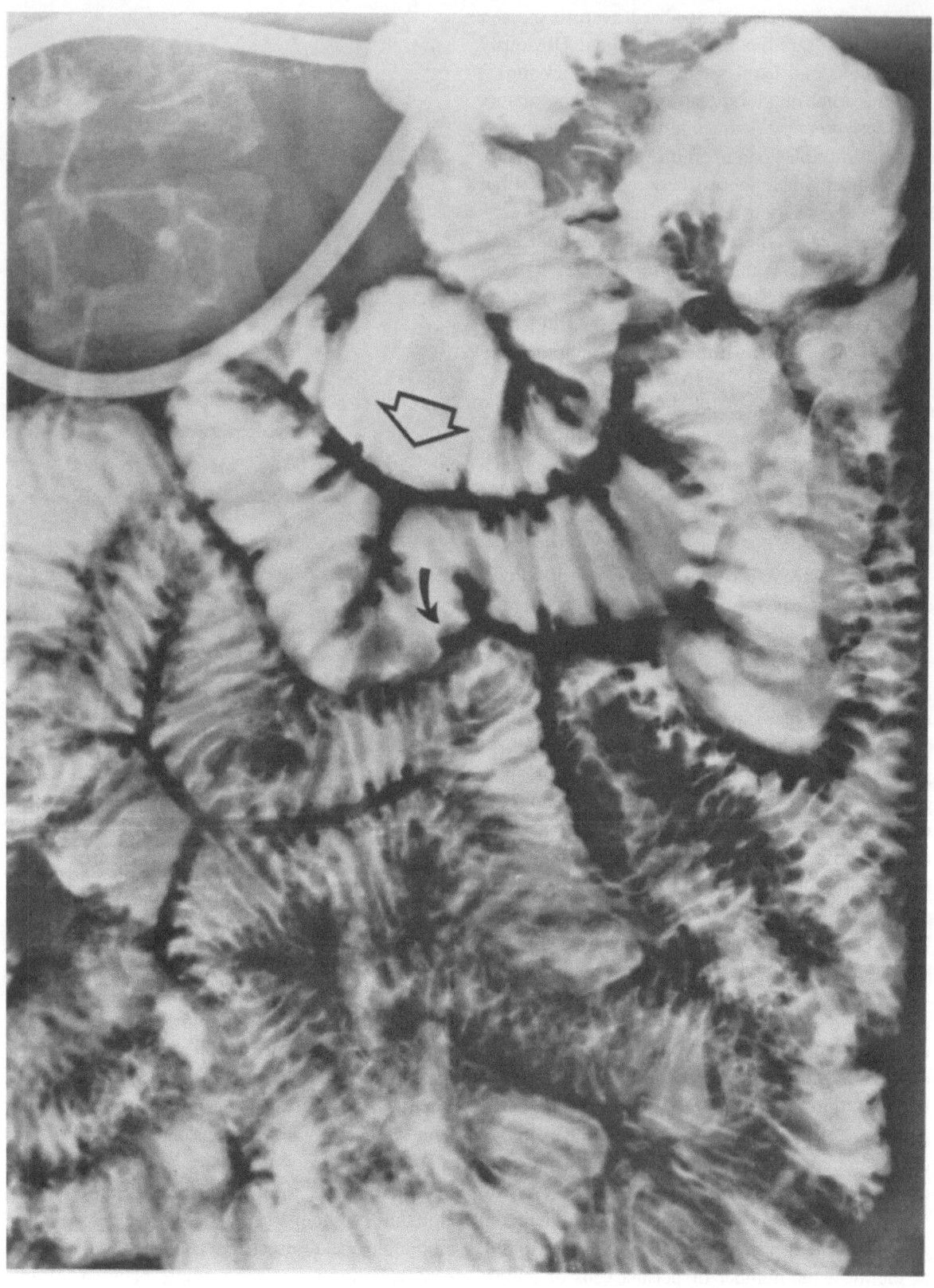

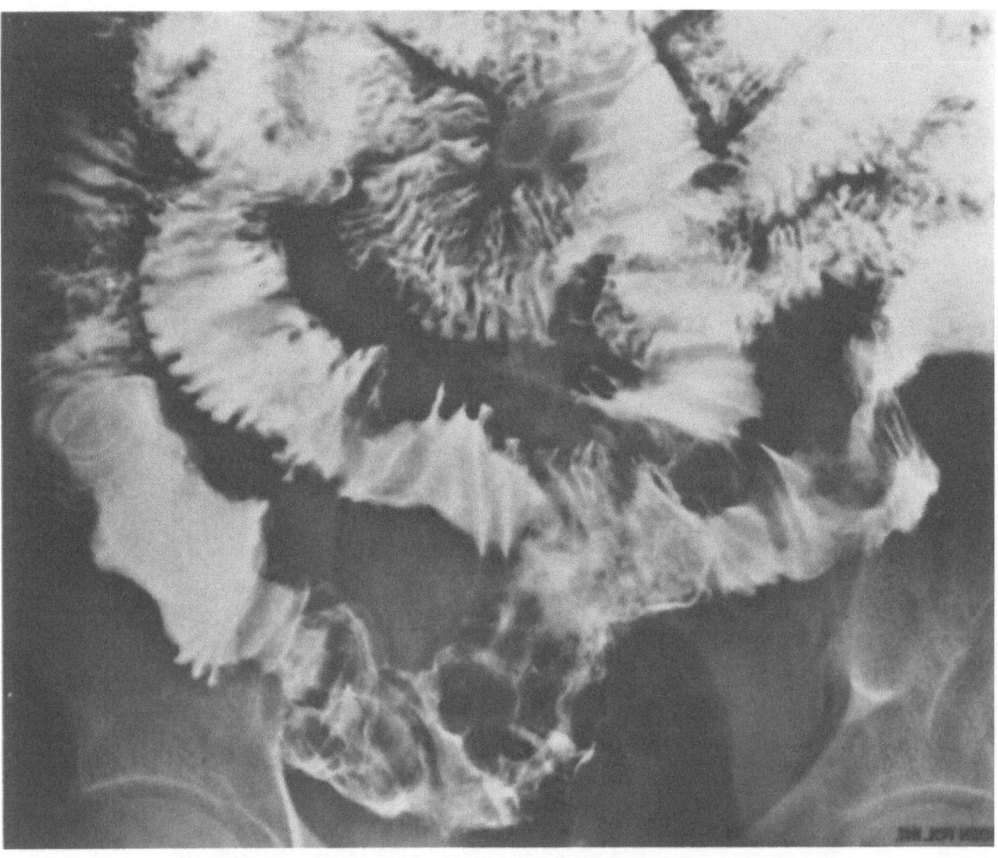

Fig. 10.30
The same patient (20-year-old male) as in fig. 10.29, about 6 months later. Now even in the ileum, which presented no abnormalities during the previous examination, an extensive obliteration of the mucosal relief is seen.

this so-called Mediterranean lymphoma, which occurs most frequently in the duodenum and proximal jejunum, is encountered in migrant workers from Morocco, Greece and Turkey.

In the earliest stage of the disease when the lymphoma causes only edema of the mucosa over a very large area, the folds are broadened and the intestinal wall is only slightly thicker if at all (fig. 10.31). This edema cannot be distinguished from the edema resulting from hypoalbuminemia; it is also difficult to differentiate it from a moderately pronounced lymphedema whereby the intestinal wall is not yet thickened and has still retained its

←

Fig. 10.29
Malignant lymphoma in the jejunum with only slight radiological abnormalities. In the proximal jejunum, the degree of obliteration and broadening of the folds varies (⬇). There are several nodular defects (→). In the distal ileum, the folds are only swollen. No abnormalities can be seen in the ileum.

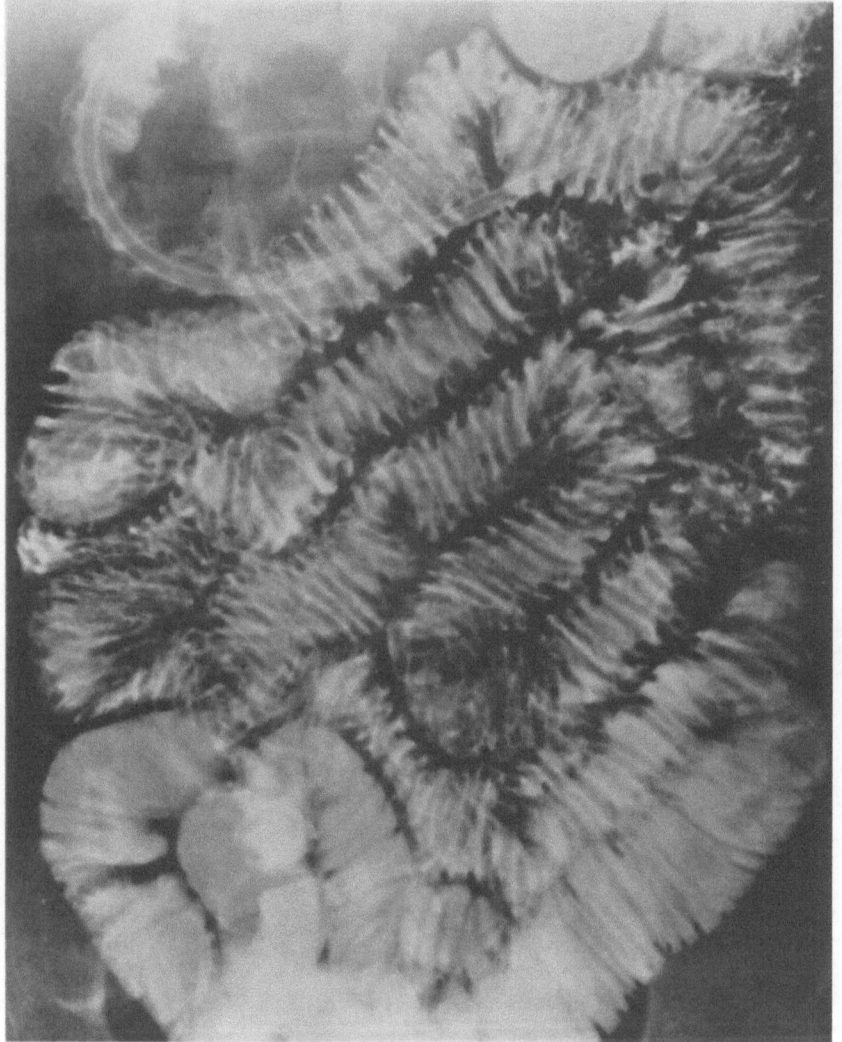

Fig. 10.31
Edematous mucosa and slightly thickened intestinal wall of the jejunum in a 24-year-old
male, not recognized at that time as a possible early malignant lymphoma.

pliancy. On the basis of our observation that this
edema can be temporary, we believe that it should
be considered a nonspecific prodromic phenomenon which presumably is due to a hypoalbuminemia. When the latter is treated, this edema disappears and in the course of the subsequent months,
sometimes even years, nodular elevations and thick
ridge-like mucosal swellings several centimeters in
length can develop. Like the edema these nodules
can also disappear temporarily or become less apparent. This is seen mainly in those parts of the
small bowel which contain the most lymphoid tissue,
such as the distal ileum, duodenum and proximal

jejunum (fig. 10.32). In this stage, the differential
diagnosis certainly should include Crohn's disease
localized in the duodenum especially when cobblestones are also seen (fig. 10.33). In addition to
granulomas in the duodenum, abnormalities are in
fact also seen in the distal ileum in one-half of the
cases. By means of biopsies, the presence of
Crohn's disease can, however, quickly be excluded.

The problems of the differential diagnosis are
much greater when a segment of the jujenum or
ileum shows very coarse, somewhat irregular
mucosal folds while the intestinal wall is not or
barely thickened and has retained a fairly good

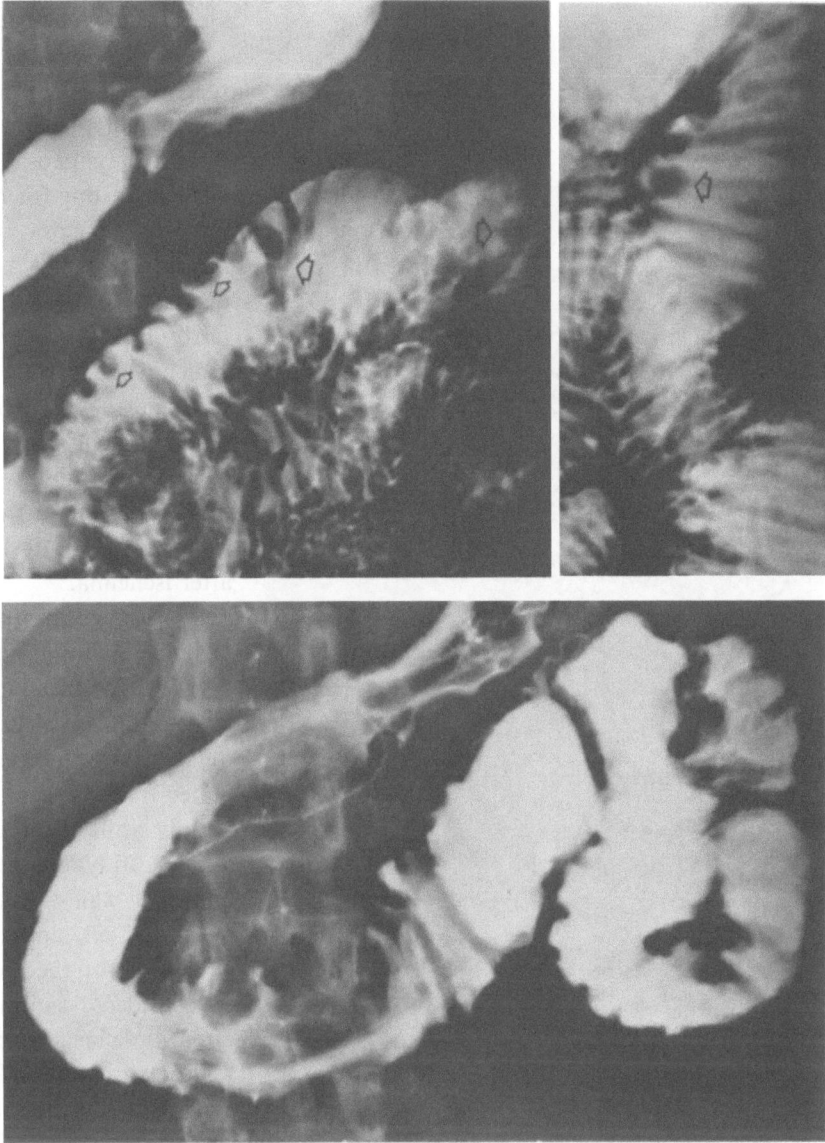

Fig. 10.32
The same patient as seen in fig. 10.31, one year later. In the duodenum and proximal jejunum the mucosal folds have disappeared for the most part and nodular lumps are seen in the lumen which may or may not originate from the folds. Crohn's disease was considered at first but the diagnosis of malignant lymphoma was soon apparent. Celiac disease was not considered because of the nodular mucosal swellings.

motility and pliancy (fig. 10.34). The mucosal surface can show multiple small ulcerations but it can also be completely intact if the spread of the lymphoma is submucosal. It is impossible to differentiate such a case, irrespective of whether there are mucosal ulcerations or not, from the changes which are due to a moderately pronounced ischemia. Although the very different set of complaints and the clinical course of these two diseases as well as the age of the patient can already form an important indication of the correct diagnosis, the solution to this dilemma is not produced until a follow-up examination is carried out 4–6 weeks later. In the case of ischemia, obvious changes are always seen: the abnormalities have disappeared or fibrosis is evident. If there are multiple ulcerations, the differential diagnosis may also include an enteritis but here adequate treatment will certainly produce a

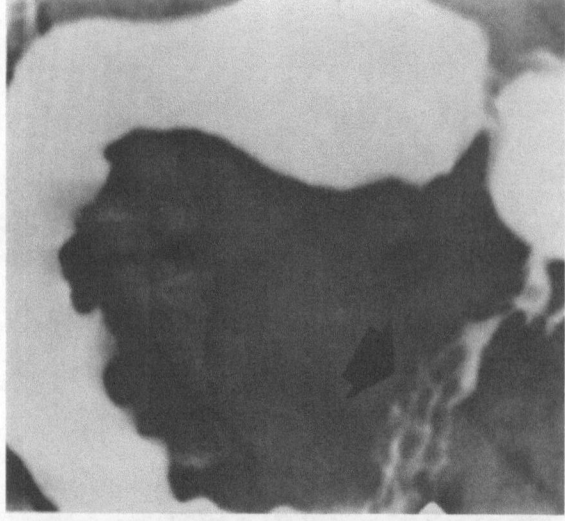

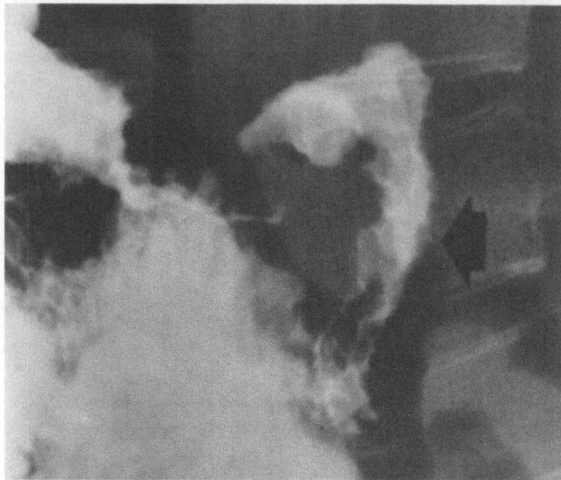

Fig. 10.33
Two patients with cobblestones in the duodenum due to
lymphosarcoma.

change for the better in 4–6 weeks. If, on the other
hand a lymphoma is involved then quite frequently
there is little or no change, even if the follow-up
examination is 2 or 3 months later. The complaints
can be few and may only be due to the fact that
malabsorption has led to several nutritional deficiencies. Adequate treatment of these deficiencies
can cause the superficial ulcerative changes to
decrease; they may even temporarily disappear for
the most part. Mainly because of the clinical well-
being of the patient and the fact that the biopsies
only show signs of chronic infection and aggregates
of plasma cells and lymphocytes in the lamina
propria, the diagnosis of lymphoma is often barely
considered.

A third manifestation of lymphoma which can
cause considerable problems in the differential
diagnosis is when a superficial spread over a large
segment of the intestine has caused total obliteration of the mucosa (fig. 10.35). The process can be
chronic, lasting for many years. A large area of the
intestinal mucosa can be covered with small ulcerations causing a close resemblance to Crohn's
disease in the acute stage. The intestinal wall is
fairly stiff, but only slightly thickened and the
lumen is moderately dilated. No contractions can be
seen and the loops lie in orderly fashion in the abdominal cavity with a minimum number of coils,
curves and folds. Due to the superficial character
of the ulcerations, there is no fibrotic shriveling and
stenoses do not develop, as in Crohn's disease and
after ischemia.

If the mucosa in the duodenum or jejunum have
atrophied, an alternative possibility could be celiac
disease. However, an eventual secondary infection
in conjunction with this latter disease reacts quite
quickly to the proper treatment augmented with a
gluten-free diet. The ulcerations then disappear
rapidly while the intestinal wall becomes obviously
thinner. In lymphoma the ulcerative changes in the
intestinal wall will disappear only with difficulty
or not at all, and they also recur very soon. A
lymphoma of the small intestine should therefore
be considered seriously if there are extensive and
often ill-defined changes in the intestinal wall in a
patient with relatively few complaints. Sometimes
in the event of prolonged uncertainty, a diagnostic
laparotomy is unavoidable.

6. Metastasis

Although metastatic tumors in the small intestine
or invasion of the mesentery are demonstrated
radiologically even less frequently than primary
tumors, they are frequently found at autopsy. In
our patient material, too, metastases were demonstrated in less than one-fifth of the total number of
patients with a benign or malignant tumor in the
small bowel. Almost half of these cases of metastatic
tumors involved metastasis of melanoma. This
high percentage is probably due to the fact that this
group of patients is subjected to periodic follow-
ups and whenever occult rectal bleeding occurs, an

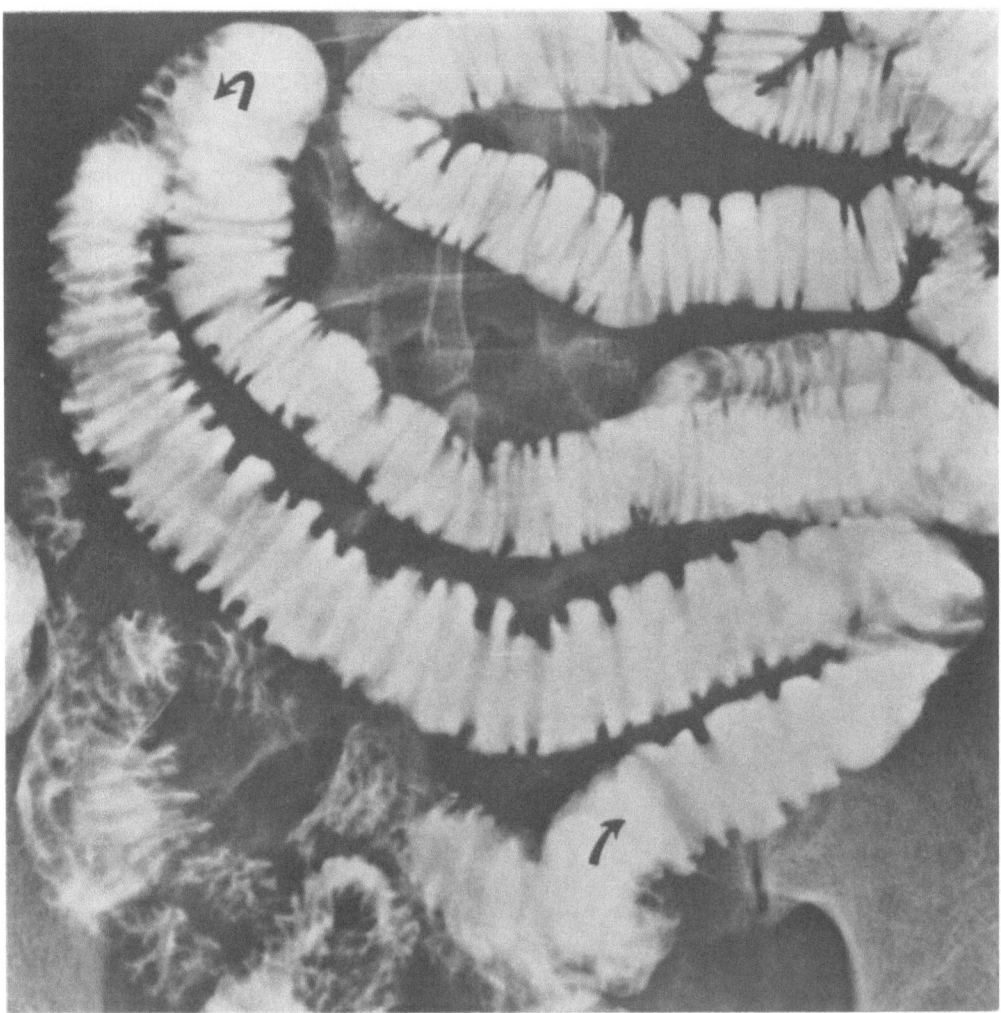

Fig. 10.34
Patient with a probable lymphoma of the ileum growing along the surface. The intestinal wall is thickened and the mucosal folds are irregular and obviously broadened; motility is fairly well-preserved. Clinically there was a clear malabsorption and a fairly marked loss of weight. The mucosal biopsy showed an increase in the number of plasma cells in the lamina propria. Only little progress of the abnormalities 6 months later. Patient has since refused further follow-up examinations.

examination of the small intestine is performed automatically.

On the other hand it is certainly possible that metastases from tumors are only demonstrated sporadically because the complaints due to the primary tumor or metastases in other organs dominate markedly or have already led to death before the metastasis in the small intestine produces definite complaints. In addition to direct invasion from adjacent organs such as pancreas, colon or stomach, metastasis is also transmitted to the small intestine by the bloodstream or lymphatic system. The primary tumor can therefore be found

in these organs but also in the esophagus, lungs, mammae, kidneys, uterus or ovaries. Metastasis from the ovary in particular can be extensive in the intestine, mesentery and peritoneum. In contrast to the malignant primary tumors of the intestine, which cause obstruction within a relatively short time, most metastases do not as a rule give rise to such complaints until much later. Metastases spread from the mesentery into the intestinal wall or grow intramurally from the subserous vascular network on the opposite side. Although they not only grow from the intestinal surface outwards but also bulge into the lumen, they only cause obstruction phenom-

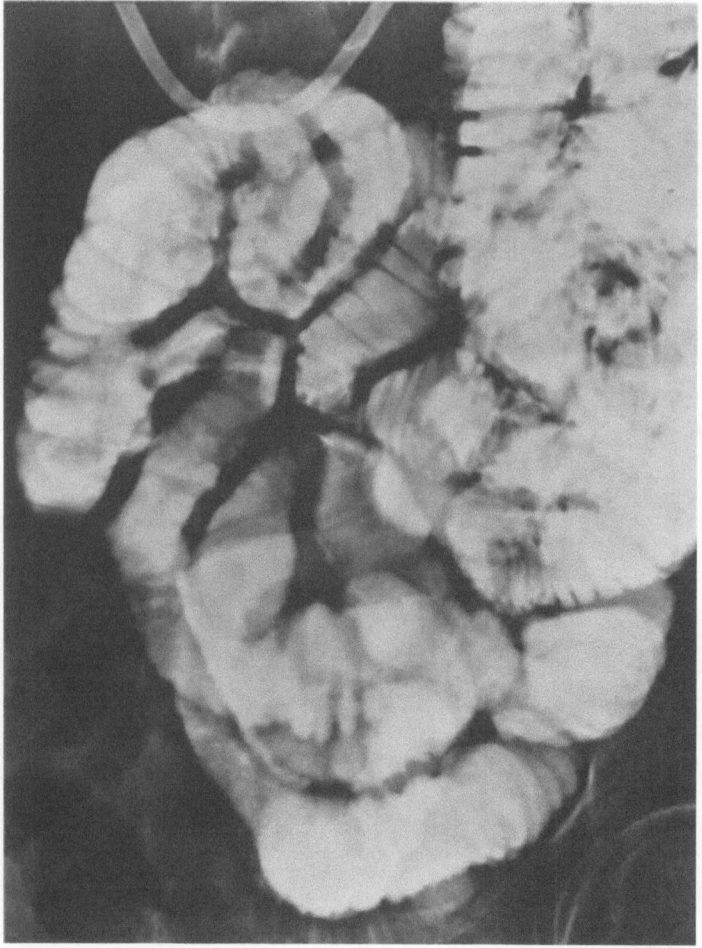

Fig. 10.35
Malignant lymphoma involving almost the entire ileum with thickened rigid intestinal wall and obliterated mucosal folds. The lumen of the intestine is slightly dilated.

ena in a much later stage (fig. 10.36). Metastases cause ulcerations and central necrosis more often than primary tumors do and fusion with adjacent organs or tissues is also more extensive (fig. 10.37). Metastasis localized in the mesentery cause a compression effect on the intestine which is only accompanied by stretching of the mucosal folds or flattening of the mucosal contours when the growing tumor is fused with the intestinal wall. Diffuse metastasis in the mesentery causes the mesentery

to become thicker as well as stiffer and shorter. The intestinal loops attached to the shortened mesentery also become – of necessity – shorter; the mucosal folds along this traject are then very close together. Moreover, these loops lie in a more or less stretched, very organized fashion and are visualized without interference from other loops.

Diffuse carcinomatosis in the abdominal cavity is as a rule not a difficult diagnosis (fig. 10.38);

                                                                                    ⟶

Fig. 10.36
Diverse examples of metastases in the small bowel. The x-rays and the pathology specimen show that they bulge out from the intestinal wall as well as into the lumen.

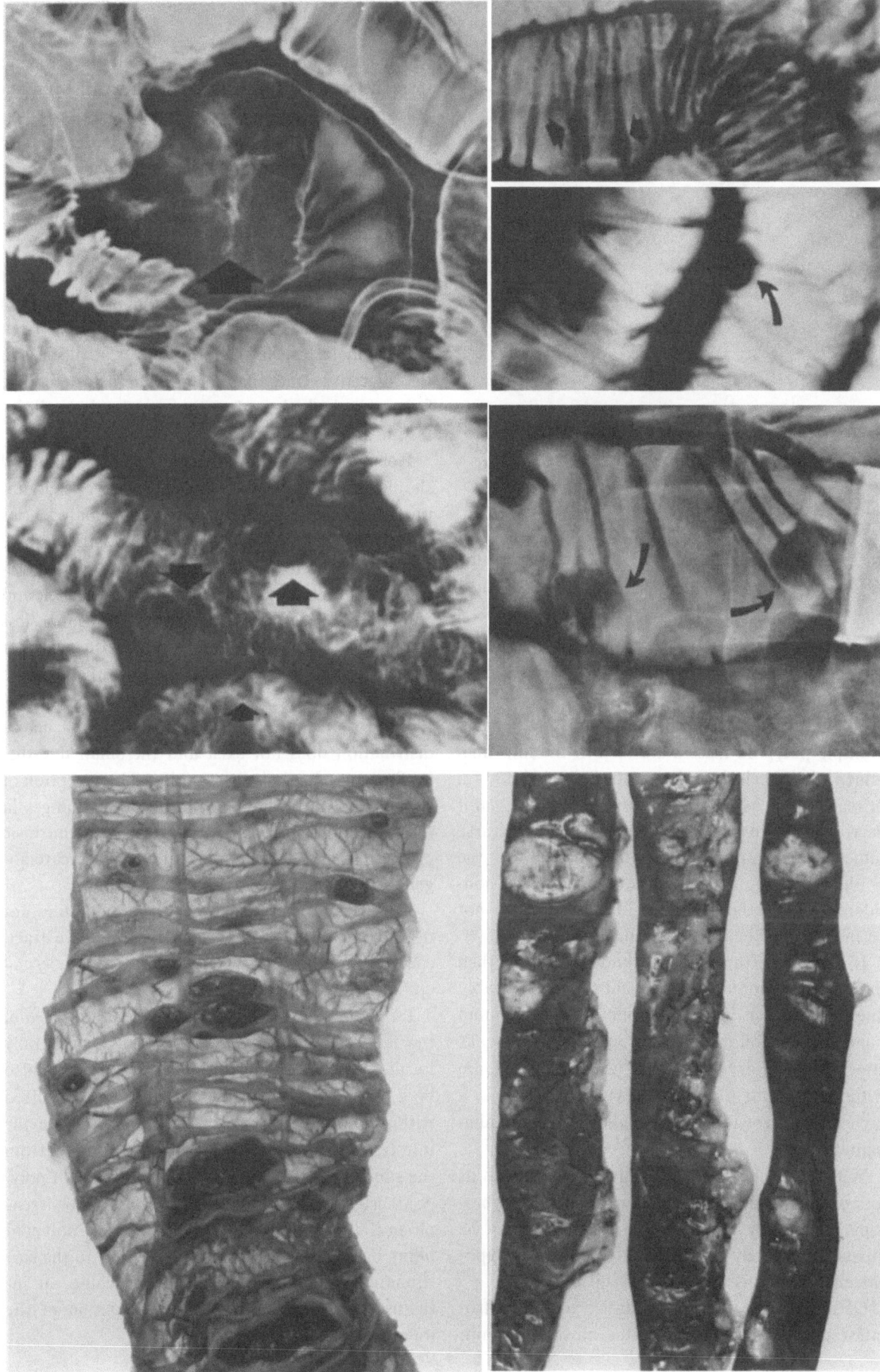

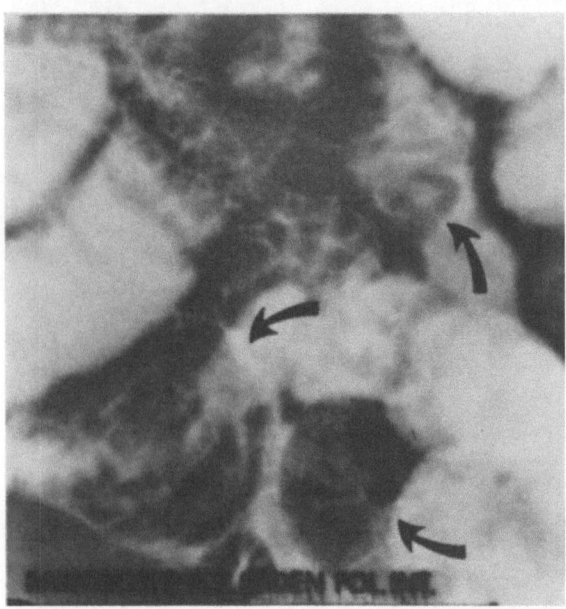

Fig. 10.37
Metastases of a reticulum cell sarcoma, one with central necrosis.

the characteristic radiological abnormalities cannot be confused with those of any other disease, not even a generalized lymphosarcoma. Whenever multiple polypoid masses are seen in the intestinal lumen, the conclusion of metastasis is obvious if a primary tumor is known to exist elsewhere. Even if necrosis and ulcerations are observed in these tumors, a lymphoreticular malignancy of the nodular type or a leiomyo(sarco)ma can be considered, but benign polypoid formations need not be included in the differential diagnosis.

If a primary tumor is not known to exist then the multiple nodular abnormalities are probably due to metastasis if they have increased in size and number on a follow-up examination several weeks later. For solitary metastases as well, which are without a doubt the most difficult to diagnose, a high rate of growth is highly indicative of a malignant disease.

With the exception of general symptoms such as loss of weight, malaise and anorexia, clinical symptoms of metastasis in the small intestine may be missed completely or may be due solely to hypochronic anemia as a result of occult blood loss.

Of the tumors which metastasize to the gastrointestinal tract, melanoma is the most important.

The complaints caused by metastasis in the small intestine can be the first signs of an as yet unrecognized melanoma. Sometimes metastases are encountered in the digestive tract while the primary tumor cannot be demonstrated. In such cases it is assumed that the metastasis originated from a primary site on the skin which disappeared spontaneously. Autopsy of patients who died of melanoma has shown that the frequency of metastasis to the small intestine is 58%, somewhat less than that for the lungs (70%) and the liver (60%). Even without metastasis to the lung or liver, metastasis in the digestive tract has been demonstrated. The frequency is highest for the proximal small intestine and decreases distalwards.

Roentgenological examination of the small bowel should therefore be carried out whenever it is important to establish the presence of hematogenous metastases. If metastases via the bloodstream have already been proven, then there is no indication for the examination. Metastases in the stomach and colon, as well as other organs, are seen much less frequently (25%). The ratio of the frequencies for stomach, small intestine and colon is in the same proportion as their respective surfaces, which is typical of melanoma. For other tumors such a distribution does not exist and the small intestine is often spared, relatively speaking. The exception of melanoma is attributed to the fact that changes in the immunological defence decrease the intrinsic protection of the small intestine against carcinogenous influences.

In general it is assumed that melanoma does not occur as a primary disease in the digestive tract, since no melanoblasts are found in the entodermal epithelium of the digestive tract.

In metastasis transmitted by the bloodstream, the lesions are usually multiple and are generally localized on the antimesenteric side. There can also be a number of metastases of equal size localized within a specific area of the arterial supply in the intestine. The metastatic melanoma spreads from the submucosa into the lumen as a nodular or polypoid, usually amelanotic growth. Thus the roentgenological aspect is that of a nodular or polypoid filling defect. Since there is no adhesion to the surroundings these nodules can easily cause an intussusception and intermittent obstruction of the intestine.

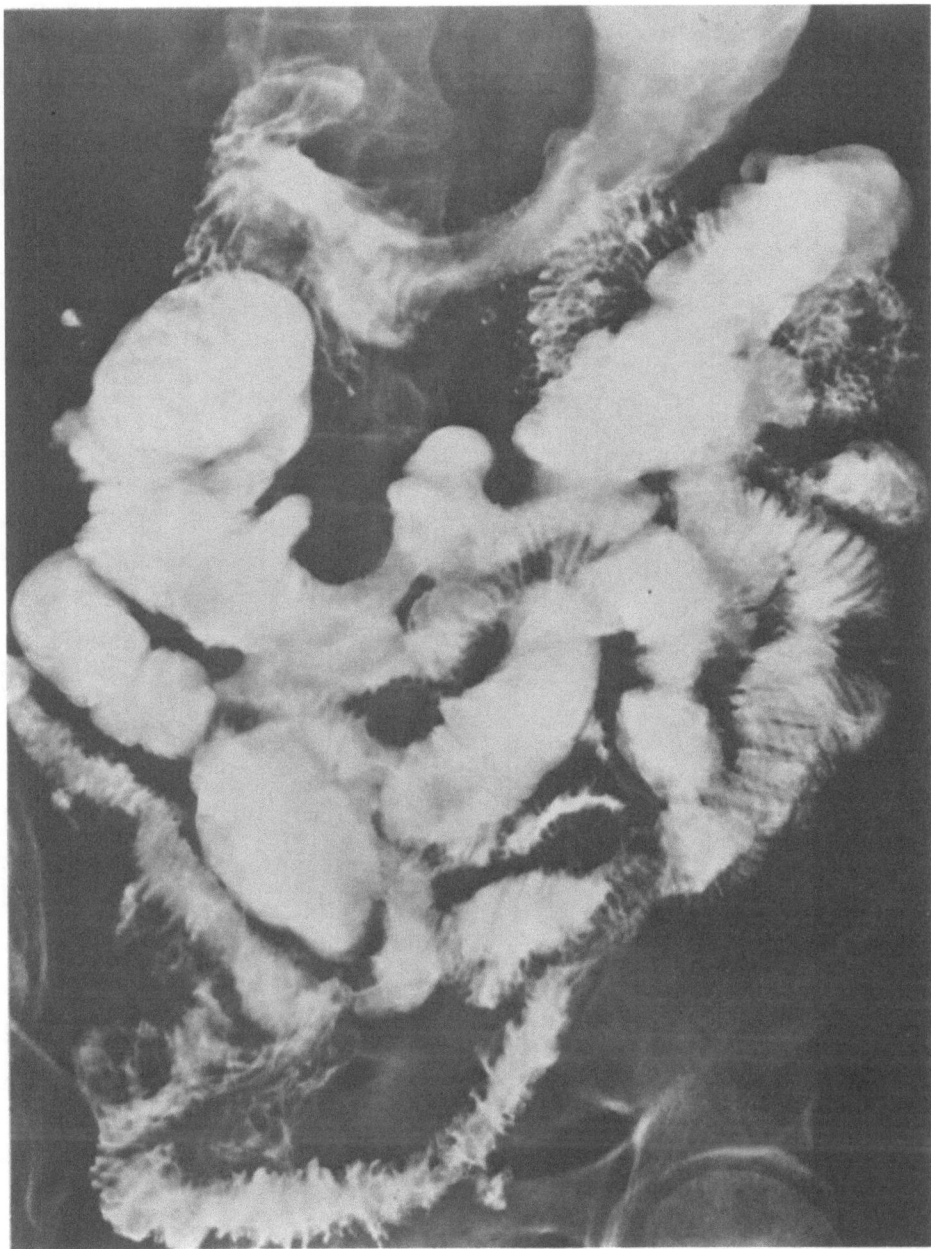

Fig. 10.38
Tumor of the stomach with an extensive peritoneal carcinomatosis.

Central ulceration in a metastasis is seen frequently and can, if it is deep, give the characteristic roentgenological aspect of a 'target lesion' or 'bull's eye' (fig. 10.39). If the ulcerations are superficial, then they are difficult to recognize radiologically. Diagnosis will include leiomyoma and leiomyosarcoma, as well as nodular lymphosarcoma and metastasis from a Kaposi's sarcoma – a fairly rare vascular tumor with a high risk of hemorrhage. If the central ulcerations are missing, then carcinoid lesions must be considered in addition to metastasis of carcinoma. In contrast to metastasis of melanoma, carcinoids are, however, much more likely to be found in the distal part of the intestine.

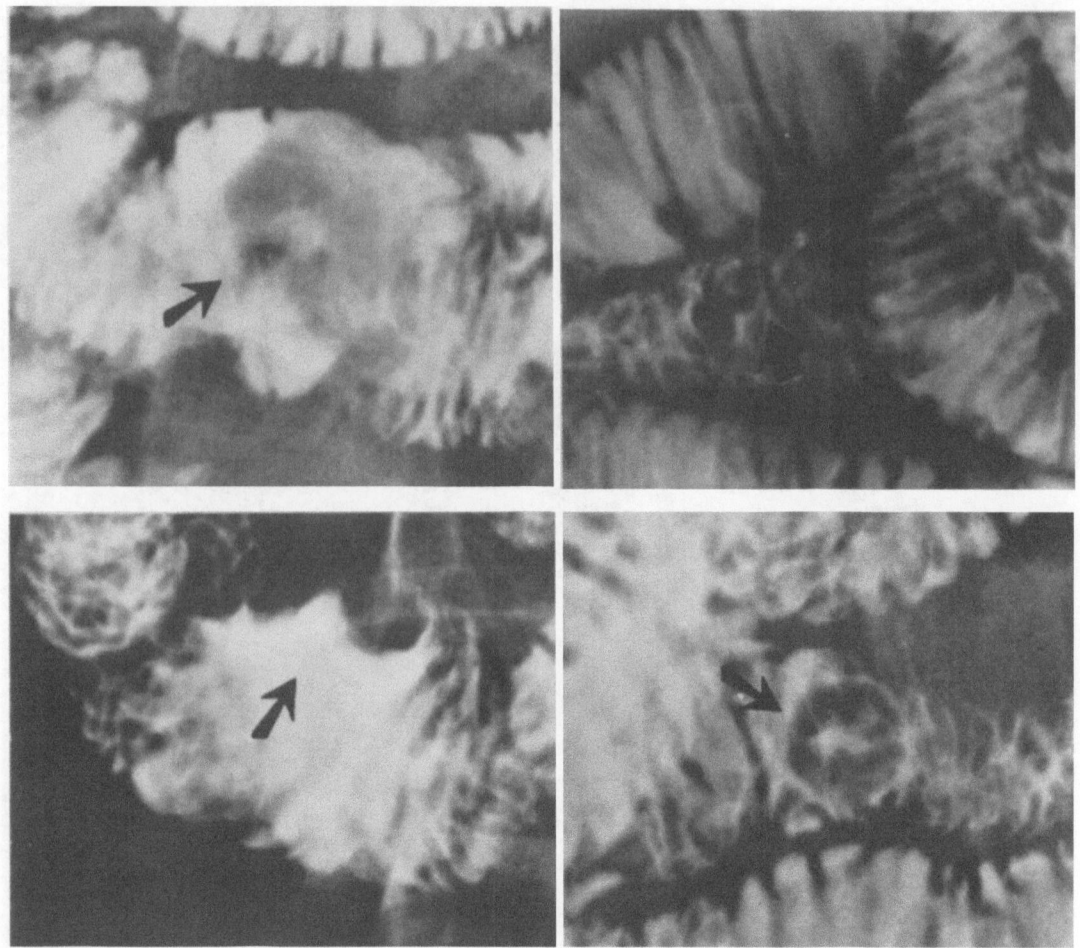

Fig. 10.39
Several examples of melanotic metastases including one very small one with central necrosis. On the left, a so-called 'bull's eye' is seen en face (above) and in profile (below).

Bibliography chapter X

HODES PH. J.; STEIN G. N.; FINKELSTEIN A. K. (1973) Tumor atlas of the gastro-intestinal tract. *Year Book Medical Publishers.* See also the nrs. 26–78–91–132 and 237 of the bibliography on pages 164 and following.

XI

VASCULAR DISEASES

Although certainly not rare, abnormalities of the small intestine resulting from an impaired circulation are often not recognized as such; fortunately some improvement in this situation can be observed. The failure to establish this diagnosis can be attributed not only to the fact that the radiological examination techniques are frequently inadequate and the mucosal changes caused by this type of lesion are not sufficiently well-known, but also to the fact that the clinician often does not consider the possibility of a vascular disorder – not even when it is quite serious. Finally this disorder may sometimes be characterized either by a very mild course or by sudden very severe episodes which are, however, so short that the patient does not consider it necessary to consult a physician. In a number of these cases the abnormalities which persist after such an accident eventually give rise to definite complaints and the roentgenograms then made are 'silent witnesses' of that which occurred several weeks or months before.

Obstructions of the blood flow in the intestinal wall can, depending upon the manner in which they develop, be classified as arterial or venous disorders or hemorrhage. Such a differentiation is, however, not always straightforward since a combination of causes is also possible.

1. Ischemia due to impaired arterial flow

a. The most common cause of a reduction in arterial flow is without a doubt arteriosclerotic changes in the wall of the superior mesenteric artery (fig. 11.1B). If the constriction due to arteriosclerosis develops gradually, there will be sufficient time for the formation of collaterals with the celiac trunk, inferior mesenteric artery and the vessels in the abdominal wall; thus occlusion of the superior mesenteric artery need not lead to serious complaints.

b. Mechanical obstruction of the intestine due to adhesions or bands, volvulus or internal hernia is usually also accompanied by obvious impairment of the circulation, arterial as well as venous (fig. 11.2).

c. After surgery involving the major vessels in the abdomen, there may be a temporary decrease in the blood flow through the superior and inferior mesenteric arteries (fig. 11.3). In addition it is occasionally necessary to sacrifice the latter vessel which sometimes plays a prominent role in the collateral circulation to the vessels in the small intestine.

d. Microemboli, occurring in polycythemia vera or as a result of valvular disease, atrial fibrillation or a myocardial infarction, can cause sudden occlusion of the generally relatively small vessels (fig. 11.4).

e. Vasculitis in arteries or small veins, as seen in Buerger's disease, Schönlein-Henoch disease (fig. 11.6) or rheumatoid arthritis, causes thrombosis and multiple occlusions in these vessels (figs. 11.4 and 11.5). This can also occur in many collagen diseases, accompanied by abnormal skin conditions, such as periarteritis nodosa (fig. 11.7), lupus erythematosus or dermatomyositis.

f. Vasoconstrictors, such as for instance ergomatine preparations, can also cause a temporary reduction in the blood supply in the intestinal wall.

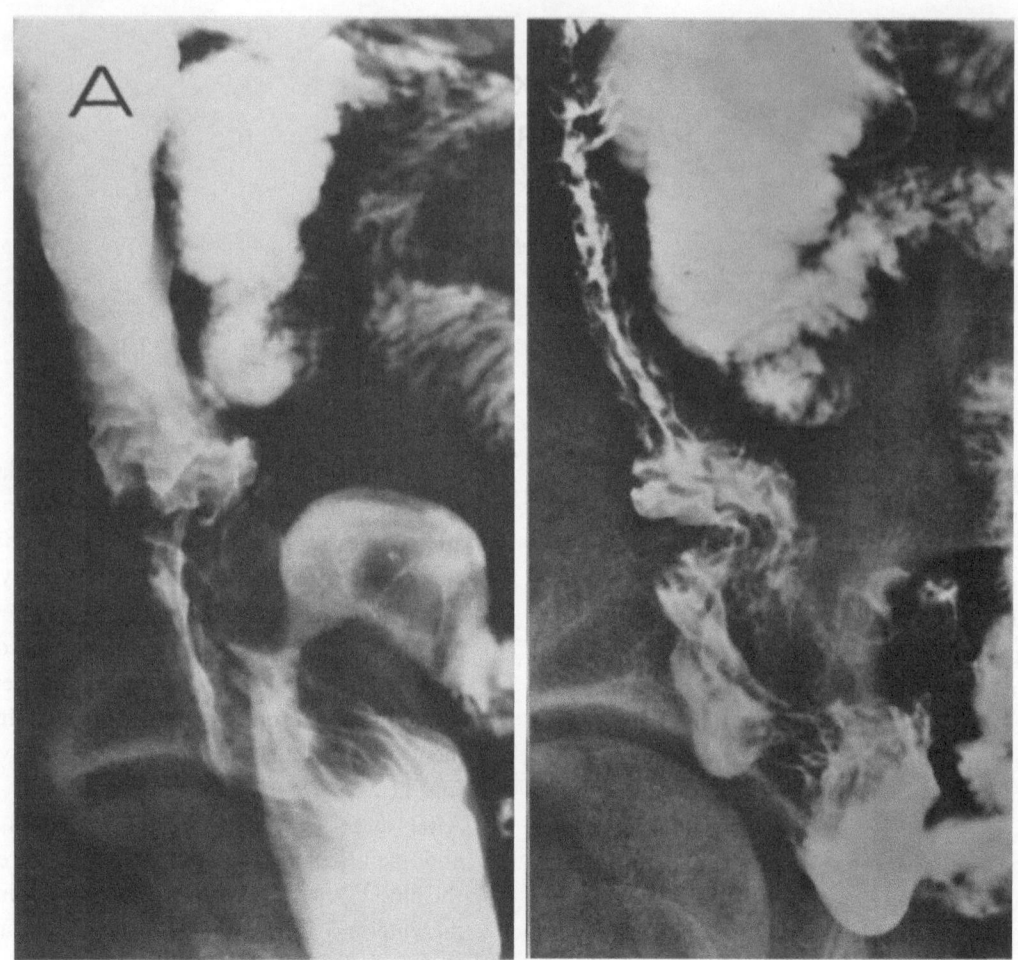

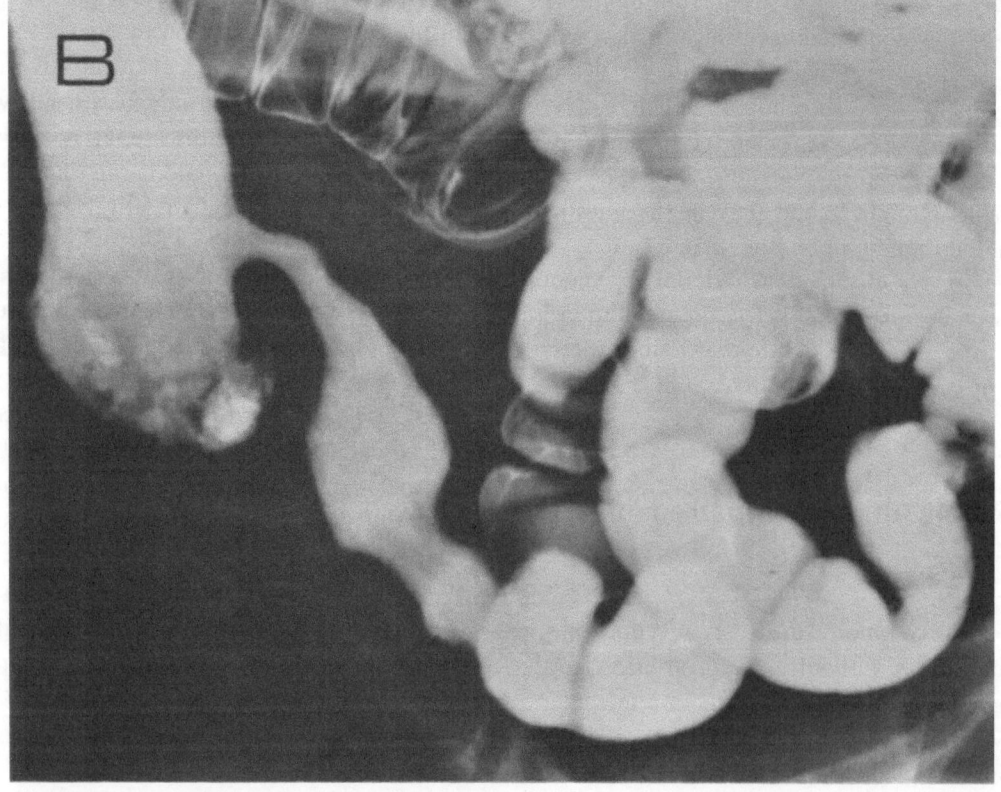

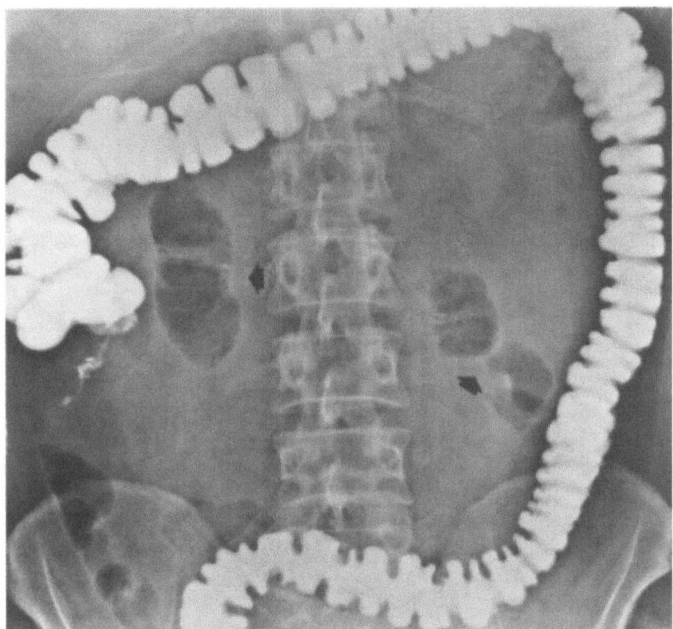 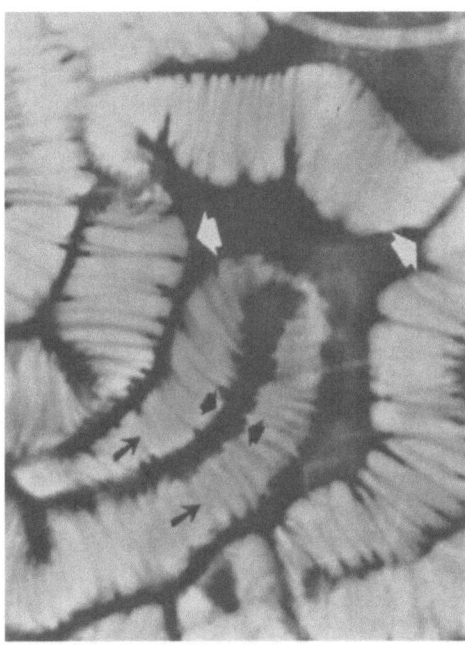

Fig. 11.2.
Two cases of vascular abnormalities as a result of constricting bands crossing over the intestine.
A.   An examination of the colon was performed because of vague abdominal complaints (left). All films showed two intestinal loops which were filled with gas and slightly dilated. Abnormalities in the small bowel were suspected and an enteroclysis examination was performed (right). This showed a band (→) at the site of the gas accumulation on the left. The intestinal loop here has an obviously thickened wall with subtle signs of 'thumbprinting' (→←). On the distal side of the gas accumulation on the right, the wall is thickened over more than 10 cm while the folds are edematous and swollen.
B.   see p. 278.

←

Fig. 11.1
Two patients after recovery from ischemia.
A.   A 50 cm segment of the distal ileum shows pathological fold relief as well as multiple deformations and fusion with adjacent loops. Surgery and subsequent pathological examination revealed a vasculitis and an ulcer 30 cm long. Because of the youth of the patient a vascular disease was not considered.
B.   Smooth wall in a 50 cm segment of the cecum and distal ileum. Wide open Bauhin's valve no longer functions. In this case especially differentiation from Crohn's disease on the basis of radiological examination is impossible.

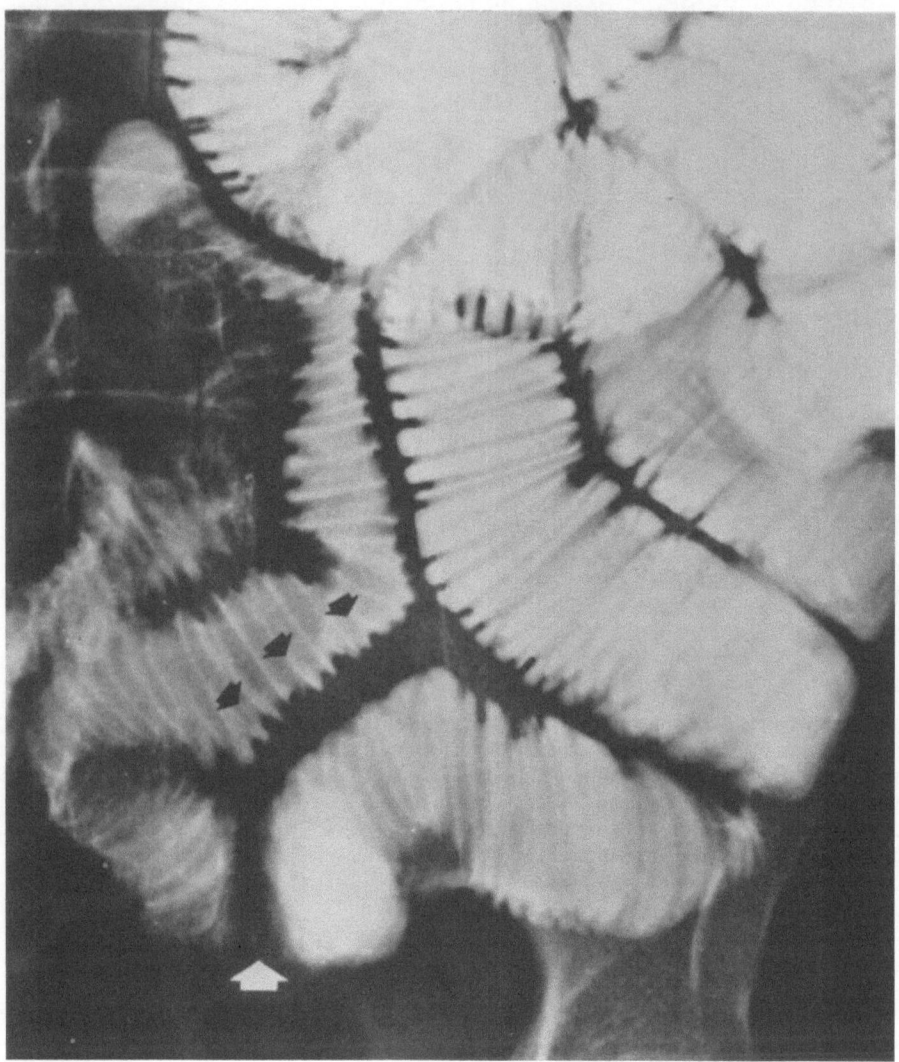

Fig. 11.2
B.   Ileus due to bands (→). In this case the intestinal mucosal folds are only clearly thickened on the distal side of the band ($\overset{\rightarrow}{\rightarrow}$)
so that it most probably is the venous flow which is disturbed.

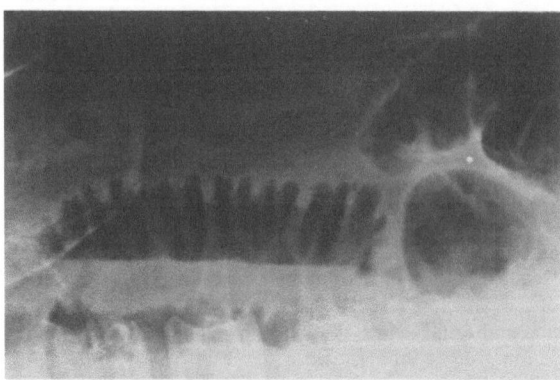

Fig. 11.3
Ileus after bifurcation of a prothesis. Markedly swollen
mucosal folds, possibly due to ischemia of the intestine
since recovery was spontaneous.

Fig. 11.4.

Vascular accident in the small bowel of a patient with atrial fibrillation.

A. There were clear signs of an ileus, both radiologically and clinically.

B. In the distal jejunum one loop contains highly edematous swollen mucosal folds; this is called 'thumbprinting'. The bowel wall is obviously thicker. No peristaltic movements could be seen in this region.

C. Several weeks later a definite clinical recovery was apparent. The roentgenograms now showed complete obliteration of the mucosal relief in the involved segment. The intestinal lumen is slightly narrower, thickening of the wall is reduced and signs of peristalsis could be seen during fluoroscopy.

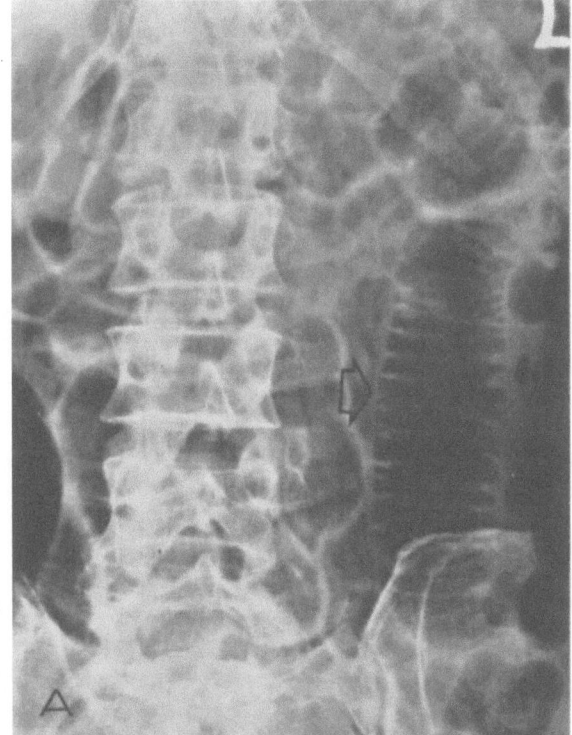

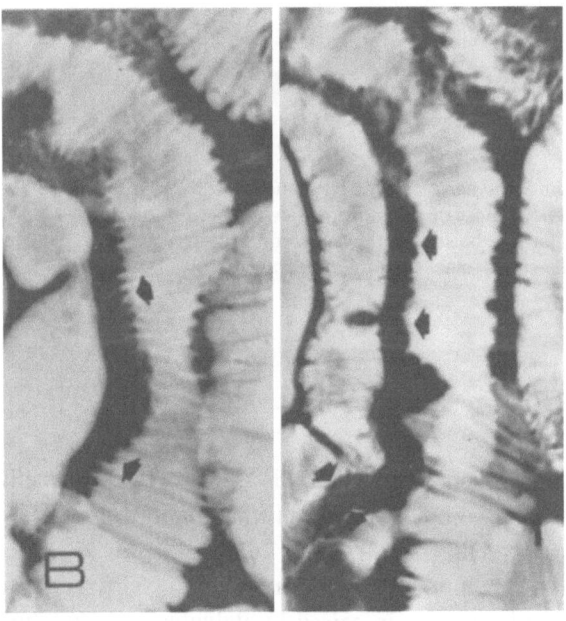

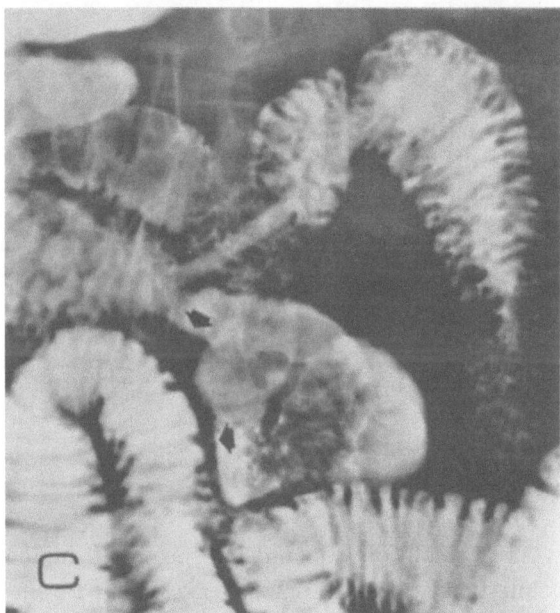

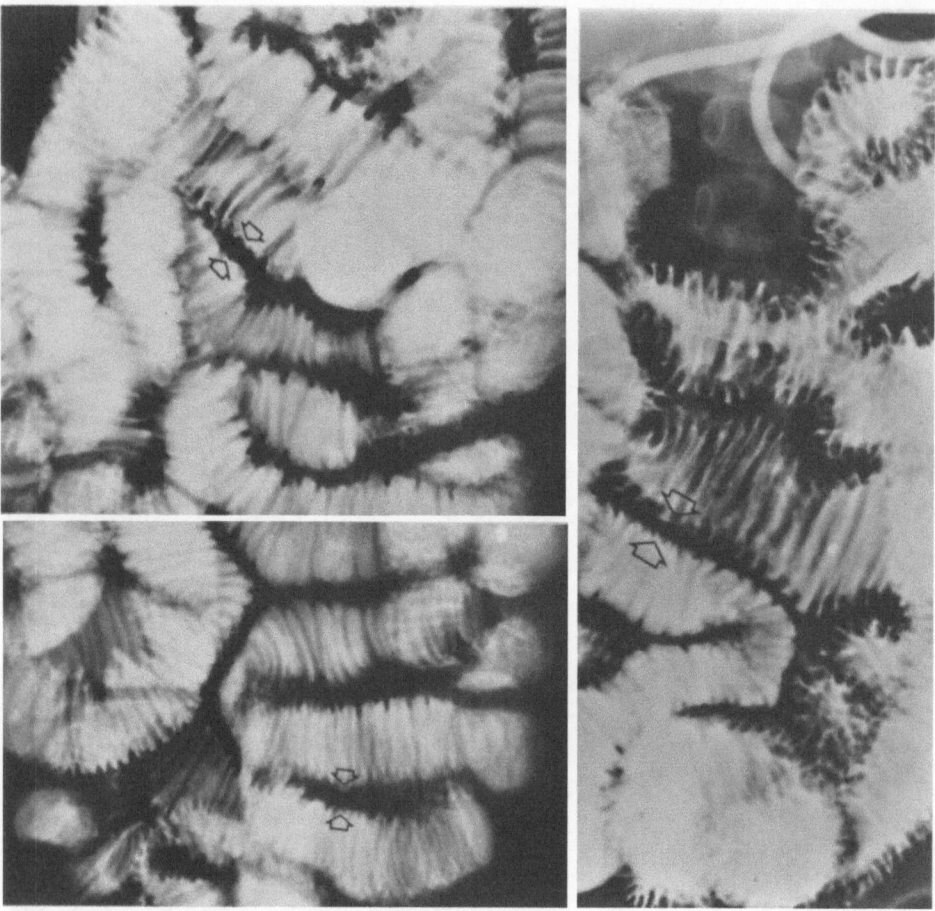

Fig. 11.5
Mesenteric arteritis of unknown origin, found during surgery, in a 10-year-old boy. The mucosal folds are moderately broadened and the wall is thickened throughout most of the intestine ($\rightarrow \leftarrow$). For comparison, the thickness of a normal bowel wall in youngsters can be seen at the right. In this child, the mucosal folds lie so close together that they have the so-called 'stacked coin' appearance.

2. Impaired venous flow

a. As a result of inflammatory processes in the intestinal wall or the mesentery, venous thrombosis can occur. In this region, however, a venous thrombosis is less common than an arterial thrombosis (fig. 11.8).

b. The blood flow can also be impaired when the veins in the mesentery are constricted by compression or invasion of cysts or tumors in the mesentery. In general such processes grow slowly and there is therefore sufficient time for an adequate collateral circulation to develop. Swollen mucosal folds therefore are usually caused by lymphedema when tumors or cysts are present.

c. The blood flow in the efferent veins is more likely to be impaired by volvulus, strangulation or an internal hernia than the flow in the arteries in the same intestinal segment.

d. Finally, severe congestive heart failure or portal hypertension due to liver cirrhosis can also cause a serious reduction in the venous flow (fig. 11.9). Obviously in these cases there will be no chance for adequate collateral circulation to develop.

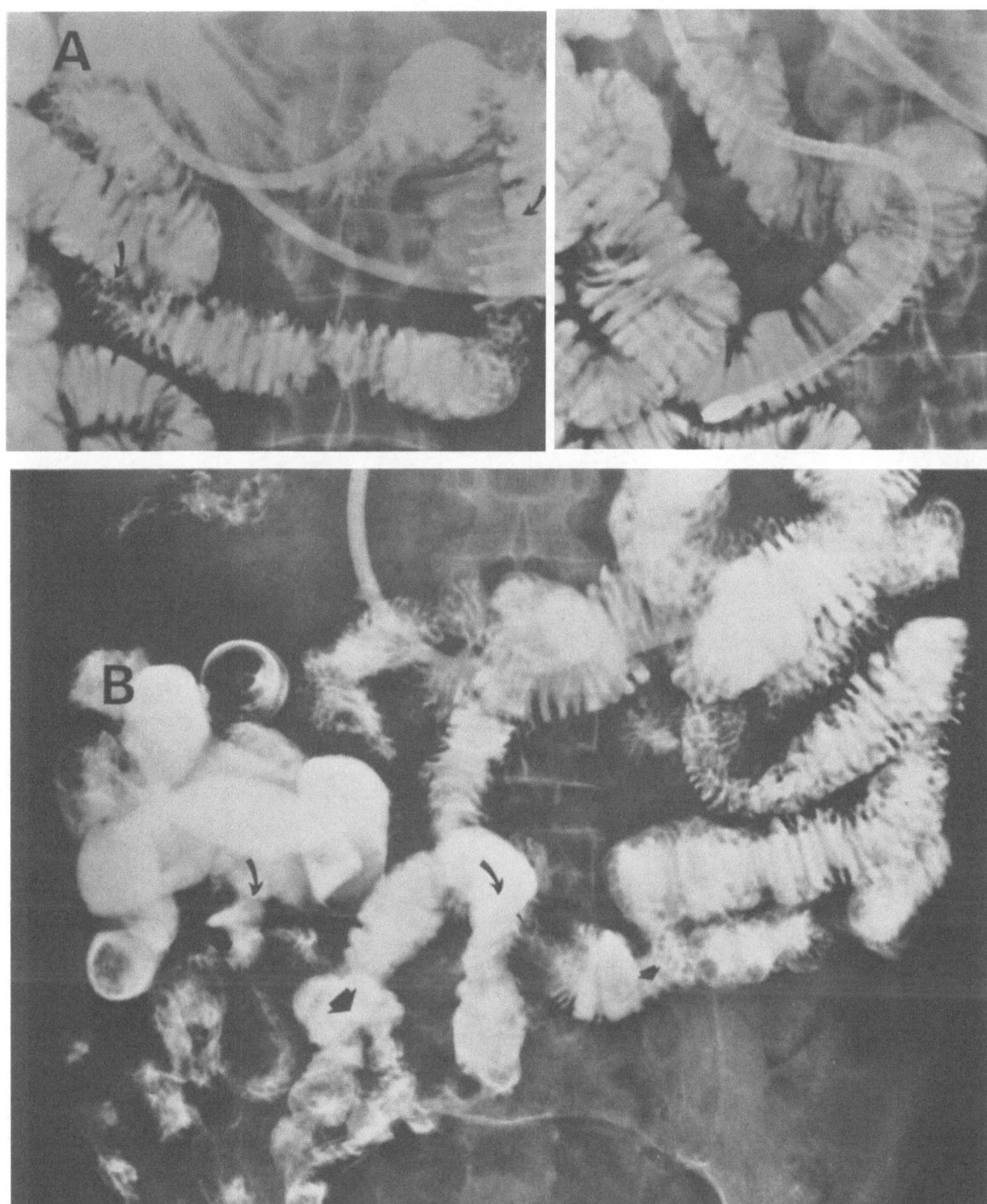

Fig. 11.6
Two patients with rectal bleeding due to Schönlein-Henoch disease.
A. Several decimeters of highly edematous swollen mucosal folds in the proximal jejunum (left), probably to diffuse sub-mucosal bleedings only. As so often in these patients, recovery was spontaneous and the mucosa already appeared normal two weeks later (right).
B. The abnormalities can, however, also be more widespread as well as more pronounced so that complete recovery does not follow. Then the mucosal relief in several areas will be pathologically changed or completely absent and there will be an obvious hypermotility in the proximal ileum in the lower right quadrant. Similar abnormalities can be encountered in other diseases which are accompanied by arteritis such as for instance dermatomyositis (see fig. 12.24).

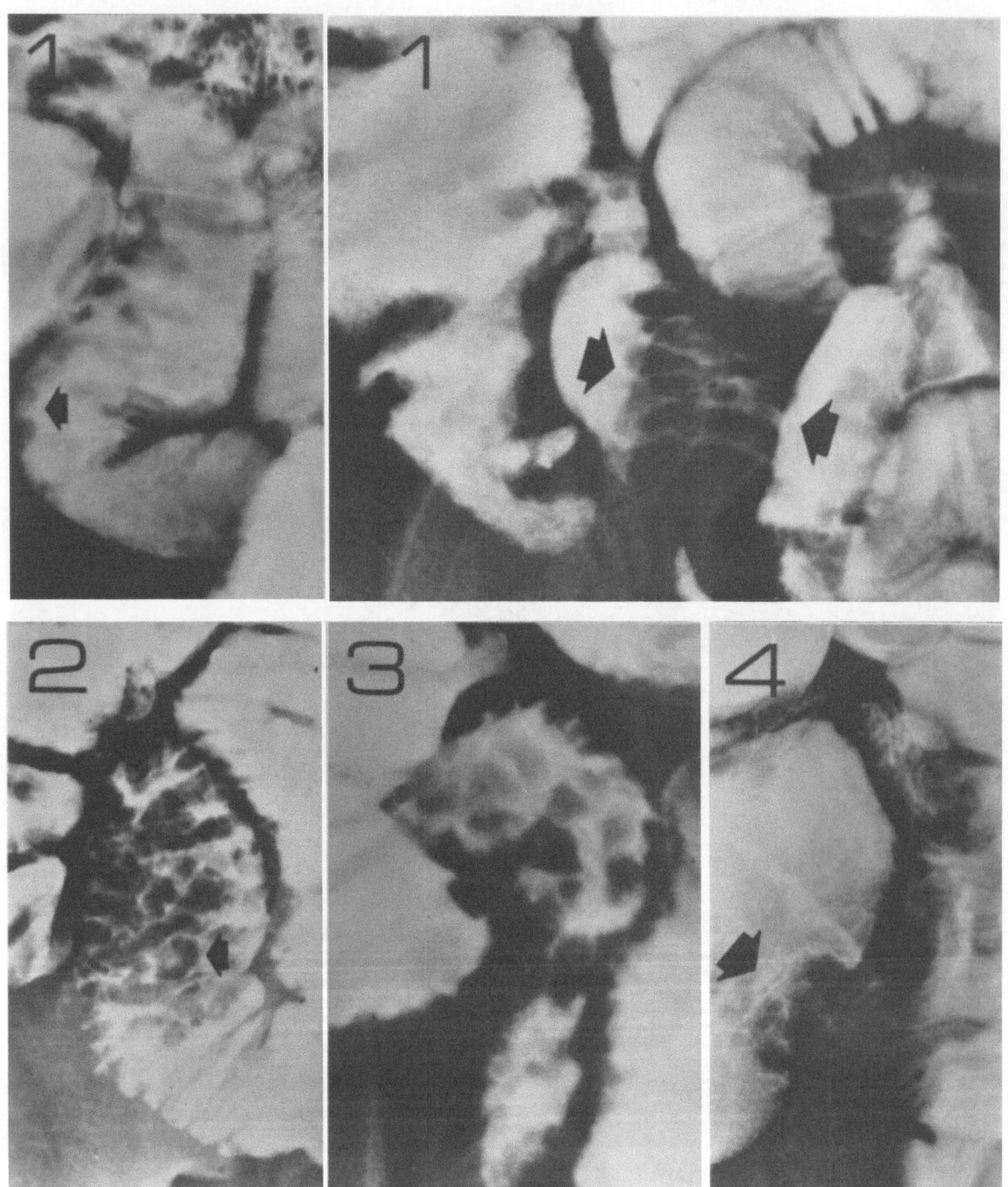

Fig. 11.7.
Four cases of periarteritis nodosa with coarse mucosal folds and granuloma-like abnormalities, some possibly even with a central ulcer crater. Several months later, one of the patients (no. 1) showed a cobblestone pattern which could not be distinguished from that seen in Crohn's disease.

→

Fig. 11.8
Thrombosis of the superior mesenteric artery. Acute abdomen for two days. Bloody diarrhea and fever. The abdominal survey film showed gaseous distention, especially in the colon. Multiple nodular defects in the ascending colon. 24 hours later the abnormalities had obviously increased (upper right). The distance between the loops of the small bowel, which now were also filled with gas, had definitely increased (not shown). The colon examination performed the next day showed multiple defects arising from the wall which must be hematomas in the mucosa. The hematomas were not palpable during surgery; we have found that this is not uncommon.

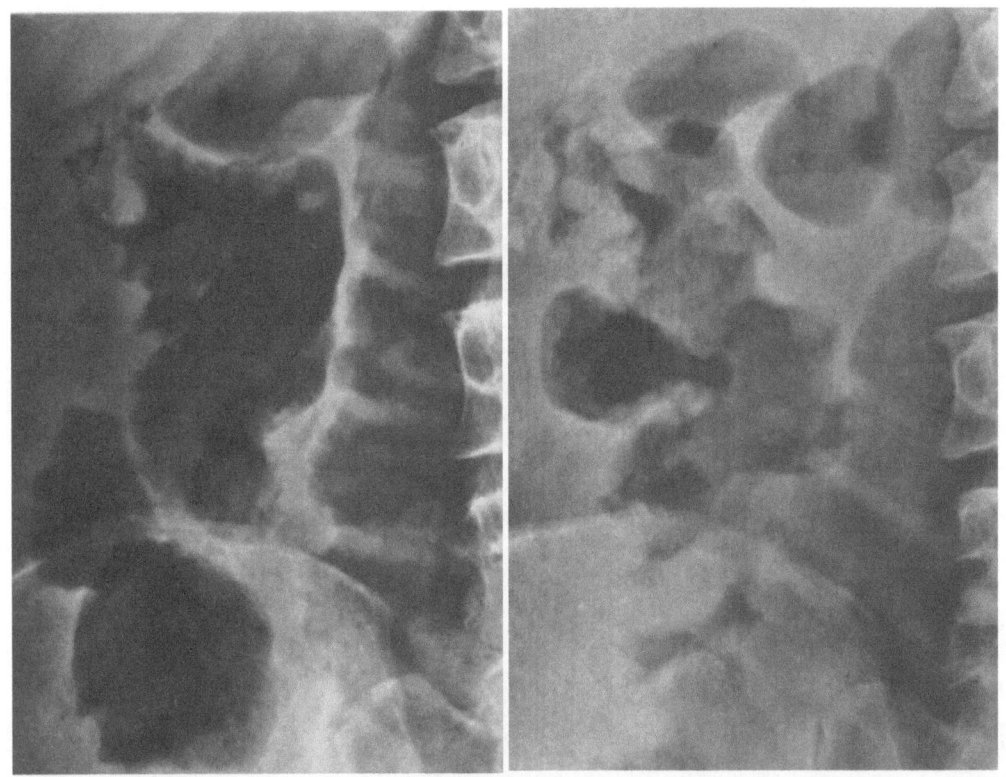

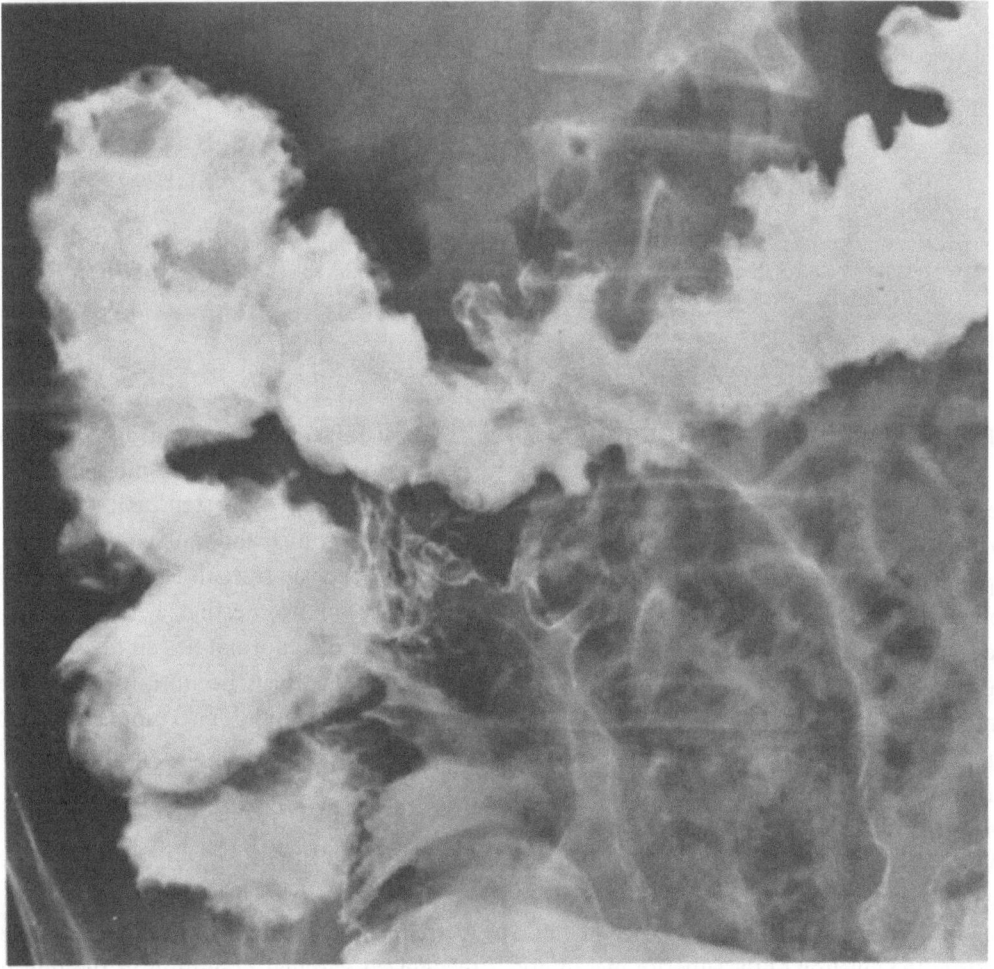

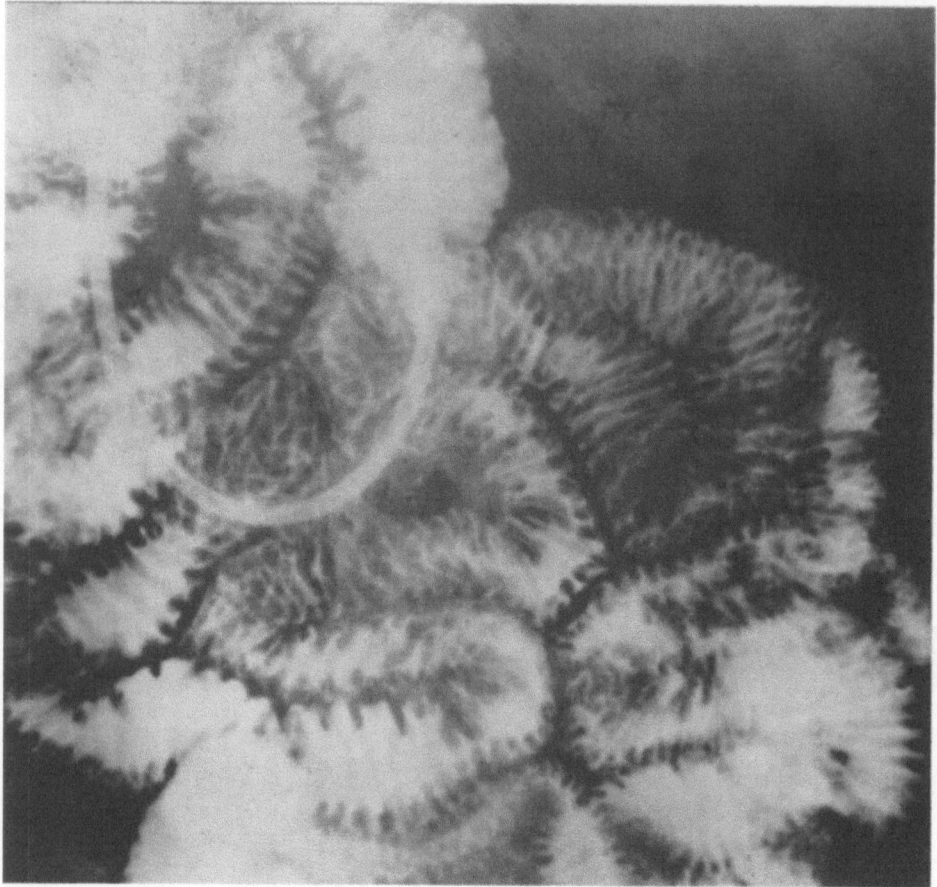

Fig. 11.9
Edematous swollen omega-shaped mucosal folds throughout the small bowel due to a pronounced impairment of the venous flow as a result of liver cirrhosis. The liver is very small; the spleen is greatly enlarged.

3. Periodic vascular insufficiency

a. A decrease in the heart minute volume, due for
   instance to hypertension, can lead to abdominal
   complaints as a result of an inadequate blood
   supply in the intestinal wall, particularly if this
   decrease is temporary and a marginal circulation
   already exists because of an arteriosclerosis or
   some other disorder.

b. After a copious meal, a pre-existing critical
   blood flow in the intestinal wall can suddenly
   become inadequate causing severe abdominal
   cramps; this is called 'intestinal angina'. Such a
   marginal circulation in the intestinal wall is
   usually due to the simultaneous occurrence of a
   stenosis at the junction of the superior mesenteric

artery and the celiac trunk. Not only an arteriosclerosis but also a fibromuscular hyperplasia
can cause such a stenosis. To establish the
diagnosis, an abdominal aortography with
lateral exposures is necessary. An examination
of the small intestine with a contrast fluid
reveals no abnormalities in these patients; the
complaints which occur 1–2 hours after eating
are too short and also not severe enough to
cause visible changes in the mucous membrane.

4. Hemorrhage

A frequently occurring but often completely unrecognized vascular condition in the intestinal wall

is the intramural hematoma. The hematoma can be very small and heals either spontaneously or within several weeks after treatment is initiated without persistent abnormalities (fig. 11.10). However, if the diagnosis is not recognized, the hematoma can become very large and cause total obstruction of the intestinal lumen. The intestinal wall may then become necrotic and perforate, usually causing the death of the patient. The most common cause of hematomas in the intestinal wall is a disturbance of the coagulation mechanism due to treatment with anticoagulants or the use of drugs containing aspirin (fig. 11.11). Much less common is bleeding due to a hemorrhagic diathesis such as hemophilia or a vitamin K deficiency. Although a blunt trauma of the stomach in itself is a frequent cause of hematomas in the intestinal wall, it is also often a concurrent cause in patients with a pre-existing enhanced bleeding tendency. Because it is fixed against the spinal column, the second half of the duodenum is the most vulnerable part of the small bowel and hematomas are indeed encountered in this segment more often than in any other. Polypoid mucosal swelling due to the hematoma can, especially in the proximal part of the small intestine, enhance peristalsis markedly and thereby cause an intussusception of the intestinal loop containing the hematoma into the proximal loop.

Hemorrhage occurs not only in the intestinal wall but also in the mesentery where it causes a local but marked increase in the space between adjacent intestinal loops; the resulting roentgenogram resembles that of the mesenteric cyst. In practice, however, differentiation between these two disorders will never be difficult because subsequent clinical findings and the histories differ completely.

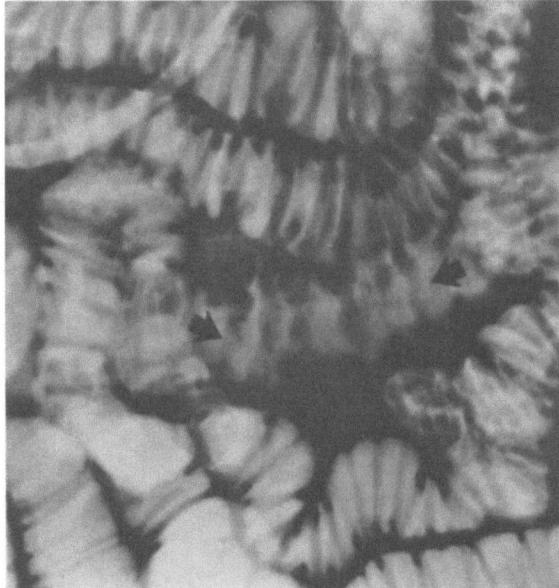

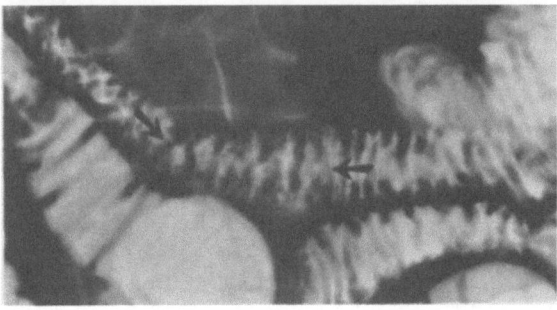

Fig. 11.10
Swollen mucosal folds in a jejunal loop which crossed the spinal column after a blunt trauma of the stomach. Complete recovery within three weeks.

a. CLINICAL SYMPTOMOLOGY

The phenomena due to a vascular accident can vary considerably according to the length of the involved intestinal segment and the rate at which the occlusion develops. Here, too, an important factor is whether or not the collateral circulation can and will develop rapidly. Arterial occlusion occurs more frequently than venous occlusion, develops fairly suddenly and causes shock with a more or less serious ileus or subileus and severe pain in the abdomen. Quite often the history or a subsequent physical examination will clearly indicate the possibility of a vascular accident, such as atrial fibrillation or an advanced arteriosclerosis. The pulse rate can sometimes be of immediate value. A venous thrombosis can cause the same complaints but they usually develop much more gradually. If the thrombosis develops very slowly, then there may be no symptoms at all. In general there is no doubt that the patient suffers the least from the frequently multiple but always very small ischemic occlusions caused by vasculitis. Although obstipation may occur, abdominal pain and diarrhea are the most frequent complaints. The history as well as a brief physical examination usually provides several indications of a disease accompanied by

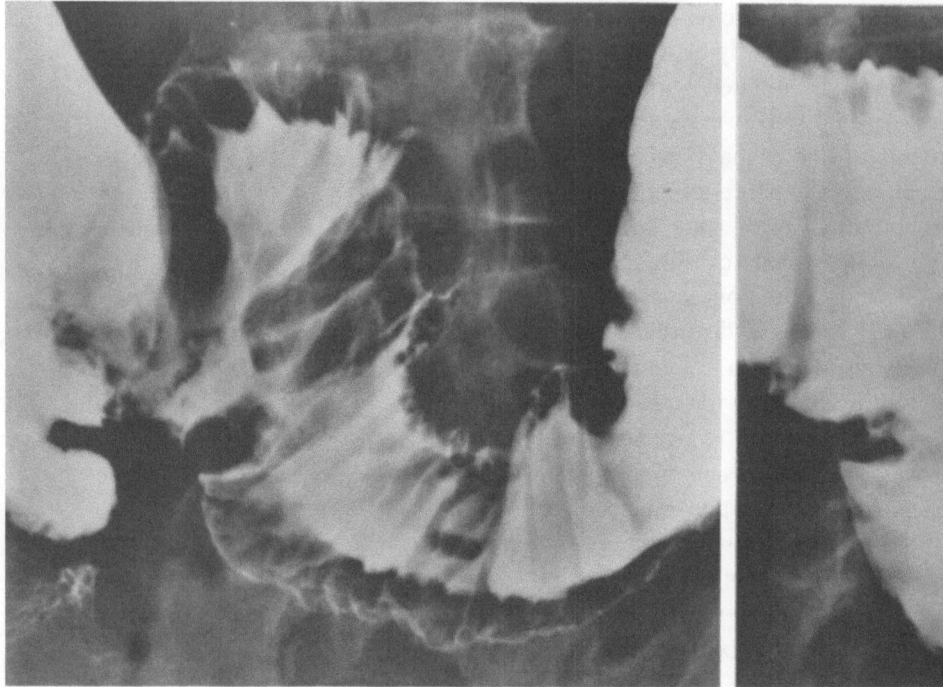

Fig. 11.11
Submucosal hematomas in the transverse colon in a patient with an enhanced bleeding tendency as a result of incorrect anticoagulant therapy. Complete recovery two weeks later.

vasculitis. Thus for instance an examination of the skin and inquiry about complaints of the joints can be quite useful.

In contrast to vascular occlusions which occur in the colon somewhat more frequently than in the small bowel, mucosal bleeding is seen in the small intestine more often than in the colon. The complaints due to hemorrhage can differ even more than those caused by a vascular occlusion. In mild cases there is only a slight discomfort in the abdomen; in a severe case there will be obstruction with vomiting and rectal bleeding. In the event of a hematoma, these complaints are fairly subacute – thus they develop more gradually than those of an arterial occlusion and more acutely than in most cases of venous occlusion.

b. ROENTGENOLOGICAL SYMPTOMS

Venous thrombosis causes a hemorrhagic infarct in the intestinal wall which as a result becomes thicker and stiffer. The x-rays reveal an increase in the space between the infarcted intestine and the ad-

jacent intestinal loops. The mucosal folds become very swollen due to the increased venous pressure and the subsequent development of edema. As a result the spaces between the folds in the jejunum where they are very numerous become so thin that they resemble the thorns on a rose bush – sharply pointed at the tips and concave on either side (fig. 11.12). In the involved intestinal loop these thorny protrusions, which enclose the swollen folds, are found on both sides of the lumen at approximately equal distances from one another. The impressions of these broadened mucosal folds on the contrast column are also called 'thumbprinting'. In the ileum the folds are so scarce and so much shorter that the pattern is that of a stiff tube with smooth walls. The average caliber of the intestine decreases somewhat in the jejunum as well as the ileum because of the thickening of the wall. Under fluoroscopy it can be seen that the peristaltic movements in the pathological loop are clearly diminished or even completely missing. In a somewhat later stage, peristalsis also decreases in the rest of the intestine, sometimes resulting in a total paralytic ileus.

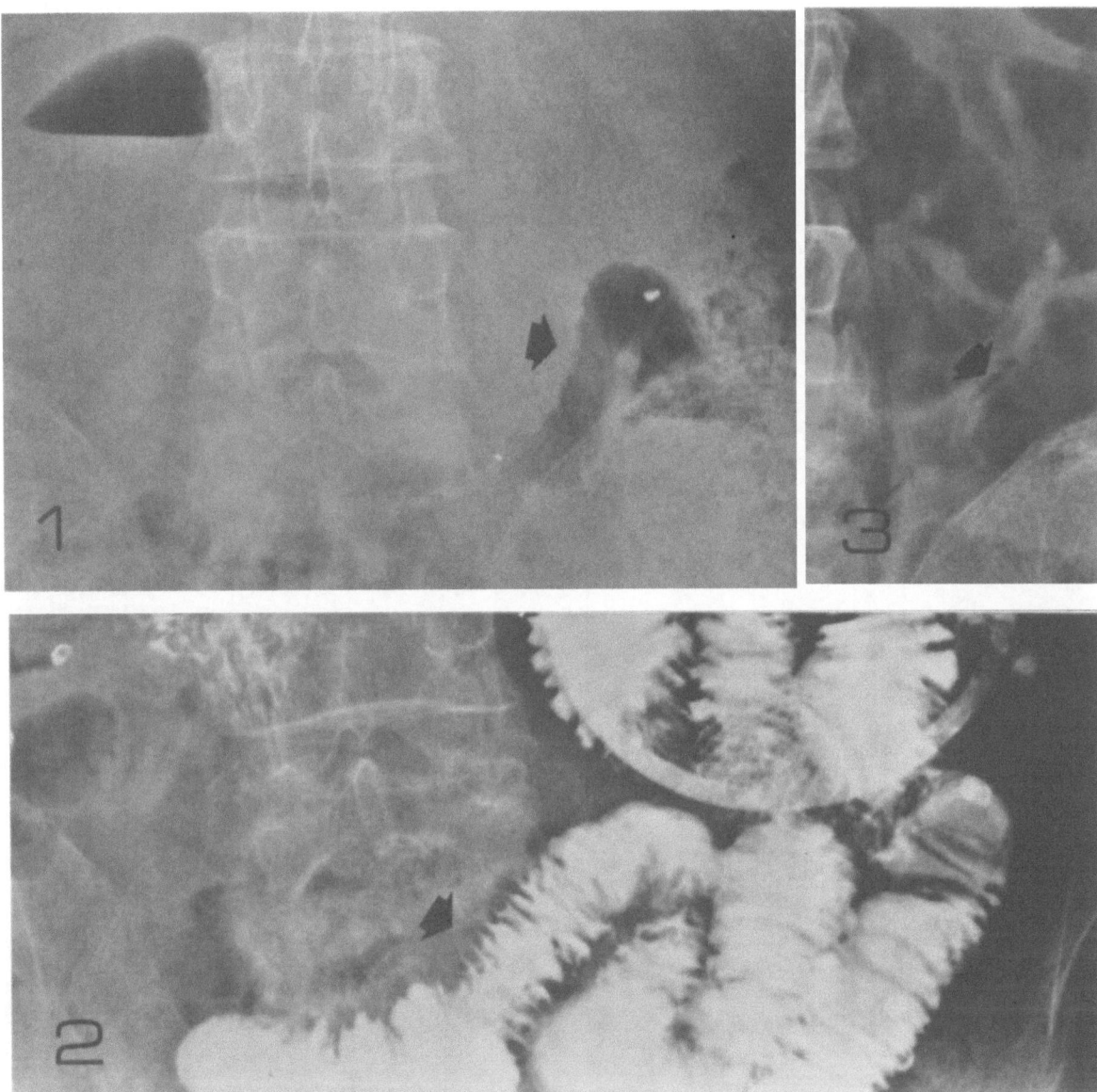

Fig. 11.12
Intestinal loop filled with gas in a patient with acute abdominal pain. The mucosal folds are flattened and obviously broadened. The enteroclysis examination performed the following day shows the same abnormalities in the same loop; the swelling of the mucosal folds has possibly even increased. Several days later an abdominal survey film revealed an intramural film of gas in the intestinal wall at the same site, apparently as a result of local necrosis with limited perforation. Fortunately, because of the very contained nature of the lesion, recovery was complete.

The first radiological examination of patients with abdominal complaints resembling those due to a vascular accident is often a plain abdominal survey film without administration of a contrast fluid, sometimes with a supplementary exposure using a horizontal beam. In the early stages these films already show a solitary air-filled loop of the small bowel which quite obviously can contain the abnormal mucosal folds described above. Another characteristic is that this gas-filled loop remains unchanged, because of the local absence of peristalsis, on repeat films taken several hours later.

The increased vulnerability of the intestinal wall, a result of the vascular insufficiency, can lead to secondary infections and mucosal ulcerations. The

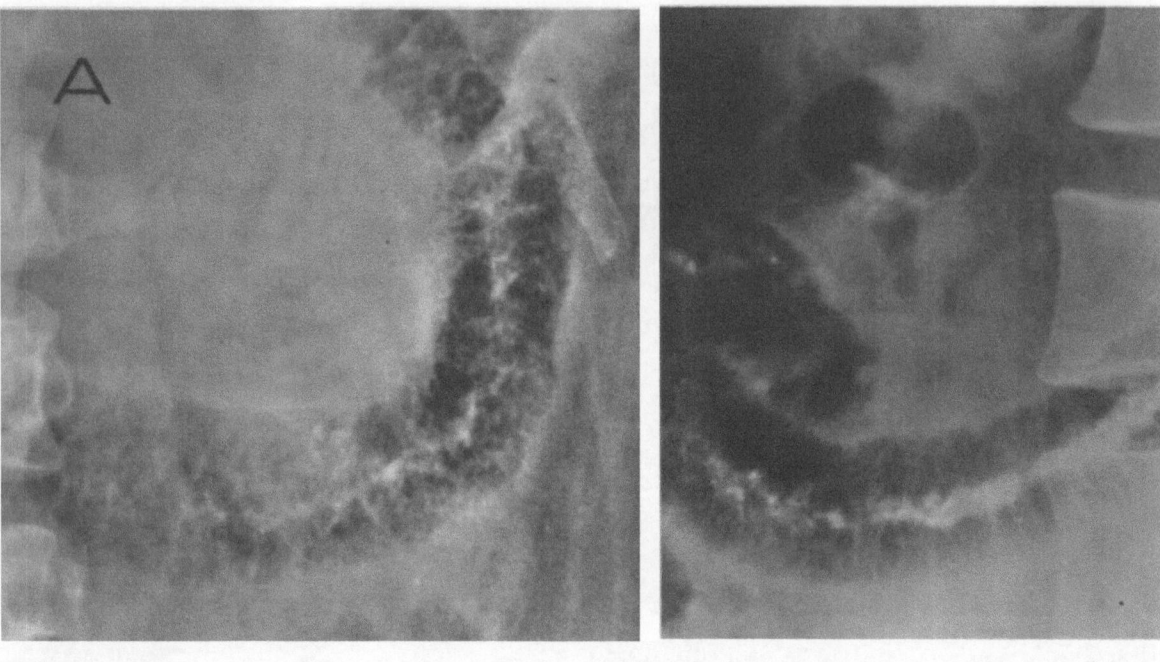

Fig. 11.13
Erratic intramural gas accumulations (A) and large pseudotumors bulging out into the intestinal lumen (B) as a result of submucosal hematomas in a patient with mesenteric thrombosis.

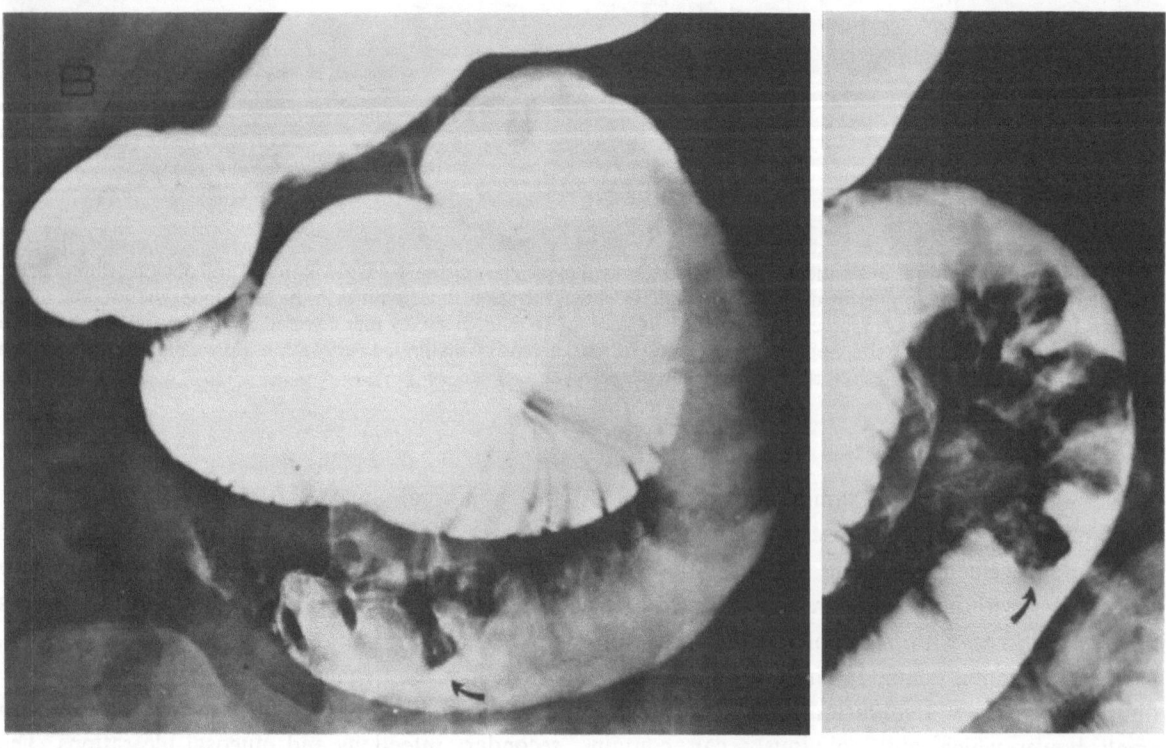

ulcers develop very quickly and are at first so superficial that they usually cannot be visualized on the roentgenograms. As a result of damage to the muscle bundles, after the mucosa the most vulnerable to lack of oxygen, local dilatations can occur which do not result from a stenosis. Later still, the necrosis and the inflammatory process will spread further to the less sensitive connective tissue of the submucosa and subserosa. The pliability of the wall of the bowel although changed by edema, is only slightly diminished. The mucosal folds can disappear completely or become more irregular. This irregularity can be enhanced by lesions in the vessel walls which cause intramural hemorrhage; they develop as a result of the necrotizing enteritis.

We can also find multiple polypoid filling defects due to hemorrhages in a still intact mucosa. These hemorrhages can be massive and cause pseudotumors which bulge far out into the intestinal lumen (fig. 11.13B). As a result of gas-producing intestinal bacteria or open communication with the intestinal lumen, accumulations of gas may become visible within the intestinal wall (fig. 11.13A); they can be differentiated from the gas seen in pneumatosis intestinalis because the latter develops in an intestinal wall of normal thickness and with a normal mucosal pattern. If there are only small quantities of gas, then they appear on the x-ray as thin lines or crevices; a large accumulation of gas can assume the most bizarre shapes.

Total necrosis of the intestinal wall with perforation to the free abdominal cavity as well as a continuation of the gas accumulation until it passes via the intestinal veins into the portal vein and the liver are conditions which are always fatal.

The radiological characteristics of an arterial obstruction can only be differentiated from those of a venous thrombosis in the early stages. Arterial occlusion causes a termination of or a decrease in the blood supply whereas the efferent blood flow remains unimpaired. The intestinal wall is then not thickened but is normal or even thinner and is pale when examined during surgery. The motility is not limited and in fact is locally enhanced. During the roentgenological examination this hypermotility and spasticity prevent sufficient filling of an intestinal loop which has recently become ischemic and dilatation of this loop cannot be visualized. However, this pure arterial pattern does not last long

because the intestinal wall rapidly becomes thickened due to necrosis with inflammatory reactions, hemorrhage and edema; differentiation from a venous thrombosis is then no longer possible, at least radiologically.

In Schönlein-Henoch disease, an acute arteritis which is accompanied by pain in the abdomen and the joints, purpura and nephritis, there is a submucosal edema with moderately swollen mucosal folds. The larger arteries in these intestinal loops, which appear red during surgery, remain unimpaired so that circulation is barely disturbed and as a rule no necrosis or ulcerations will develop. Here, too, motility is enhanced but it encompasses a larger segment than in the early stages of an ischemic infarct. The caliber of the intestine is normal or only slightly decreased.

The etiology of Schönlein-Henoch disease is unknown. For years it was thought to be an allergic disease but today it is considered more likely to be one of the collagen diseases. Unusual for this group of diseases is the fact that Schönlein-Henoch disease is a recurrent disease; in addition the relationship with the concomitant Streptococci infection is unknown. Schönlein-Henoch disease also differs from the other collagen diseases in that it is self-limiting and usually disappears without persistent abnormalities (fig. 11.6A). Recently, however, it has become evident that this differentiation is not clear-cut and that residual abnormalities can in fact be seen (fig. 11.6B).

Although there are good arguments for including the collagen diseases in this chapter on vascular diseases, it was decided that since motility disorders are so common they should be included in the chapter on disturbed motility. An exception has been made for Schönlein-Henoch disease for historical reasons.

Hematomas in the intestinal wall due to hemorrhagic diathesis heal in one or two weeks and, in contrast to hematomas of a vascular accident, with restitutio integrum. Radiologically, however, a simpel hematoma is not always easy to differentiate from hemorrhage due to a vascular accident. A common hematoma is indicated by the presence of a mesenteric mass due to the hemorrhage in the mesentery; in addition the caliber of the intestine does not change and peristalsis remains normal.

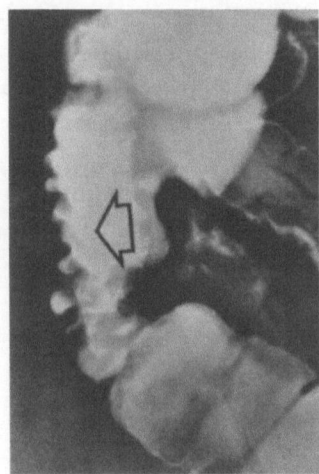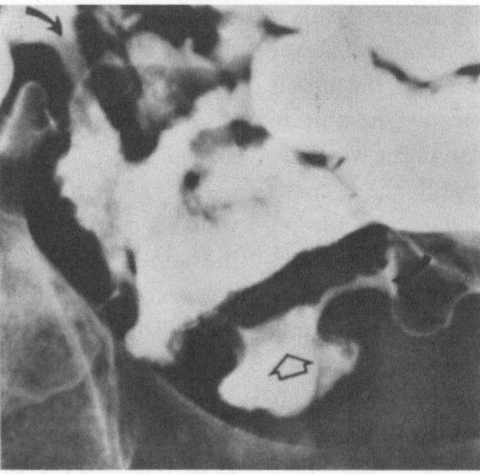

Fig. 11.14
Fibrous remnants after a vascular accident with pseudodiverticula (left), long smooth
stenoses and asymmetrically shriveled ulcers (right). Differentiation from Crohn's
disease by means of radiological examination is usually not possible.

C. PROGNOSIS

The results of ischemia, immediately as well as
later, depend upon the location, the extent, the
rate of development and the total duration.

Anatomically circulation in the intestinal wall
in the distal part of the intestine differs from that
in the proximal part. In the ileum the afferent
vessels lie in the subserosa, thus on the outer side
of the intestinal surface. From here numerous perpendicular branches extend straight through all
layers of the intestinal wall in the direction of the
lumen. In an intestinal segment with this type of
circulation the afferent terminal vessels are not
constricted as quickly by the swelling and compression due to edema and hematomas as those in
the jejunum where both the large and the small
afferent vessels form a network deep in the submucosa and tunica muscularis. An ischemic attack
lasting about 3 hours causes necrosis of the mucosa
but the muscularis usually remains intact. The
mucous membrane becomes totally atrophied as a
result of the necrosis and the mucosal relief disappears; months later, however, there can be a recovery of the mucosa. Then, adhesions or fusion
with adjacent intestinal loops is often seen since a
fibrinous layer coats the intestine as a result of the
ischemia.

An anoxia lasting 5–6 hours also causes damage
to the muscle bundles. Both the inner and the outer
intestinal wall now show necrotic changes and
ulcerations; the latter heal with the formation of
connective tissue and lead 1–3 months later to
shriveling and stenoses. Ischemic stenoses are
usually about 2–5 cm long, have smooth walls and
increase in caliber gradually at the transition to the
healthy intestine on each end (fig. 11.15). In the
case of a tumor, the stenosis is often shorter, has
more irregular margins and the transition to the
normal intestine is much more abrupt.

After ischemia, just as after ulcerations in
Crohn's disease which heal with fibrotic shriveling,
pseudo-diverticula and sacculations can develop on
the antimesenterial side of the intestine with a
straight smooth-walled shriveling on the opposite
side (fig. 11.14). In the colon a persistent abnormality of this type is, however, more common than in
the small bowel. Ischemic episodes lasting 8–9
hours, or longer, cause total necrosis of the intestinal
wall with perforation into the free abdominal
cavity. The nerve cells are the least sensitive to
anoxia so that intestinal motility remains as a rule
unchanged after an infarct.

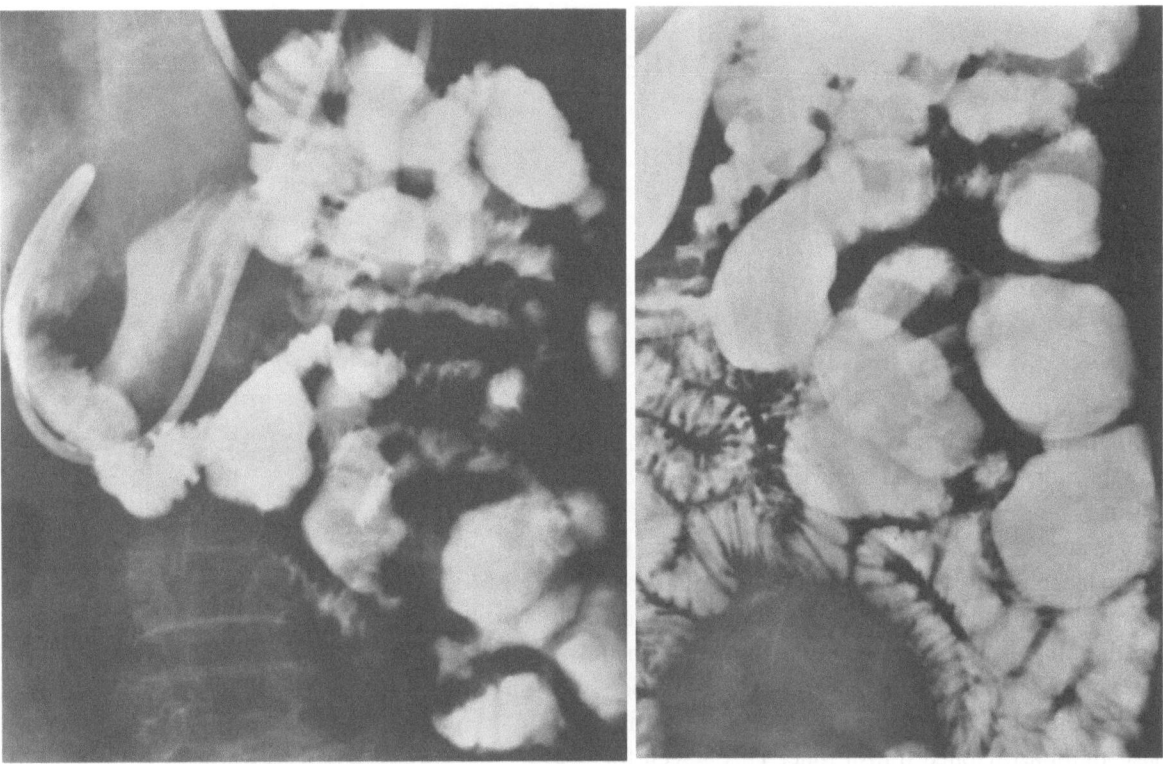

Fig. 11.15
Elderly male with multiple ischemic stenoses several centimeters in length in the jejunum. The mucosal pattern has disappeared in the intestinal segments between the stenoses. Although an angiographic examination revealed a vascular insufficiency in this part of the small bowel and the appearance of the vessels indicated that the mesentery was shriveled, it is not possible to distinguish here between a state after remission of an inflammatory process, for instance Crohn's disease, and a primary vascular disease. Because of the stenoses, a biopsy instrument could not be introduced so that celiac disease with atrophy of the mucosa and ulcerations also could not be excluded – at least not in this manner.

Bibliography chapter XI

BOLEY S. J.; SCHWARTZ S. S.; DONALDSON R. M. (1971) *Vascular disorders of the intestine.* Butterworths, London.
REUTER S. R.; REDMAN H. C. (1972) Gastrointestinal angiography. Monographs in *Clinical Radiology*, Saunders, Philadelphia.
Vascular diseases of the alimentary tract. *Clinics in gastroenterology*, Saunders, Philadelphia. (1972).
VOEGELI E. (1974) *Die Angiographie bei Dünndarm und Dickdarmerkrankungen.* Thieme, Stuttgart.

XII

DISTURBED MOTILITY

Although many highly divergent diseases can be accompanied by changes in the motility in the small bowel, understanding and knowledge of the mechanism responsible for these motility disorders can be considered no more than rudimentary. The infusion technique has shown that motility is disturbed much more frequently than is generally assumed. On the other hand we have also found that when the contrast medium is administered orally hypermotility is sometimes incorrectly diagnosed on the basis of an accelerated transit time. This is seen for instance in achylia gastrica or may be due to hyperperistalsis of the stomach. In both cases there is an accelerated gastric emptying and therefore a shorter transit time. The elimination of this variable factor, the gastric emptying time, in the enteroclysis examination has increased the possibilities of comparing the transit time through the small intestine (see page 27).

The greatest contribution toward establishing the diagnosis of disturbed motility is without a doubt the fact that during this examination the contrast column is followed under intermittent fluoroscopy so that very local changes in motility are as a rule no longer overlooked (figs. 12.1 and 12.2).

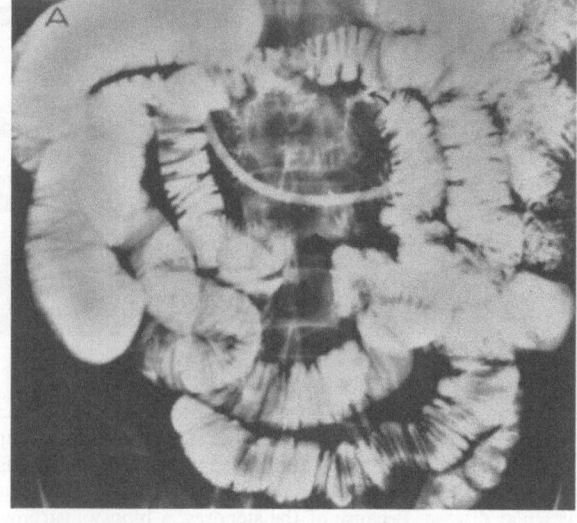

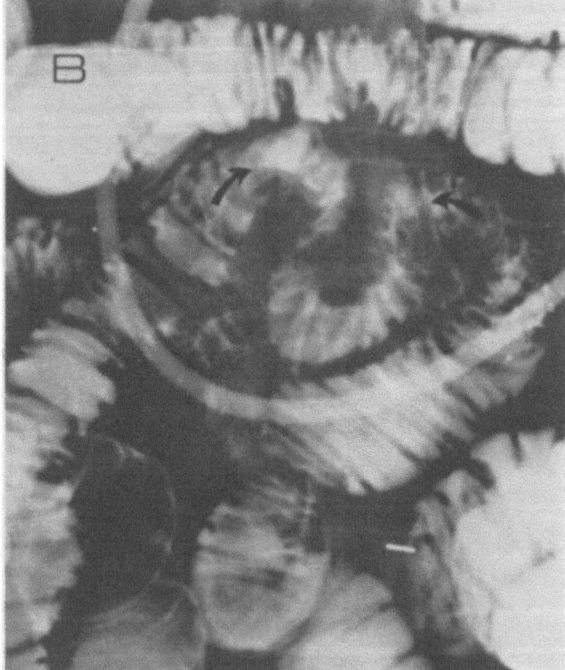

Fig. 12.1
X-rays of a patient with very local enhanced motility of the small bowel without visual abnormalities of the mucosal folds.
A. Radiation enteritis, shortly after irradiation for Hodgkin's disease. After a laparotomy staging procedure, the involved intestinal loops fused with the surroundings and as a result were more susceptible to x-ray damage.
B. A follow-up examination two years later showed that the position of the involved intestinal loop has not changed; now, however, mucosal changes can be seen. The fold relief has become irregular, the intestinal wall is thickened and rigid, and total dilatation is no longer possible.

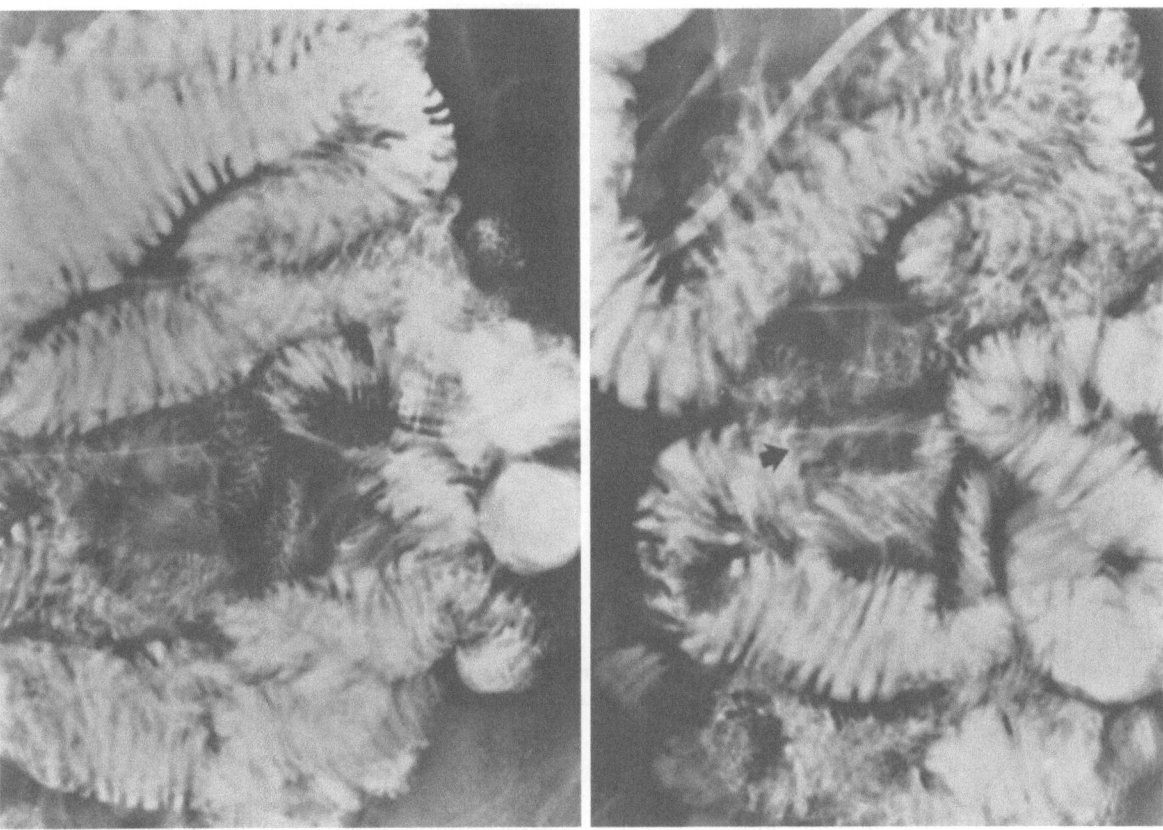

Fig. 12.2
Adhesions after abdominal surgery; displacement of these loops by means of compression and palpation was not possible. In one of the two segments in the contraction phase, the feathered mucosal pattern (→) is clearly visible.

Some diseases are accompanied by the strange phenomenon of either an enhanced or a decreased motility, such as for instance the collagen diseases and diabetes mellitus. Thus not only a hypomotility is signalized but also a hypermotility; the latter is due to a mild anoxia of the intestinal wall. In the collagen diseases, this anoxia is due to a vasculitis; in diabetes it is the result of an insufficiency of the peripheral circulation due to arteriosclerotic changes in the walls of the arteriolae. If there is a diabetogenic diarrhea, then as a rule there will also be a retinopathy and the kidney and pancreas functions will be disturbed. The impaired functioning of the pancreas can be such that resorption of diverse food substances is disturbed resulting in a pancreatogenic steatorrhea.

If motility is not sufficient to propel the contrast fluid distalwards quickly, as indicated by the fact that very few intestinal loops are in a state of contraction, the barium suspension will flocculate almost immediately (fig. 12.3).

On the basis of the number of patients and also the number of causative factors, a decreased motility occurs in the intestine more frequently than a hypermotility. As far as the latter is concerned, an enhanced motility throughout the entire small bowel is seen more often than a local hyperperistalsis. Although seemingly paradoxical, most states of hypomotility alternate with periods of hypermotility. In fact these attacks of hyperperistalsis cause most of the patient's subjective complaints and lead him to consult a physician. The causative factors of a disturbed motility of the small intestine can be grouped in several major categories:

A. neurogenic or humoral
B. mechanical obstruction; ileus

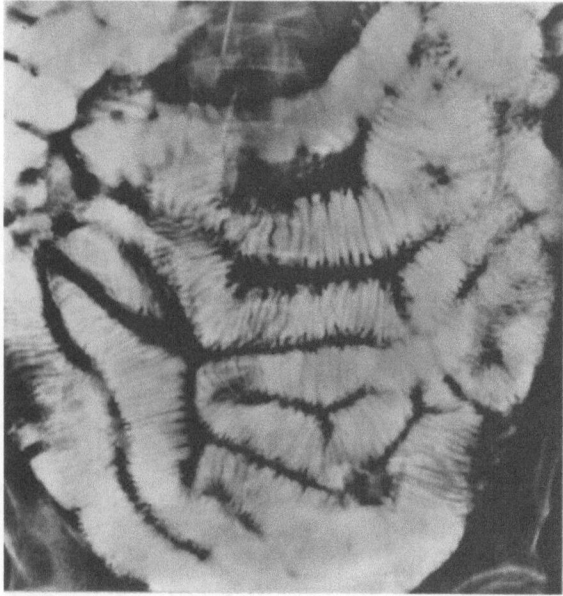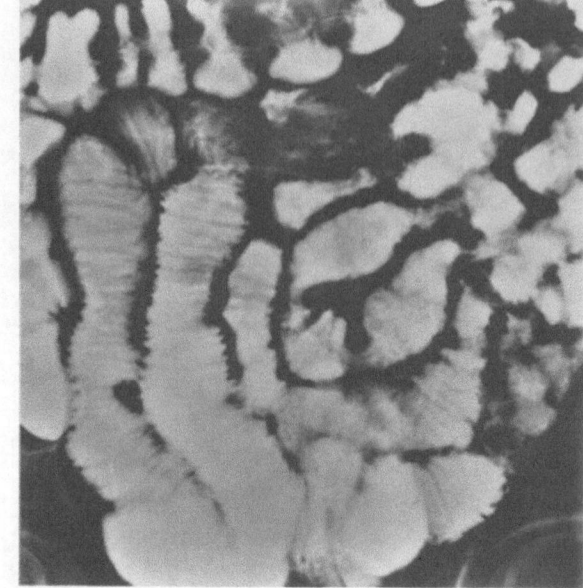

Fig. 12.3
Pancreatogenic steatorrhea with some dilatation of the intestinal lumen wihout an increase in motility. (Under the influence of drugs?) Since the contrast fluid cannot be propelled distalwards quickly in this case, a marked flocculation develops within several minutes (right).

C. diseases affecting the intestinal wall
D. inflammatory processes
E. allergic reactions
F. anoxia
G. disturbed resorption.

A. NEUROGENIC OR HUMORAL FACTORS

Carcinoid lesions and states of fear or emotion cause a pronounced increase in peristaltic movements; this is due to the elevated adrenalin production. The mechanism of the diarrhea which tends to accompany a hyperparathyroidism is unknown; it is possible that a reduced production of gastric acid and the accelerated gastric emptying which is in part the result of the former play a role.

Many of the diseases in this group, however, lead to a decrease in peristaltic movements. The most common cause is without a doubt prolonged medication with tranquillizers, sedatives or antispasmodics (see page 306). Other factors are diabetic neuropathy, amyotrophic lateral sclerosis, multiple sclerosis, chronic alcoholism, myoedema, pregnancy, severe abdominal pain and peritonitis.

Dilatation, which is sometimes quite pronounced, and reduced peristalsis, particularly in the proximal part of the small intestine, are also encountered in Naish's syndrome (fig. 12.4). This disease, described by Naish and his associates in 1960 (GUT, 1, 62), is due to degenerate changes in the myenteric plexus. The course is chronic, gradually increases in severity and is characterized by periods of temporary exacerbation or abatement of the complaints. Inadequate mixing of the digestive juices with food substances in the proximal jejunum impairs digestion; in this section of the bowel rapid flocculation of the barium suspension is also often seen (fig. 12.5). Periods of severe abdominal pain can occur as a result of segmented nonpropulsive contractions in the small intestine; histological examination shows that these contractions are due to such a marked hypertrophy of the innermost layer of smooth circular muscle in the intestinal wall that the thickened wall is even obvious macroscopically.

Differentiation between this disease and drug-induced atony of the intestine, some cases of amyloidosis or scleroderma will not always be possible by means of the radiological examination alone. To establish the diagnosis in such cases it is particularly important that the history be complete and accurate

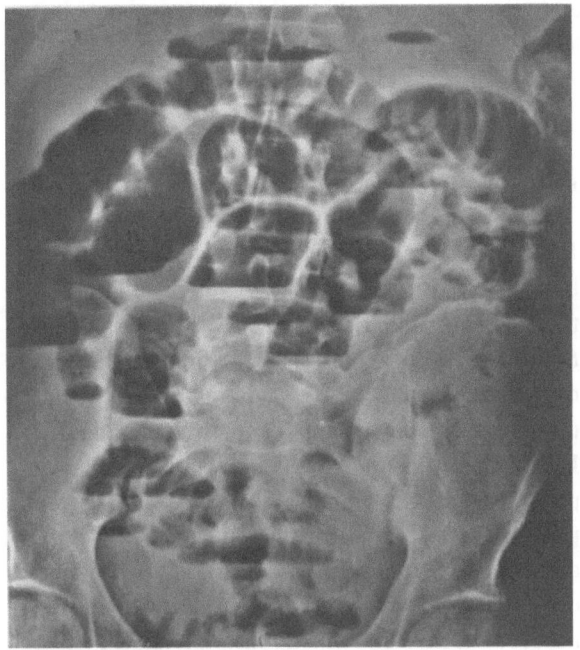

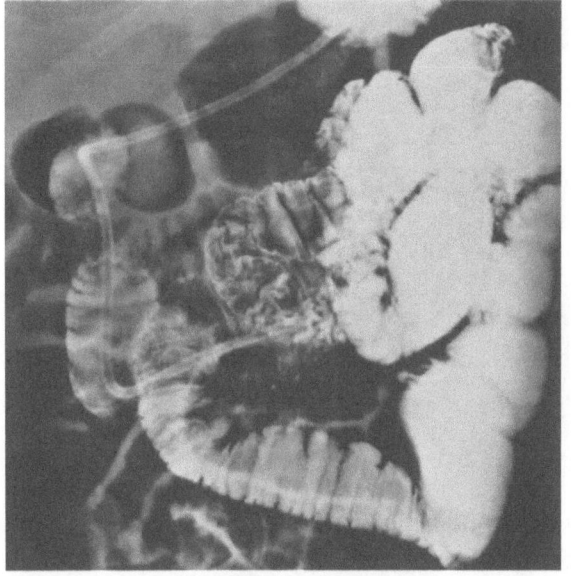

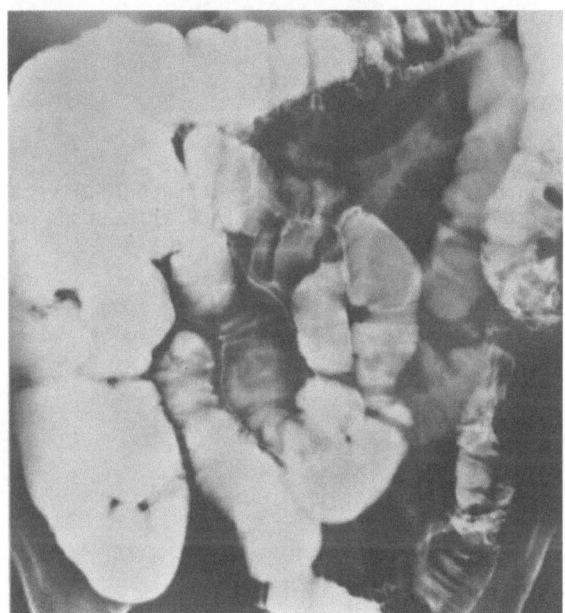

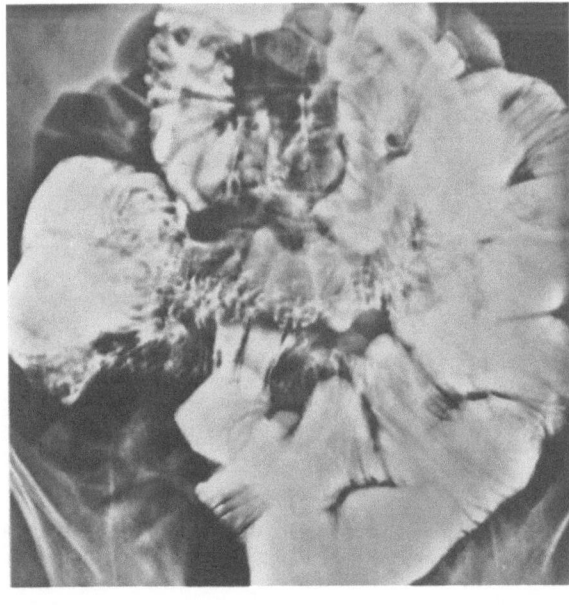

Fig. 12.4
Two patients with degeneration of the nerve cells in the wall of the bowel (Naish's syndrome). Although the intestinal loops are markedly dilated in both patients, contracted segments can still be seen. Numerous fluid levels were observed in the erect position.

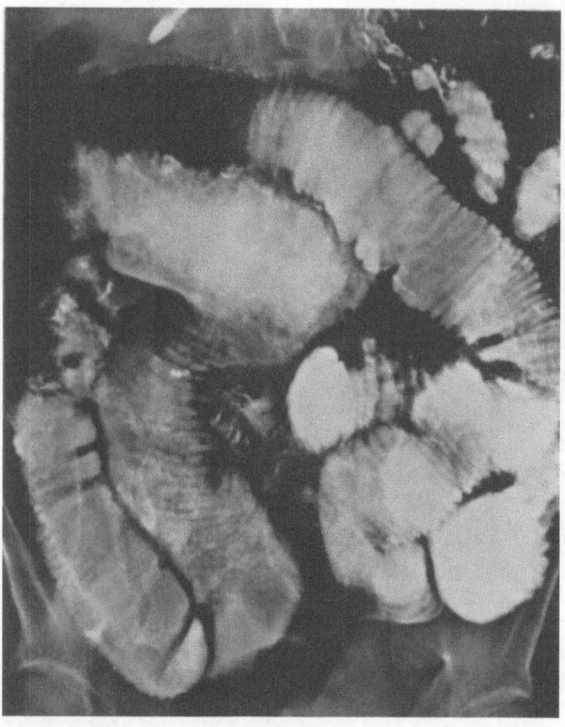

Fig. 12.5
Pronounced flocculation of the contrast fluid in Naish's syndrome. The intestinal loops are highly dilated, as in the patients in fig. 12.4.

and that mucosal biopsies be examined histologically.

B. MECHANICAL OBSTRUCTION

Mechanical obstructions due to stenotic processes, bands or multiple adhesions cause a dilatation of the intestine which increases as the distance from the obstruction decreases. In the first instance these obstructions cause a pre-stenotic hyperperistalsis; the peristaltic movements decrease in a later stage. Even when this latter phenomenon is observed, peristalsis has not changed in the most proximal part of the bowel where the caliber of the loops is also entirely normal (fig. 12.6). This finding is extremely important for differentiation from drug-induced atony, in which case peristalsis in the proximal intestine is also clearly reduced. When a subileus gradually deteriorates, becoming a manifest ileus, dilatation also spreads in the proximal direction so that ultimately the peristaltic movements will be decreased in this area too, and

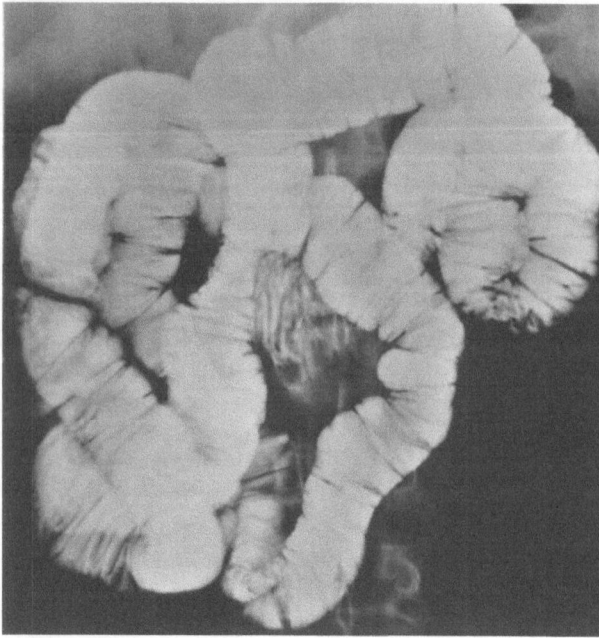

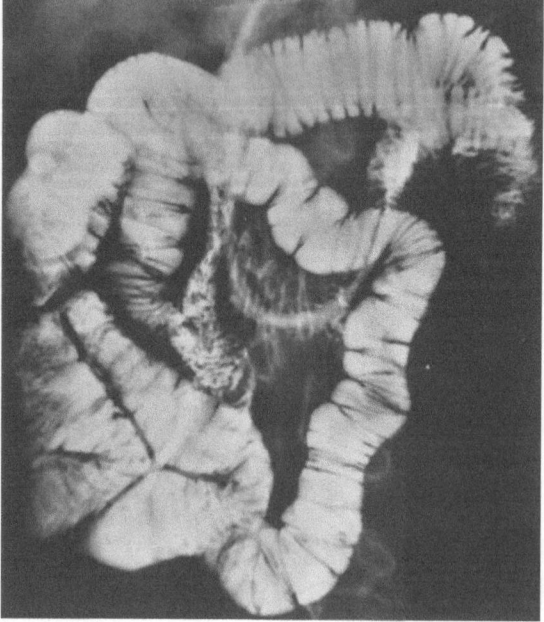

Fig. 12.6
Dilated intestinal loops due to a mechanical obstruction in the distal ileum. Although in this stage of the enteroclysis examination intestinal segments can no longer be seen which are in a state of contraction, the contractility was completely normal at the beginning of the examination (right).

differentiation from a drug-induced atony becomes more difficult.

As long as peristalsis still exists and the obstruction is therefore not total, it is certainly worthwhile to try to demonstrate by means of the enteroclysis examination the reason for and the location of the obstruction. Thickening of the barium suspension in the small intestine, feared for so many years, never occurs; on the contrary the contrast fluid becomes rather highly diluted so that in the case of an ileus the s.g. of the first dose of contrastfluid must be slightly higher than normal. In addition it is recommended that the rate of flow be somewhat lower than normal since the administration of large amounts of fluid (2–2½ liters) will soon cause a decrease in the remaining peristaltic movements, especially when transit through the bowel is markedly restricted. We have found, however, that such large quantities of contrast fluid will pass through the small intestine very rapidly, and through the thinnest stenosis within 8–12 hours. Before an enteroclysis examination of a patient with ileus, the possibility that the obstruction is localized in the colon must be excluded since then resorption of fluid from the contrast column will certainly cause thickening of the barium suspension on the proximal side of the stenosis. In case of doubt or difficulties, retrograde enteroclysis can be considered (fig. 12.7).

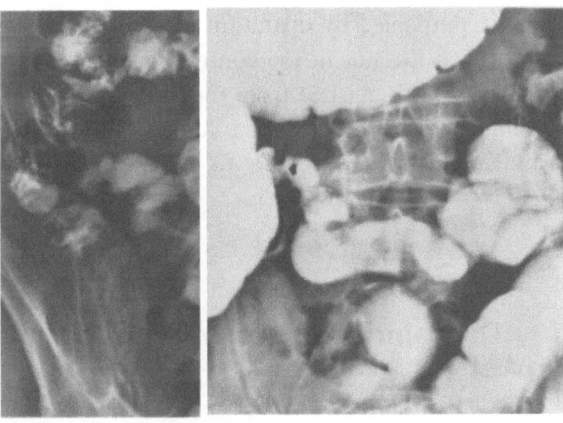

Fig. 12.7
Obstruction in the ileum several centimeters proximal to Bauhin's valve, due to a chronic nonspecific inflammation. It was not possible to reach the site of the obstruction in spite of the administration of 2½ liters of contrast fluid; this was, however, achieved quickly during a colon examination with rectal filling.

C. DISEASES AFFECTING THE INTESTINAL WALL

It will be obvious that diseases affecting connective and muscular tissue as well as those characterized by diffuse amyloid deposits will severely impede normal functioning of the musculature. Some of the collagen diseases (see page 275) and amyloidosis (see page 323) can be accompanied by a clearly decreased motility and an increased caliber which may be very local or can involve large segments or even the entire intestine. As mentioned elsewhere (page 298), the collagen diseases are frequently accompanied by vasculitis which can eventually also give rise to a local anoxia of the intestinal wall and therefore a hyperperistalsis. In amyloidosis, too, motility can be enhanced; in this case, however, it is due to stimulation of the peristaltic movements by abnormal stretching of the intestinal wall as a result of the meteorism which can develop in this disease.

A pronounced decrease in motility without a dilatation of the intestinal loops is also seen in an acquired generalized lymphedema. The intestinal wall is then so thick and rigid that persitalsis has become impossible, even if the musculature is intact.

D. INFLAMMATORY PROCESSES

Extensive inflammatory processes in the wall of the small bowel can impair the normal function of the musculature mechanically, but can also damage the muscle layers themselves. As mentioned previously (page 202) motility in the distal ileum can also be reduced if there is a right-sided ulcerative colitis with an inadequate Bauhin's valve. In none of these cases is there a marked dilatation of the lumen. Inflammatory processes on the other hand can also cause a local hyperperistalsis or spasms in (usually) nearby sections of the small bowel or colon. The origin and the action of these reflex mechanisms are not known precisely.

Chemical enteritis usually causes a decrease in motility; this is seen for example in lead poisoning and uremic enteritis. A disturbed kidney function, whether due to diabetes or not, can lead to an in-

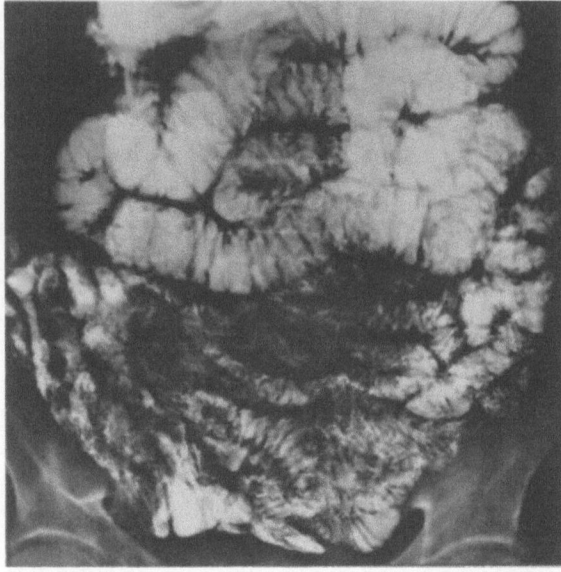

Fig. 12.8
Pronounced hypermotility of the entire ileum with some stagnation of the contrast fluid in the jejunum as a result of numerous fusions and adhesions in the distal half of the small bowel. Compression showed that all ileal loops were totally fused.
  The patient complained of considerable rumbling in the stomach and attacks of pain, especially when he assumed certain positions. Occasionally a subileus developed with numerous fluid levels.

creased urea concentration in the blood. The urea can then diffuse into the lumen of the intestine where urea enzyme causes the formation of ammonia leading to a chemical enteritis, sometimes accompanied by ulcerations. It should be noted that ulcerations in the intestinal wall of kidney transplant patients are not due to a chemical enteritis but are the result of changes in the vessels caused by immunosuppressive therapy. The chemical enteritis caused by gastric acid in Zollinger-Ellison disease (page 235) also results in hypermotility, probably because the content of the intestine is considerably enlarged as a result of hypersecretion and severe malabsorption.

E. ALLERGIC REACTIONS

Infestations by worms (ascaris) and parasites (Giardia lamblia) as well as allergic reactions to food substances such as for instance milk can cause violent, sometimes very local, peristaltic movements with a pronounced narrowing of the intestinal lumen. A very local hypermotility can also be encountered in Schönlein-Henoch disease, a possibly allergic vasculitis which as a rule disappears without persistent abnormalities.

F. ANOXIA

In all cases involving a mild anoxia of the intestinal wall, motility can be enhanced locally. The lumen of the intestine is then always significantly smaller and the mucosal folds lie very close together. Examples of such diseases are vasulitis as in for instance collagen diseases, radiation enteritis, intestinal angina and vascular insufficiency due to adhesions (fig. 12.8).

G. DISTURBED RESORPTION

Diseases belonging to this category are pancreatogenic steatorrhea, Zollinger-Ellison disease (see page 235) and adult celiac disease (see page 311).
  Impaired resorption of food substances, sometimes accompanied by dilution of the contrast fluid, causes an increase in the contents of the intestine and as a result an enhancement of the peristaltic movements. This 'intestinal hurry' is often accompanied by dilatation of those intestinal loops which are not in the contraction phase; it is then easily distinguished from the 'intestinal hurry' accompanied by a decreased lumen as seen for instance in anoxia or due to allergic reactions (fig. 12.9).

1. Drug-induced atony of the small bowel

It is known that disturbed motility in the colon may develop in patients in psychiatric clinics as a result of the medication prescribed. Serious obstipation may then follow which sometimes even leads to a complete ileus. In general the radiological examination reveals a very long dilated colon which

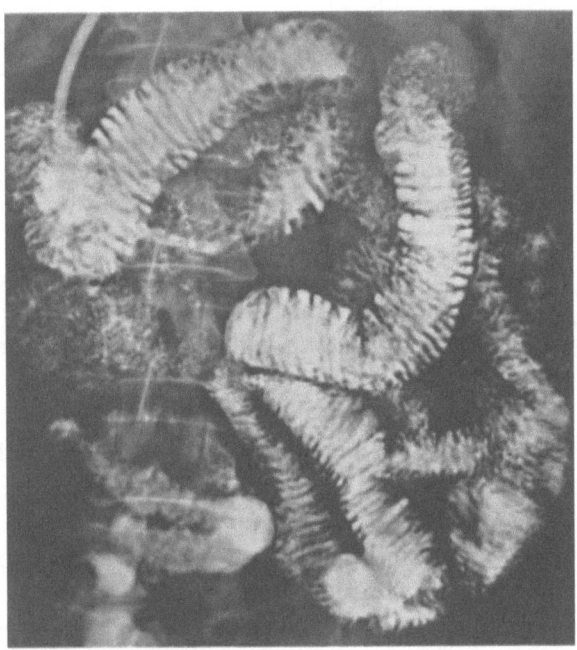

Fig. 12.9
Active motility of the intestine in a patient with pancreatogenic steatorrhea. The loops in the rest phase have an exceptionally large caliber.

empties only partially or not at all. It is seldom or never possible to determine whether the long dilated colon used to be completely normal or that a pre-existing dolichocolon was perhaps a predisposing factor. To prevent frequent recurrence, surgical shortening of the sigmoid is often necessary.

Although it is clear that the small intestine will react in a similar manner to the administration of such drugs, very few publications on this subject are known in radiological literature and only very brief reports have appeared in surgical journals. This can probably be explained by the fact that such abnormalities cannot be demonstrated adequately in this part of the digestive tract by means of the conventional examination techniques. The reason for this is that the dosage and the rate of flow of the contrast medium in a small bowel examination differ completely from those used in the colon examination.

Since the introduction of the enteroclysis technique whereby the rate of flow is the same in all patients, we have noted that in a number of patients a strikingly large dose of contrast fluid is required before the cecum is reached. In fact in some

patients even with our maximum dosage of 1200 cc barium suspension followed by 1200 cc water, the cecum is only reached after 30–45 minutes. Since this technique of roentgenological examination is executed under intermittent fluoroscopy, we have also seen that the intestinal loops in these patients not only are dilated but also show a pronounced decrease in peristalsis. Moreover, in spite of a correct positioning of the Bilbao tube, reflux of the contrast fluid into the stomach occurred fairly regularly. Upon inquiry it appeared that there had been prolonged medication with tranquillizers, antispasmodics or sedatives in all cases. There was no clear difference when these drugs were discontinued several weeks before the examination.

Because of the anatomical location, and especially the patient's complaints, dilatations of the small bowel of iatrogenic origin can best be divided into those of the duodenum and those of the entire small intestine. The roentgenograms then show the following:

A: The duodenum shows rather pronounced dilatation, sometimes mainly in the distal segment (fig. 12.10). This is immediately observed during fluoroscopy in the first few minutes of the examination; at the same time it is noted that this widening

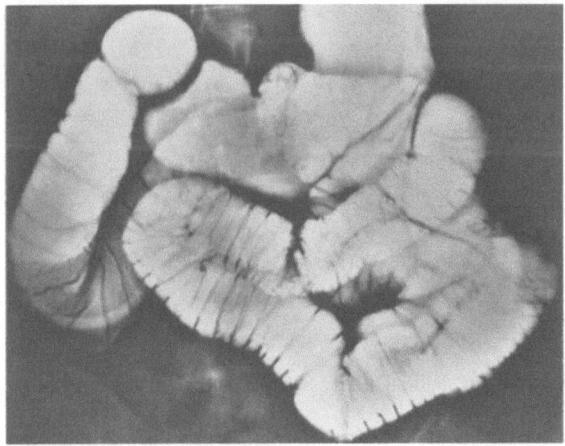

Fig. 12.10
Hypomotility and pronounced dilatation of the entire small intestine due to prolonged use of antispasmodics and pain relievers. The abnormality is already noted during the first few minutes of the examination. The impression of the aorta on the duodenum is often clearly visible in these patients. Retroperistaltic movements in the duodenum are common and there is usually marked reflux of the contrast fluid into the stomach.

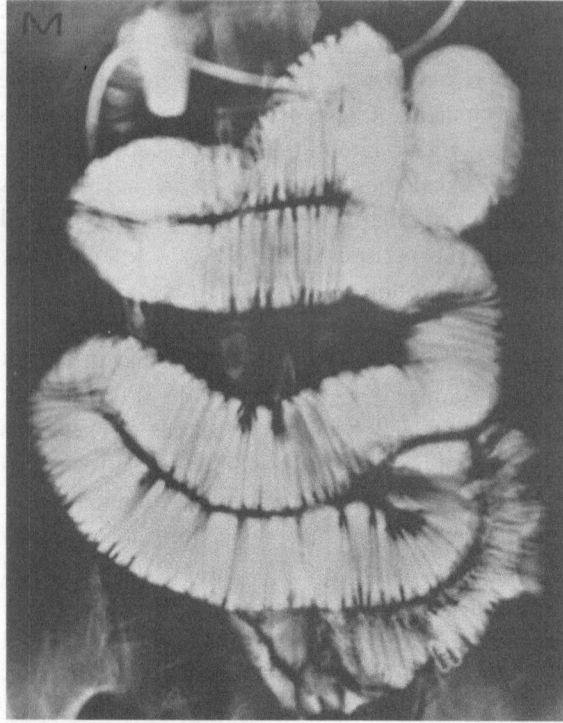

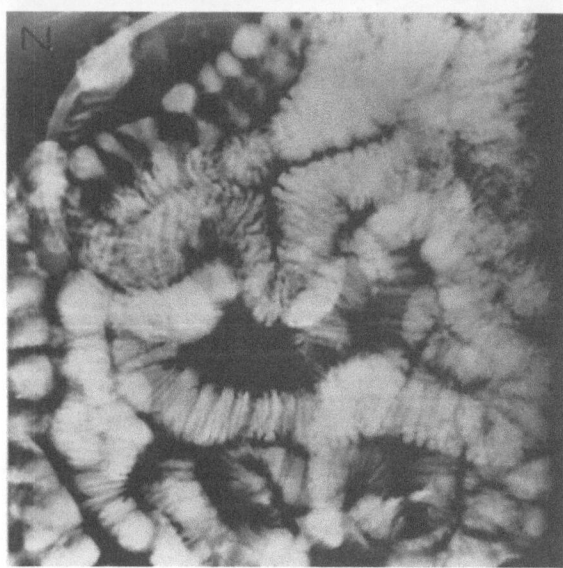

Fig. 12.11
M. Dilated jejunal loops and practically no peristaltic movements.
N. After administration of metoclopramide through the tube or by injection, the tone of the intestine usually increases, dilatation decreases and motility improves.

is accompanied by retroperistaltic pendulum movements. It may already have been discovered beforehand that the tube cannot be inserted into the duodenojejunal junction – or only with considerable

difficulty. In these patients the tube often becomes lodged at the level of the superior mesenteric artery. When it is pushed further, it curls back in the direction of the pylorus.

This apparent obstruction, obviously caused by an acute angle between the aorta and the superior mesenteric artery, is only encountered in thin patients – more especially in patients who have become emaciated within a short period of time. In such cases it makes little difference whether the patient lies on his stomach, either side or his back.

One can easily imagine that the impression of the superior mesenteric artery on a dilated and atonic duodenum would be sufficient to impede passage, certainly in very thin patients since the angle between this vessel and the aorta is already so acute. The retroperistaltic motion so often observed in such a dilated duodenum may be the cause of the reflux of the bilious duodenal contents into the prepyloric area of the stomach. The pyloric ring is after all also influenced by drugs which induce atony so that it does not close sufficiently to prevent this reflux. Just as an esophagitis may develop as a result of the reflux of gastric acid into the esophagus, an antral gastritis can be caused by the reflux of basic gall into the stomach. The superficial erosions then encountered cannot be demonstrated radiologically but are visible during gastroscopy.

The complaints of these patients are not always easy to differentiate from those caused by a duodenal ulcer although it has been noted that vomiting is a frequent symptom and that the hunger pains so classical of an ulcer are not obvious or are missing. Some patients have discovered that a certain position, usually the right or left side, will cause them the least discomfort. A light (bread) meal is in general tolerated more easily than a warm meal and small portions better than large. Although obviously indicated, it is clear that antispasmodics and psychopharmaca will have an adverse effect on the complaints – they will increase rather than decrease. Primperan (metoclopramide) is indicated in these cases; this drug causes an increase in the tone of the musculature of the abdominal and intestinal walls, enhances gastric emptying and decreases the retroperistaltic motion (fig. 12.11). Duration and dosage are of course dependent upon the severity of the complaints; in general recovery will take many weeks and sometimes even months

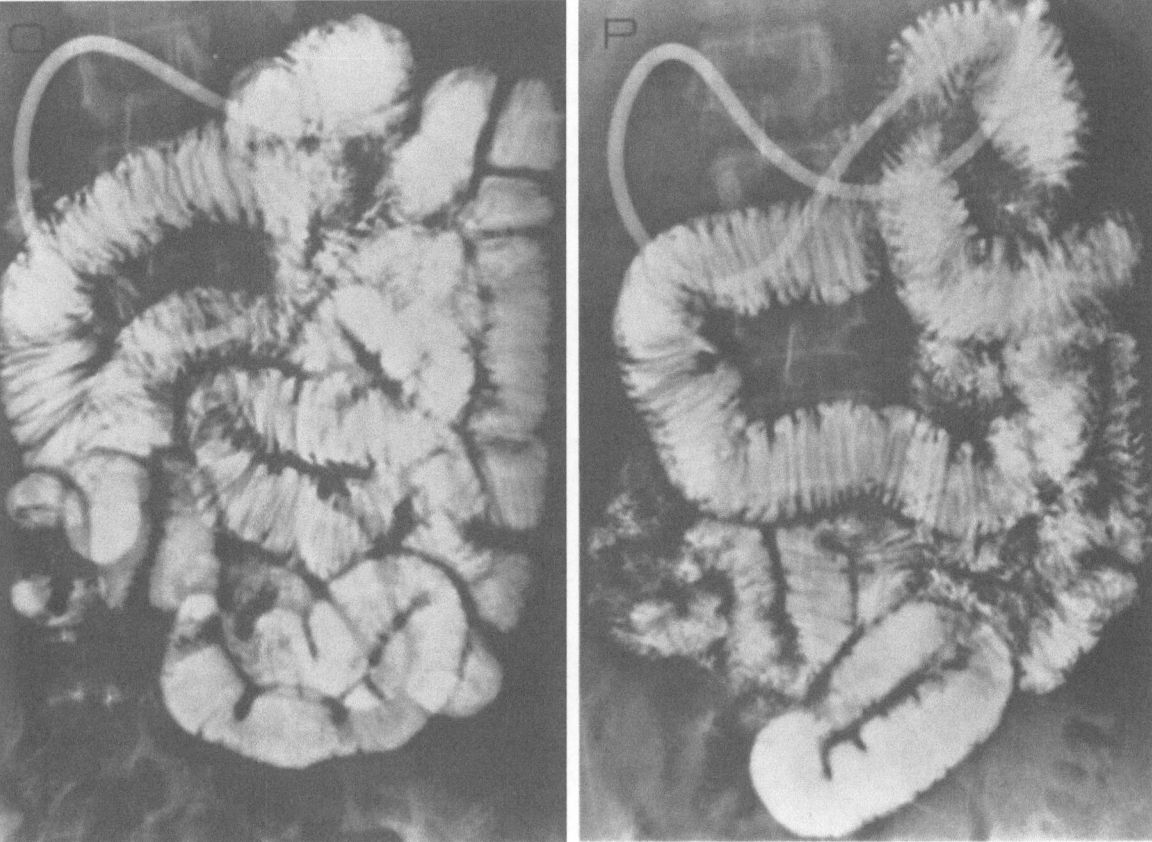

Fig. 12.12

o.   Mild case of drug-induced atony. There are fewer loops in the contraction phase than in normal cases but no dilatation of the lumen can be seen.

p.   Several weeks after the use of tranquillizers was discontinued, the number of intestinal loops in the state of contraction is again normal.

whereby it is recommended that the dosage be gradually decreased (fig. 12.12).

Another way in which the treatment clearly differs from that of an ulcer is diet. If the angle between the aorta and the superior mesenteric artery is acute, it is particularly important to improve the nutritional state of the patient and thereby increase this angle.

B: If the level of the superior mesenteric artery or Treitz's ligament can be passed without difficulty and the cause of the retarded passage appears to lie in a more distal part of the intestine, it has been found that the patient often complains of cramps or colic-like abdominal pain. Of course in these cases a recurrent obstruction must be considered, possibly caused by a benign or malignant tumor and eventually accompanied by temporary intussusceptions.

Radiologically the following may be seen:

1. Only the jejunum is dilated; the ileum is not. Usually the transition from the dilatation to the normal intestine is not gradual but quite abrupt so that sometimes there seems to be an obstruction at the ileojejunal junction (fig. 12.13). A more detailed examination of the intestinal loops in this region reveals no anatomical basis for this assumption and one must therefore speak of a 'pseudo-obstruction'. It is peculiar that this stagnation in the flow of the contrast fluid often suddenly disappears completely; the ileum then fills very rapidly and the cecum is quickly reached. It is highly doubtful whether there is always a true atony in these last cases, certainly if the number of contractions becomes normal in a later stage of the examination (fig. 12.14).

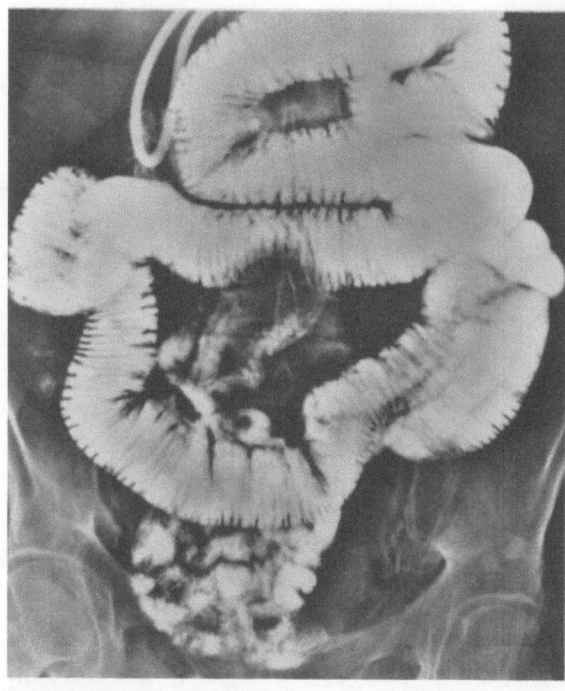

Fig. 12.13
Atony of the small bowel accompanied by pronounced dilatation of the jejunum only. The tone in the ileum is presumably not high and the apparently normal diameter is probably the result of very inadequate filling. In the region of the ileojejunal junction there is probably a physiological bottleneck which either is not found in every intestine or only impedes transit under certain conditions.

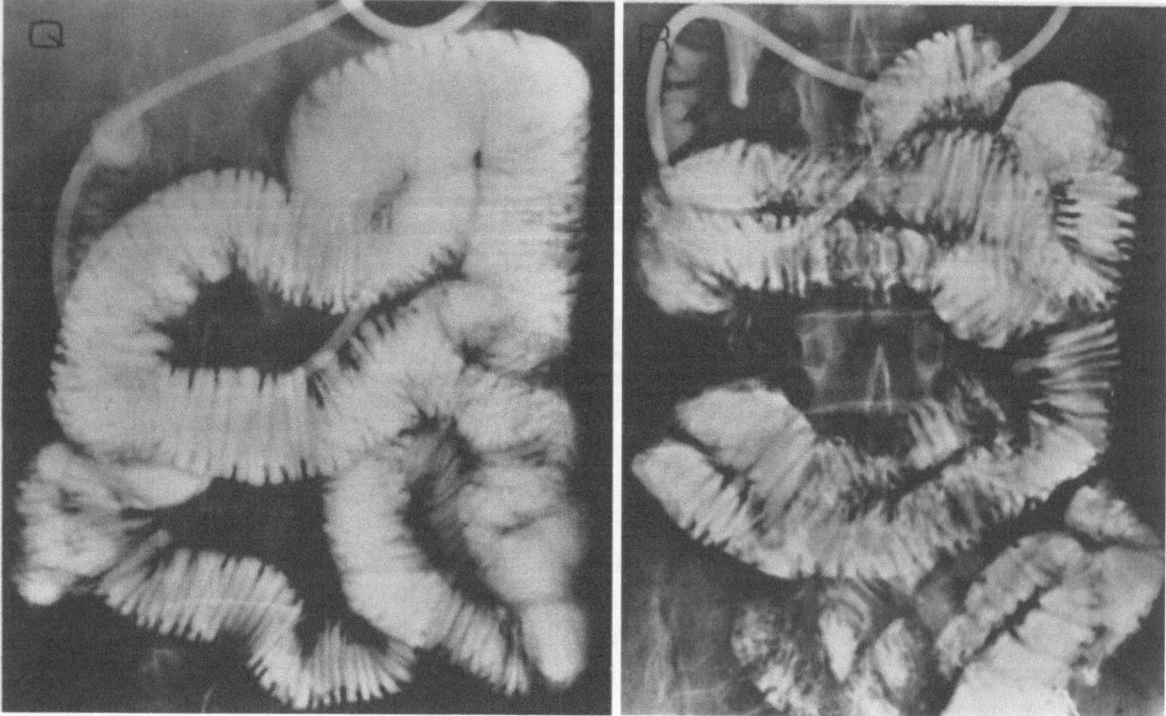

Fig. 12.14
Q. Dilated jejunal loops and stagnation of the passage to the ileum of unknown origin.
R. Several minutes later the stagnation suddenly disappeared. Although there are fewer intestinal loops in the contraction phase than normal, an antony is not at all certain.

2. Both the ileal and the jejunal loops are dilated; the temporary stagnation in the ileojejunal junction is missing in these cases (figs. 12.15 and 12.16).

3. The ileal loops are dilated more than the jejunal; this is the least common form. Because the dilatation increases in the distal direction, a mechanical obstruction is considered the most likely possibility in these cases. And to some extent the obstruction does in fact exist because in these patients the ileum always contains food remnants which definitely impede passage of the contrast fluid (fig. 12.17). Fortunately by means of radiological examination, the obstruction caused by a space-occupying process can in general easily be differentiated from a pseudo-obstruction due to the administration of drugs. In the former case the average caliber of the proximal intestinal loops can be completely normal and peristalsis may be undisturbed or sometimes even increased. If the obstruction is pronounced, then the caliber of the intestine will increase distalwards and just before the site of the obstruction there may be a clear prestenotic dilatation (fig. 12.18). A moderate dilatation and a decrease in the peristaltic movements in the ileum, sometimes also accompanied by atrophy of the mucosa in the region of the ileocecal junction and normal motility in the jejunum, can also be due to the chronic use of laxatives (fig. 12.19). In a case of drug-induced atony on the other hand dilatation of the loops and lack of peristalsis already appear as dominating symptoms in the proximal part of the intestine.

Unfortunately the reason for the stagnation in the flow of contrast medium which may develop in a number of cases at the ileojejunal junction, or in the proximal ileum, is still a matter of conjecture. As yet it appears to be a temporary mechanical twisting, or an eventual torsion of the intestine.

In the small bowel there may appear to be highly different obstructions, apparently physiological in origin, which impede an accelerated flow of contrast medium. It is obvious that this is also true of adhesions and bands which develop after surgery. The latter are, however, easily demonstrated on

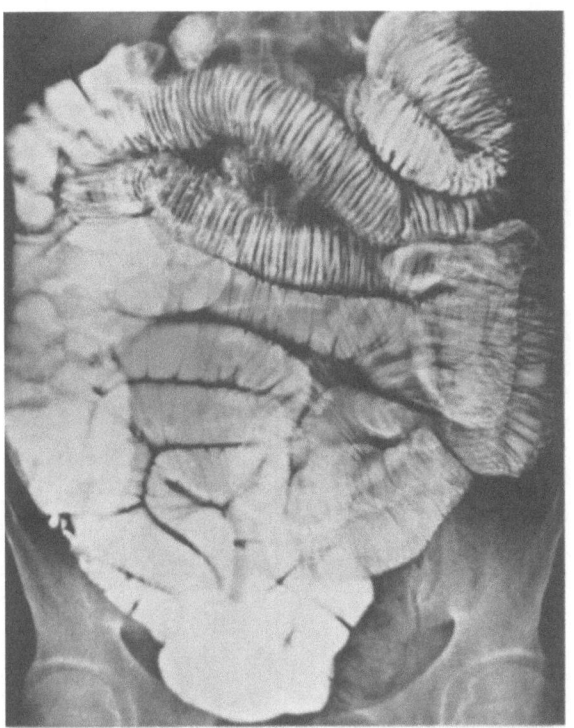

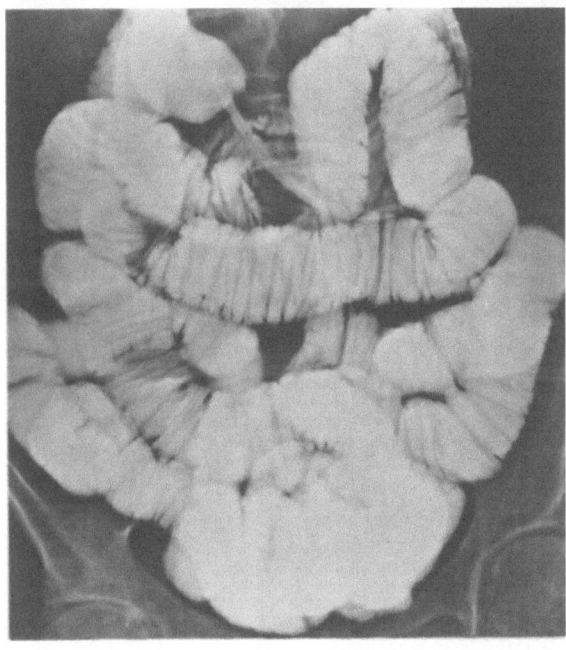

Fig. 12.15
Two clear-cut cases of atony of the entire small bowel, as a result of prolonged medication with vagotonic agents.

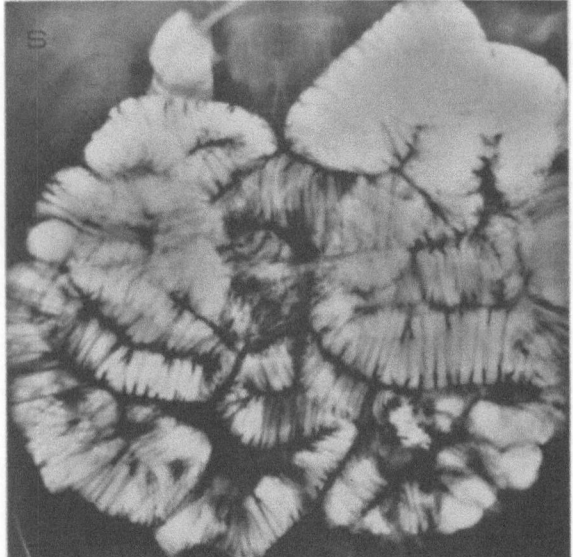

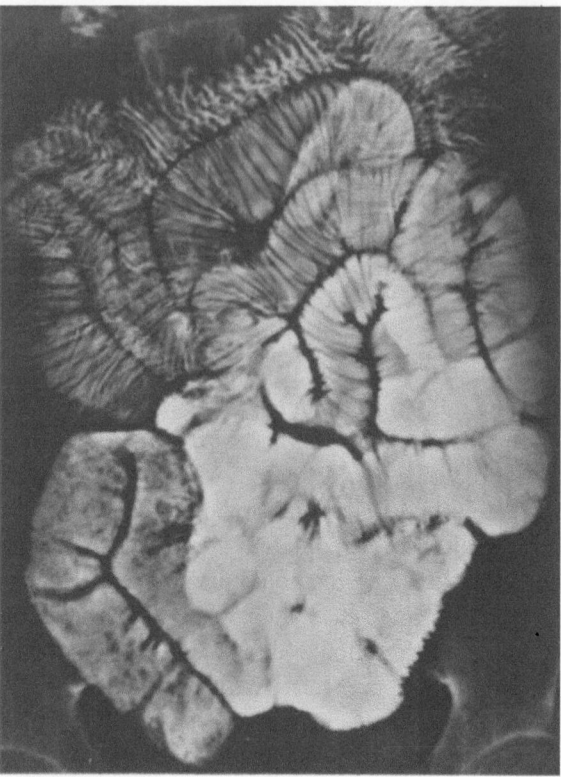

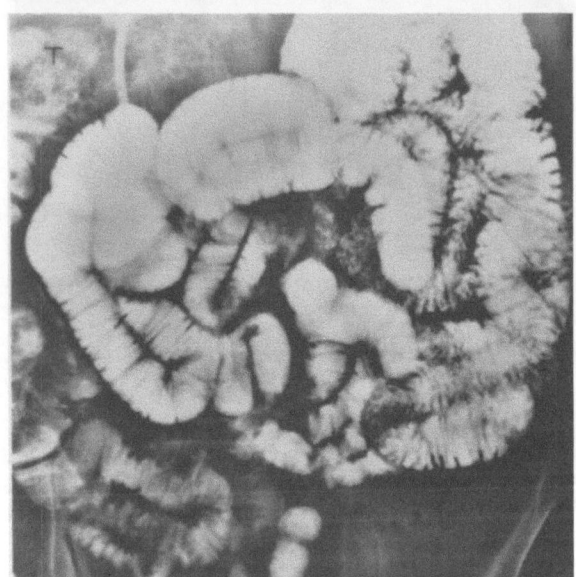

Fig. 12.17
Drug-induced atony of the intestine. In the distal ileum there
are food remnants from the previous day which act as an
extra mechanical obstruction and impede passage.

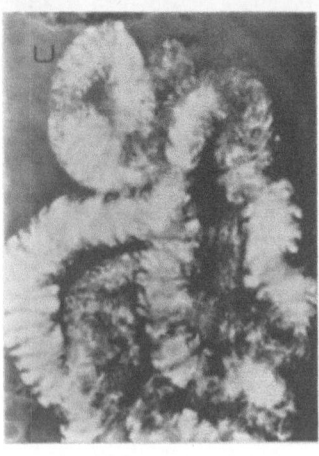

Fig. 12.16

s. Moderately pronounced atony of the small intestine due
to prolonged medication with tranquillizers. Because
the patient complained of recurrent attacks of abdominal
pain, antispasmodics were prescribed and the complaints
increased.

t. All drug therapy was discontinued for three months; at
the end of this period some improvement in the motility
could be observed. Subjectively, however, the complaints
had already diminished considerably. For the previous
examination 1300 cc contrast fluid were required to
reach the cecum; this time only 900 cc were used.

u. 1½ years later a follow-up examination showed that
peristalsis and the caliber of the intestine had become
completely normal. We have found that an improvement
in motility always precedes normalization of the tone of
the intestine. The patient's complaints almost always
disappear sooner than the radiological abnormalities.

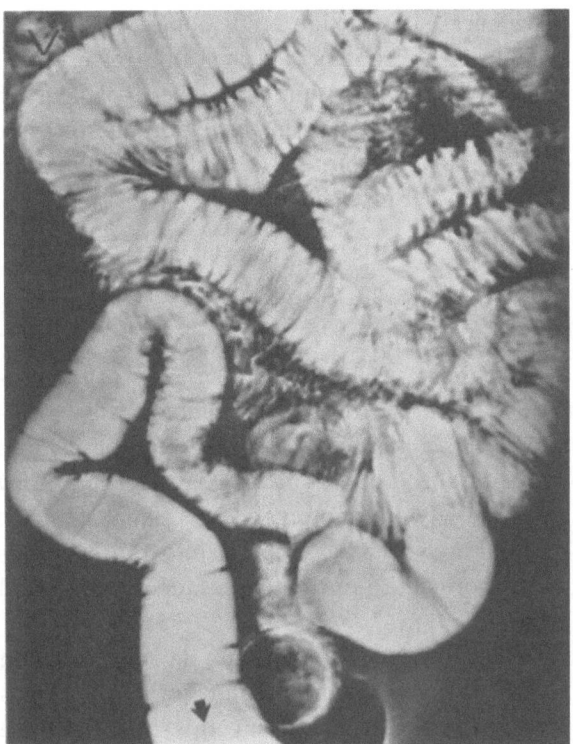

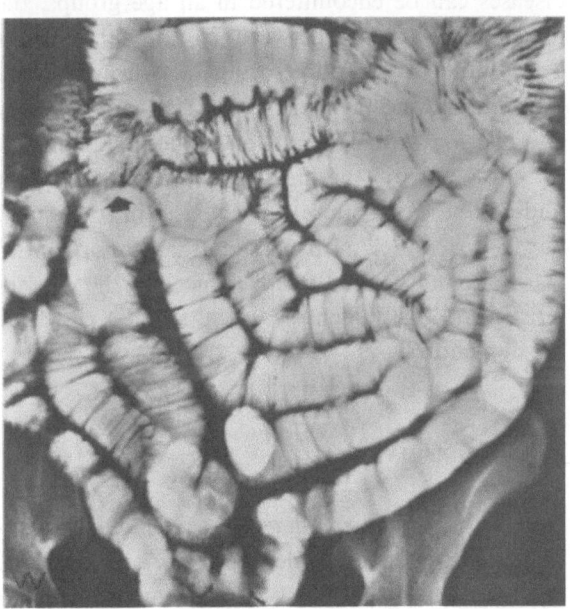

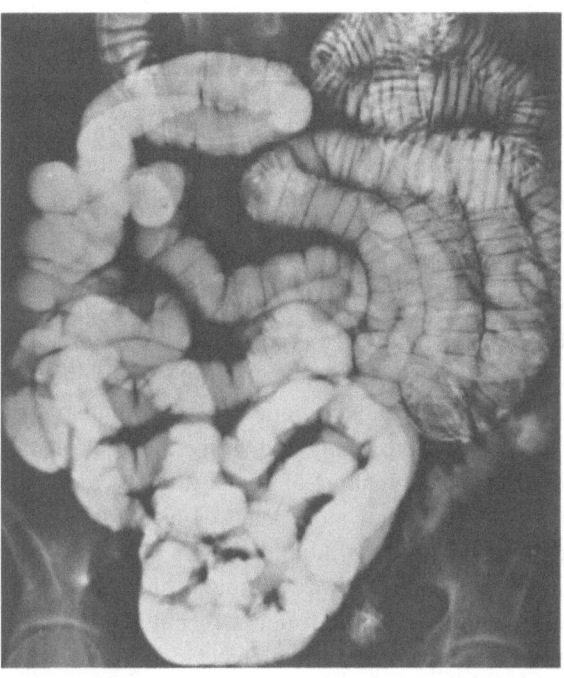

Fig. 12.19
In rare cases a diminished peristalsis in the ileum can be due to the chronic use of laxatives. In the classical case, atrophy of the fold relief is seen which extends to the cecum; moreover, dilatation is not as pronounced as in patients who use spasmodics. In the beginning of the examination contractions in the jejunum are completely normal; this was also the case in this patient. As soon as large quantities of contrast fluid are required to reach the cecum (here 1000 ml barium suspension followed by 1000 ml water), the loops in the jejunum also became dilated and peristalsis decreases (enteroenteral reflex mechanism).

Fig. 12.18
v. Strikingly pronounced increase in dilatation in the distal ileum which appeared to be due to stagnation of the flow of contrast fluid due to a tumor in the cecum. Motility in the jejunum was completely normal.
w. Patient with subileus due to mechanical obstruction of the transit through the small intestine due to bands in the lower abdomen (→ ←). Although more difficult to recognize than in patient V, it can be seen that dilatation is more pronounced in the ileum than in the jejunum and also that the jejunum still shows states of contraction, especially in the upper right quadrant (→).

spot films. The function of the radiological examination by means of enteroclysis may perhaps best be compared with that of a water loaded urography for the urinary tract. In pyknics the small intestine is as a rule shorter than in asthenics; the mesentery is shorter and also contains more fat. As a result the loops of the small bowel lie in a very orderly fashion with respect to one another. The physiological potential sites of obstruction may then be absent; specifically we have never seen a stagnation of the flow at the level of the superior mesenteric artery nor at Treitz's ligament in pyknics.

The significance of these radiological findings (dilatation and decreased motility) should now be obvious in many cases; in other cases – those patients with few or vague complaints – this question is not yet answered. It is possible that the 'unphysiological' rapid flow of the contrast medium causes the temporary stagnation.

However, this stagnation often correlates so closely with the complaints of the patient that it prabably does not only occur during enteroclysis but is in fact a true representation of an actual phenomenon. Our experience with two patients in our series supports this assumption; they underwent a conventional gastrointestinal examination one week before enteroclysis. The enteroclysis examination lasted 40–45 minutes – which is exceptionally long, in spite of the administration of 1800 cc contrast fluid. During the oral gastrointestinal examination of these patients when the rate of flow was more physiological, we noted that in spite of the administration of passage accelerating drugs it was 8 hours (instead of the normal 1–2 hours) before the cecum was reached. Under comparable physiological conditions, such as after the consumption of a normal meal, it can therefore apparently take quite some time before the small intestine is empty. Our observation that transit in patients with a dilated intestine and decreased peristalsis impeded by food remnants from the previous day can therefore now also be explained.

It is known that tranquillizers, sedatives and antispasmodics tend to decrease the tone and peristalsis in the intestine quite effectively and that excessive and prolonged use of these medications can even lead to a total ileus. Of course the transition from a normally functioning intestine to a pseudo-obstructing ileus is not sudden and there must be a period in between characterized by a gradual increase in the radiological abnormalities as well as the complaints. Although the tolerance to the above-mentioned drugs and thus the occurrence of these abnormalities in the digestive tract apparently differs greatly among individuals, this undesirable side-effect should certainly be considered when abdominal complaints are encountered in chronic users of these drugs. A radiological examination of the small intestine by enteroclysis can be a very important tool for this diagnosis when it is seen that peristalsis in the intestine is greatly diminished and the diameter of the lumen is clearly increased. In the case of a subileus or an ileus, an unnecessary operation can be prevented since the presence of a mechanical obstruction can almost always be excluded by means of a technically well-executed enteroclysis examination. For these patients in particular, this is exceedingly important since the post-operative restoration of the intestinal function is sometimes a problem.

2. Collagen diseases

Collagen diseases are systemic diseases of the connective tissue, probably immunologically determined. Since connective tissue is found throughout the body, this group of diseases is characterized by a wide variety of symptoms such as skin conditions, mucosal abnormalities, complaints of the joints and abnormalities of the lungs, kidneys, heart and vessels.

Collagen diseases are not rare; the most common are scleroderma, periarteritis nodosa (PAN), lupus erythematosus and dermatomyositis. Although these diseases can be encountered in all age groups, the patients are usually between 20 and 40 years of age. With the exception of PAN, which is more common among men, these diseases – particularly scleroderma – are generally encountered in females. Manifestations in the digestive tract are a frequent finding (50% or more); incidence in the small bowel varies. It is also possible that abnormalities will be found in the digestive tract but the characteristic and easily identified skin conditions will be missing entirely.

a. SCLERODERMA

The most common collagen disease, often recognized at a glance, is scleroderma. As a result of fibrosis, the skin becomes very smooth and tightly stretched so that the face resembles a mask. A sharp prominent nose and a mouth which is smaller than normal are the most striking features. Hyperpigmentation can often also be seen and hard thick subcutaneous patches of calcium deposits can be felt.

In the internal organs, the same sclerosing process can cause for example fibrosis of the myocardium or the lungs with the accompanying symptoms.

Fibrin deposits in the intima of the walls of the small arteries cause stenoses and therefore ischemic necrosis in for instance the finger tips (Raynaud's phenomenon) and diverse internal organs, including the small bowel. In the digestive tract the layers of smooth muscle become atrophied and are replaced by fibrous tissue. This leads first to a decrease in peristalsis, then hypotonic dilatations and finally sometimes stenoses.

The most well-known characteristic, occurring in 80% of the cases, is reduced peristalsis and a slight dilatation of the esophagus. Less well-known but still encountered in one-half of the patients is a decreased peristalsis and dilatation in the small intestine; the degree of dilatation can vary and is sometimes so local that sacculations are observed (fig. 12.20). In this stage the patients complain of a 'full stomach' and an irritating flatulence. Obstipation can be so marked that obstruction sometimes develops. The duodenum and jejunum are affected the most so that in a later stage malabsorption may also occur and obstipation may be replaced by steatorrhea. Less common and, if the other classical symptoms of the disease are missing, often not recognized as such, are the abnormalities of the stomach. In most cases, a definite atony is seen with dilatation of the stomach and a decrease in peristaltic movements, just as in the esophagus. On the other hand a change in the wall of the stomach due to scleroderma can resemble a linitis plastica or even a very local stenosis in the pars antralis or the pylorus. An uneven dilatation of the jejunum together with sacculations need not be due to scleroderma; we have seen this combination once in a chronic alcoholic with Wernicke's syndrome (fig. 12.21).

b. PERIARTERITIS NODOSA

In this disease, which in contrast to the other collagen diseases occurs predominantly in males, the skin conditions consist of red spots and subcutaneous nodules mainly on the dorsal side of the hands and feet, the tensor side of the extremities and on the face.

Pathologically the disease is characterized by an inflammatory process in the walls of the medium-sized and small arteries causing occlusion and necrosis.

Erythrocyte sedimentation rate and temperature are obviously increased; there is leukocytosis with a shift to the left and sometimes also an esosinophilia. Various organs can be involved; often abnormalities of the kidneys, heart and lungs are also found. In about one-half of the cases manifestations also occur in the small intestine; in contrast to scleroderma, however, the abnormalities here are localized in the distal jejunum and the ileum. The radiological characteristics are highly similar to those of vascular occlusion: they consist of edema, ulcerations, hemorrhage and sometimes also perforation (fig. 12.22). Partly because of the localization, differentiation from Crohn's disease is sometimes impossible; this can persist for some time since these two diseases can have highly similar courses. As in Crohn's disease the appendix may also be involved; in fact this occurs fairly frequently in periarteritis nodosa (see fig. 11.7).

c. (SYSTEMIC) LUPUS ERYTHEMATOSUS (SLE)

The skin abnormalities in this disease include a butterfly-shaped exanthem around the eyes and across the bridge of the nose. The skin there is scaly and atrophied and during exacerbation of the disease, the exanthem may become slightly elevated or even bullous. In one-half of the patients, there is a polyserositis, lymphadenopathy or abnormalities of the internal organs such as the kidneys, heart, spleen, liver or intestine due to a constricting arteritis. In three out of four patients there are complaints of the joints and certain multinucleate leukocytes will contain the LE bodies characteristic of this disease. Quite often there is also a hyperglobulinemia. Occasionally Raynaud-like abnormalities are seen on the fingers similar to the skin conditions on the face. Abdominal complaints can be due to a peritonitis as well as an arteritis.

If the vascular abnormalities are only slight, then we will only observe a hypermotility as a result of anoxia (fig. 12.23).

If the abnormalities are more serious then in the distal ileum they can only be distinguished from those seen in Crohn's disease with difficulty or not at all.

As in scleroderma and drug-induced atony of the bowel, the duodenum can be markedly dilated

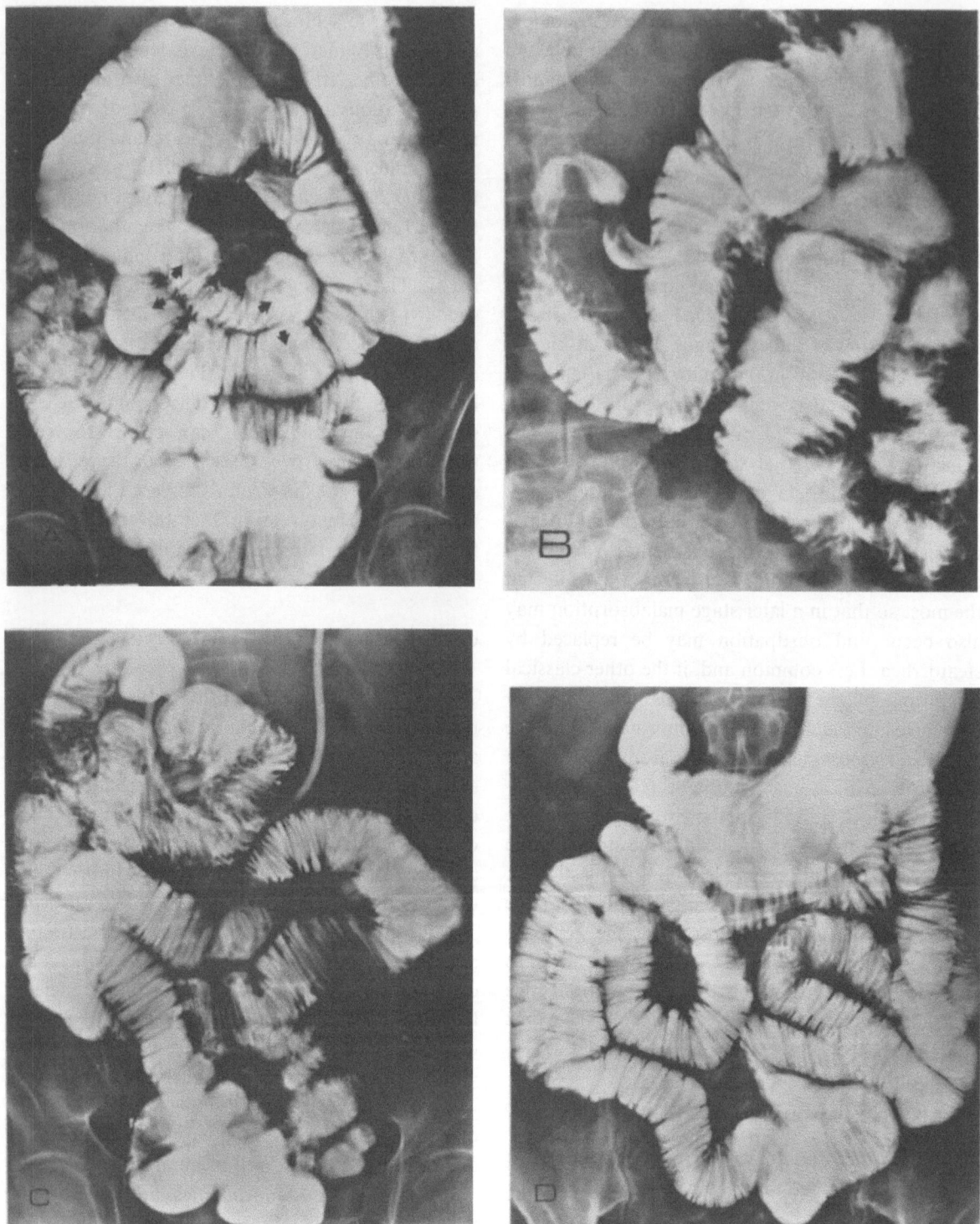

Fig. 12.20

Six patients with scleroderma and the resulting abnormalities encountered in the small intestine.

A. Very large stomach with pronounced dilatation of the descending limb of the duodenum. The jejunum, which is also dilated, shows several local sacculations (→) but there are also contractions in the upper right quadrant. This patient also had abnormalities of the skin and the esophagus.

B. Sacculations in the jejunum.

C. Unequal dilatations in the jejunum but also many contracted loops (in contrast to a drug-induced atony where this is not seen). In this patient there were also abnormalities of the hands and esophagus.

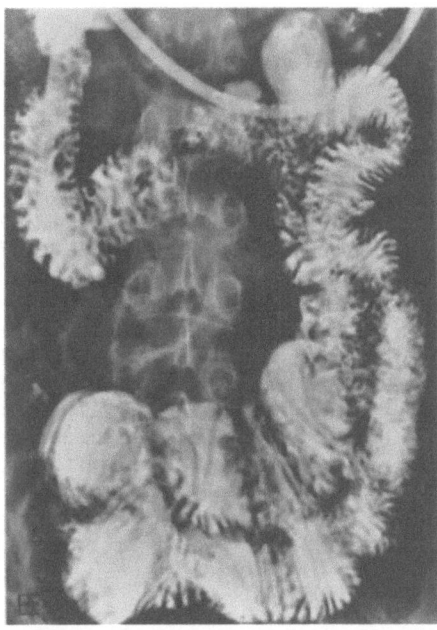

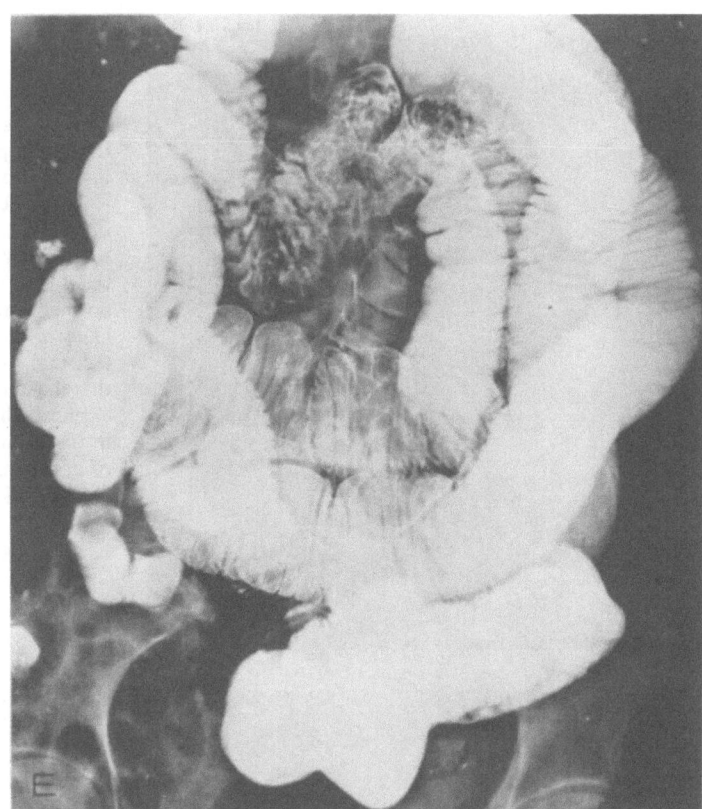

Fig. 12.20

E. Sacculations in the jejunum. Motility was fairly normal at first but became clearly disturbed within several minutes. In this patient, abnormalities of the skin, hands and esophagus were also seen.

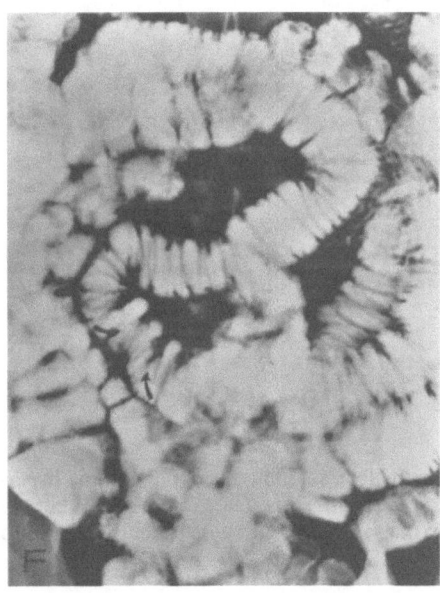

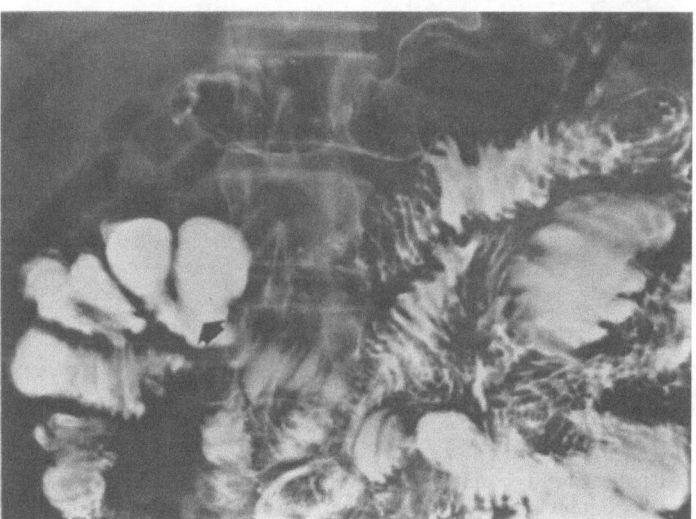

Fig. 12.21

Unequal dilatation of the jejunum and the ileum with sacculations (→) in a chronic alcoholic with Wernicke's syndrome. Normal stomach. Mucosal folds in the proximal jejunum are broadened; this is a normal finding in alcoholics which we have never encountered in patients with scleroderma.

F. Minimal sacculations (→ ←) in the jejunum in a patient with scleroderma. It is of course not possible to establish whether this configuration is incidental, and thus should be considered normal, or shows subtle abnormalities due to scleroderma.

←

D. Abundant reflux into a stomach of normal size. Dilatation of the duodenum and jejunum without sacculations or contracted intestinal segments. This patient also had abnormalities of the esophagus; differentiation from a drug-induced atony of the small bowel is not possible.

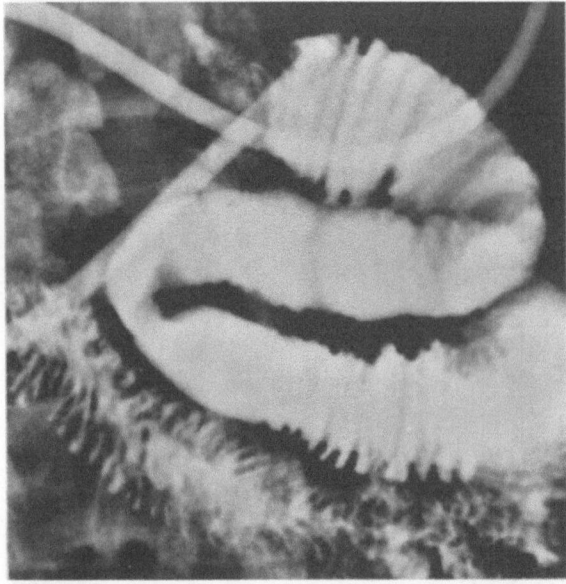

Fig. 12.22
Periarteritis nodosa in a 16-year-old girl. Mucosal folds have disappeared and the wall of the proximal jejunum is thickened over a length of about 20 cm.

The differentiation between ischemic abnormalities and infiltration of the mucous membrane by a lymphoreticular malignancy is almost impossible. The rather abrupt edges of the lesion, the lack of nodular swellings and the completely normal mucosa in the rest of the small intestine are more likely to indicate a vascular origin of the abnormalities. The fact that thickening of the intestinal wall is only local and that the mucosa in the duodenum is normal (not visible here) exclude celiac disease. Because of the lack of cobblestones in the jejunum – otherwise so numerous – and the absence of an edematous swollen mucosa at the edges of the lesion, Crohn's disease also need not be considered.

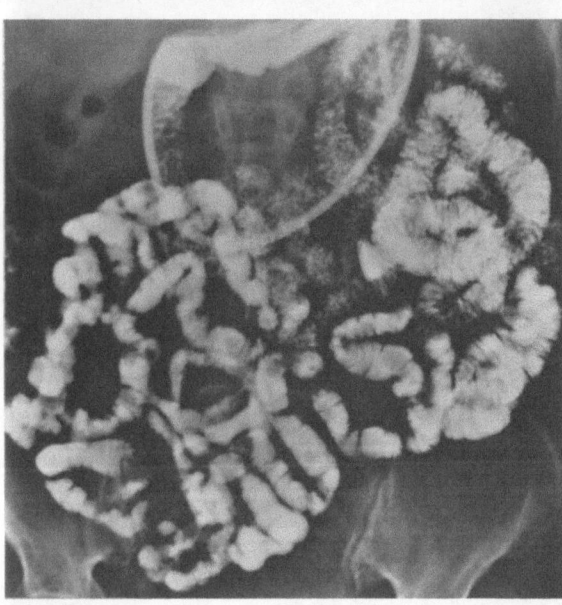

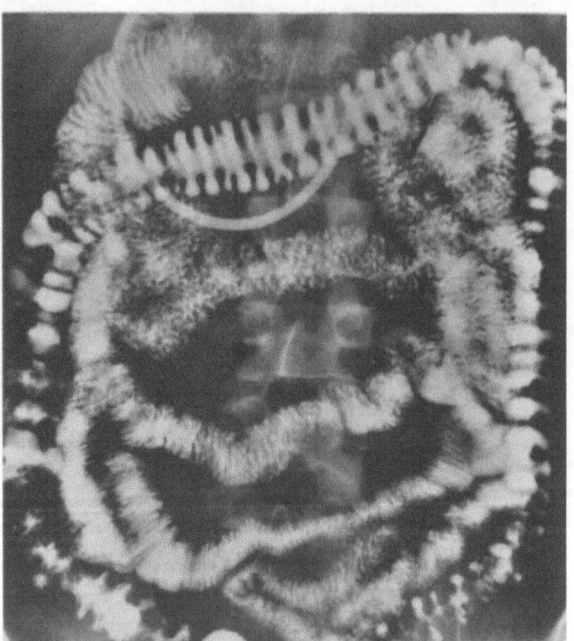

Fig. 12.23
Two patients with chronic abdominal cramps as a result of SLE. The loops of the small bowel show a very pronounced hypermotility but no ischemic mucosal lesions can be found. Many of the loops are in the contraction phase and the lumen of the intestine is obviously smaller than normal. Since the colon can also be quite spastic, it is sometimes possible in these cases to fill both the large and the small intestine with only 400 cc barium suspension.

leading to the development of a superior mesenteric syndrome.

The prognosis of the disease is rather poor; many of the patients die as a result of severe damage to the liver or kidneys.

d. DERMATOMYOSITIS

In addition to erythematous and edematous changes of the skin, characterized in particular by periorbital edema, inflammations of the transverse striated muscles which lead to necrosis are the major symptoms of this frequently fatal disease. The muscles affected most frequently are those of the pelvis, shoulder and neck. Rapid fatigue of the eye muscles sometimes causes double vision, and if the diaphragm and the intercostal muscles are involved, a pronounced dyspnea will develop. One-half of the patients also have deglutitory complaints; if accompanied by Raynaud-like abnormalities on the hands, differentiation from scleroderma can sometimes be difficult – especially if the skin changes are similar to those of scleroderma.

The gastrointestinal abnormalities are characterized by diffuse ulcerations and hemorrhage which can spread out over a large area (fig. 12.24). These vascular lesions are due to a disseminated thrombosis of the small vessels. Microscopically we then find thickening of the intima of the small arteries in the mucosa or submucosa. A specific part of the intestine is not preferred. In 10–15% of the cases, a malignancy will develop somewhere in the digestive tract but also quite frequently in other organs.

3. Adult celiac disease (W. F. H. Müller)

Celiac disease is encountered in small children as well as adults; the classical case is characterized by fatigue, loss of weight and diarrhea.

The stools are usually pulpy, voluminous and pale, and will float in water. Watery diarrhea can,

however, also develop. The steatorrhea can be latent; there are also cases known of patients with obstipation. These patients very frequently present completely different symptoms such as pain in the joints and neurological abnormalities.

As a result of a marked decrease in the Ca resorption osteomalacia can develop and tetanic cramps can occur. A defective vitamin K resorption can cause purpura, a vitamin B_{12} deficiency, a megaloblastic anemia and a decreased Fe absorption and iron deficiency anemia.

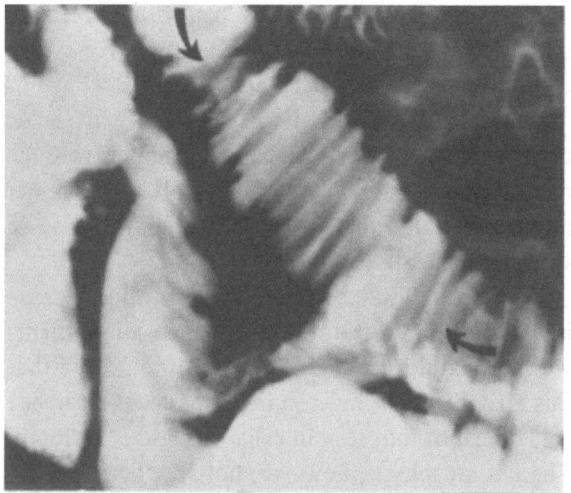

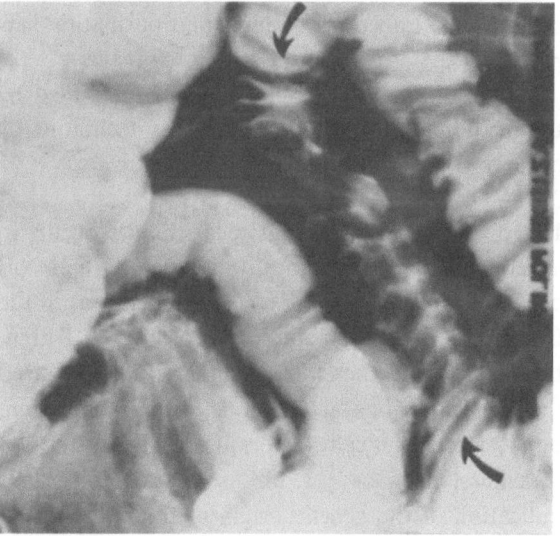

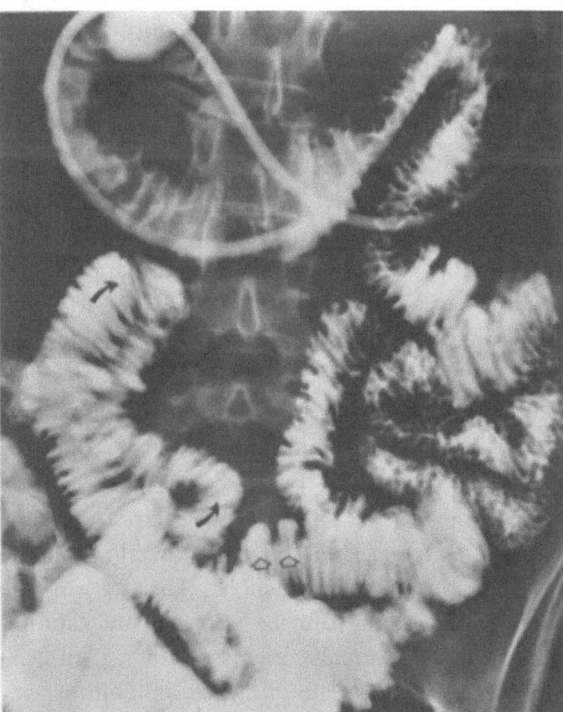

Fig. 12.24
Diffuse vascular abnormalities in the small intestine of a patient with dermatomyositis.

Coarse and also irregular mucosal relief in the region of the ileojejunal junction ($\rightarrow \leftarrow$). In the duodenum, too, the folds appear fairly coarse; the degree of filling here is, however, moderate. As in the patient with scleroderma in fig. 12.20F, a number of small sacculations can also be seen ($\uparrow\uparrow$).

Abdominal pain, often resembling the dyspeptic complaints of a duodenal ulcer, is also a frequent complaint. Obviously these highly variable atypical symptoms make it difficult to establish a diagnosis.

The symptoms can be acute, for instance after traveler's diarrhea, pregnancy or a stress situation, but the course of the disease can also be very stealthy so that the patient himself often does not even realize that he is sick since he has learned to live with his complaints. The fact that the nature of this illness was not recognized in the past has led to a multitude of terms, including celiac disease, adult celiac disease, idiopathic steatorrhea, primary malabsorption, sprue, celiac sprue, free-gluten disease and gluten-induced enteropathy.

In 1953 Dicke showed that children with celiac disease improved when wheat was omitted from the diet, and together with Weyers and Van de Kamer he demonstrated that it was the gluten fraction in wheat which caused the symptoms.

A second milestone in the history of celiac disease is Pulley's demonstration of flat mucosa in patients with idiopathic steatorrhea (1954). It appeared that this atrophy of the mucosa in idiopathic steatorrhea is identical to that seen in celiac disease in children. The flat atrophy is, however, not specific for celiac disease; it is also seen in kwashiorkor, tropical sprue, some infectious diseases and dermatitis herpetiformis.

Finally diagnosis was considerably simplified by the introduction of the peroral biopsy technique by Shiner.

It is a well-known fact that celiac disease occurs in several members of one family and that the diagnosis can be established in 10–18% of the relations in the first degree of each patient. According to Rubin, this disease is therefore definitely not acquired through exogenous factors alone, specifically gluten, but is also genetically determined. The pattern of transmission is as yet unknown. An important indication of the genetic origin of the pathological reaction to gluten may be the frequent occurrence of the histocompatibility antigens HL A1 and HL A8 in patients with celiac disease. But, since antigens can also be found in normals, other factors must also be involved.

The frequency of celiac disease in England is 1:2000; in West Ireland it is 1:300 (1973). No exact figures are available for the Netherlands but at the Celiac Symposium held in 1974, it was estimated at about 1:1000. This means that there are approximately 1300 patients with celiac disease in the Netherlands.

RADIOLOGICAL APPEARANCE

In 1953 Mackie was the first to describe the radiological abnormalities of the small bowel in nontropical sprue; he observed an abnormal nonpropulsive peristalsis. In 1934 Snell and Camp described smooth contours in the jejunum and duodenum. In subsequent years diverse publications appeared describing flocculation and segmentation of the barium suspension; Golden called this phenomenon the 'deficiency pattern'. However, flocculation and segmentation are not at all specific for celiac disease but are also encountered in numerous other diseases even when a so-called 'high stable' barium suspension is used.

By administering larger quantities of the barium suspension, Schwishuk et al. and Marshak were able to visualize the mucosal pattern as well as the dilatation more clearly. Ishell et al., however, found that in spite of using a non-flocculating suspension for patients with celiac disease, flocculation and segmentation were still observed more frequently than dilatation of the small intestine. With the enteroclysis method, a large dosage of contrast medium is administered very rapidly and this irritating disintegration of the barium suspension can be avoided under all conditions, even if the preparation is not particularly stable. However, rate of transit of the contrast fluid in patients with celiac disease can be so accelerated that it is still impossible to obtain adequate filling of the intestinal loops even with enteroclysis. Therefore when celiac disease is suspected it is essential that the rate of flow of the contrast fluid be even greater than the normal 80–100 ml/min. For this purpose the barium suspension must be diluted with water so that the viscosity is reduced and it will flow through the infusion system more quickly. The s.g. of the barium suspension can be reduced by dilution from 1.25 for normal patients to an s.g. of 1.20 without objection. The decrease in contrast intensity which results from the decrease in s.g. can

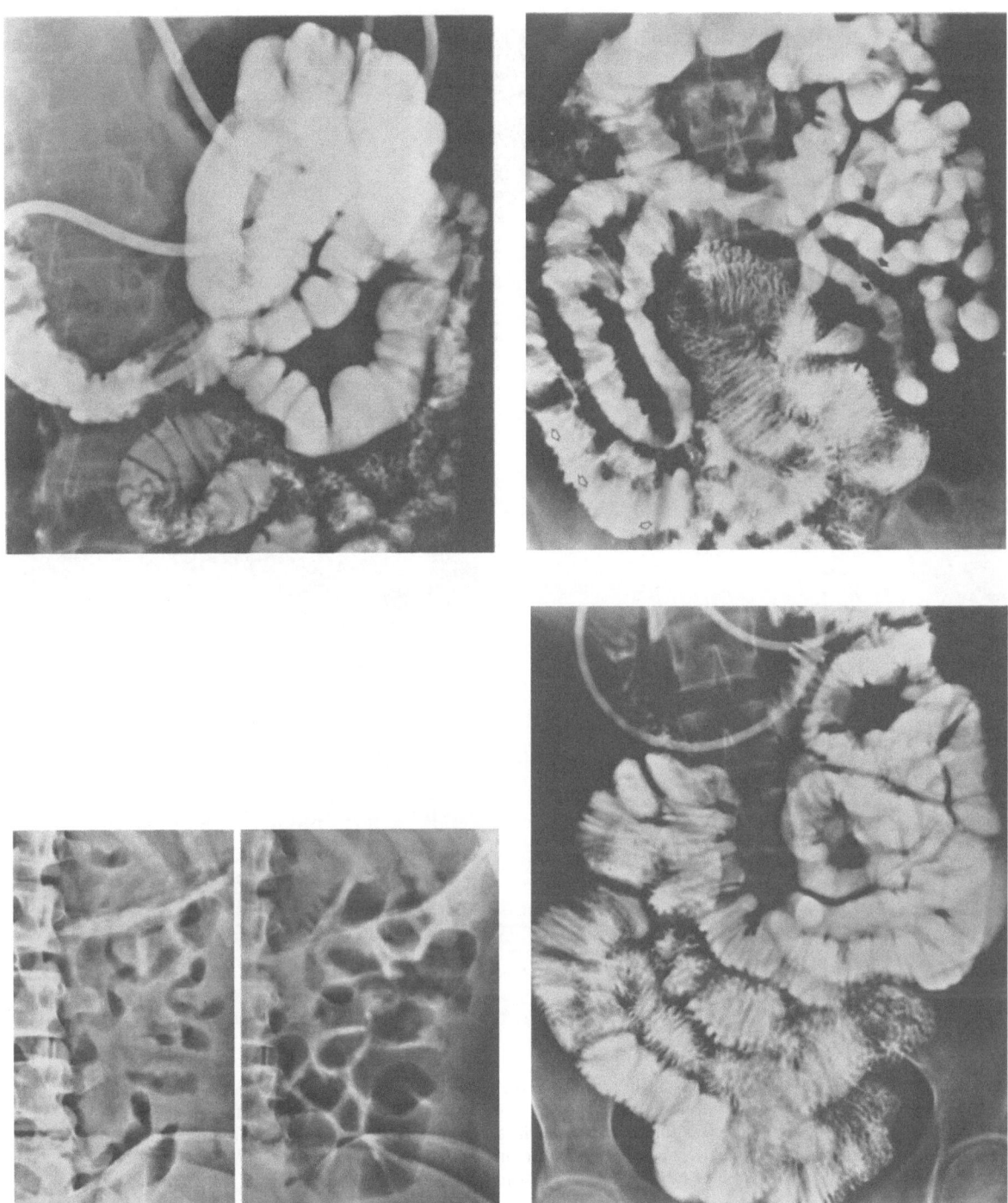

Fig. 12.25

Two patients with celiac disease showing the 'moulage' sign in the jejunum due to atrophy of the folds of Kerkring.

The patient on the right, who was not aware that she had celiac disease, also had a hypoalbuminemia, possibly due in part to a secondary infection acquired while on a camping trip. It is quite obvious that the walls of the jejunum are markedly thickened (→←) and that the mucosal folds further distalwards in the intestine are greatly broadened (↑↑). After treatment of the hypoalbuminemia, the thickness of both the intestinal wall and the mucosal folds was again normal; the pattern of an uncomplicated celiac disease remained (lower-right). It is interesting that the improvement could already be seen on the abdominal survey film (lower-right: after treatment; lower-left: intestinal gas pattern upon admission to the hospital).

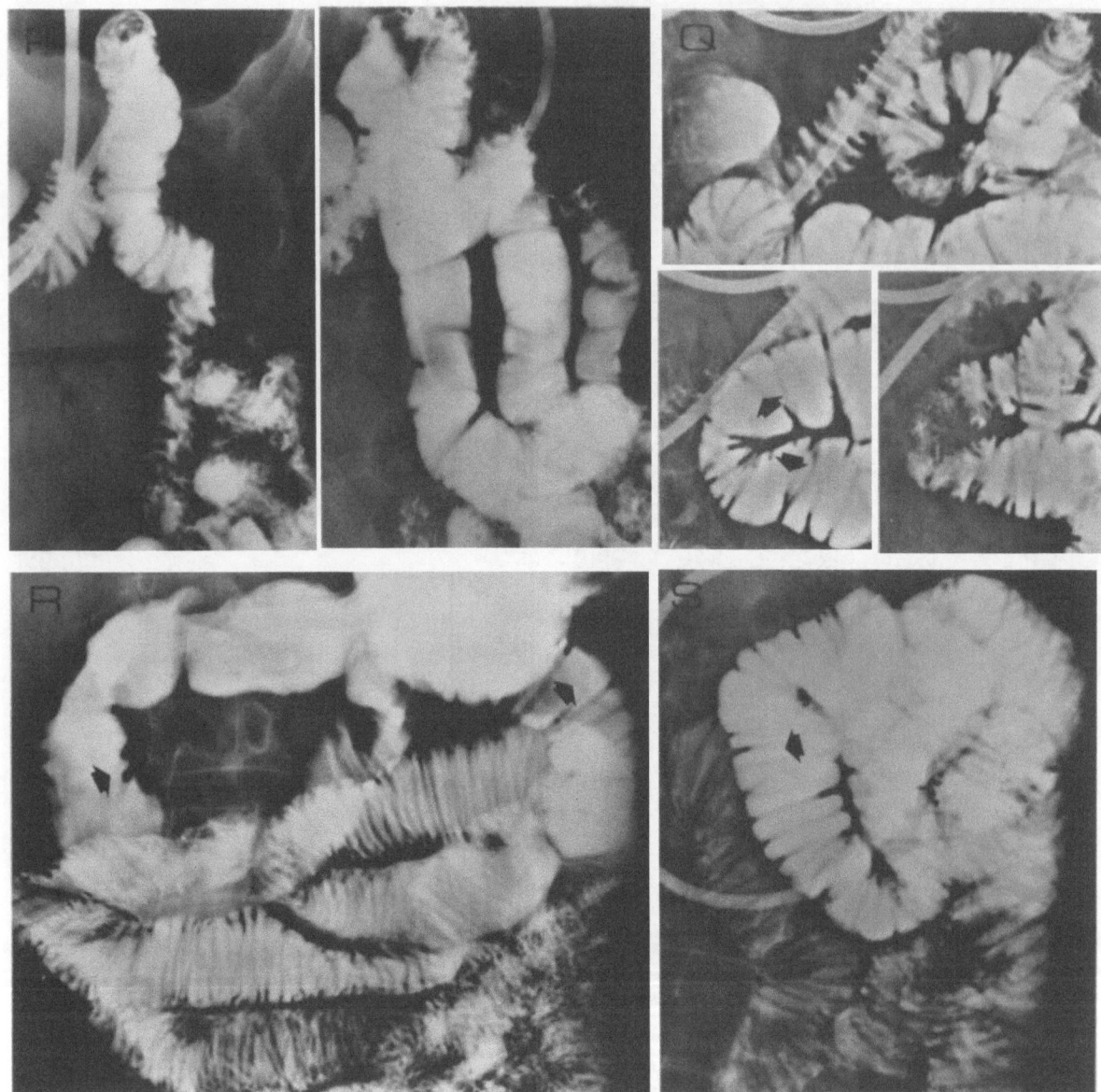

Fig. 12.26
Four patients with celiac disease with only slight atrophy of the mucosa in the jejunum. It is interesting that for all of these patients the presence of this disease was discovered by means of the roentgenological examination (the celiac disease provocative test). In patients P and Q, it is clear that the abnormalities are only visible when the intestine is well-filled. The slight atrophy of the folds in patient S in highly similar to that seen in the patient with amyloidosis in fig. 12.35–1. Localization of the abnormalities in the most proximal part of the jejunum led us to consider celiac disease first.

be compensated for by lowering the exposure voltage 10 or 20 kV. A characteristic of celiac disease is smooth margins in the jejunum; it is always easiest to discover these smooth contours in a well-filled segment of the bowel (fig. 12.25).

The importance of a rapid contrast medium flow when trying to detect a slight decrease in the number and flattening of the mucosal folds, which would

suggest celiac disease, is demonstrated in fig. 12.26. It would be obvious that the radiologist's tentative diagnosis would have been missed with the slower rate of flow inherent in the oral administration of the contrast medium.

In some cases a well-filled jejunum can show the haustral-like pattern seen in the colon; these structures are caused by spasms (fig. 12.27). In celiac

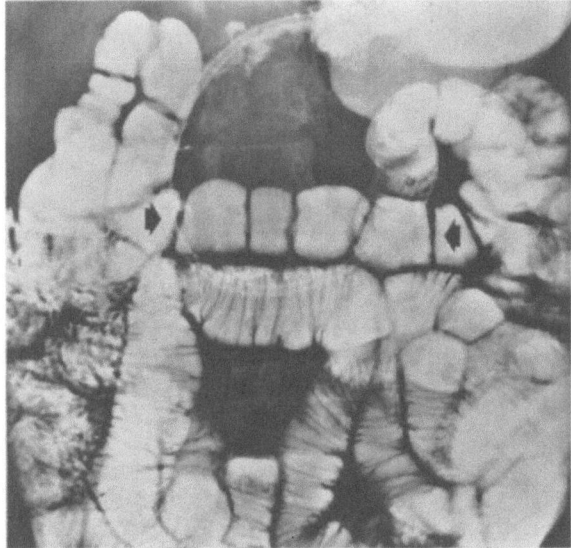

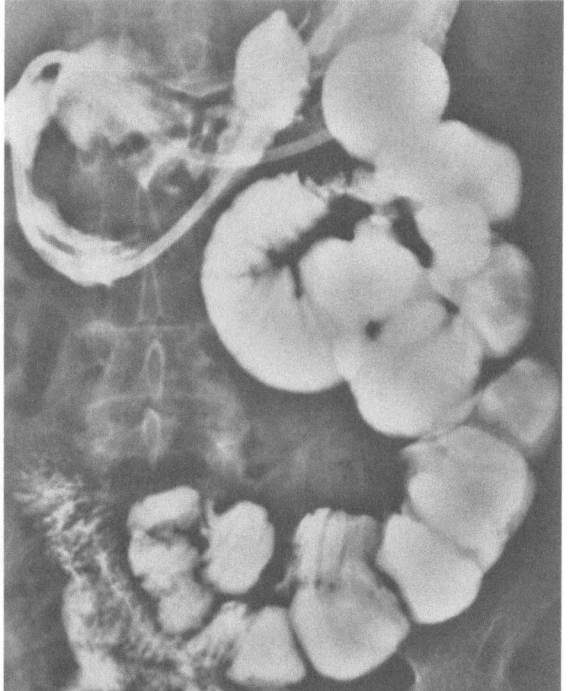

disease, a gastric examination shows that the folds in the duodenum are often coarse and asymmetrically thickened; this is in itself hardly specific and is therefore not sufficient to establish this diagnosis, especially if there are no mucosal abnormalities in the jejunum at all. An enteroclysis examination of this same duodenum would, however, obviously reveal the flattened folds and thus the probable diagnosis, certainly when a good case history is available.

A disadvantage, albeit of little importance, of the infusion method is that the duodenum often cannot be visualized in a well-filled state since the tip of the Bilbao tube should be located at Treitz's ligament in order to avoid reflux into the stomach.

The mucosal folds in the jejunum in patients with celiac disease can show interesting variations. We have observed the following groups of abnormalities.

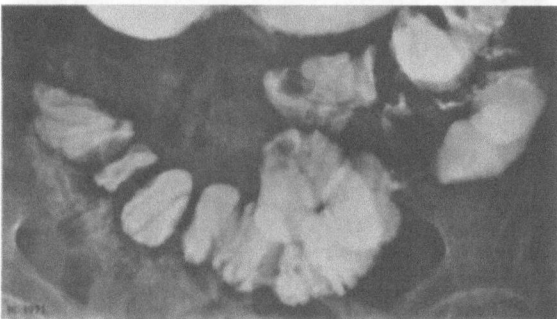

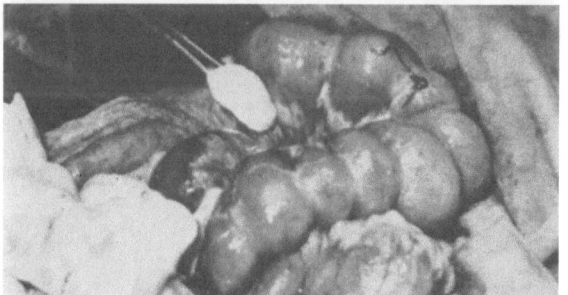

Fig. 12.27
Two patients with a colon-like haustration in the jejunum. The abnormalities seen in the patient on the right, which closely resemble the ischemic abnormalities in fig. 11.15, appeared during surgery to be due to spasms and cicatrization at the site of circular ulcerations. These stenotic ulcerations possibly resulted from atrophy of the vascular system in this patient. On the surgical films not only the colonization pattern is clearly visible but also, in the open intestine, the atrophied mucosal relief in the jejunum.

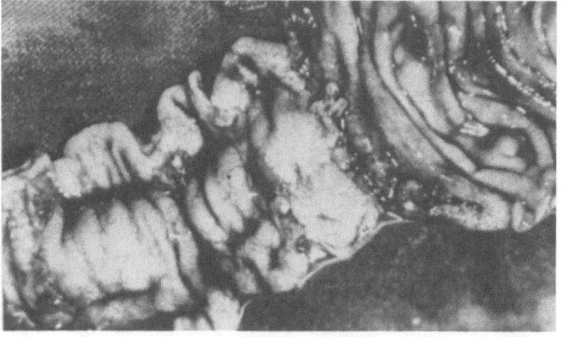

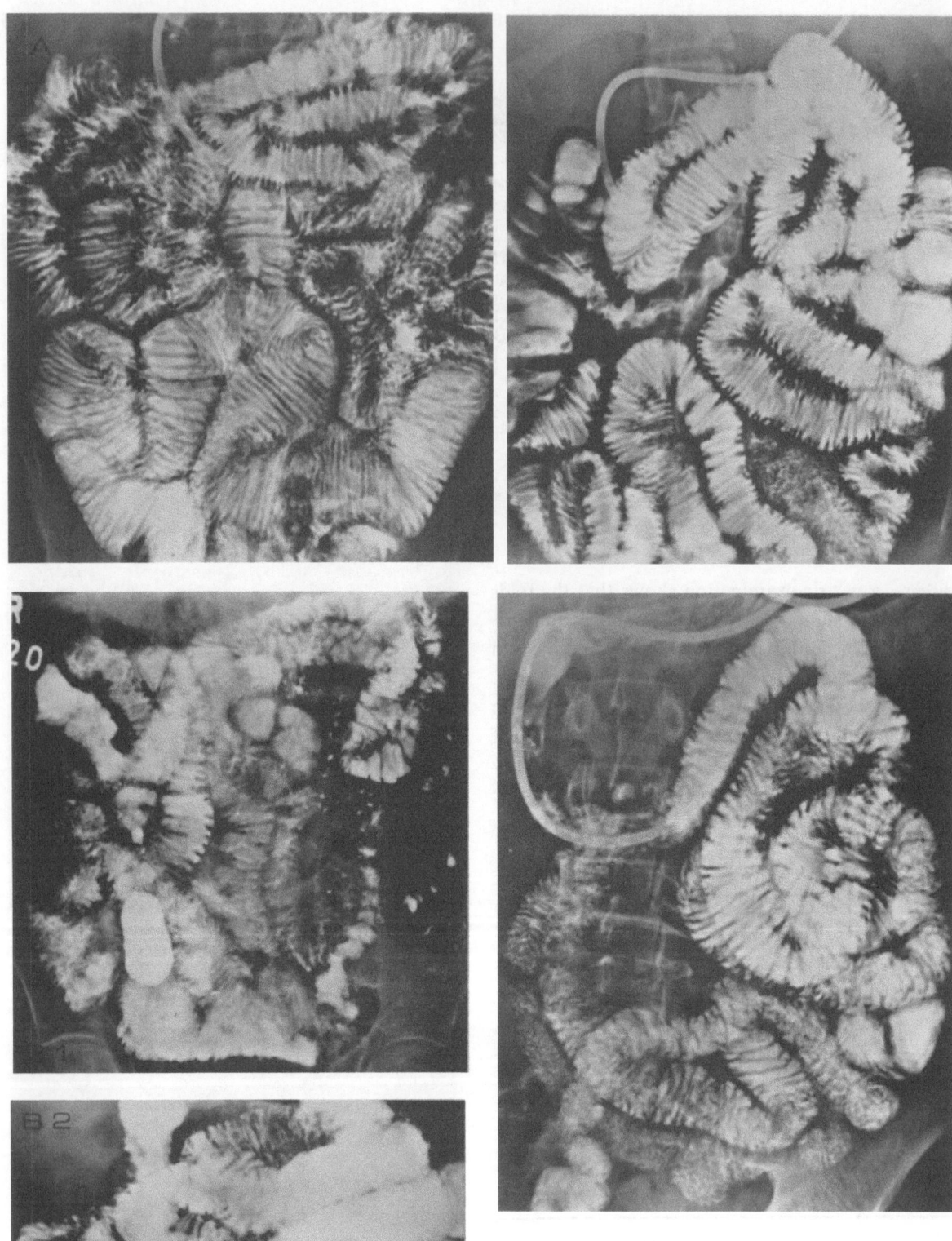

Fig. 12.29

Four patients with celiac disease (A, B, C, D) with highly dilated loops in the jejunum and especially the ileum. Transit was so rapid that it was not possible to fill the intestine adequately. Patients A, B & C also showed considerable radiological improvement after treatment (right column). There was no follow-up examination of patient D, a 10-year-old child. Patient B, one of our first cases after the introduction of the (at that time not yet perfected) enteroclysis method (2), had been examined shortly beforehand by the conventional passage technique (1) which produced very pronounced flocculation and dilution of the contrast fluid.

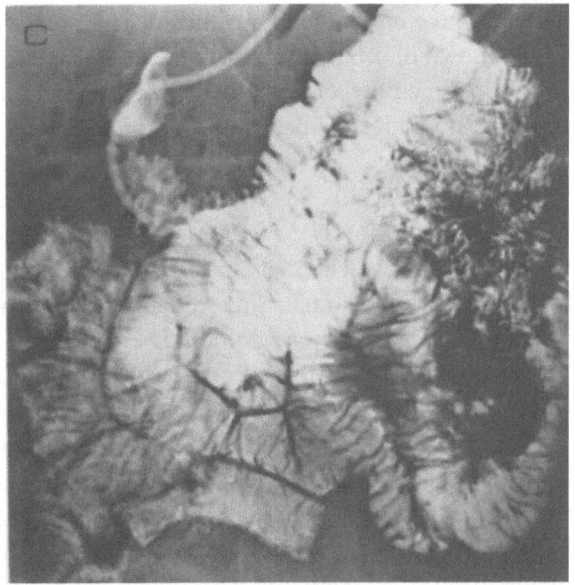

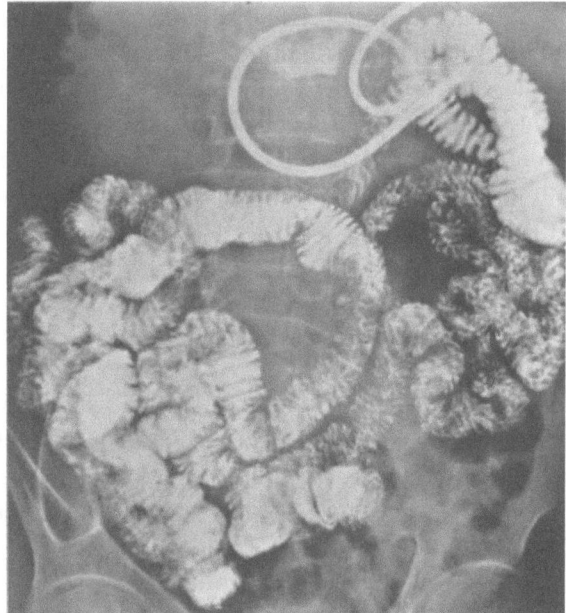

thickening of the contrast medium, such that visualization of the mucosa which still exist is no longer possible. As a result of a positional anomaly (malrotation) of the small intestine (see page 326) ileal loops may be found in the upper left quadrant; pronounced filling of these loops produces fairly smooth contours and this misleading pattern must be differentiated from that described above for celiac disease (fig. 12.28).

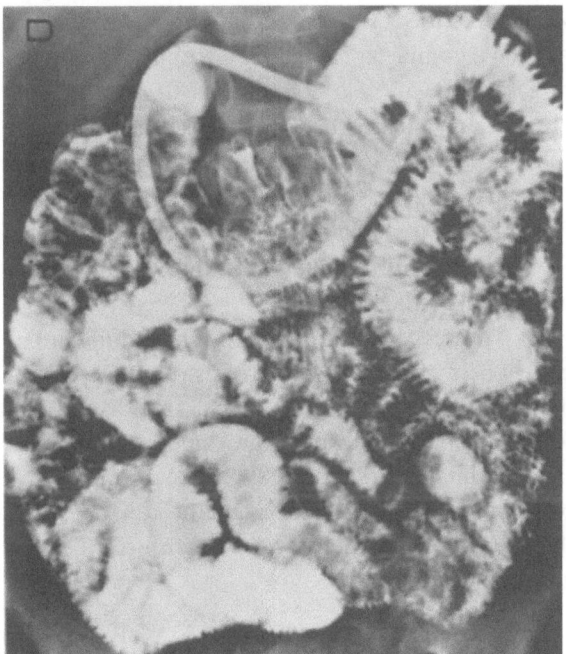

GROUP I

In about one-half of the patients with celiac disease the mucosa in the duodenum and the jejunum is very smooth. This could be due to a flattening of the circular folds which have become shorter and an increase in the distance between the folds. This is the so-called 'moulage' sign, a true representation of atrophied mucosa (fig. 12.25); in contrast 'pseudomoulage' (see fig. 5.7AB) which also shows a smooth mucosal surface is due to stasis and

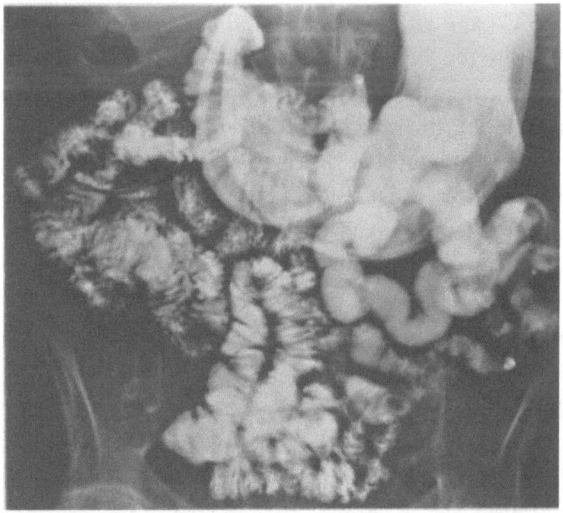

Fig. 12.28
Misleading pattern suggesting celiac disease: it is due to the abnormal position in the upper left quadrant of the ileum which at this moment shows few mucosal impressions (disintegration of the beginning of the contrast column!).

In celiac disease peristalsis in the smooth atrophied jejunal loops is abnormal and non-propulsive. The ileal loops are frequently dilated with numerous mucosal folds. It is possible that this should be considered as an attempt to compensate for the decrease in the mucosal surface in the jejunum ('jejunization', fig. 2.4).

GROUP II

In about one-quarter of the patients with celiac disease we have seen a striking dilatation of both the ileal and the jejunal loops (fig. 12.29). The diameter of the jejunum as well as the ileum may even be 40-55 mm (in enteroclysis the normal value is a maximum of ± 35 mm). Peristalsis is very active and the intestine is highly contractile so that the transit time is exceedingly short (the cecum can be reached within 5 minutes). In spite of a high rate of flow of the contrast medium it is difficult to obtain adequate filling of the intestinal loops. A pronounced dilution of the barium suspension occurs as a result of the excess of intestinal juices in the intestinal lumen. It is possible that this large quantity of fluid is not due to hypersecretion but to a disturbed water resorption. Patients in this group, like those of group 1, usually have the most severe clinical symptoms. There is a definitely disturbed resorption of diverse food substances such as fats, Fe, Ca and vitamin B_{12} as well as a marked protein loss in the digestive tract. This so-called protein-losing enteropathy is accompanied by a generalized edema of the mucosal folds in the small bowel. These swollen folds are clearly visible on the x-rays; in addition it is noted that the thickness of the intestinal wall has also increased.

GROUP III

In the remaining 25% of the patients with celiac disease, rapid transit and dilatation of the intestinal loops can also be found, but they are not as pronounced as in group II and therefore are not specific for celiac disease. The diagnosis in these cases generally cannot be established by means of radiology. It is interesting to note that these patients have only mild complaints. There are even cases known of celiac disease in which the diagnosis was confirmed by biopsy but the roentgenograms revealed no abnormalities at all.

For this group of patients in particular, the radiological abnormalities cannot be differentiated from those seen in dermatitis herpetiformis. In the latter disease, which is characterized by bilateral itching there are papular and vesicular lesions on the tensor side of the extremities. The transit time is also exceptionally short. In some cases almost the entire small intestine is in a state of contraction, a phenomenon which can also be encountered in carcinoid (fig. 12.30). Strangely enough the risk that patients with dermatitis herpetiformis will also have a concurrent celiac disease is statistically fairly high. Aside from this there are also many points of similarity between these two diseases. For example we can find the full range of flat villi – from normal to even a complete 'snowflake' atrophy. As in celiac disease, we will also see various degrees of malabsorption, steatorrhea and thickened mucosal folds due to the loss of protein. It is peculiar that these abnormalities of the digestive tract also react favorably to a gluten-free diet; we have found that the skin conditions likewise improve although a number of authors disagree.

It is, however, not always possible to differentiate clearly between these three groups of celiac patients nor between celiac disease and dermatitis herpetiformis. Thus for instance the smooth contours in the proximal small bowel typical of group I can be found together with the numerous dilatations in the jejunum and especially the ileum described for group II (fig. 12.31).

There is usually a rapid clinical improvement after gluten is omitted from the diet; this is, however, more often true in children than in adults. The mucosal lesions may obviously improve; in adults this recovery can be incomplete.

For a number of patients in our series, a follow-up examination of the small intestine was carried out 2 months to 2 years after the gluten-free diet was instituted (fig. 12.29). In all our cases dilatation, hypersecretion and mucosal edema when present had disappeared or diminished (mainly patients

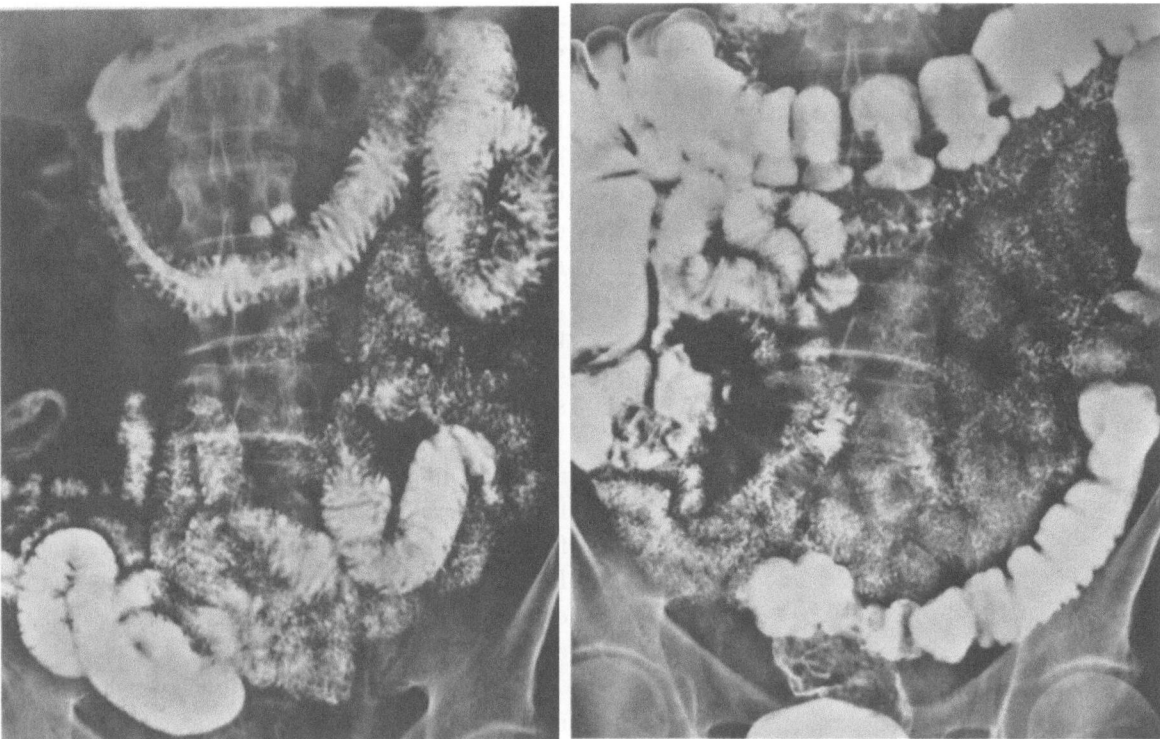

Fig. 12.30
Two stages of the examination of a patient with dermatitis herpetiformis. Transit was exceptionally fast, almost the entire small bowel is in a state of contraction. The loops are not dilated and there is no atrophy of the mucosa in the jejunum.

from group II) but an essential recovery of the smooth mucosal surface (mainly patients from group I) was never seen. Apparently therefore the mucosal folds never reappear once an intestinal loop has become atrophied.

COMPLICATIONS

a. MALIGNANCIES

Since the publications by Golden in 1936 and Mackey and Fairley in 1937, it has been known that there is some connection between steatorrhea and the development of malignant lymphoma. At first steatorrhea was thought to be secondary to the infiltration of malignant cells into the intestinal wall and occlusion of the lymphatic channels in the small intestine. In 1962 Golden and his associates suggested that intestinal lymphoma could develop as a complication of adult celiac disease. This was confirmed by Harris who examined 250 patients with celiac disease and found 40 cases of malignancy. 16 of these 40 patients had carcinoma of the digestive tract; the esophagus was the most common localization, relatively speaking. It is interesting to note that although the greatest turnover of cells occurs in the proximal part of the small intestine, carcinoma seldom develops in the duodenum and jejunum. Four patients had malignancies elsewhere in the body. There were 20 patients with lymphoma, 1/3 of them did not originate in the intestinal wall. The malignancies occur more frequently in males than females. It also appeared that within one family the number of patients with adult celiac disease in conjunction with a malignancy was larger. If a gluten-free diet is followed for at least 12 months, the risk of carcinoma will decrease but not that of lymphoma. A tumor must always be included in the differential diagnosis when the patients do not improve on a gluten-free diet or have new complaints after a temporary remission.

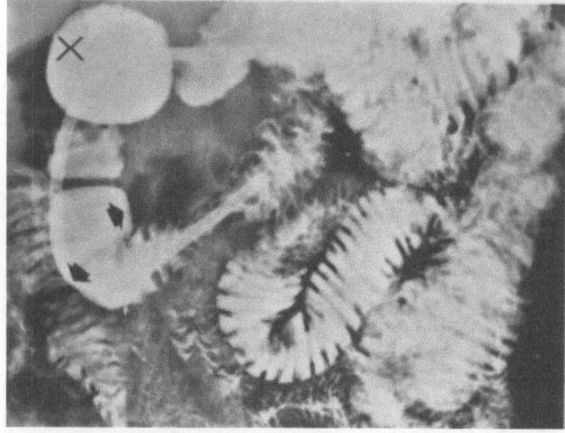

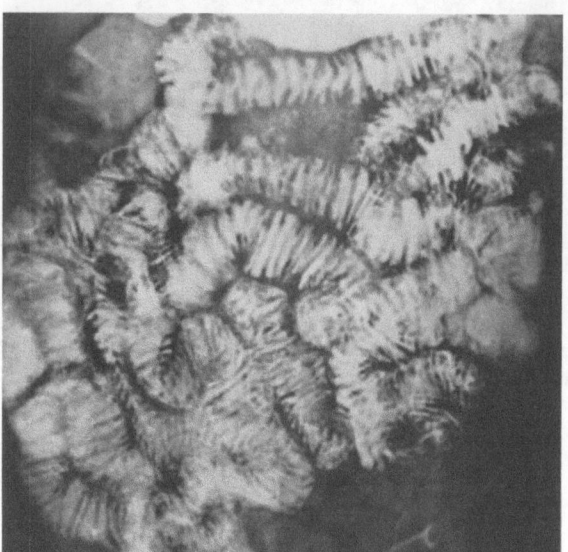

This is also the case when, in addition to symptoms such as loss of weight, diarrhea and skin conditions, there is obstruction or perforation. In celiac disease both humoral and cellular immunological disorders are known. From the above, it can be seen that these factors, whether genetically determined or not, could play a role in the development of a malignancy.

Biochemical parameters indicating incipient lymphoma are a low albumen concentration, a high alkaline phosphatase content and an increased serum IgA level.

There are reasons to assume that an immature or abnormal immune system is a predisposing factor for the development of malignancies due to the failure of the so-called 'immunological surveillance'. Potential neoplastic cells which develop due to errors in cell division are not recognized as such and are therefore not removed.

To discover mucosal abnormalities caused by malignancies in celiac disease at an early stage, it is essential that the examination is not thwarted by flocculation or segmentation of the contrast medium. More so than for any other disease of the small intestine, the use of enteroclysis is therefore here an absolute necessity.

b. ULCERATIONS

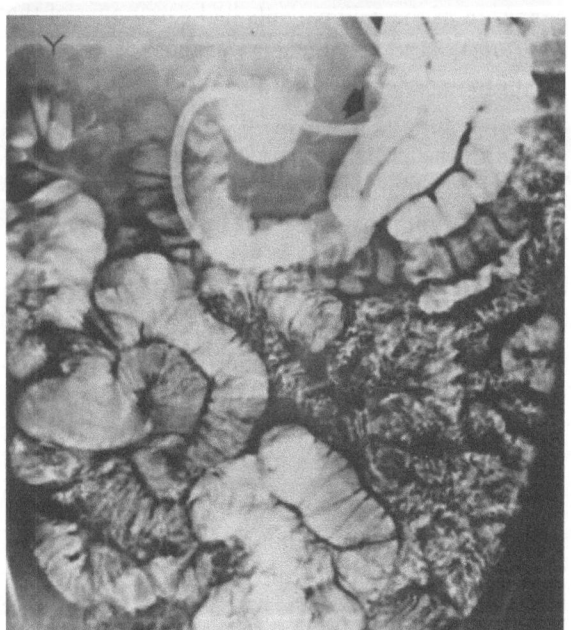

If patients with celiac disease no longer react favorably to a gluten-free diet, then not only malignancy but also ulcerations must be included in the differential diagnosis. In addition to the symptoms of the malabsorption, these patients may also complain of vomiting and severe pain in the upper abdomen. The ulcerations may be solitary or multiple and, as a result of spasms or fibrotic

Fig. 12.31
It is not always possible to classify the abnormalities found in patients with celiac disease in one particular group. Transitional forms are also encountered. The differentiation between a dermatitis herpetiformis and celiac disease is likewise difficult; furthermore these two diseases often develop together, as in these two patients. Here the radiological aspect of group II (pronounced dilatations in the proximal jejunum) is found together with an atrophy of the folds of Kerkring in the proximal duodenum which is characteristic of group I.

shriveling, can cause a haustral-like pattern in the jejunum. The most dangerous complications are hemorrhage and perforation; eventually transit may also be impaired. The disease is usually fatal in such cases unless the ulcerous and stenotic section of the jejunum is removed in time and the patient follows a gluten-free diet.

c. INTUSSUSCEPTIONS

According to the literature, non-obstructing intussusceptions may develop – possibly causing the colic-like pain in the abdomen. This hypothesis in itself seems highly unlikely and in fact the roentgenograms illustrating these reports show that probably all of these cases were incorrectly interpreted because of inadequate filling and misleading patterns. In any event we have never been able to demonstrate this phenomenon in our patients with the enteroclysis method.

d. RESULTS OF MALABSORPTION

The disturbed resorption of a number of food substances causes deficiences which can lead to the following complications:

1. In some cases rather severe hemorrhaging in the intestinal wall or the retroperitoneal cavity as a disturbed coagulation mechanism due to a vitamin K deficiency.
2. A reduced Ca resorption can give rise to tetanic cramps and an osteomalacia.
3. Several cases can be found in the literature of volvulus as a result of a marked increase in the size of the colon (fig. 12.32). Enlargement of the colon in patients with celiac disease can be due to:

A. an increase in the bulk of the feces as a result of malabsorption
B. a decrease in the muscular tone due to a K deficiency.

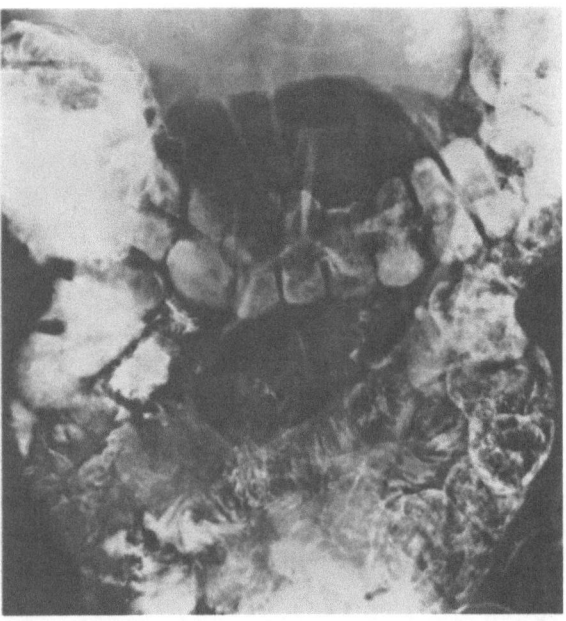

Fig. 12.32
A dolichocolon, a very long and voluminous sigmoid which is filled with gas in this x-ray, has caused volvulus. The development of volvulus is a common complication in celiac disease. It is not known exactly whether the increase in the volume of the sigmoid is due to an increase in feces or to changes in the tone of the musculature of the large and the small intestine as a result of the disturbed mineral resorption.

4. Amyloidosis

Amyloid is a protein substance which can be deposited in tissue by an as yet unknown mechanism without demonstrable cause. It is assumed that an immunologically determined disturbance of the function of the plasma cells is involved. In addition to this so-called primary amyloidosis, there is also a secondary amyloidosis whereby amyloid deposits occur in conjunction with various diseases such as chronic infections, multiple myeloma and lymphoreticular malignancies. Amyloid deposits can be local but may also be spread diffusely throughout all layers of the wall anywhere in the digestive tract. Furthermore the deposits can be very small but also quite large; in the latter case they can form nodular masses and bulge out into the contrast column such that differentiation from lymphoreticular malignancy can be difficult (fig. 12.33). Depending upon the localization of the

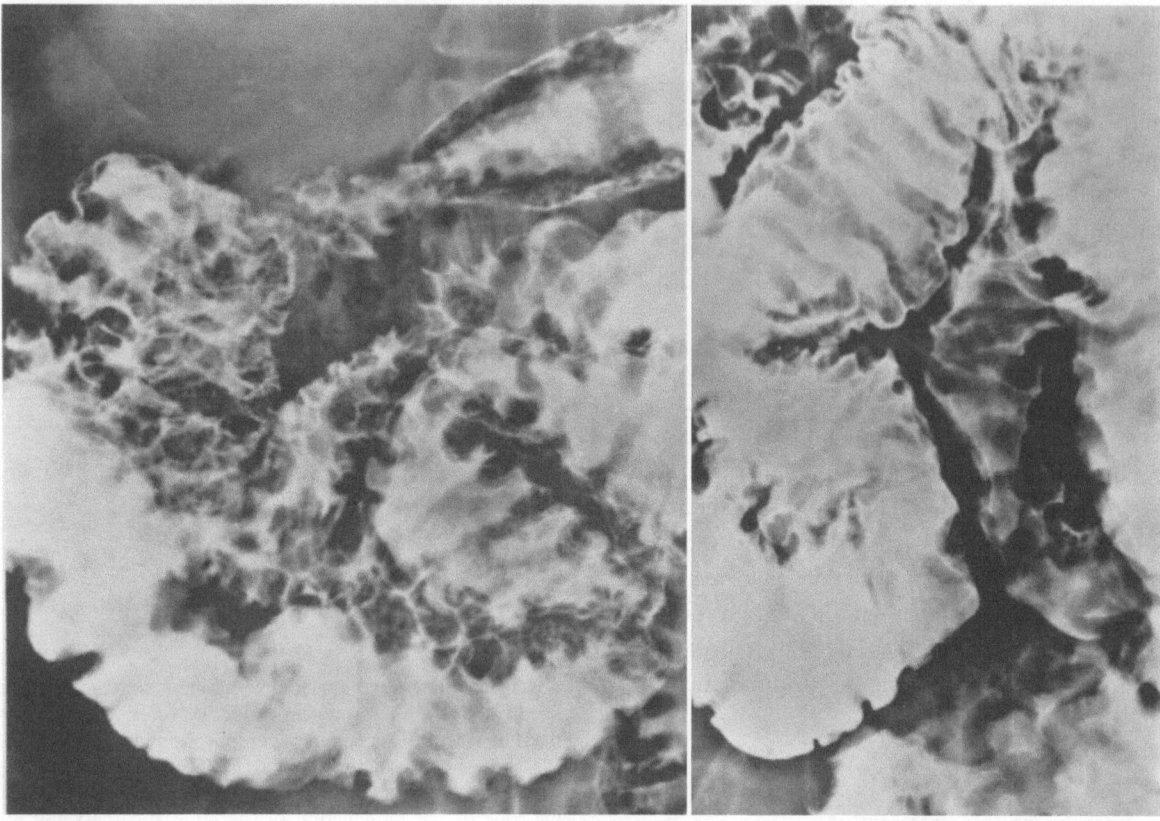

Fig. 12.33
Primary amyloidosis of the small intestine. Both the obviously thickened intestinal wall and the markedly broadened mucosal folds, which can still be recognized here and there, contain numerous pea and marble-sized lumps. The lumen of the intestine shows multiple unequal dilatations without stenoses. In a lymphoreticular malignancy either there are no pronounced dilatations at all or they are due to a stenosis; in addition in patients with this disease larger spaces between the intestinal loops are to be expected.

deposits, resorption and motility can become seriously disturbed leading to a malabsorption syndrome and fairly severe meteorism. The complaints due to localization in the small intestine consist mainly of painful cramps accompanied either by diarrhea as a result of gas accumulation or by a pseudo-obstruction due to the severely disturbed motility (fig. 12.34). The lumen of the small intestine can be obviously dilated, the intestinal wall thickened and the mucosa atrophied. If atrophy of the mucosal folds is moderate, they become broadened and flat so that the mucosal surface appears lightly undulatory (fig. 12.35). A severe atrophy of the mucosa in the ileum produces a completely smooth mucosal surface without folds as seen in a case of reflux ileitis in ulcerative colitis or after remission of Crohn's disease (fig. 12.36). Smooth walls in the jejunum are usually due to celiac disease; then there is definitely no dilatation of the lumen since the muscular layers are intact.

In amyloidosis the lumen may be dilated; if it is not, then differentiation from celiac disease may cause difficulties and must be based on the aspect of the ileum (fig. 12.36). In the colon atrophy of the mucosa cannot be distinguished roentgenologically from the destruction caused by the chronic use of laxatives. Amyloidosis can only be differentiated radiologically from ulcerative colitis because there are (almost) no ulcerations in the former.

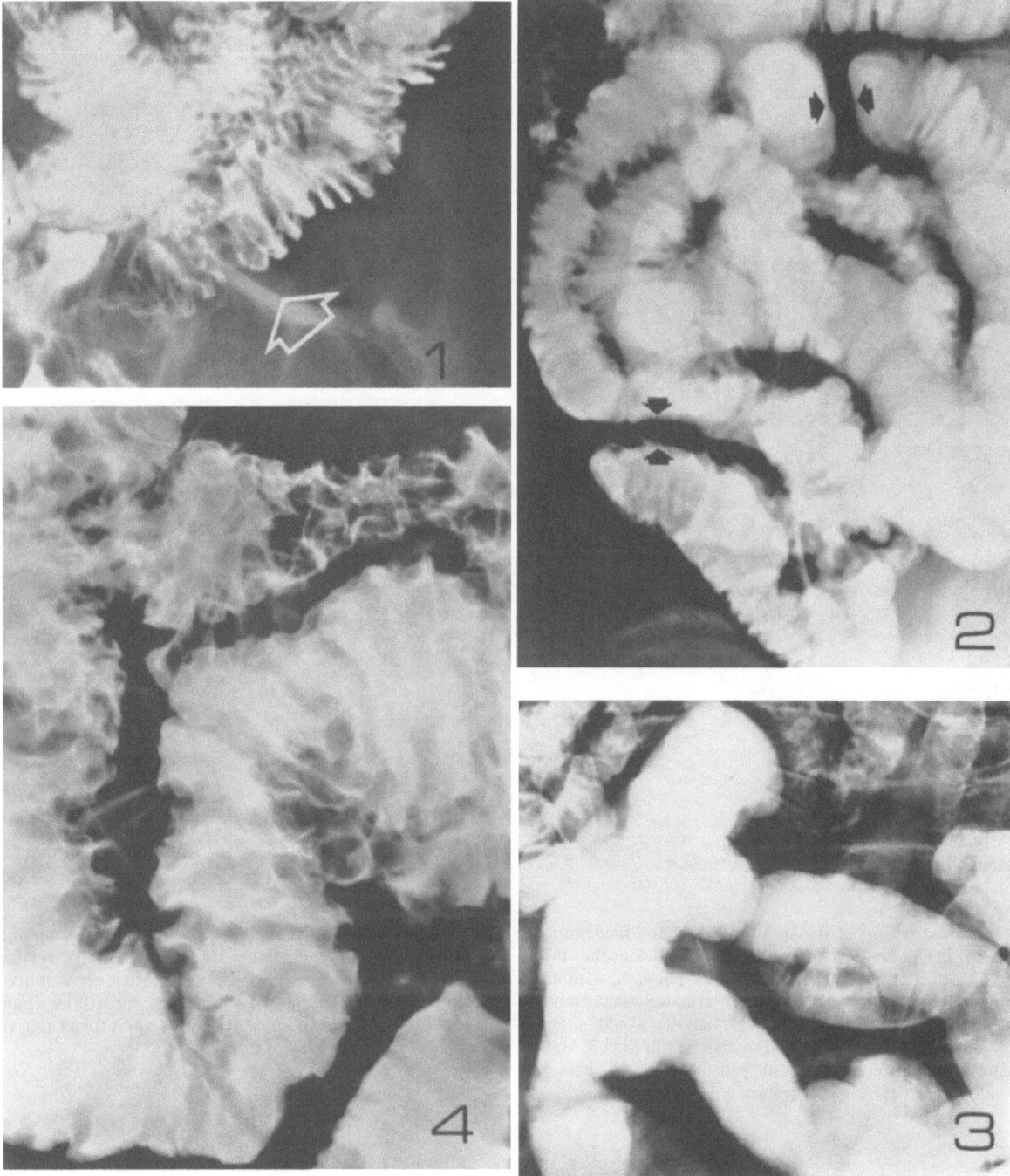

Fig. 12.35. Abnormalities, increasing in severity, in four patients with primary amyloidosis of the small intestine.
1. Decreased motility in the small bowel and mucosal folds with a slightly undulant course in some regions (→).
2. No clear-cut abnormalities in the jejunum (not shown). In the ileum the mucosal relief is flattened and the intestinal wall is thickened. Differentiation from a lymphoma (compare fig. 10.35) is not really possible. After remission of Crohn's disease the intestinal wall is neither as thick nor as rigid (stiff).
3. Flat mucosal relief throughout almost the entire small bowel (detail of the patient shown in fig. 12.36).
4. Highly thickened intestinal wall and very broad irregular mucosal folds which in places can no longer be recognized. Multiple nodular amyloid deposits and unequal dilatation of the intestinal lumen (detail of the patient shown in fig. 12.33).

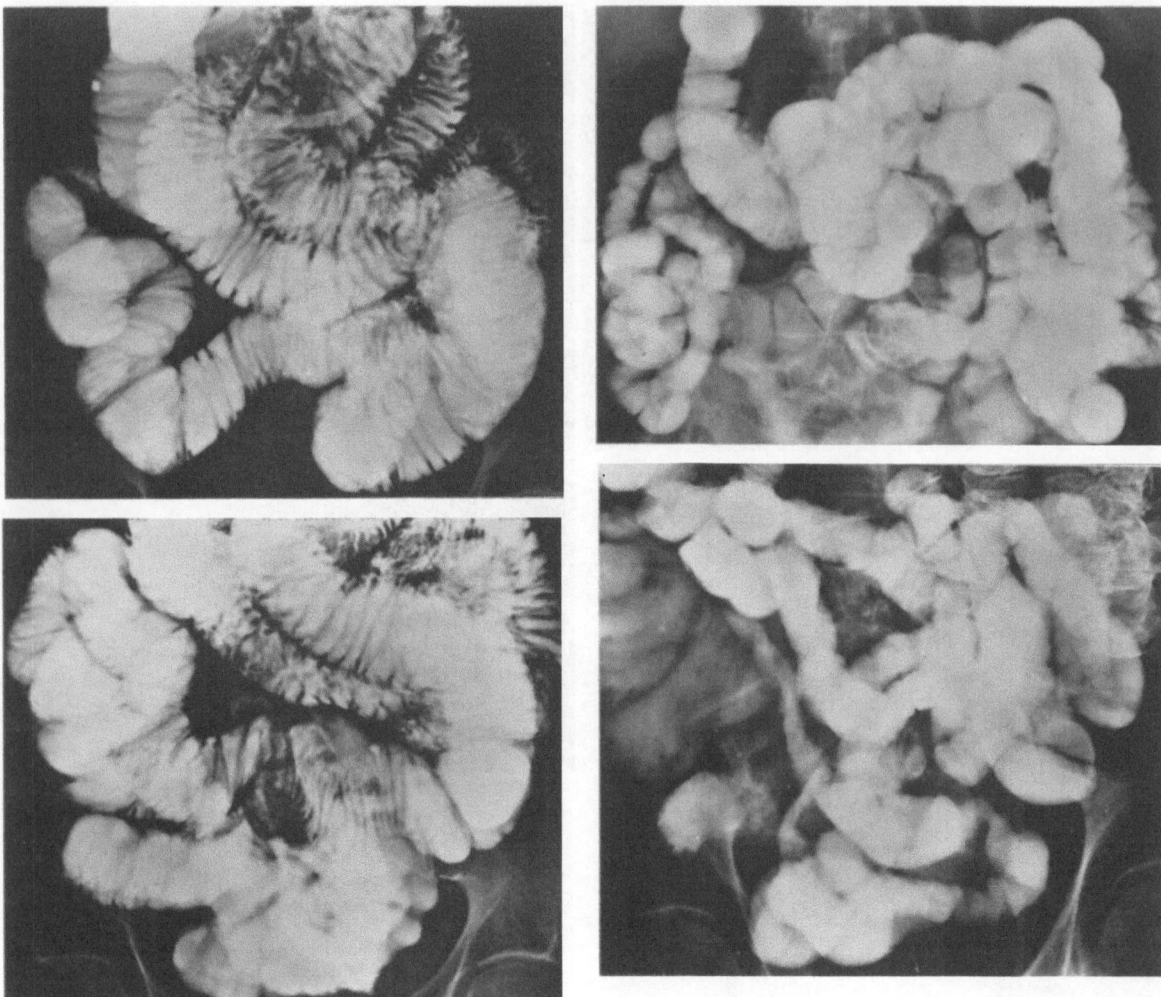

Fig. 12.34
Pseudo-obstruction of the small intestine due to disturbed motility in a patient with amyloidosis. It is obvious that there are diverse contractions, especially in the jejunum. Although differentiation from scleroderma or drug-induced atony is very difficult, the presence of sacculations would suggest scleroderma; this degree of dilatation of the ileum and a more pronounced decrease in peristalsis in the jejunum would indicate a drug-induced atony.

Fig. 12.36
Flat mucosal relief in the duodenum, jejunum and ileum of a patient with primary amyloidosis. In the differential diagnosis lymphoma should also be considered. After remission of Crohn's disease and in celiac disease, the abnormalities would be less extensive and the rigidity and unequal thickening of the wall seen here would be missing.

Bibliography chapter XII

CUMMINGS J. H. (1974) Laxative abuse. *Gut 15*, 758–766.

DYER N. H.; DAWSON A. M.; SMITH B. F.; TODD I. P. (1969) Obstruction of bowel due to lesion in myenteric plexus. *Brit. med. J.* I, 686.

MALDONADO J. E.; GREGG J. A.; PAGREEN A. L.; BROWN N. J. (1970) Chronic idiopathic intestinal pseudo-obstruction. *Amer. J. Med. 49*, 203.

MOSS A.; GOLDBERG H. I.; BROTMAN M. (1972) Idiopathic intestinal pseudo-obstruction. *Amer. J. Roentgenol. 115*, 312.

NAISH J. M.; CAPPER W. M.; BROWN N. J. (1960) Intestinal pseudo-obstruction with steatorrhoea. *Gut 1*, 62.

SEAMAN W. B. (1972) Motor dysfunction of the gastro-intestinal tract. *Amer. J. Roentgenol. 116*, 235.

Literature about celiac disease can be found in: MÜLLER W. F. H. (1976) Radiological examination of the small intestine in celiac disease. Leiden.

See also the nrs. 3–8–11–13–27–33–41–48–53–60–76–91–166–177–178–188–213–221 and 242 of the bibliography on pages 164 and following.

XIII

CONGENITAL ANOMALIES

1. Abnormal positioning of the entire small bowel: disturbed rotation or fixation

In 90% of the adults, the jejunum is located in the left upper quadrant and the ileum in the right lower quadrant of the abdomen (fig. 13.1); according to Zimmer, a small convolution usually lies in the middle forming the transition between these two segments of the intestine. The lack of this 'intermediate convolution' may be the most common anomaly.

The small intestine usually leaves the retroperitoneal space and enters the abdominal cavity to the left of the spinal column; however, in rare cases it can also lie in the middle in front of the spinal column or even to the right of the latter (fig. 13.2).

Variations in the normal position of the mass of intestinal loops are frequently encountered and are probably dependent upon the size of the liver at the time of the reduction of the physiological herniation (fig. 13.3). If during this reduction, the jejunum does not pass behind the superior mesenteric artery into the left half of the abdomen but instead remains on the right side, then we are confronted with an inversion of the small intestine. In these cases the ileum lies in the middle or to the left in the abdominal cavity (fig. 13.4). If the ileum is found on the left side, the distal segment can lie in the lower, middle or upper abdomen. It is therefore possible that the last ileal loop coming from the left will cross the abdomen diagonally to end up at the cecum in the lower right quadrant (fig. 13.5).

If the entire colon is found in the left half of the abdomen, then the second stage of the rotation phase did not occur at all and the radix mesenterii will extend more or less vertically from top to bottom. Usually the entire mass of jejunal loops is

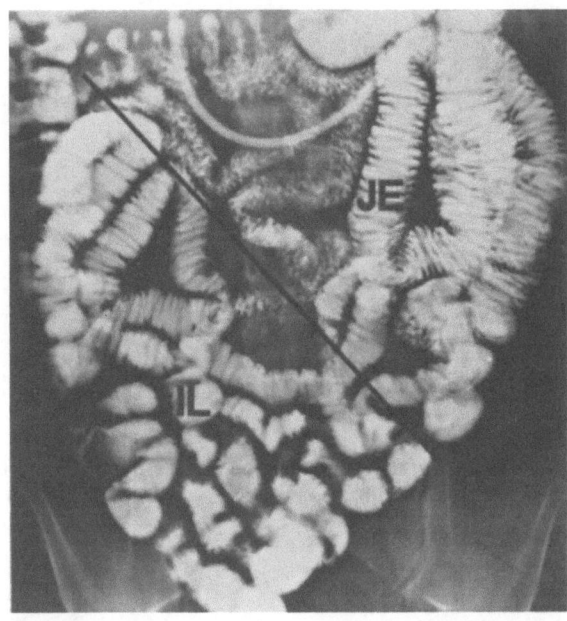

Fig. 13.1

Most common position of the small bowel. Jejunum in left upper quadrant; ileum in right lower quadrant. The line separating these two convolutions is diagonal, running more or less perpendicular to the radix mesenterii which extends from the upper left to the lower right.

then located in the right half of the abdomen and the duodenojejunal junction is approximately in the center (fig. 13.6). An even more unusual situation is when only part of the jejunum passes behind the superior mesenteric artery into the left upper quadrant and Treitz's ligament is also in the normal position to the right of the spinal column (fig. 13.7).

If the omphalomesenteric duct is far removed from Bauhin's valve, most of the ileal loops may end up in the right half of the abdomen during second stage of rotation (fig. 13.8) and, if the ascending colon does not drop, the cecum may also be found in the upper right quadrant. The relationship between the failure of the ascending colon to

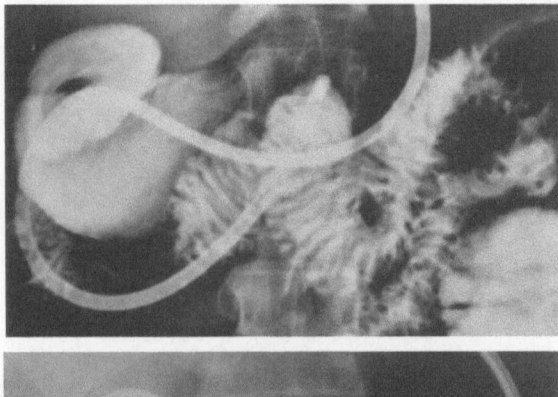

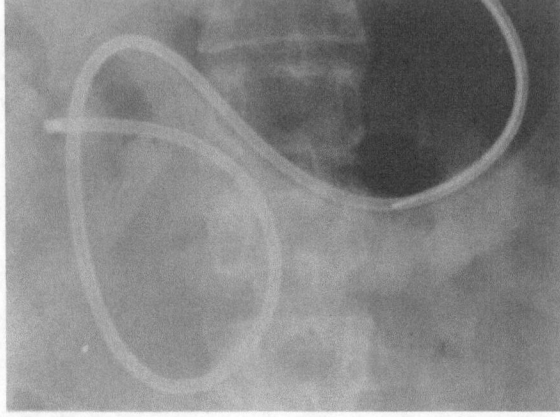

Fig. 13.2
Treitz's ligament may also be found in the center in front of the spinal column (upper) or next to it on the right (lower).

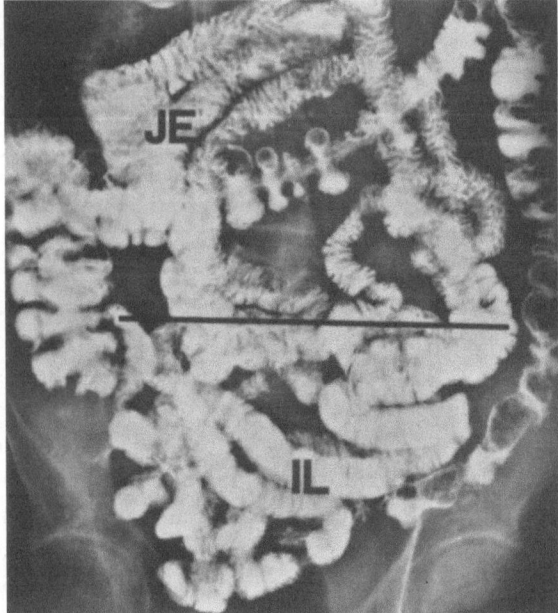

Fig. 13.3
A fairly frequently encountered variation in the position of the mass of loops of the small intestine is when the jejunem lies more or less in the middle of the upper abdomen with the ileum almost directly underneath.

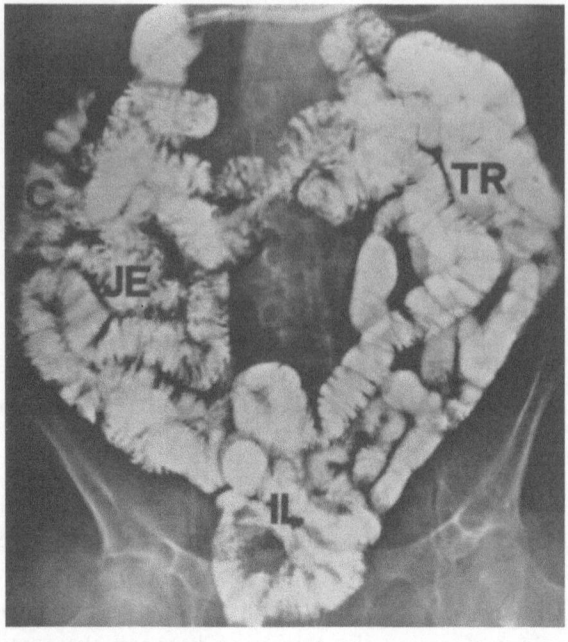

Fig. 13.4
If after reduction of the physiological herniation the jejunal loops do not pass behind the superior mesenteric artery to the upper left quadrant but remain on the right, then the ileal loops are forced to lie more or less in the left half of the abdomen. In this case the transition (= tr) between the jejunum and the ileum is in the upper left quadrant. In contrast to a total inversion, the duodenum and the cecum are in the normal position here. Furthermore in this patient, the ascending colon barely descended so that the cecum (C) is in the right upper quadrant.

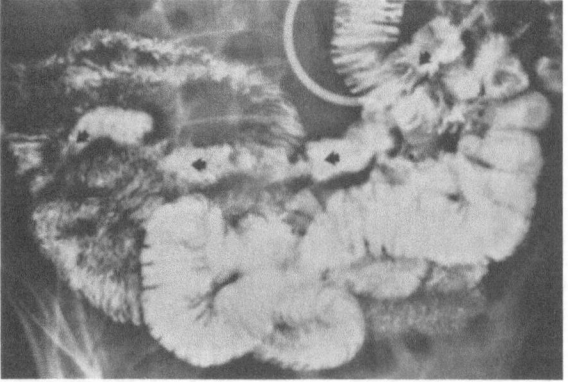

Fig. 13.5
The jejunum is in the right half of the abdomen and the ileum in the left. The distal ileum crosses the abdomen diagonally from left to right (→ →).

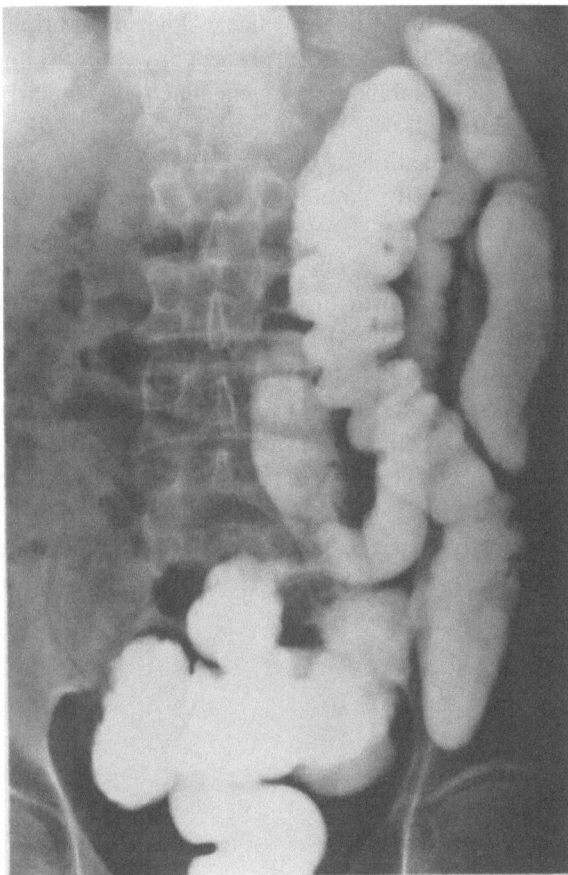

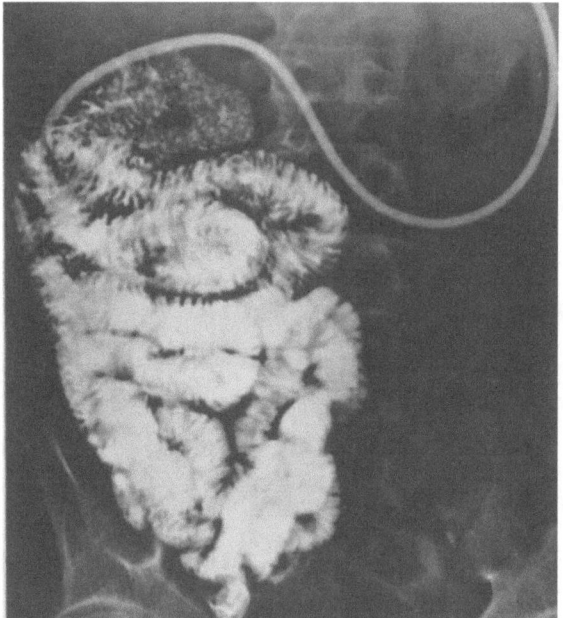

Fig. 13.6
Lack of rotation of the mesentery and the intestine. The colon lies on the far left in the abdomen and the small bowel on the right. Treitz's ligament is in the middle.

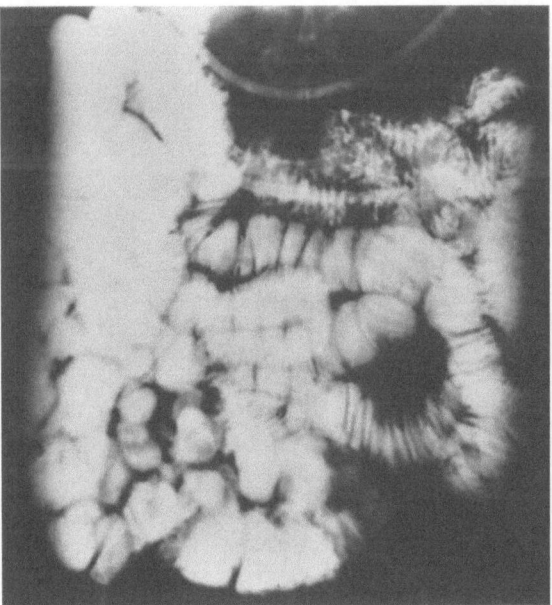

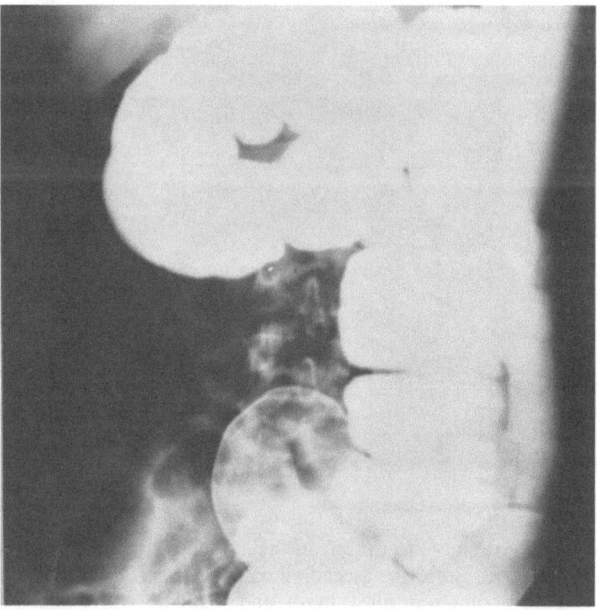

Fig. 13.7
Although the intestine failed to rotate as in fig. 13.6 the proximal jejunum was displaced during reduction of the physiological herniation to the upper left quadrant. Possibly a liver of unusual size or a difference in the timing of the reduction of the physiological herniation played a role of the abnormal course of events in fig. 13.6 and 13.7.

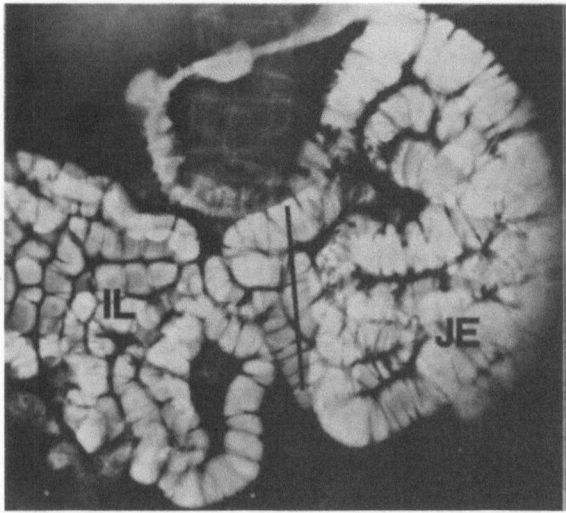

Fig. 13.8
If the omphalomesenteric duct is far from the cecum, there is an increased risk that during reduction of the physiological herniation a large section of the ileum will end up in the right half of the abdominal cavity.

drop and a distal ileum which is high in the right upper quadrant is not clear. It is in any case striking that this combination is encountered regularly (fig. 13.9).

Lack of fixation of the cecum after descent can lead to excessive mobility of this organ and eventually to a lateral Bauhin's valve (fig. 13.10). When fixation of the cecum is retarded, it may show pronounced growth in length. A very low cecum may develop if in the final stage descent of the ascending colon continues too long. In all of these cases the cecum can end up deep in the pelvis minor and may in addition become very voluminous (fig. 13.11). If the cecum and the sigmoid then become filled with feces, they can block the pelvis minor so completely that the ileum is severely compressed (fig. 13.12).

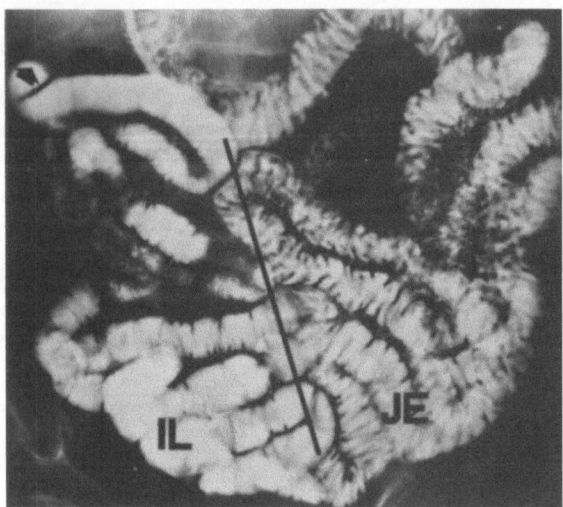

Fig. 13.9
A. The jejunum is to the left in the abdomen, the ileum to the right. Since the ascending colon failed to drop, the cecum (not yet filled here) and Bauhin's valve are situated under the liver in the upper abdomen.
B. Ileum in the right upper quadrant and incomplete descent of the cecum. The jejunum was in the left half of the abdomen and the transition between the two parts of the intestine was found in the middle of the lower abdomen.

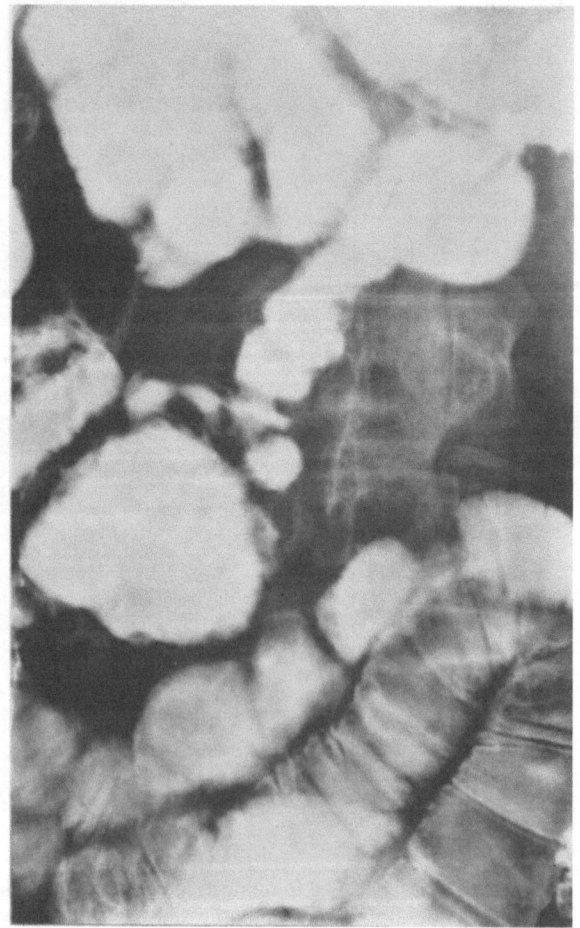

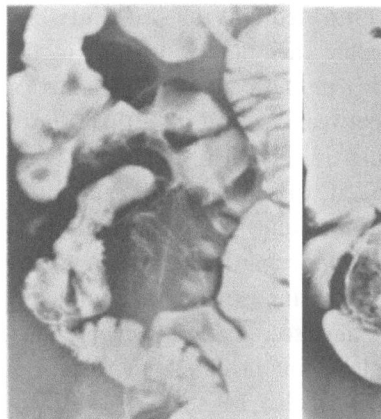
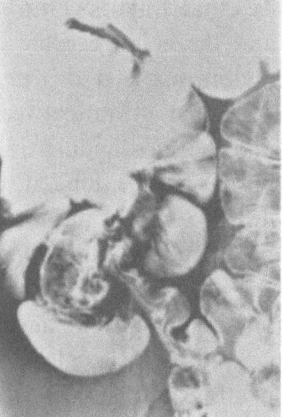

Fig. 13.10
Excessive mobility of the cecum; Bauhin's valve will then sometimes assume a lateral position.

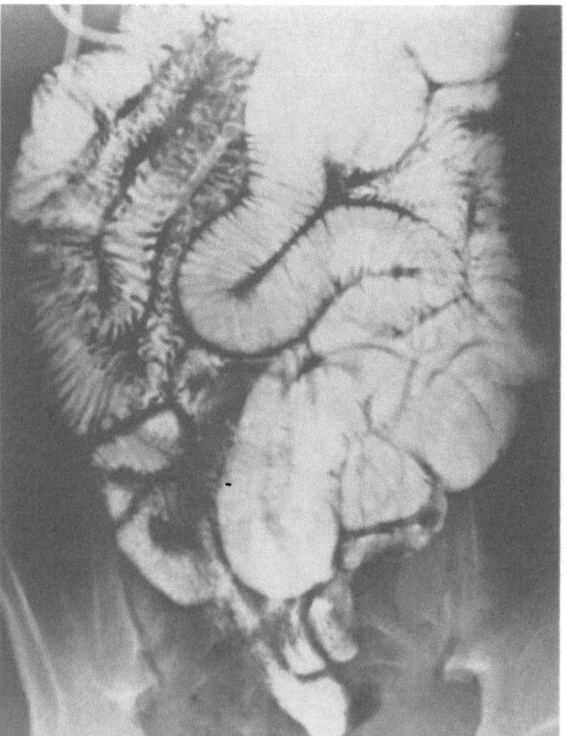

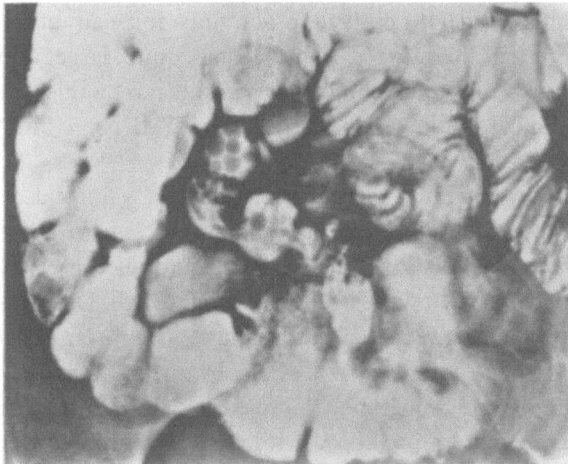

Fig. 13.11
Excessive lengthwise growth of the cecum because descent of the ascending colon lasted too long; this may sometimes be accompanied by abnormal fixation. See also fig. 7.30.

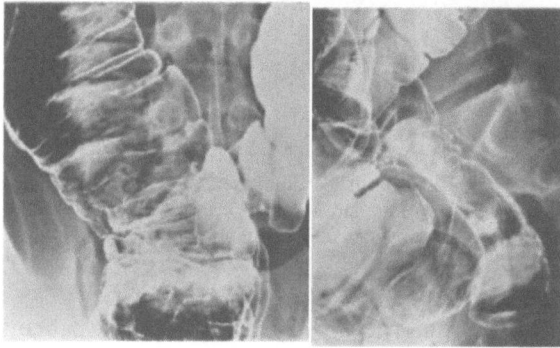

Fig. 13.12
If the sigmoid and a deep-seated voluminous cecum both contain large quantities of feces, they can block the entrance to the pelvis minor such that the distal ileum will become somewhat constricted and temporary obstruction phenomena can develop; this is recognized by dilatation of the ileal loops which increases in the distal direction.

Quite rare are the cases of total stomach-intestine inversion or the anomaly whereby the jejunum lies in the middle of the upper abdomen, the ileum in the middle of the lower abdomen and the stomach and the cecum to the left.

Although it is a very striking abnormality, malrotation during embryonal development is often overlooked, or is at least not included in the reports. Fortunately this negligence seldom has consequences since most developmental anomalies do not give rise to complaints. This is, however, not always true since some inversions can be reduced rather easily and can cause intermittent complaints.

In particular temporary inversion of the most proximal jejunal loops sometimes occurs (fig. 13.13). Probably as a result of some torsion of the involved intestinal segment, slight vascular disorders may develop. The ease with which temporary inversions can occur increases as the length of the intestinal mesentery increases and that of the radix mesenterii therefore decreases.

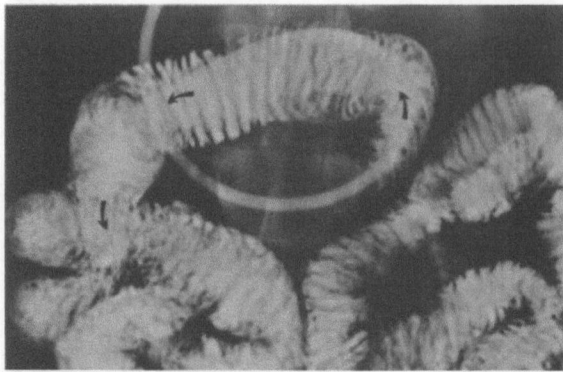

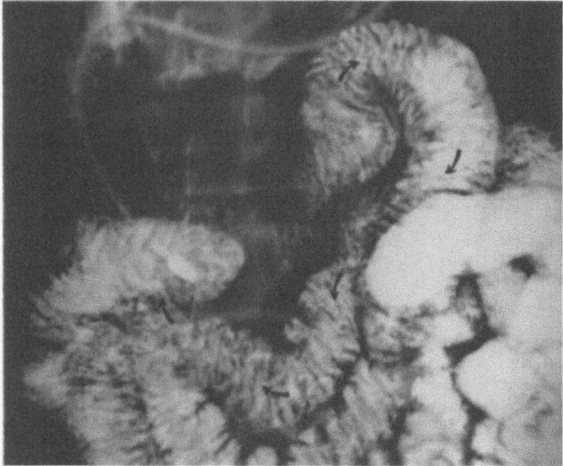

Fig. 13.13
Temporary inversion of the most proximal part of the jejunum. During the first examination this loop was located in the right upper quadrant (upper); in a subsequent examination it was approximately in the middle (lower).

Further questioning may reveal that some patients have colic-like attacks of abdominal pain whenever they assume an abnormal position, such as bending over, climbing (or descending) the stairs quickly, etc. – thus when making sharp thrusting movements. It is obvious that there must be personal contact between the physician and the patient in these cases before a correct diagnosis can be established, and that the diagnosis will certainly be missed if survey films taken by a laboratory assistent are considered sufficient.

2. Abnormal or fixed positioning of several intestinal loops: internal hernia

In about the eleventh fetal week, rotation of the digestive tract is completed and the small intestine and the colon assume their final positions in the abdomen. After this phase a number of bands or adhesions form between several intestinal loops and the surrounding tissue which serve to fix these loops in position. If these bands or adhesions develop before the intestine has assumed its final position, then the abnormalities described above can occur. If they are inadequate or completely missing then, as we have seen, pathological mobility can develop locally. An incomplete or partial fixation can, however, also be such that the intestinal loops can herniate through the resulting opening. Such hernias are found in the region of the ileocecal valve, the so-called retrocecal hernia, and in the duodenojejunal flexure, where left and right paraduodenal hernias develop (fig. 13.14). The latter type in particular accounts for half of all internal hernias; it can become quite large and cause alarming clinical signs which resemble the clinical findings of obstruction in the proximal intestine.

In the region of the ileocecal valve, a fairly deep sac can develop, especially if the mesentery of the distal ileus is long; a mass of ileal loops can easily become fixed within such a sac (fig. 13.15). Differentiation between a hernia and a deep retrocecal fossa is not always possible by means of roentgenology. Sometimes the fossa is so small that the intestinal loop trapped within it can be forced free by increasing the degree of filling (fig. 13.16). In general it is not possible to use compression or palpation to force loops out of a hernia or a deep fossa.

Herniation of the small intestine through defects in the mesentery can be left-handed as well as right-handed and can become so large that they include practically all the loops of the small intestine.

Congenital or traumatic defects in the mesentery, the mesocolon or the mesosigmoid can cause compression of a large or small segment of the small intestine; such abnormalities can also result from an inflammatory process or surgery (fig. 13.17). Another common type of herniation is that through the transverse mesocolon whereby the intestinal loops, part of the omentum or both end up behind the stomach causing a clear impression on the pars antralis (fig. 13.18).

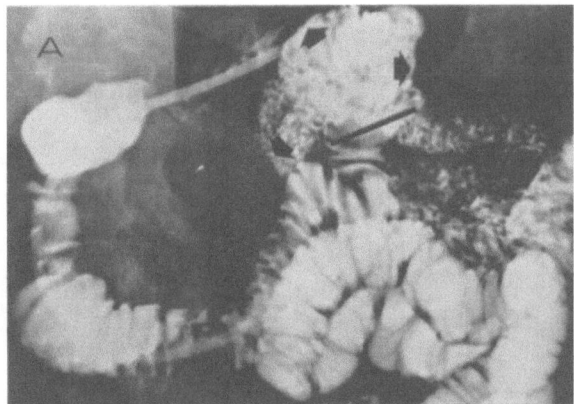

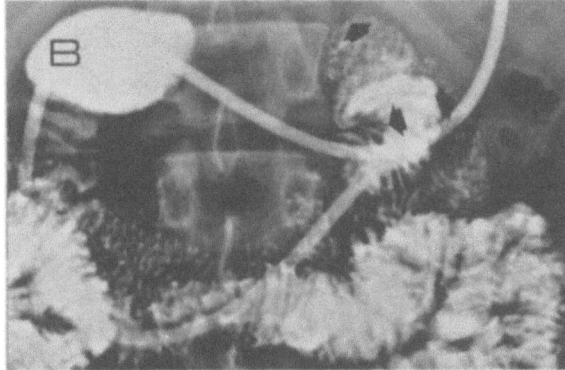

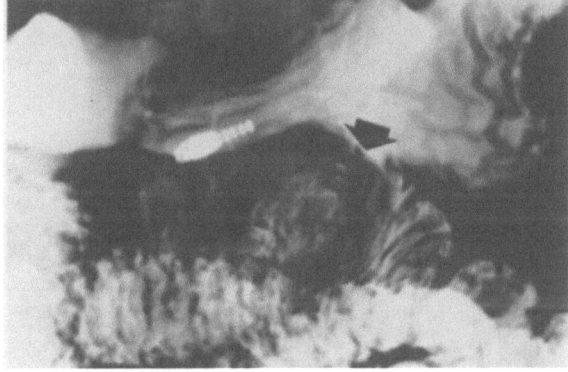

Fig. 13.14

Two cases of paraduodenal herniation.

A. Only slight intermittent complaints so that surgery was not necessary.

B. Hernia is small but the complaints were quite severe (upper). During complaint-free periods, the herniation was not visible (lower).

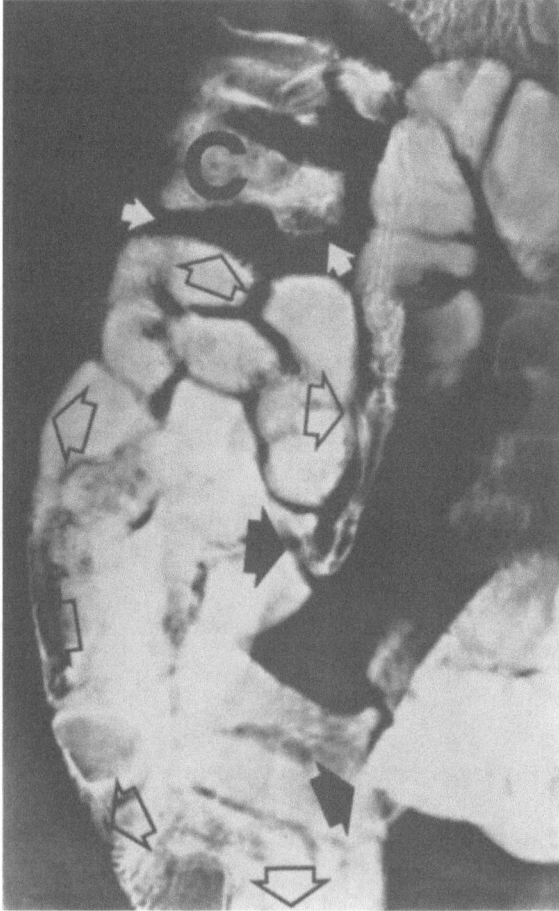

Fig. 13.15

Large sac (open black arrow) containing fixed ileal loops with air. The afferent and efferent ileal loop indicated by black arrows. C=Cecum.

Finally an inguinal or abdominal herniation may also be encountered; in addition the foramen of Winslow can be too large so that the intestinal loops pass easily into the lesser sac of peritoneum. In order to determine the diagnosis lateral exposures are often essential, especially in the event of an abdominal hernia at the site of an old surgical scar. Sometimes in this type of hernia anterioposterior exposures will reveal nothing since the orifice can be missed rather easily in this direction. It is also quite important that the contrast column be followed under fluoroscopy since intestinal motility in and in front of the hernia is often very locally but quite clearly disturbed. There may be an obstruction or locally reduced motility but usually there is a pronounced hypermotility and the patients complain of recurring colic-like attacks of abdominal pain localized exactly at the site of the hernia. Another characteristic is that the afferent and efferent loops of the compressed intestine taper slightly at the hernial orifice which is in itself invisible; they also lie close together and are absolutely fixed so that they cannot be moved by

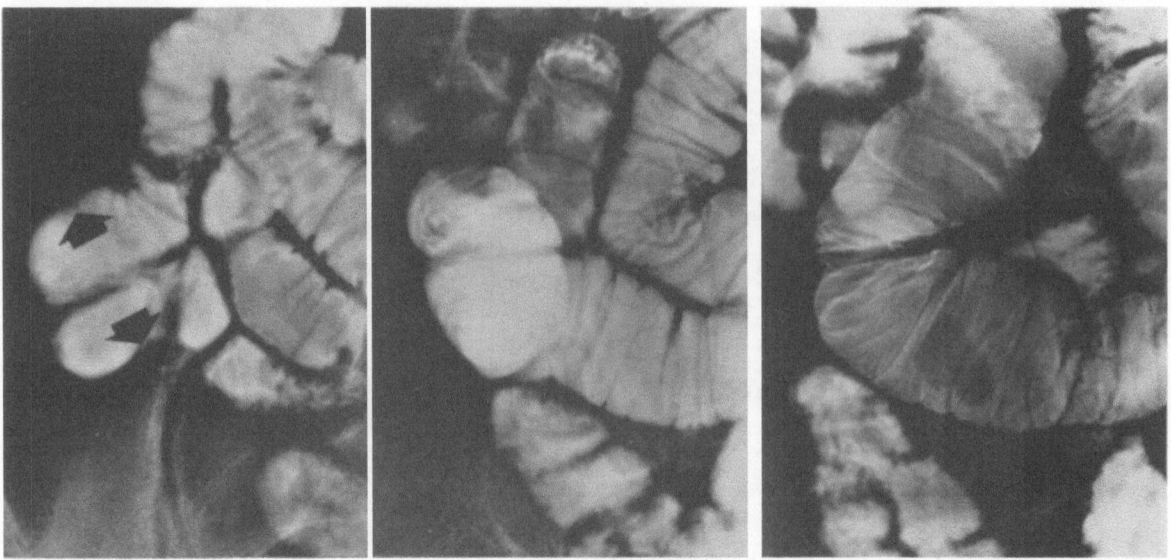

Fig.   13.16
Segment of ileal loop in shallow retrocecal fossa (← →) which was freed (from left to right) by means of maximum filling (water infusion).

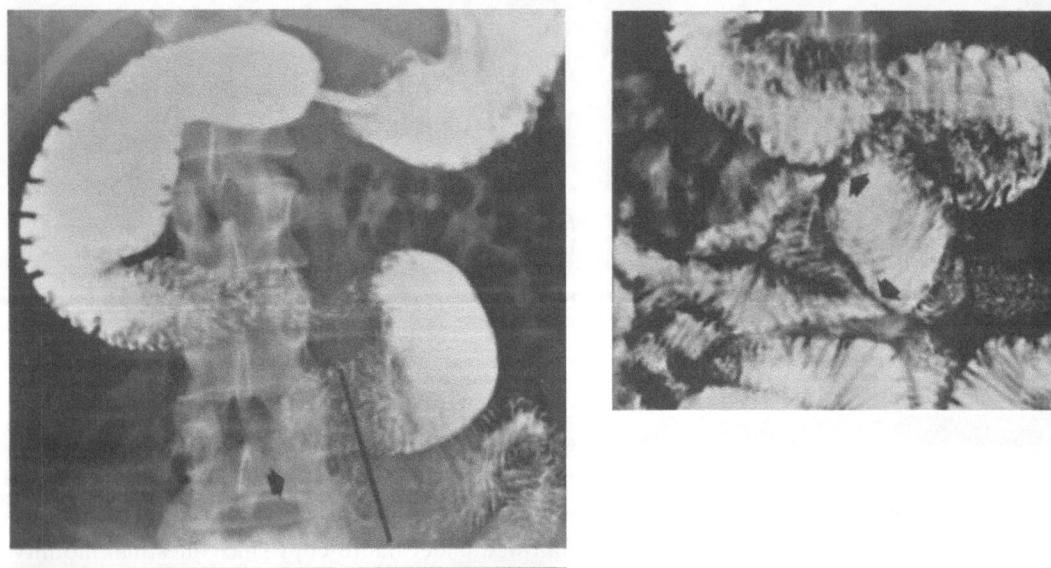

Fig. 13.17
Herniation of a segment of the proximal jejunal loop through a small defect in the mesentery (—), which developed after surgical removal of a mesenterial cyst. Proximal to the herniation is a prestenotic dilatation; on the distal side is very local pronounced hyperperistalsis which without a doubt caused the colic-like attacks of abdominal pain.

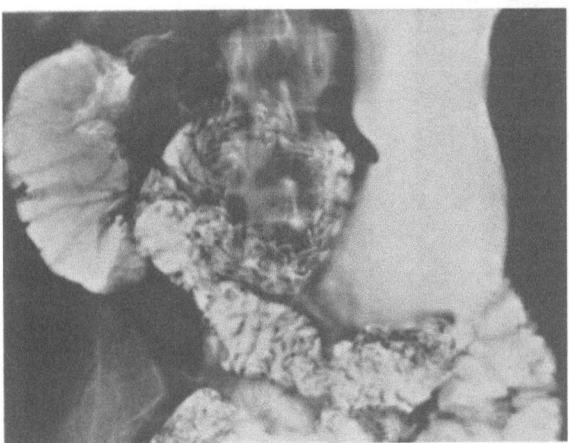

Fig. 13.18
Compression effect of proximal jejunal loop on the posterior pars antralis of the stomach which is encountered in cases of herniation through the transverse mesocolon (or through a dilated foramen of Winslow into the lesser sac). In this case there were no complaints and therefore surgical confirmation was not available.

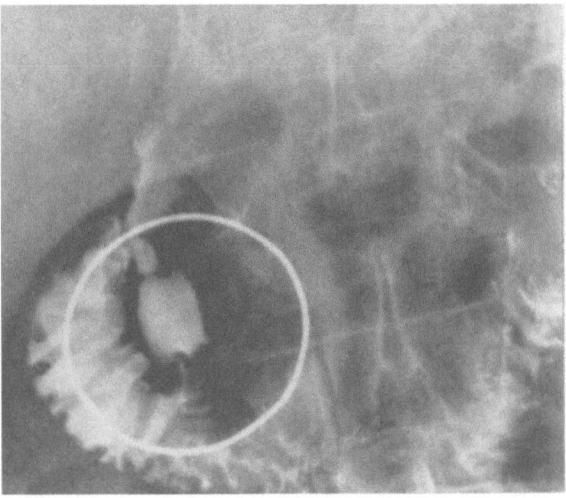

Fig. 13.19
Duplication cyst in the duodenum.

palpation. If survey photographs of the abdomen are made before the contrast medium examination, it will be noted that several intestinal loops consistently lie close together and are filled with air; moreover, when the patient stands upright, these loops show fluid levels.

According to the numerous reports in the literature, a preoperative radiological examination almost never yields a diagnosis of 'internal hernia'. We have found, however, that this disorder with its fairly classical history is easily recognized if this possible diagnosis is at least considered and if the roentgen examination is carried out using the enteroclysis technique and intermittent fluoroscopy.

3. Duplications

Although duplications can occur anywhere along the entire length of the small intestine, they are without a doubt most common in the ileum. The duplication may become filled with contrast fluid if there is an open communication with the intestinal lumen (fig. 13.19). Often, however, this is not the case and the space is enclosed. An accumulation of secretion products in this space will cause the so-called duplication cyst. Sometimes the only indication of these cysts is an impression on adjacent loops.

4. Diverticulosis

Small groups of 2–3 diverticula are frequently found in the small intestine, almost always in the duodenum. Larger groups of 4–6 localized in the proximal jejunum are a somewhat less frequent finding; in our department we have encountered this in 1 out of every 200 examinations of the small intestine (fig. 13.20). 20–30 diverticula spread throughout the entire jejunum is found in one of every 800 patients (fig. 13.21). In diverticulosis the number and size of the diverticula decrease gradually in the distal direction (fig. 13.22). A diverticulosis in the ileum is therefore a rare phenomenon; in our series this was signalized only twice in 4000 examinations (fig. 13.23). Diverticulosis seldom causes complaints; occasionally, however, a volvulus may develop as well as a diverticulitis or dyspeptic complaints due to a disturbance of the bacterial flora as a result of stasis. Mechanical complications can develop especially if the diverticula are very large. If the mesentery is fairly long, then as a result of changes in posture pronounced changes in the position of the loops can occur and torsion of a diverticulum may easily develop leading to necrosis and perforation (fig. 13.24).

Acquired diverticula are usually located on the mesenteric side of the intestine where the wall is

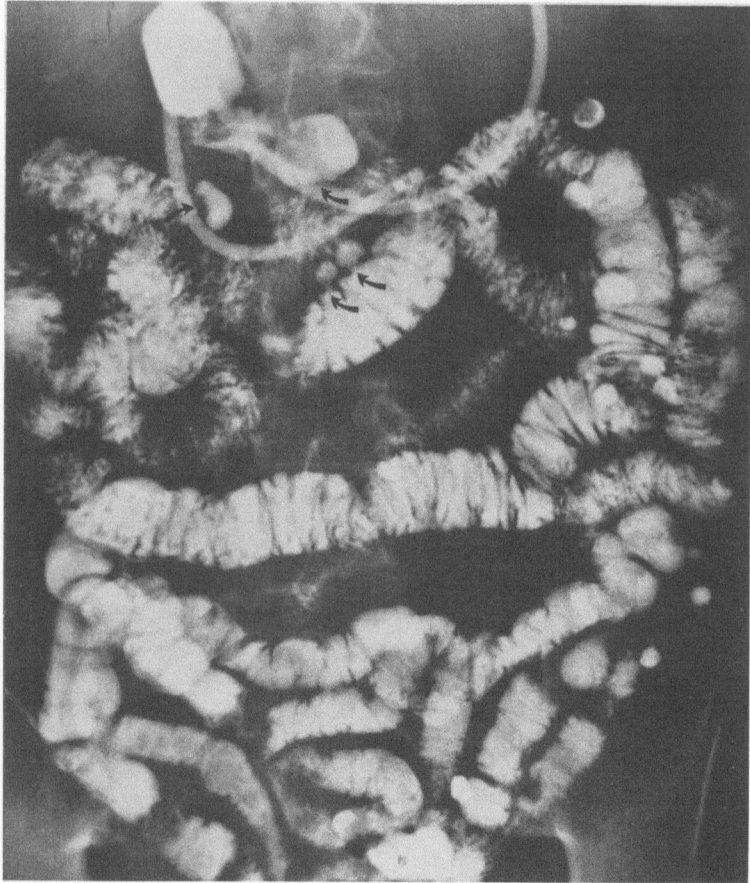

Fig. 13.20
Four diverticula in the duodenum and proximal jejunum. The more intense white round shadows in the left half of the abdomen are due to residual contrast fluid in diverticula in the left half of the colon after a colon enema 1 week prior to the enteroclysis examination.

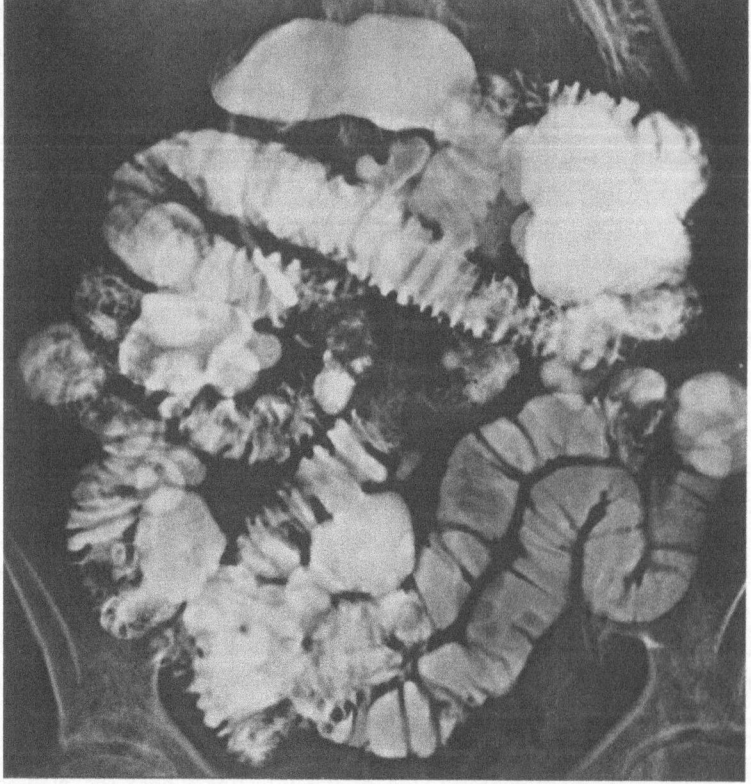

Fig. 13.22
Jejunal diverticulosis. The size and number of the diverticula decrease in the distal direction.

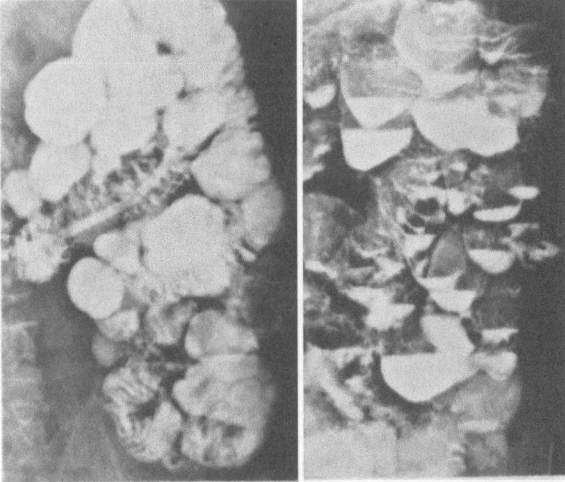

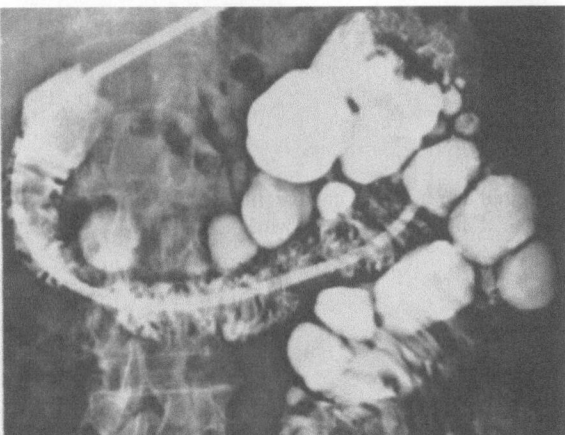

mined with certainly so that differentiation between a congenital anomaly and an acquired diverticulosis is usually not possible (fig. 13.26).

One must be careful not to consider all multiple sac-like bulges in the intestine as diverticula. One such case, for example, is illustrated in fig. 13.27: 4 or 5 diverticula-like formations are seen to originate from one point and appear to vary in size from 2–20 cm. It was found that they were due to multiple autoamputations after a hernia during adolescence which was treated surgically. It was no longer possible to determine whether erroneous ligation played a role in the development of this peculiar anatomical phenomenon.

Fig. 13.21
Numerous very large diverticula in the duodenum and jejunum; they are visualized most easily when the intestine is in the contraction phase and is therefore relatively empty. When the patient is erect, there are numerous fluid levels.

the weakest due to the presence of vascular openings. The wall of such a diverticulum is very thin and, like that of false diverticula in Crohn's disease, does not contain the muscular layer.

False diverticula in Crohn's disease are easily differentiated from other diverticula because they form in an obviously diseased intestinal wall (fig. 13.25).

Congenital diverticula are on the anti mesenteric side of the intestine; they involve the tunica muscularis as well and are therefore contractile.

The mucosal folds in the intestinal wall can be followed through the neck of the diverticulum; however, in practice this cannot always be deter-

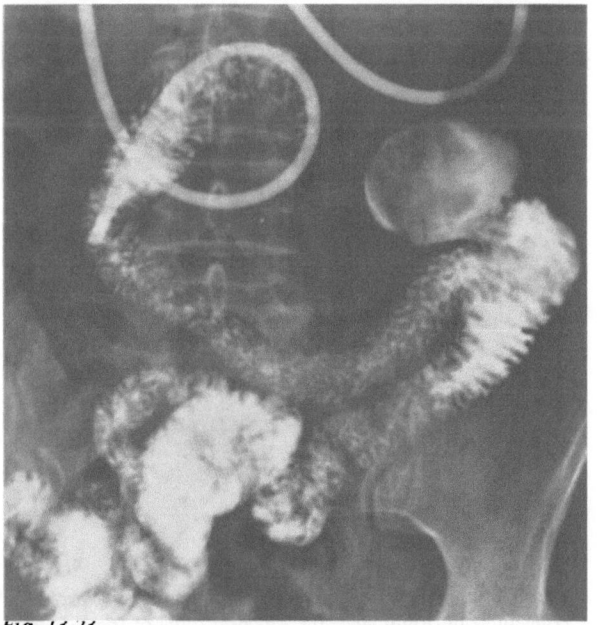

Fig. 13.23
Six small diverticula in the distal ileum. Ileal diverticulosis is a rare phenomenon.

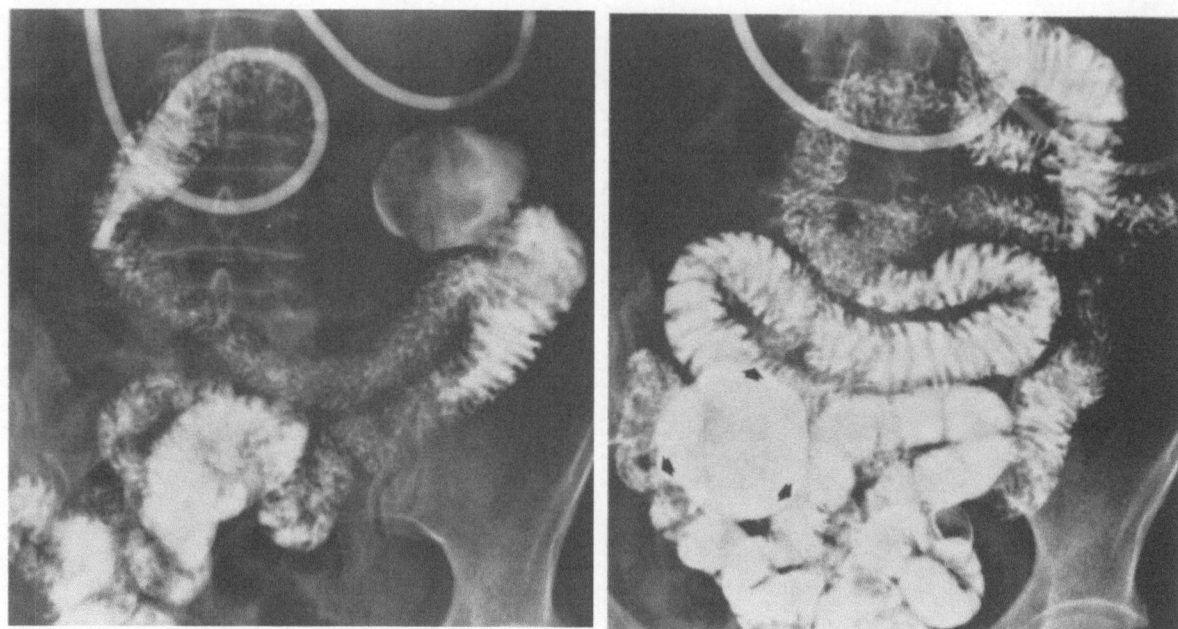

Fig. 13.24
Large highly mobile diverticulum in the proximal jejunum. As a result among others of changes in the posture of the patient, the neck of such a diverticulum can easily twist causing the symptoms of an acute abdomen with the danger of necrosis and perforation.

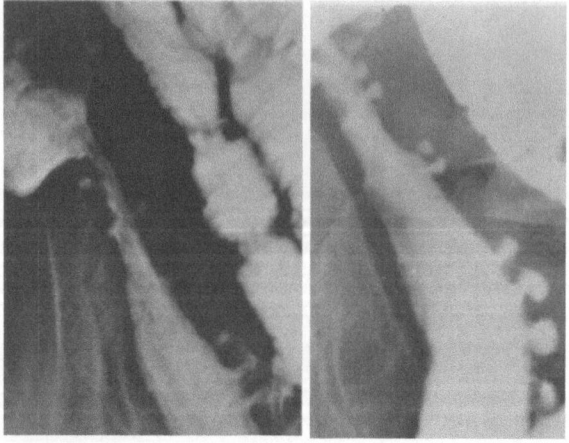

Fig. 13.25
False diverticula in Crohn's disease are easily distinguished from true diverticula because they develop in a clearly diseased intestinal wall, as in this case where mucosal folds can no longer be seen.

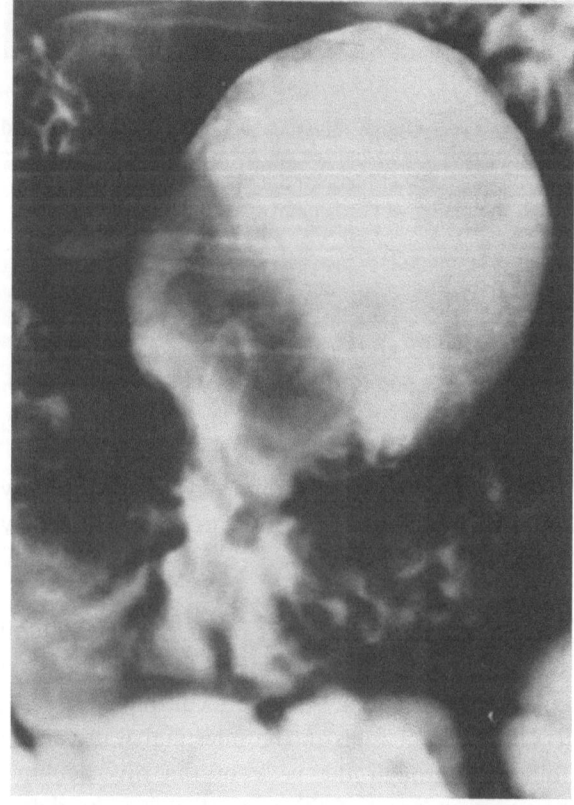

Fig. 13.26
Large solitary diverticulum in the small intestine probably congenital in origin since the mucosal folds of the intestinal wall can be followed easily through the neck of the diverticulum.

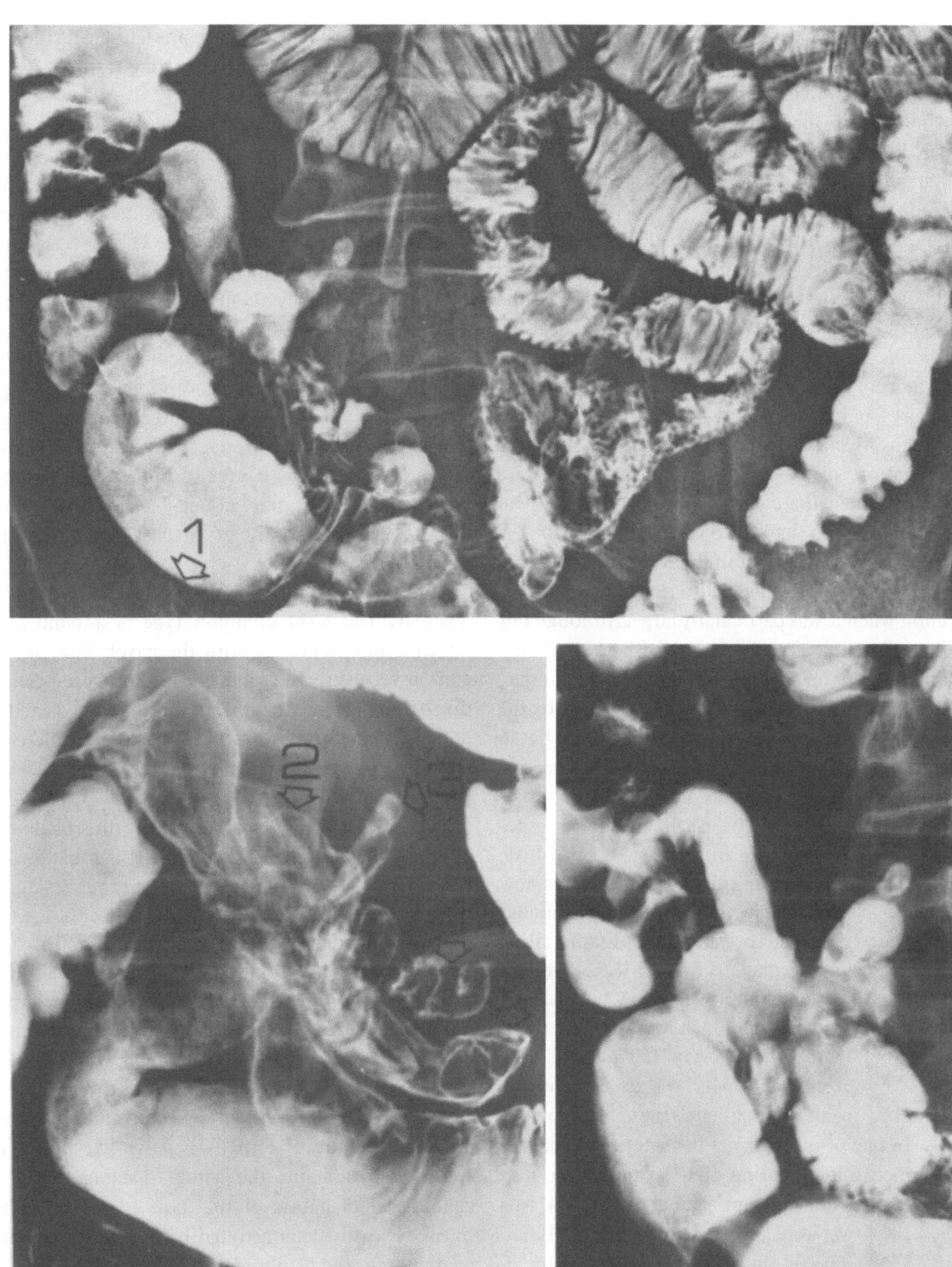

Fig. 13.27
Five sac-like bulges, extending from one point in the ileum, developed due to constrictions and autoamputation of the intestinal lumen after an incarcerated inguinal hernia was treated surgically. It is no longer possible to determine whether artificial ligation is involved here.

5. Meckel's diverticulum

Every serious radiologist is greatly disappointed if his findings are not confirmed by specialists from other disciplines: in the case of an examination of the small intestine, this means the findings of the surgeon and the pathologist.

One abnormality which is usually not identified until surgery or at autopsy and is very seldom diagnosed beforehand by the radiologist is the Meckel's diverticulum. Although all of the leading textbooks mention the Meckel's diverticulum and list the complications, the radiological illustrations are very sparse. In fact the radiologist only observed a Meckel's diverticulum during a transit examination of the small bowel in those rare instances when the contrast medium ended up in the diverticulum and also was retained in the sac noticably longer than in the rest of the intestine (fig. 13.28). He occasionally also recognized a diverticulum when it was particularly large. Although this failure of radiological diagnosis must be attributed mainly to an inadequate examination technique, the low diagnostic score is also due in part to the fact that the clinical course can sometimes be so acute that the patient must undergo immediate surgery. There was therefore no time for a radiological examination of the small intestine – especially since it had proven in the past to be of little value. Since the gastrointestinal examination is now no longer carried out in the conventional manner but by means of enteroclysis, these disappointing results regarding the diagnosis of a Meckel's diverticulum have certainly improved. Now by means of roentgenological examination, a Meckel's diverticulum is found in 1 out of every 150 patients. We believe, however, that a Meckel's diverticulum is overlooked in an approximately equal number of cases. In one of our patients this happened because we concentrated during the examination too heavily on a concomitant jejunal tumor; in two other cases we were diverted by Crohn's disease (fig. 13.29). This is understandable, especially in one of these cases where a very local dilatation was

incorrectly assumed to be a prestenotic dilatation because of the presence of the string sign.

A Meckel's diverticulum develops because the proximal end of the omphalomesenteric duct remains open; it is found at autopsy in 1–2% of the adults. Normally this duct atrophies during an early stage of fetal development. The diverticulum is always located on the antimesenteric side of the intestine. It is usually about 80 cm from the ileocecal valve although this distance can range from 20 to 100 cm. The Meckel's diverticulum can be very small (fig. 13.30) or several centimeters long (fig. 13.31); in extreme cases it can even be 30 cm long. In general, however, it does not exceed 10 cm. Depending upon the degree of obliteration and/or persistence of the omphalomesenteric duct, there are 3 types (fig. 13.32) of Meckel's diverticulum (Arey 1947).

Type A. The most common type is a blind sac which is not connected with the navel. The x-rays can be very surprising and misleading because the diverticulum is free to move in the abdominal cavity and will therefore always be projected in different positions on successive photographs (fig. 13.33).

Type B. This type of Meckel's diverticulum, which is encountered less frequently, is a blind sac which is attached to the navel by a fibrous residual band of the omphalomesenteric duct. In contrast to type A this diverticulum is always localized in approximately the same position because of its fixation. Often the tip of the diverticulum will point in the direction of the navel in all projections.

Type C. A very rare type of Meckel's diverticulum develops when there is an open channel leading outside the body. Externally a polyp-like bulge is seen which contains the fistula opening. Roentgenological diagnosis of this type is not difficult since it is easily demonstrated by injecting contrast medium into the fistulous tract.

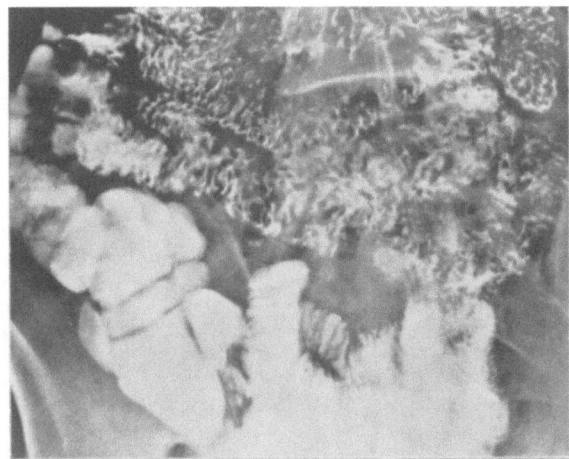

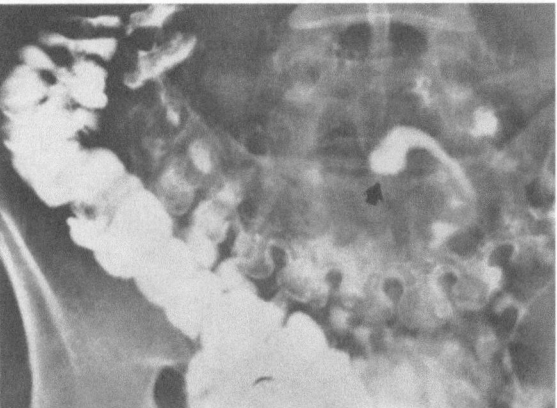

Fig. 13.28
A Meckel's diverticulum can be discovered easily, even if no effort is made to do so, if contrast fluid is retained in the sac of the diverticulum after the transit examination of the small intestine is completed (lower). On the survey film before the examination (which was at that time carried out in the conventional manner), the diverticulum was not seen (upper).

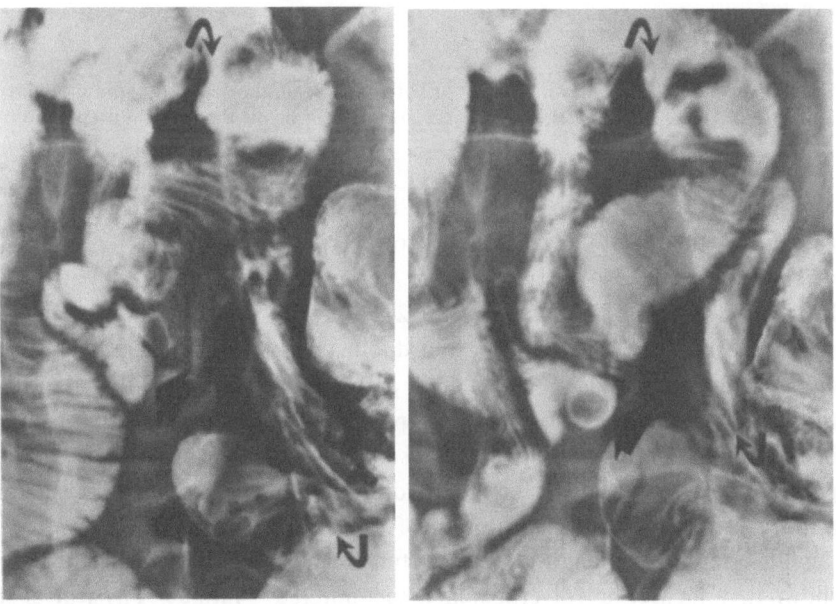

Fig. 13.29
Small Meckel's diverticulum (→) which was overlooked because attention was distracted by scar formation (→ ←) due to Crohn's disease.

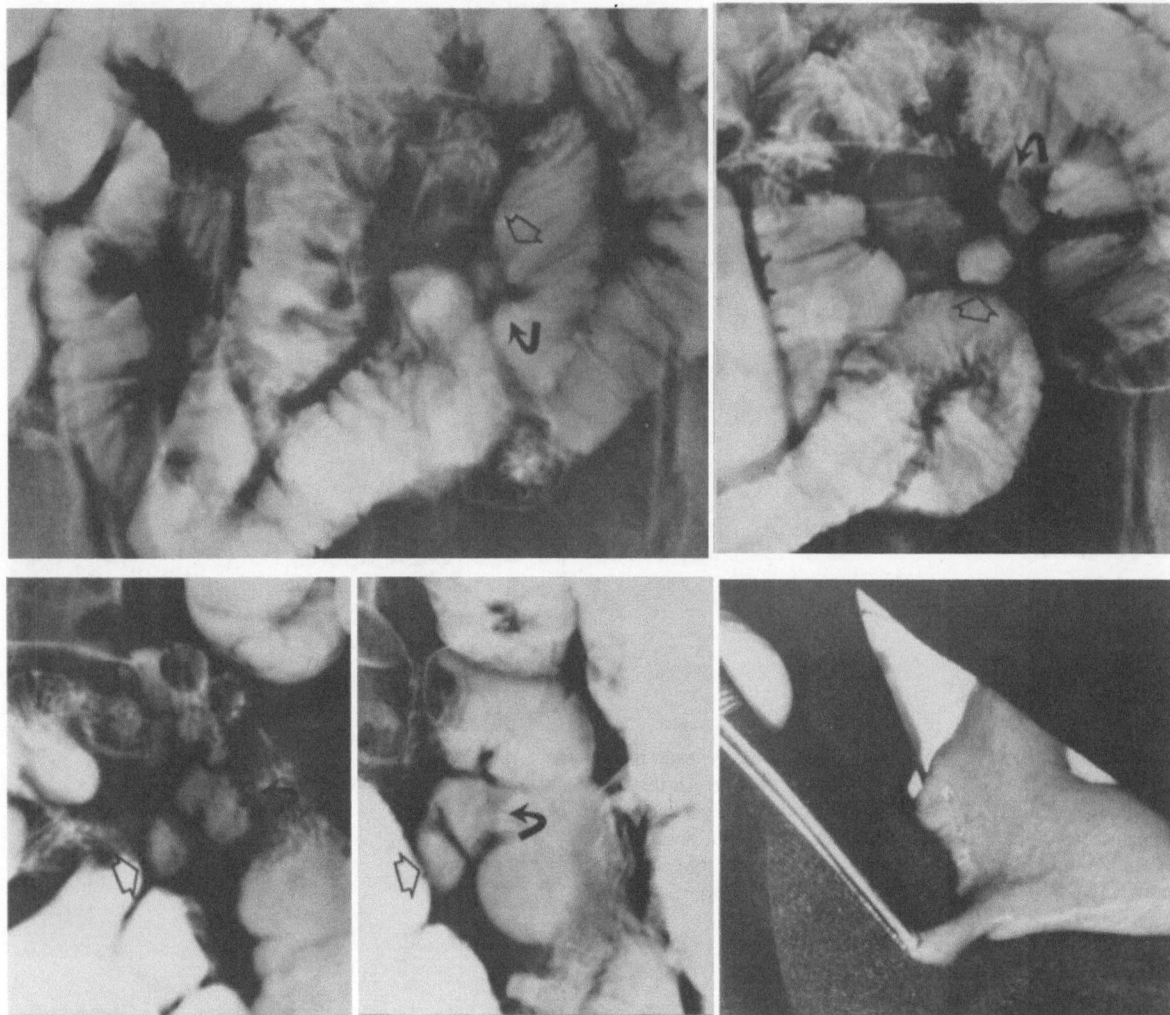

Fig. 13.30A
Small Meckel's diverticulum which is not or barely visible on the detail from the spot film (upper left) can be seen on the spot films taken with the compression technique. To the right below the surgical preparation.

In general the wall of the diverticulum is the same as that of the small bowel (70%). However, the diverticulum can also be partially or completely lined with heterotopic tissue; in 15–20% of the cases this tissue is gastric mucosa, but duodenal or colonic mucosa is also encountered and sometimes even pancreatic tissue (4%). A peptic ulcer in a Meckel's diverticulum is not an unusual finding; pathologists have known this for more than a century. Tumors in and calcification of the diverticulum are rare findings. Autopsy studies have shown that the Meckel's diverticulum is encountered in men more frequently than in women in a ratio of 3:1; it has also been established that it often occurs in combination with other congenital anomalies.

a. CLINICAL SYMPTOMS

All of our patients with a surgically confirmed Meckel's diverticulum were clearly anemic; in most cases there was even visible rectal bleeding. In addition it was striking that almost all of these had had complaints for years and had for this reason been examined radiologically several times although a satisfactory explanation had yet to be established. Some patients complain of abdominal pain or recurrent high temperatures, others only of fatigue. Physical examination often reveals a site which is sensitive to pressure; sometimes resistance is also encountered during palpation. A Meckel's diverticulum can be present without ever causing complaints; on the other hand a sudden perforation or peritonitis can also cause life-threatening situations.

b. RADIOLOGICAL EXAMINATION

Many suggestions have been made in the past concerning the technique of the small bowel examination aimed towards improving diagnostics and thus also increasing the chance of visualizing a Meckel's diverticulum. A large group of radiologists hoped to solve this problem by fractional oral administration of the barium suspension (Prevot 1936; Mendelsohn 1952; Bischoff & Stampeli 1955; Berne 1959). They believed that the diverticulum was almost never visualized because it was hidden by other intestinal loops. Others (Grossman et al. 1950; Wagner et al. 1955; Arcomano et al. 1962; Grollman and Sachs 1965) preferred a colon examination; by means of retrograde filling of the distal ileal loops the diverticulum would be filled (fig. 13.34). Obviously the diverticulum can be visualized more easily in this manner since other intestinal loops are no longer projected over the diverticulum. But even with these methods most radiologists were convinced that numerous Meckel's diverticula were still overlooked. If a diverticulum is inflamed and the mouth is swollen by edema, it is logical that closure can occur. The number of such cases will, however, be quite small and it does not explain the failure to identify the many Meckel's diverticula which are present but never cause complaints. Some contend that because the diverticulum is contractile, it is not continuously filled and is therefore overlooked on the roentgenograms (Elias et al. 1950; Lewitan 1953; Berne 1959). The presence of feces or intestinal contents could also prevent filling with contrast medium. Alvary (1951) believes that diverticula with a small mouth will in general be well-filled because the contrast fluid is probably retained longer. A diverticulum with a large mouth will indeed fill more easily but will subsequently also empty quickly. Because of this rapid filling they are interpreted on the x-rays as a loop of the small bowel (Alvary 1951; Berne 1959).

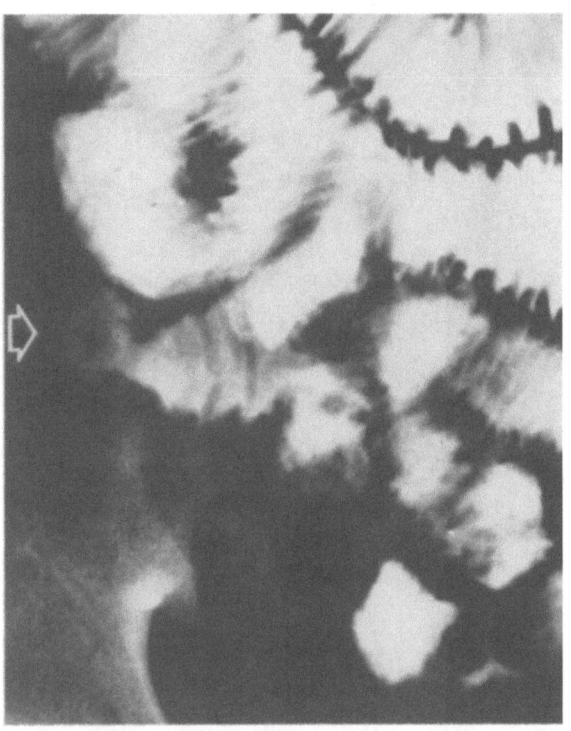

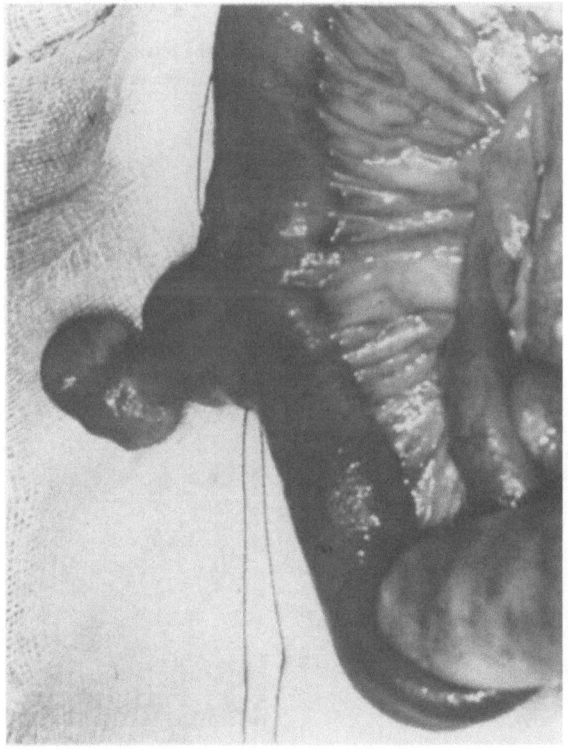

Fig. 13.30B
Small Meckel's diverticulum with a short omphalomesenteric duct.

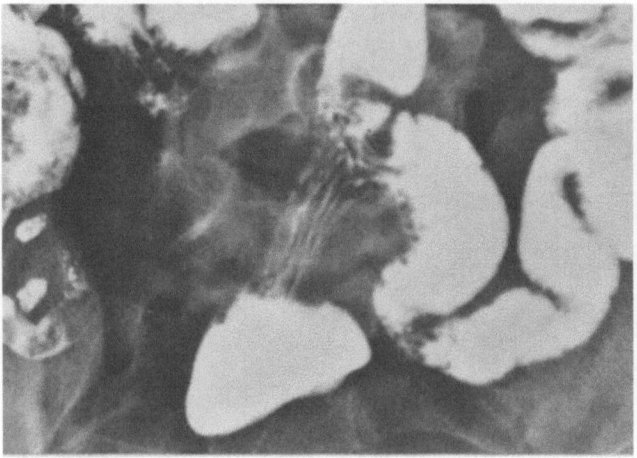 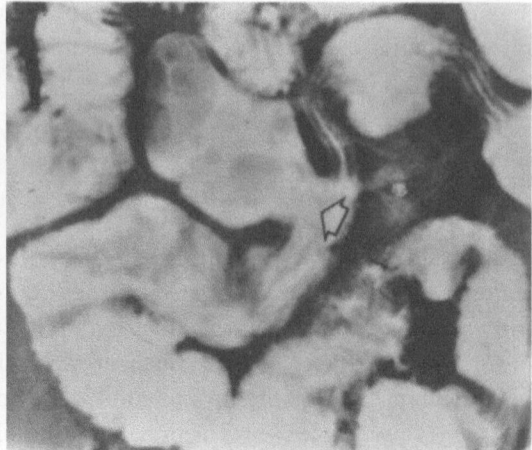

Fig. 13.31
Two medium-sized Meckel's diverticula.

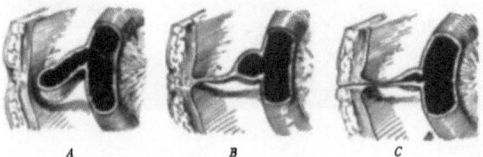

Fig. 13.32
The three types of Meckel's diverticulum (Arey 1947).
A. Moving freely in the abdominal cavity. This type is by far the most common.
B. Attached by means of a band to the navel.
C. The lumen of the omphalomesenteric duct is not yet completely obliterated.

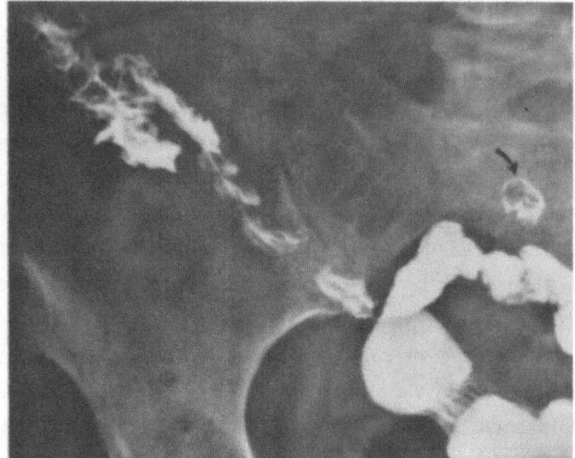

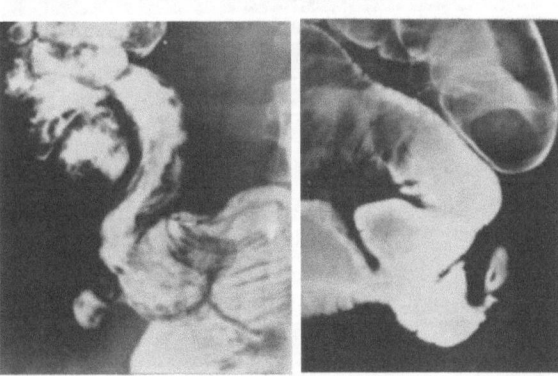

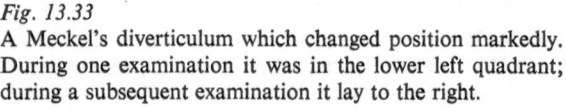

Fig. 13.33
A Meckel's diverticulum which changed position markedly. During one examination it was in the lower left quadrant; during a subsequent examination it lay to the right.

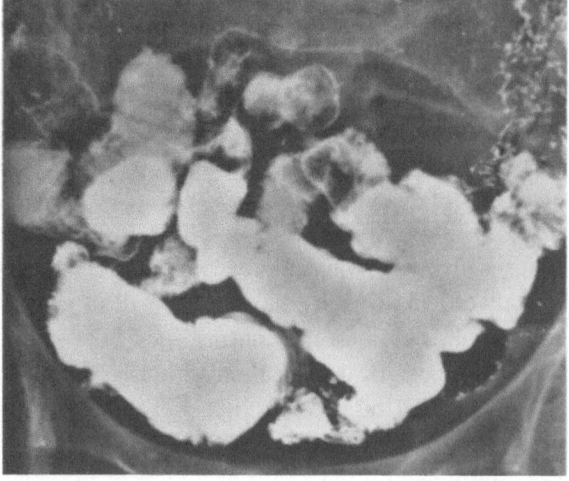

Fig. 13.34
Diagnosis of Meckel's diverticulum in the manner propagated in the past; retrograde filling of the small intestine via a colon enema (upper). The diverticulum was not recognized during the transit examination (lower).

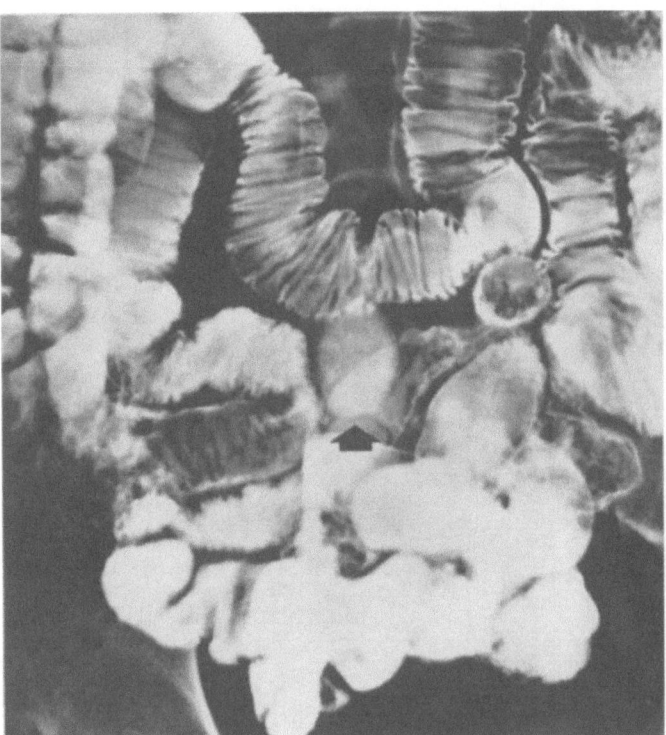 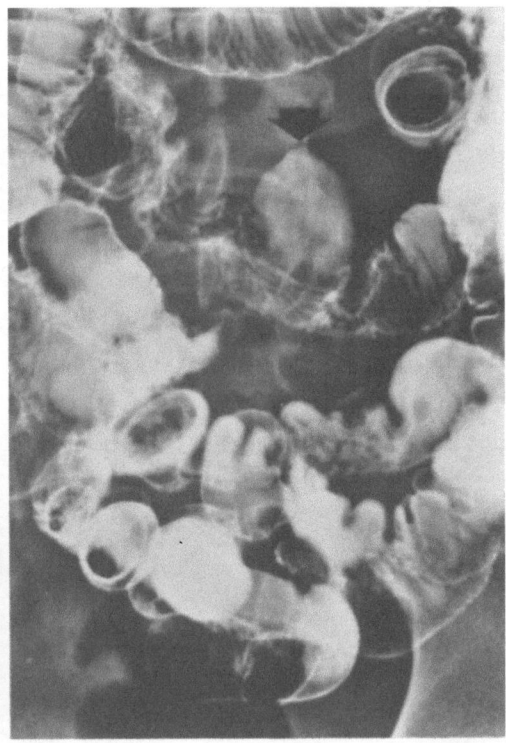

Fig. 13.35
This Meckel's diverticulum (→) was not recognized on the survey film before an enteroclysis examination performed elsewhere (left). The spot films taken later also clearly showed a round shadow with no signs of mucosal folds (right). There is an approximately 6 cm long omphalomesenteric duct (on the photo to the right below the diverticulum, although poorly visible).

Films taken during fluoroscopy have shown that the latter assumption is indeed true in most of our patients. The roentgenological examination occupies a key position in the establishment of a diagnosis so that this examination should be executed with the greatest care. We agree with Dalinka et al. (1973) who are convinced that the failure to recognize a Meckel's diverticulum is due solely to an inadequate examination technique. If a diverticulum has a wide mouth and can therefore be well-filled, it is important to provide such an abundant supply of contrast medium that this filling does indeed occur. We have found that for this purpose the enteroclysis technique is the only method for examination of the small intestine which is quick and certain. Merely administering the contrast fluid through a tube into the duodenum is in itself not a sufficient guarantee of an adequate radiological examination. The examination with the enteroclysis method must be carried out accurately; it must be remembered that in order to discover a Meckel's diverticulum it is essential that several spot films be made of the diverse ileal loops in different projections using a good compression technique. During the examination these films must be studied carefully so that further detailed studies can be carried out in the case of doubt. If this is not done, then one can be sure that most of the Meckel's diverticula, even the very large ones, will be overlooked and therefore not diagnosed. In particular the presence of a diverticulum should be suspected if suggestive configurations are visualized which show no signs of mucosal ridges (fig. 13.35).

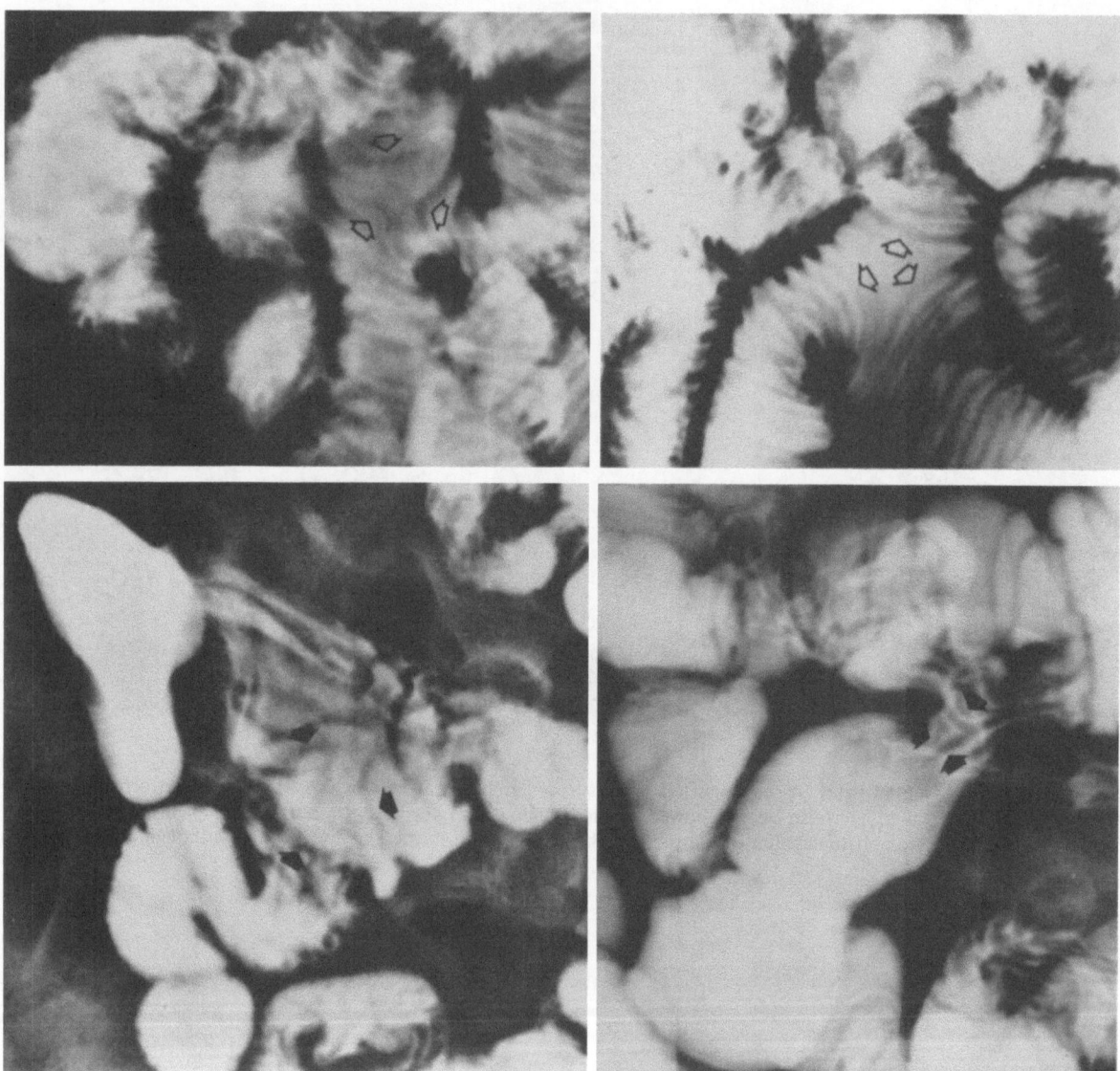

Fig. 13.36
Four different cases of Meckel's diverticulum, all more or less recognizable. The triangular plateau between the mucosal folds indicates the site of the exit of the omphalomesenteric duct.

If a triangular shadow, as seen in fig. 13.36, is encountered anywhere in the mucosal patterns of the intestinal loops then one can be sure that this is the junction with the omphalomesenteric duct and that a Meckel's diverticulum is therefore present, even if it cannot be visualized further on the x-rays.

A frequently encountered misleading pattern is the round diverticulum-like shadow which is in fact an axial projection of an intestinal loop (fig. 13.37). Another misleading pattern is the configuration which resembles a blind sac but is actually

the front of the advancing column of barium suspension. Moreover, in this apparent blind sac mucosal folds are often missing due to the disintegration and increased viscosity of the contrast fluid at the front as a result of the mucin and juices in the intestinal lumen (fig. 13.38).

A highly unusual misleading pattern is seen in fig. 13.39 where a configuration resembling a small diverticulum is caused by the partial superposition of two intestinal loops.

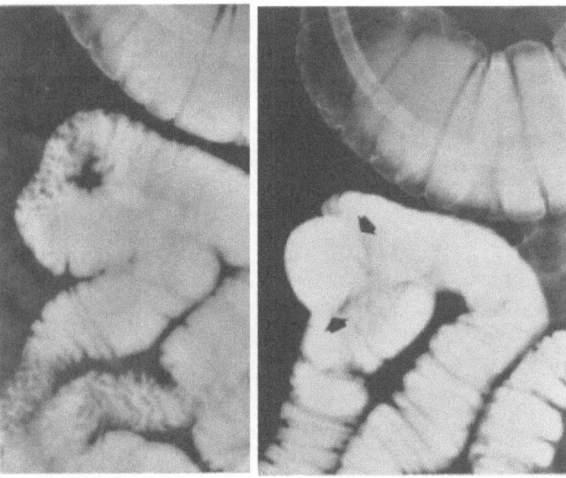

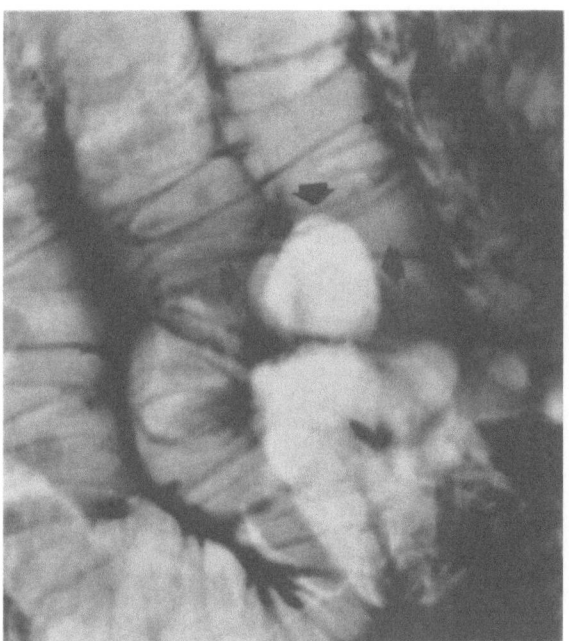

Fig. 13.37
Two patients with a diverticulum-like shadow in the mass of intestinal loops which was found to be due to an intestinal loop taken in axial projection. To confirm this a repeat examination was necessary for the patient in the right photograph.

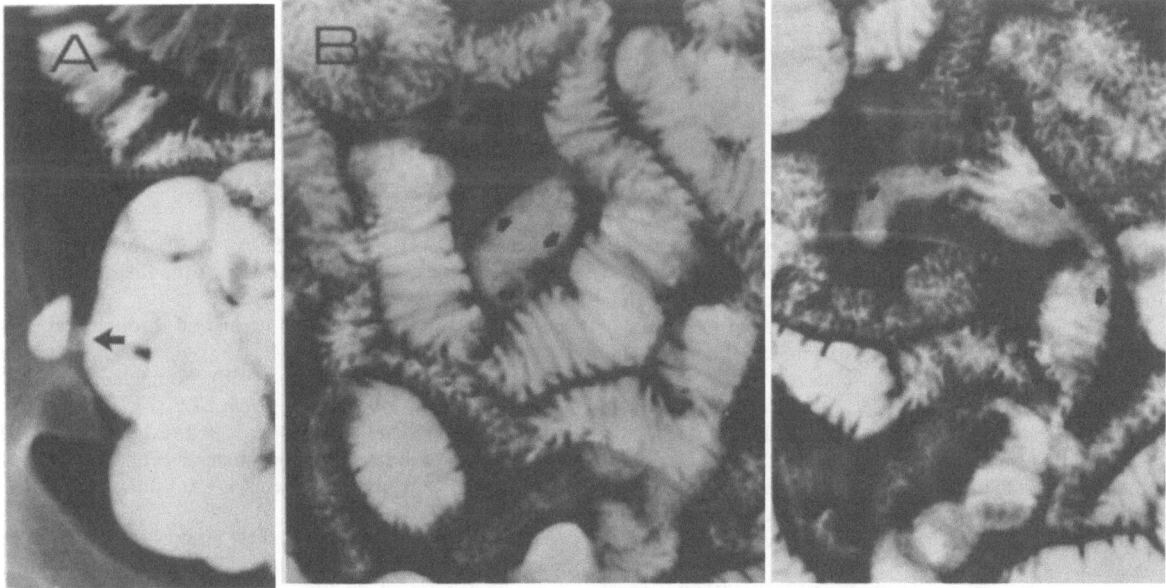

Fig. 13.38
Two patients with a misleading pattern suggesting a (Meckel's) diverticulum. In both cases this is in fact the front of the contrast column. In patient B, disintegration of the contrast fluid is clearly visible. The photograph of this patient on the left shows an isolated round shadow similar to that seen in fig. 13.35, but a second exposure taken almost simultaneously revealed that this was a normal segment of the intestine.

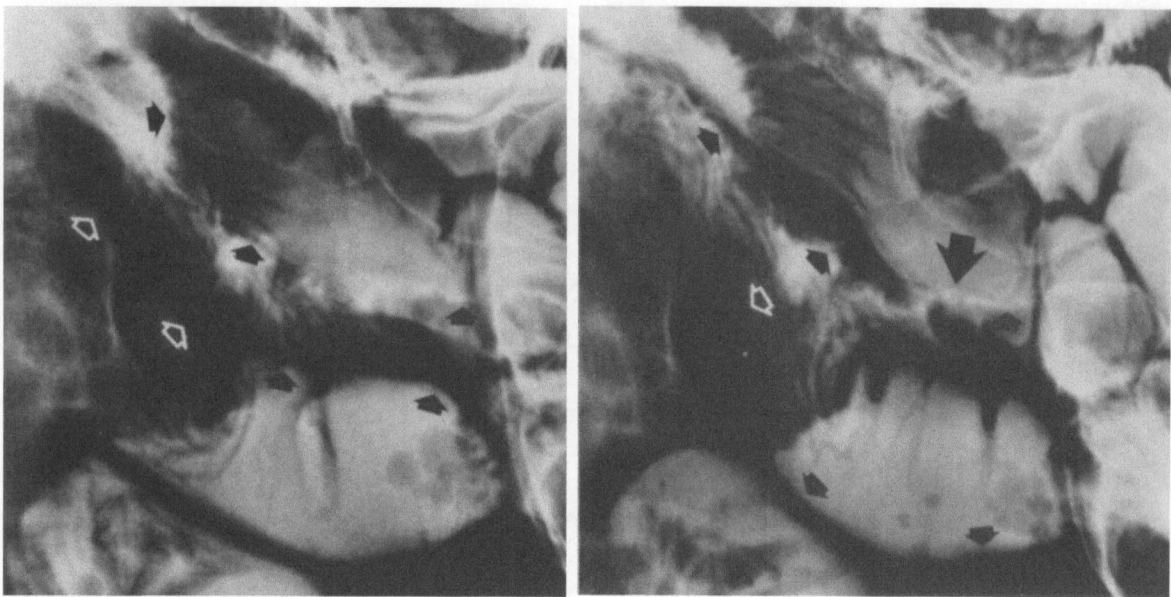

Fig. 13.39
Misleading pattern suggesting a small (Meckel's) diverticulum due to an air bubble and the partial superposition of two intestinal loops. As so often a second exposure taken almost simultaneously provided the explanation.

Bibliography chapter XIII

AREY L. B. (1947) *Developmental Anatomy.* A textbook and laboratory manual of embryology. Saunders, Philadelphia.

BISCHOFF M. E.; STAMPFLI W. P. (1955) Meckel's diverticulum with emphasis on roentgendiagnosis. *Radiology 65*, 572.

CUTLER G. D.; SCOTT H. W. (1944) Transmesenteric hernia. *Surg. Gynec. Obstet. 79*, 509.

DALINKA M. K.; WUNDER J. F. (1973) Meckel's deverticulum and its complications, with emphasis on roentgenologic demonstration. *Radiology 106*, 295.

DUSZYNSKI D. O.; JEWETT T. C.; ALLEN J. E. (1971) Tc 99 m Na pertechnetate scanning of the abdomen with particular reference to small bowel pathology. *Amer. J. Roentgenol. 113*, 258.

GROSSMAN J. W.; FISHBACK C. F.; LOVLACE W. R. (1950) Hemorrhage from a Meckel's diverticulum as a cause of melena in infancy. *Radiology 55*, 240.

FIDDIAN R. V. (1961) Herniation through mesenteric and mesocolic defects. *Br. J. Surg. 49*, 186.

HENKE F.; LUBARSCH O. (1929) *Handbuch der pathologischen Anatomie IV/3*, 158–179.

HANSMANN G. H.; MORTON S. A. (1939) Intraabdominal hernia. Report of a case and review of the literature. *Archs Surg. 39*, 973.

KING E. S. J. (1935) Intestinal herniation through a mesenteric hiatus. *Br. J. Surg. 22*, 504.

MOCK C. J.; MOCK H. E. JR. (1958) Strangulated internal hernia associated with trauma. *Archs Surg. 77*, 881.

ROONEY J. A.; CARROLL J. P.; KEELEY J. L. (1963) Internal hernias due to defects in the meso-appendix and mesentery of small bowel, and probable Ivemark syndrome. *Ann. Surg. 157*, 254.

STEIN G. N.; BENNET H. H.; FINKELSTEIN A. (1958) The preoperative Rö-diagnosis of Meckel's diverticulum in adults. *Amer. J. Roentgenol. 79*, 815.

WAGNER F. B.; SHALLOW T. A.; EGER S. A. (1955) Gastroenterological aspects of Meckel's diverticulum. Analytical review of 100 cases. *Amer. J. Gastroent. 23*, 195.

XIV

ILEUS - FUSION - BANDS - VOLVULUS - INTUSSUSCEPTIONS — INCISIONAL HERNIA

1. Ileus

When there is an obstruction in the small intestine, then even if no fluid is administered orally, the contents of the loops on the proximal side of the stenosis will increase as a result of secretion and exudation products from the intestinal wall. This causes an increasing dilution usually accompanied by flocculation of the contrast fluid in the loops proximal to the obstruction – and not dehydration as generally feared. In all literature not one single publication concerning experiments with animals or patients can be found which reports thickening of the contrast medium in the loops on the proximal side of an obstruction in the small intestine. As a result of the increased tone, the peristaltic movements are initially enhanced; if the obstruction persists, peristalsis decreases gradually.

Sloan et al. (Radiology 76; 407–414; 1961) carried out an excellent series of experiments with 60 dogs; they showed that the increased fluid and the distended loops proximal to a stenosis will develop within several hours and that the radiologist may only suspect a diagnosis of ileus when gas is also seen in these loops. This gas consists of 68% ingested air, 12% gas caused by bacteria and 20% gas from the blood via the intestinal wall. During the same experiments it appeared that the length of the distended segment proximal to a stenosis increases gradually with time and that the viscosity of the contrast fluid decreases. It was found that several hours after an obstruction had been induced, the radiological diagnosis 'ileus' could be established more easily in well-hydrated dogs than in dehydrated dogs. In a later stage significant differences between these two groups could no longer be seen.

About 1960, an attempt was made to use water-soluble contrast media containing iodine to localize the obstruction radiologically in what was assumed to be a safer way.

Many radiologists believed that Gastrografine would be ideal when barium failed due to flocculation or was contra-indicated. The following contra-indications are mentioned in the literature:

1. atresia or fistulas in the tracheo-esophageal area (danger of aspiration);
2. diagnosis of certain pre-operative and post-operative disorders of the digestive tract such as bleeding ulcers, suture leakage or perforation;
3. partial obstructions which the barium cannot penetrate or whenever dehydration and thickening of the barium suspension might occur.

It was found that Gastrografine is generally a satisfactory contrast medium both as far as the reproduction of gastric mucosa is concerned and because of the greater ease with which a pyloric stenosis can be diagnosed or a fistulous tract filled. However, all authors discovered that dilution of the contrast medium in the small intestine was so great that morphological evaluation of this area was absolutely impossible. In addition no-one succeeded in making acceptable double-contrast exposures, and some authors reported that more than 50 ml can cause abdominal cramps, vomiting and diarrhea. Reasonably satisfactory colon films can, however, be made because absorption of fluid causes an increasing thickening in this region. Thus it was often possible to obtain good filling of that part of the colon on the proximal side of a stenosis which the barium could not penetrate from the distal side. It remained impossible to localize tumors in the small intestine, although the diagnosis 'obstruction' could often be made on the basis of the presence of dilated loops.

Some radiologists believed that if the Gastrografine had not yet reached the colon 4 hours after oral administration, a post-operative ileus must be due to an obstruction and not a paralysis. Gastrografine may, however, be visible in the colon within 15 minutes even when a definite obstruction does exist in the small intestine. This thin liquid contrast medium can even pass through a very narrow stenosis of 1 or 2 mm easily. In approximately 2% of the patients, some of the iodine contrast medium is excreted into the urine. This is believed by some to indicate the presence of an obstruction, perforation or other pathological condition in the digestive tract. Although surgical confirmation has often supported this line of reasoning and Tosch (Fortschritte R. 95/2; 189–222; 1961) has shown with radioactive Gastrografine that it can indeed occur, disappointment and false-positive diagnoses have also been reported.

Gastrografine has strong hyperosmotic characteristics and this may be dangerous in the case of an intestinal obstruction. Since the osmotic pressure of 50 ml 70% Urokon is equal to that of 15 gm magnesium sulfate, a dose of 6 ml per kg body weight can cause such excessive fluid withdrawal that the circulating plasma volume can be reduced by 15–30%. The osmotic pressure of Gastrografine in isolated intestinal loops can be so great that the circulation in the intestinal wall is seriously disturbed. In addition the vomiting and diarrhea caused by Gastrografine can further disturb an already critical electrolyte balance. It has therefore become clear that in the event of a suspected obstruction in the small intestine Gastrografine is quite unsuitable as contrast medium. If still considered desirable, then it must in any event be handled with extreme caution and may be used only when the clinical condition of the patient does not form a contra-indication. Furthermore it must be realized that Gastrografine does not adhere easily and that therefore reliable morphological information can only be obtained when the loops are well-filled. In addition Gastrografine is such a thin liquid that fistulous tracts or perforation may not be discovered because the contrast medium flows past such abnormalities so rapidly that there is not enough time for penetration. In 1960 Shehadi

wrote that the introduction of the aqueous iodine contrast medium could be considered a milestone for diagnostics involving the digestive tract (Am. J. Roentg. 83; 933–941). Fortunately since then the use of Gastrografine has lost some of the ground it had taken by storm; however, a new landmark in the diagnostics of the digestive tract will be reached when use of this medium is only a rare exception.

The development of an adequate diagnostic technique for patients with ileus has continuously been impeded not only by the exaggerated value attributed to Gastrografine, but also by a second factor which appears to be equally as insurmountable. The majority of radiologists as well as almost all referring colleagues from other disciplines still believe that when an ileus is suspected, the most adequate approach is an abdominal survey film with horizontal beam. Although there is no danger in this method and even the inexperienced clinician can usually see very easily on such an x-ray that his clinical suspicion is confirmed, namely by observing fluid levels, its value can be considred dubious. It is apparently not or insufficiently realized that:

1. An ileus can exist without visible fluid levels. As described above this is certainly true in the beginning stages when there may as yet be insufficient gas or when the intra-abdominal pressure is so high that the accumulation of gas is greatly retarded or even prevented.

2. Fluid levels form as a result of the presence of gas as well as thin fluids in the digestive tract. It is obvious that this combination is not at all rare and is even pronounced in patients with diarrhea or malabsorption accompanied by hypersecretion or retarded resorption. Abdominal survey films of an erect patient who for some technical reason has been allowed to eat before the examination are not often encountered so that it probably is understandable that many will have acquired little or no experience in recognizing this particular phenomenon.

3. Even the presence of fluid levels together with dilated intestinal loops need not necessarily indicate an ileus; this can also be encountered in a number of the diseases discussed in Chapter

VI such as drug-induced atony, scleroderma, amyloidosis or certain forms of celiac disease.

4. An x-ray of an erect patient taken with a horizontal beam may demonstrate the presence of free intra-abdominal air below the diaphragm but actually such films should not be considered adequate for this purpose. Often the x-ray is assumed to be satisfactory if the diaphragm is just visible along the upper edge of the roentgenogram. It should be remembered, however, that only larger quantities of gas will be seen on such films; small and therefore narrow sickle-shaped pockets of air between the liver and the diaphragma are not visualized by an oblique beam. If it is necessary to demonstrate the presence of smaller gas accumulations below the diaphragm, then the diaphragm should lie at the level of the central beam, thus in the middle of the roentgenogram.

5. A dilatation of intestinal loops filled with gas can be established much more easily on an exposure taken with a vertical beam since the gas in the lumen spreads out over a much larger area when the patient is lying down.

In fact experienced radiologists do not need fluid levels to establish a diagnosis of ileus.

An ileus characterized by dilated loops filled with large quantities of gas is only difficult to differentiate from more or less similar patterns in patients with atony of the intestine, scleroderma, Naish syndrome or amyloidosis when the ileus is a result of any one of these diseases. If there is no nonobstructing or pseudo-obstructing ileus in conjunction with the above mentioned diseases, then the intestinal loops will show no hairpin-like configurations and the air accumulation will be highly local or will alternate with more or less normal segments. If the ileus is more advanced, then the peristaltic movements in the segment most proximal to the obstruction will be so greatly disturbed that a second x-ray taken several minutes later will show that the gas pattern in the intestine has barely changed. This local 'stillness' will not be observed in conjunction with one of the above-mentioned diseases, even if the intestinal motility is greatly disturbed. This symptom of local but total absence of peristalsis, identified by lack of change in and the persistence of even one single dilated intestinal loop filled with gas, can be considered highly significant for diagnosis; it almost certainly indicates a local obstruction or paralysis (fig. 11.2). In this stage only a subileus is involved and often it has not yet even been recognized clinically; however, further analysis of the nature of the disease is exceedingly worthwhile and the establishment of a correct or probable diagnosis is in fact almost always possible.

Only a barium suspension can be considered as contrast medium for the diagnosis of ileus, as in every other enteroclysis examination. The total amount of contrast medium required for the examination is highly dependent upon whether the obstruction is in the proximal or distal ileum as well as the stage of the ileus and the degree of motility still present. In general much more than the initial dose of 600 ml must be administered; a total dose of 2400 cc is, however, never exceeded.

As the amount of contrast fluid administered to patients with ileus increases, peristalsis decreases in a fairly long segment as stretching of the intestinal wall continues.

In order to retard this so-called 'inhibitory' reflex mechanism, it is recommended that the rate of flow of the contrast medium be decreased gradually during the examination. As in all other cases when large quantities of contrast fluid must be administered, here too the s.g. of each successive dose of 600 cc barium suspension is decreased with respect to the preceding dose. In practice this gives the following dose schedule:

1st dose of 600 ml
         s.g. = 1.30; rate of flow 100 ml/min
2nd dose of 600 ml
         s.g. = 1.25; rate of flow 80–75 ml/min
3rd dose of 600 ml
         s.g. = 1.20; rate of flow 60–50 ml/min
4th dose of 600 ml
         s.g. = 1.15; rate of flow 40–25 ml/min

In most cases the site of the obstruction is then reached in about an hour, even if it is fairly pronounced and rather distal in the small intestine (fig. 14.1). It is certainly possible to make good compression spot films after administration of this maximum dosage of 2400 ml – but a very careful and precise technique is required (fig. 14.2). If the

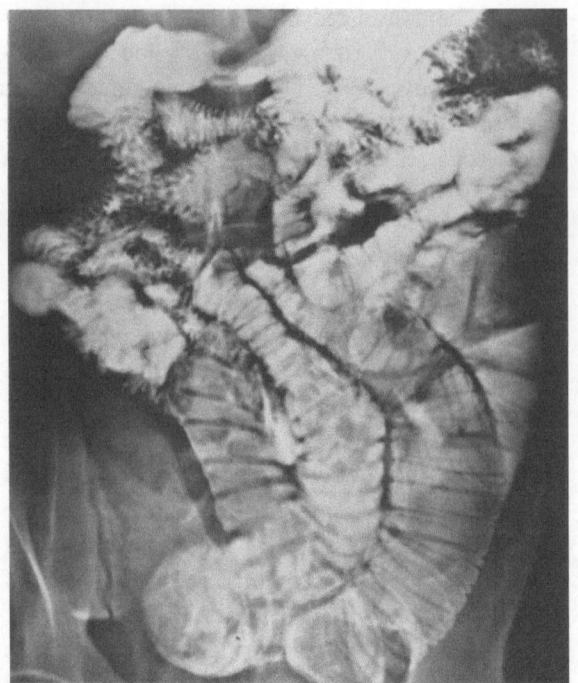

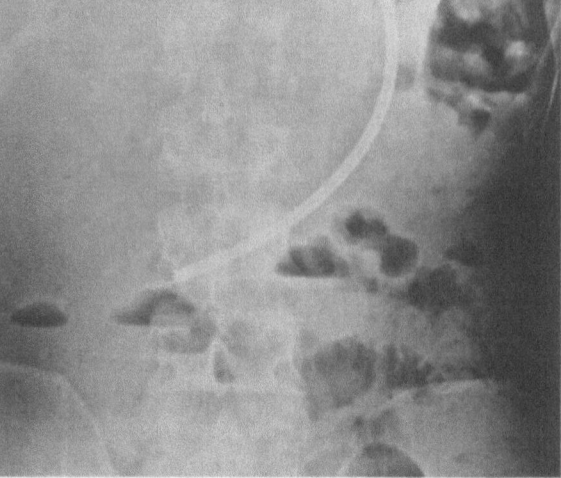

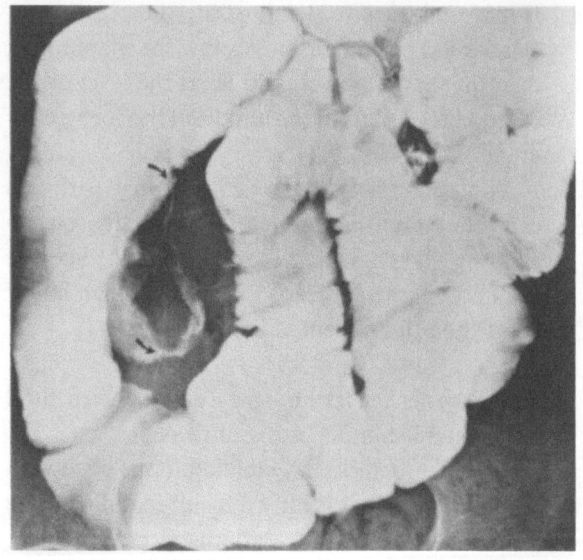

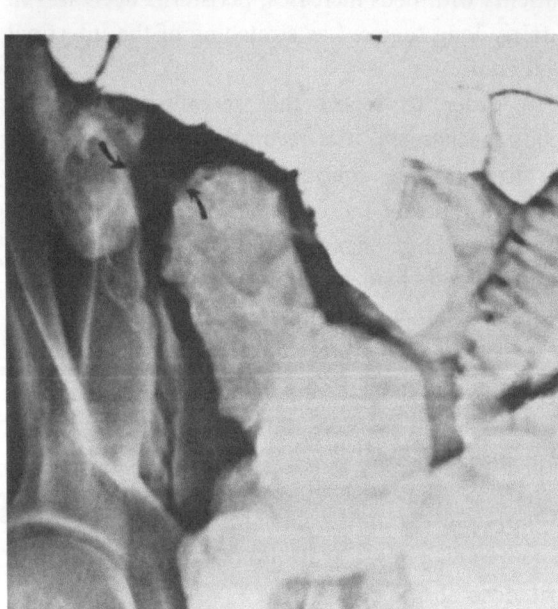

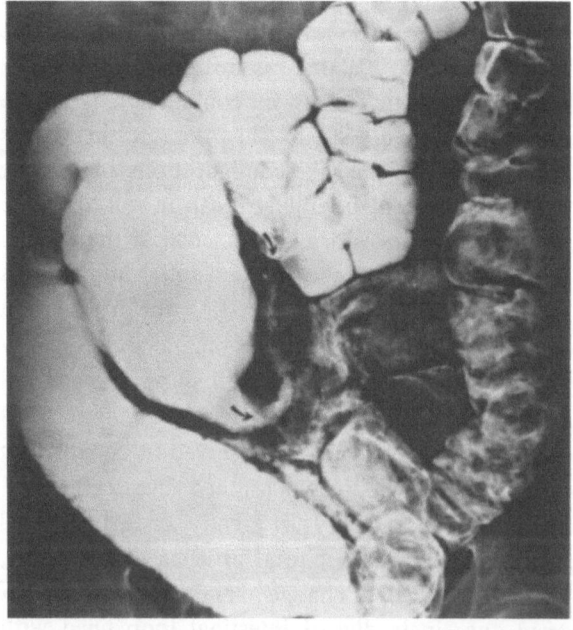

Fig. 14.1
Patient with ileus due to an obstructing stenosis in the distal ileum (Crohn's disease). In the jejunum peristalsis is still active; distalwards, however, the loops become dilated and the peristaltic movements diminish. In spite of the administration of 1800 cc contrast fluid, it was still possible to take adequate exposures with the compression technique.

Fig. 14.3
Ileus due to recurring stenosis in a patient with an ileocolic anastomosis and a 'short bowel' (Crohn's disease). In spite of the use of 1800 cc contrast fluid the small bowel was almost empty within three hours.

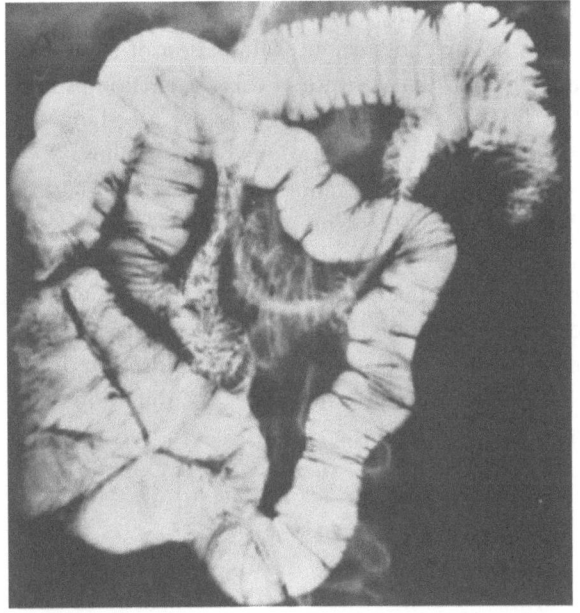

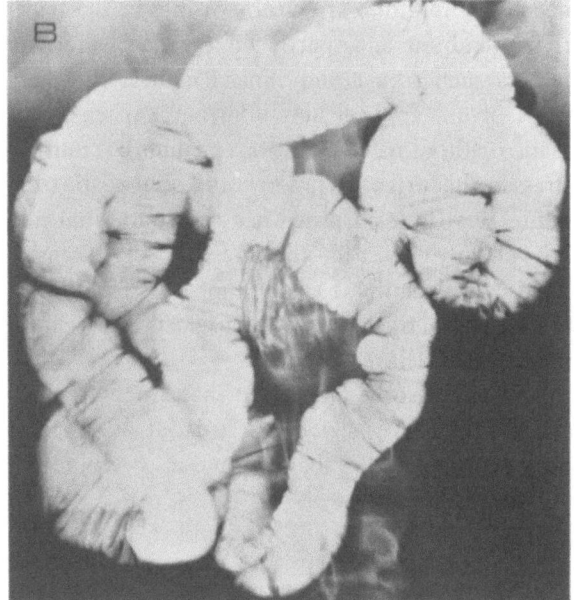

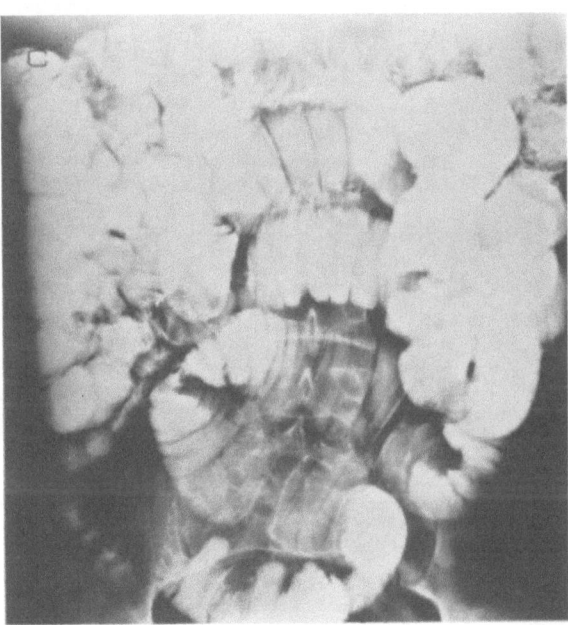

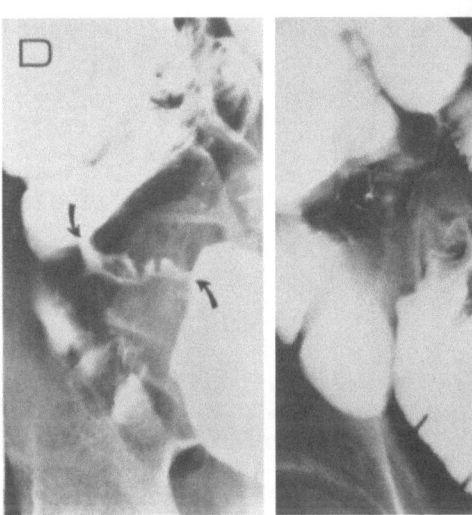

Fig. 14.2
A series of exposures of a patient with a tumor causing marked stenosis in the distal ileum.
A. Survey film after 600 ml barium suspension
B. Survey film after 1200 ml barium suspension
C. Survey film after 2400 ml barium suspension
D. Spot films with compression technique after administration of 2400 ml barium suspension showing the tumor in the region of Bauhin's valve.

obstruction is not yet reached, then we follow the conservative approach – and wait.

To our surprise it has repeatedly been shown that this large quantity of contrast medium usually reaches the colon within 6–8 hours, even in the case of very pronounced stenoses located in the distal-most part of the small intestine (see figs. 14.3 and 14.4). In a few patients with an almost total ob-struction the colon was not reached until the next morning (24 hours later). Occasionally it is possible to locate the site of the obstruction by means of the gas contours on one or more of the abdominal survey films. In other cases signs of a space-occupying infiltrate are clearly visible in the lower right quadrant and, partly on the basis of other factors such as age and clinical course, the diagnosis of an 'appendicular infiltrate' can easily be made (without using a contrast medium). It must be stressed that extensive pre-operative diagnostic techniques serve little purpose when the abdominal film has already revealed the presence of extensive bands, an ileus due to gall stones, perforation in the digestive tract or when surgical intervention must not be delayed.

It should also be mentioned that an enteroclysis examination may only be carried out after it has been determined that the obstruction is *not* located in the colon.

When evaluating the abdominal survey films taken before the barium examination, it should be remembered that the site of the obstruction usually lies further distalwards than is presumed on the basis of the gas configurations on these films.

In the case of a stenosis in the colon, there is dehydration of the contrast fluid proximal to the site of the obstruction and the barium suspension becomes so thick that barium stones develop, causing an eventual subileus to become a manifest ileus. In the event of doubt as to the location of the ileus, a retrograde enteroclysis examination may also be considered (fig. 14.5).

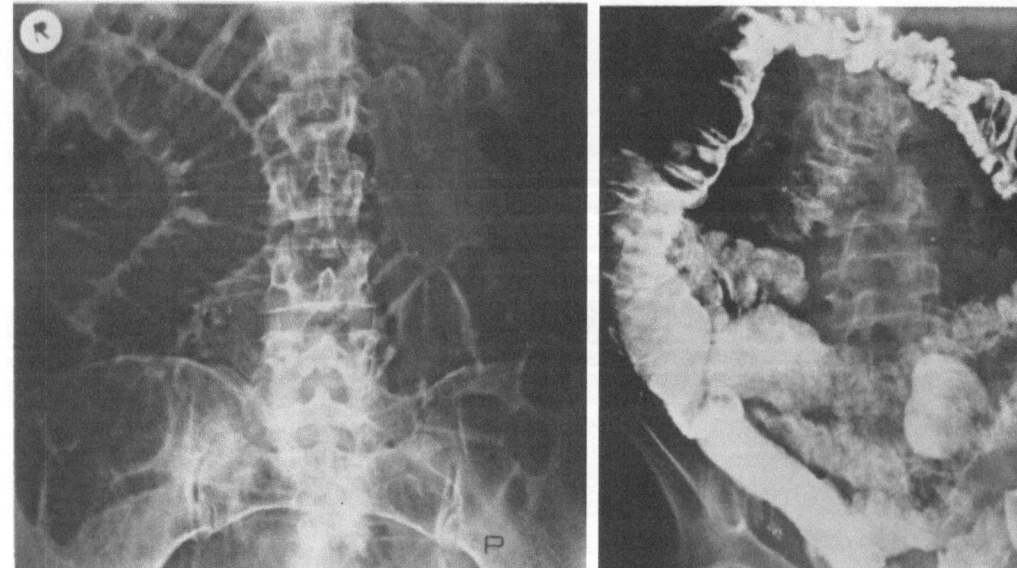

Fig. 14.4
Series of survey films of a stenotic process in the distal ileum which developed after a minor ileal resection.
P. Plain abdominal survey film showing numerous dilated intestinal loops filled with an overabundance of gas.
Q. Survey film after administration of 1200 ml barium suspension
R. Survey film after 1200 ml barium suspension followed by 1200 ml water.
The stenosis, which is several centimeters long, was visualized on the spot films with the compression technique but the cause was not identified. The obstruction turned out to be due solely to the narrow anastomosis with pronounced edema of the intestinal wall.
S. About 10 hours after initiation of the examination, which lasted 1 hour, most of the contrast fluid is in the colon.

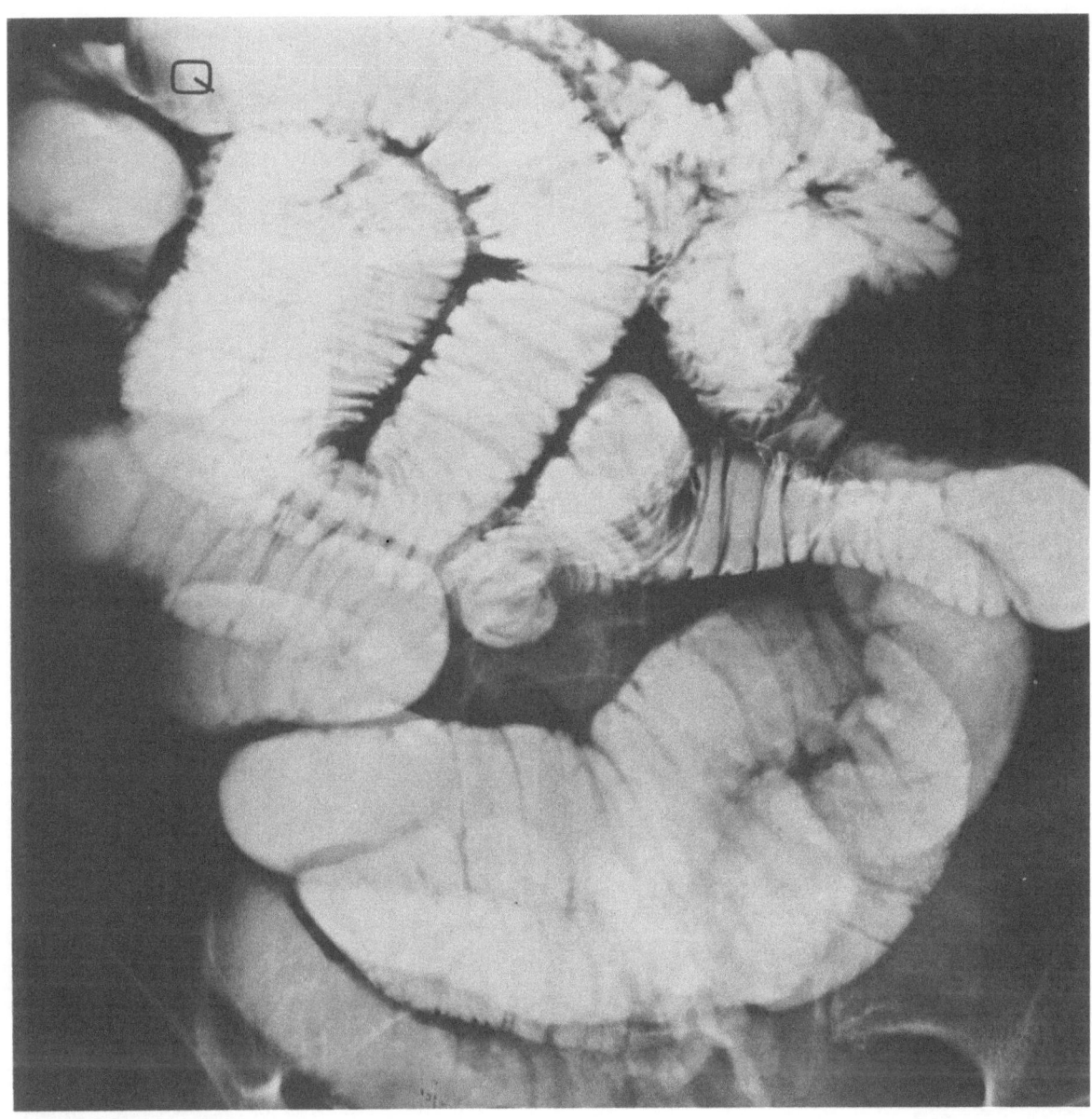

*Fig. 14.4*Q

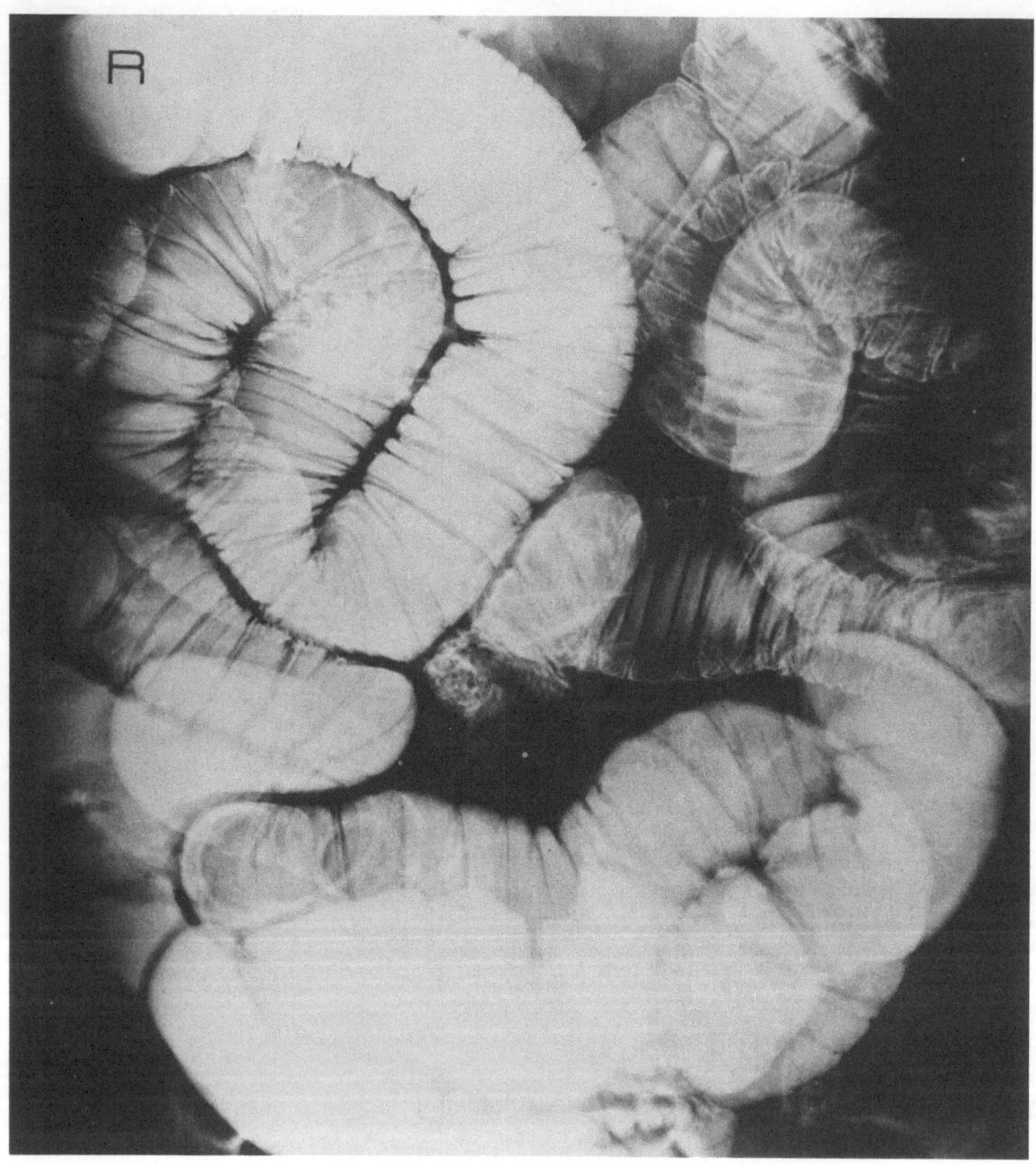

*Fig. 14.4*R

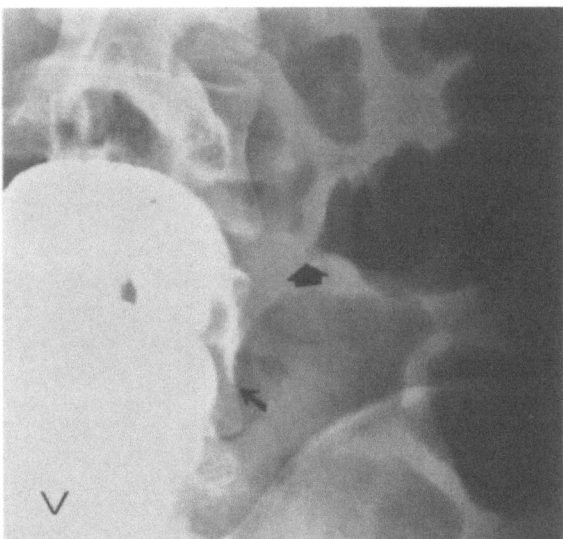

Fig. 14.5

v. Ileus which was found during surgery to be due to constriction by a band. The survey films without contrast fluid showed a cone-shaped shadow (thick arrow). By means of retrograde enteroclysis, the site of the obstruction (thin arrow) was approached from the distal direction.

w. Total obstruction due to metastases in the intestine. The site of the obstruction (→) could only be approached from the distal side. Highly swollen jejunal loops filled with air.

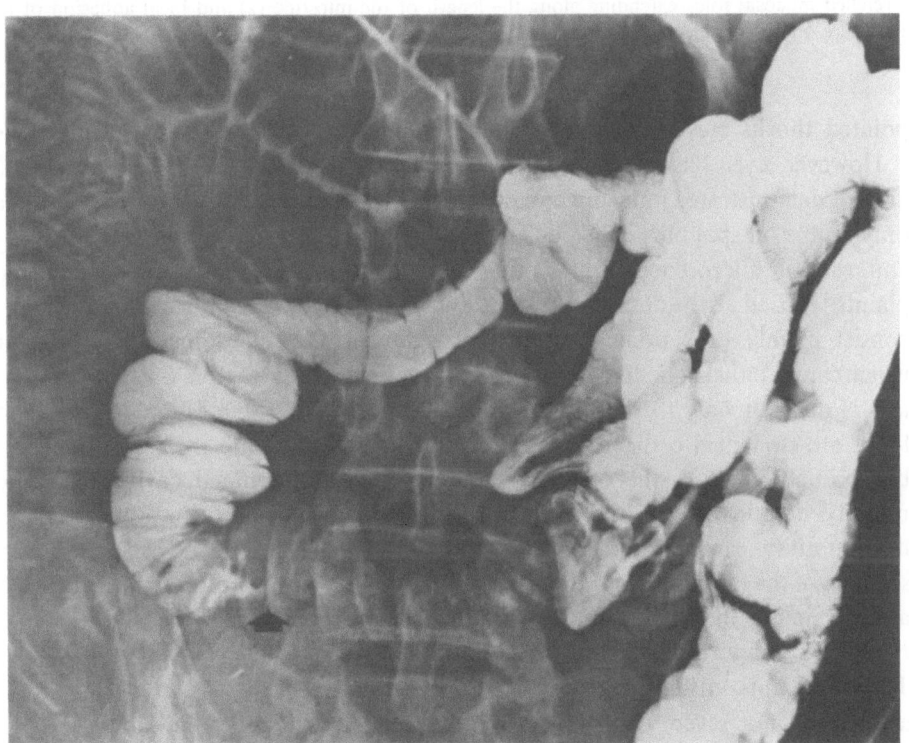

2. Fusion — Bands

Bands are almost never demonstrated by a radiological examination. In accordance with this fact and probably also as a result, guidelines for the identification of bands cannot be found in textbooks of roentgenology.

Bands are often multiple; they can develop after surgical intervention although other causes are certainly also possible. Small bands between adjacent loops can be considered more or less as very local adhesions; then the x-rays often reveal highly elongated mucosal folds locally which extend parallel to the length of the intestine (fig. 14.6). In other cases the band causes highly characteristic pointed bulges on the intestine. These bulges can be large and single (fig. 14.7) or small and multiple, in which case they generally appear as several

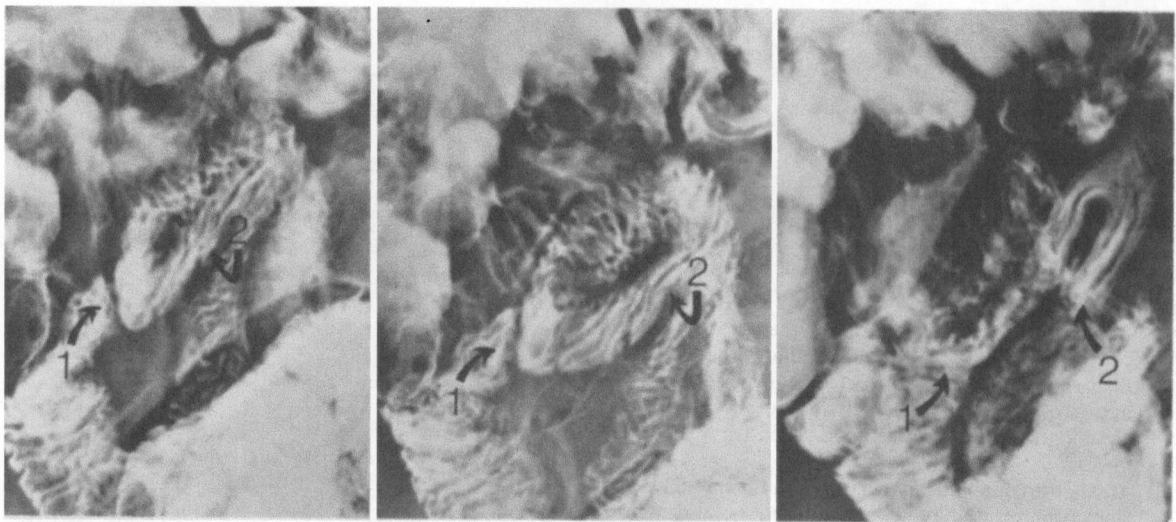

Fig. 14.6
Stretched mucosal folds extending along the length of the intestine (2) and local adhesion of two intestinal loops (1). (See elsewhere on this page).

pointed thorns clustered close together (fig. 14.8).

However, even these easily recognized adhesions are not demonstrated immediately; they are usually only visible on spot films taken during compression and careful fluoroscopic examination. The complaints caused by adhesion, fusion and bands consist mainly of periodic pain in the abdomen which can be either colic-like or sharp and thrusting; this is due not only to the fact that the intestinal loops are elongated or have sharp kinks (fig. 14.9) but probably also to the often quite pronounced motility frequently visualized (fig. 14.10). This hypermotility can encompass a large or a small segment of the intestine; it is often most pronounced after a copious meal and presumably develops as a result of a temporary anoxia in some of the loops. The complaints arising from adhesions and fusion are usually not severe enough to require surgery; they do, however, increase gradually in the course of time.

The patients suffer more from the long bands which cross several intestinal loops. Sometimes these bands may already be visualized on the abdominal survey films as long thin ribbon-like clarifications which extend straight across the abdomen. Bands are highly constricting and, in contrast to adhesions, quickly give rise to complaints of obstruction. In intestinal loops filled with contrast fluid the bands are easily identified by the indentations which they cause in the intestinal lumen (fig. 14.11). These indentations may be only on one side or may extend across one or more intestinal loops, depending upon whether the loop is in the center or at the periphery of the abdominal cavity and also on the course of the band with respect to the direction of the beam.

As will be clear the diverse symptoms described above often appear in combination. In figures 14.6, 14.7 and 14.8 these symptoms are numbered as indicated below.

1. local adhesion of two loops
2. highly elongated mucosal folds extending along the length of the intestine
3. pointed bulge due to local adhesion
4. several small thorn-like bulges due to local adhesion of the intestinal wall to the surroundings
5. indentation of the intestinal loop by a band

Fig. 14.7
Pointed bulges on elongated intestinal loops (3) due to fusion. Also visible are several indentations (5) as well as slight elongation of the somewhat thorn-like spaces between mucosal folds (4)

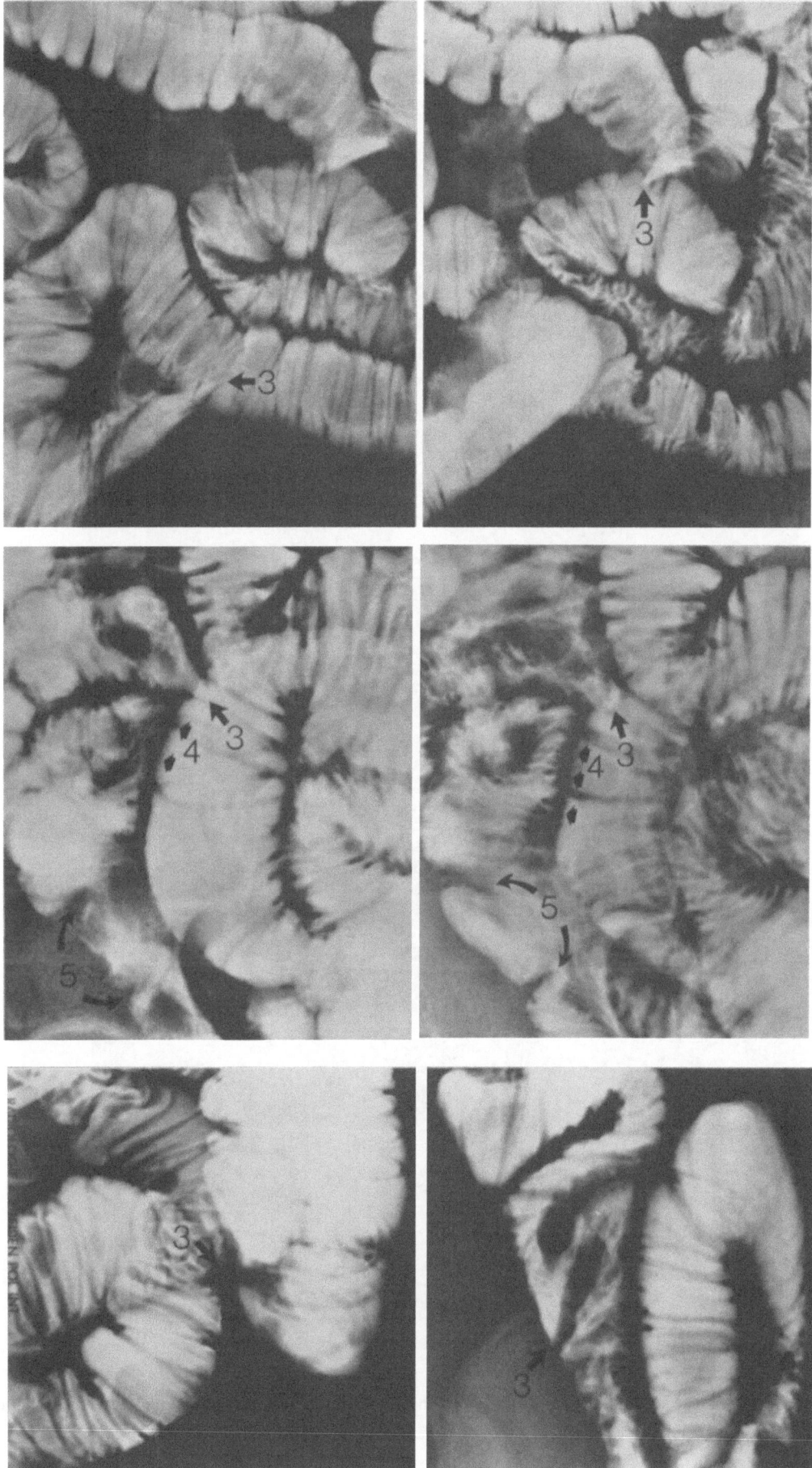

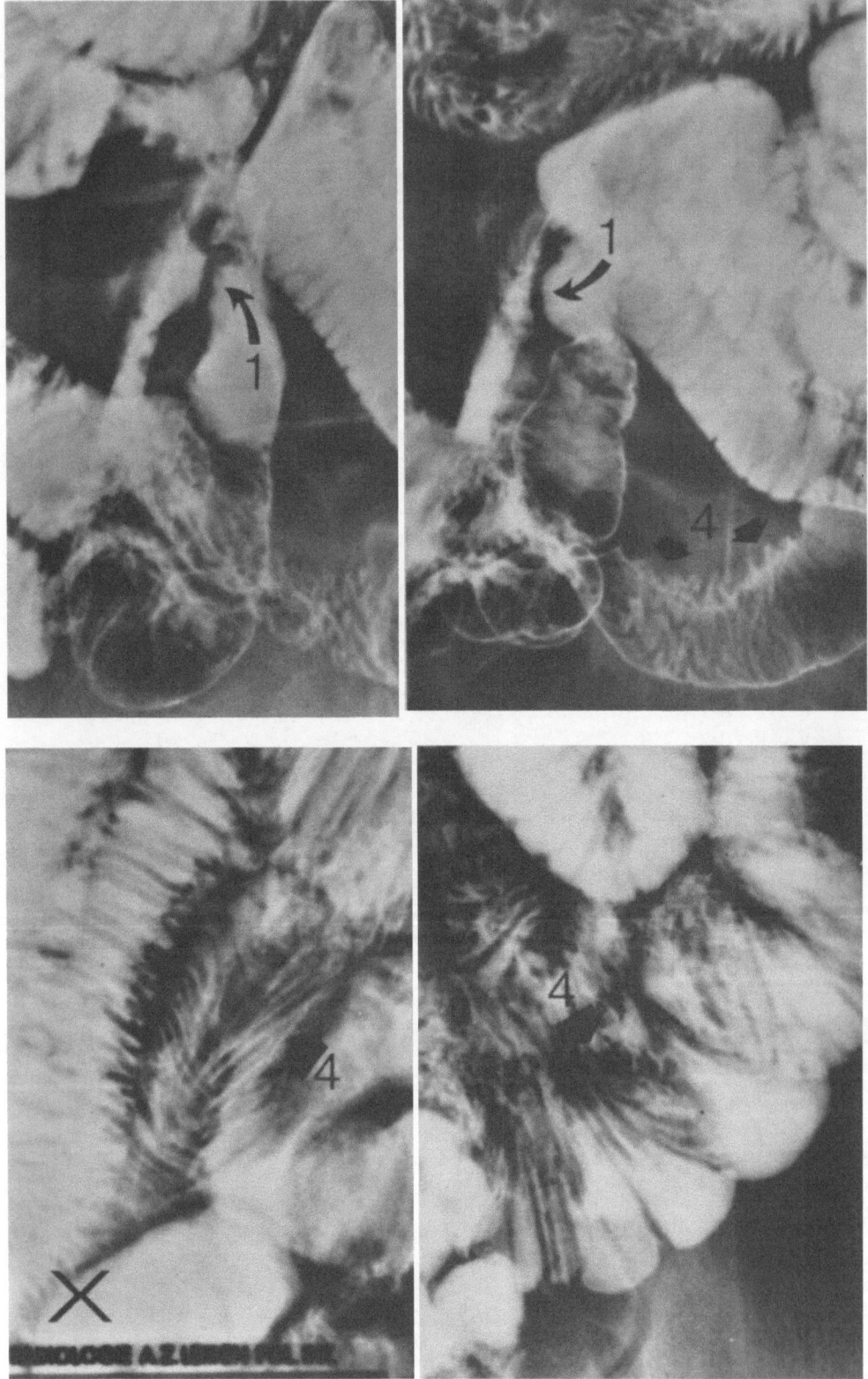

Fig. 14.8

x.   Pointed elongated mucosal folds due to local fusion of the intestinal wall with the surroundings (4); local adhesion of two
     loops (1).

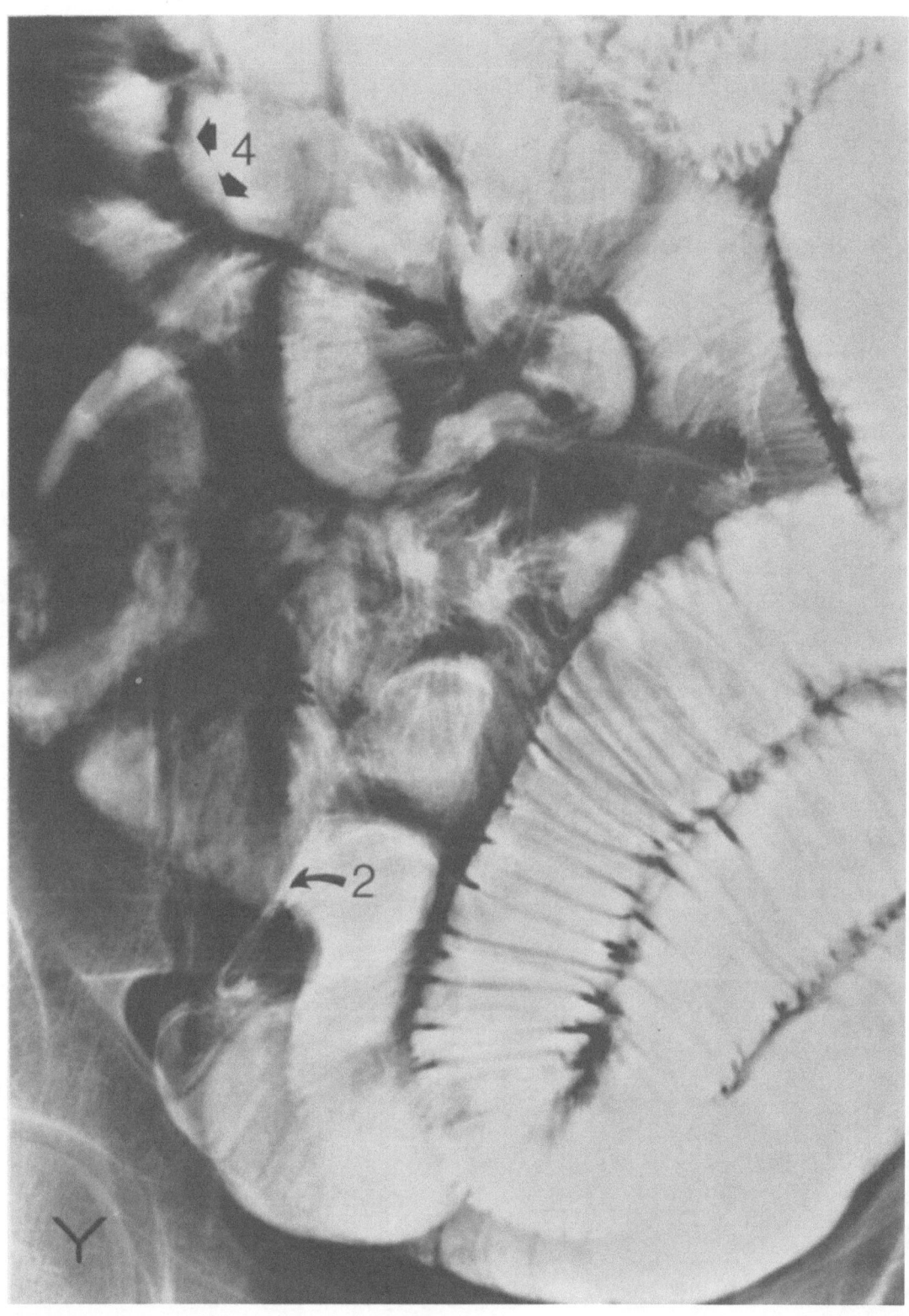

Y. Mucosal folds elongated in the lengthwise direction (2) in a patient with complaints of ileus. Extensive fusion throughout entire left half of the abdomen. (For an explanation of the numbers, see page 356).

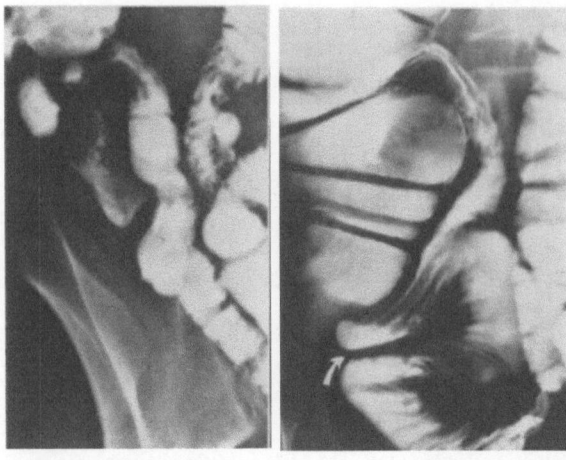

Fig. 14.9
Periodic colic-like abdominal pains which developed only
during the day were possibly due to the kink in the distal
ileum which is fused with the lowest pole of the cecum. Transit
would be impeded at this point when the patient stands erect
and the cecum is well-filled (right).

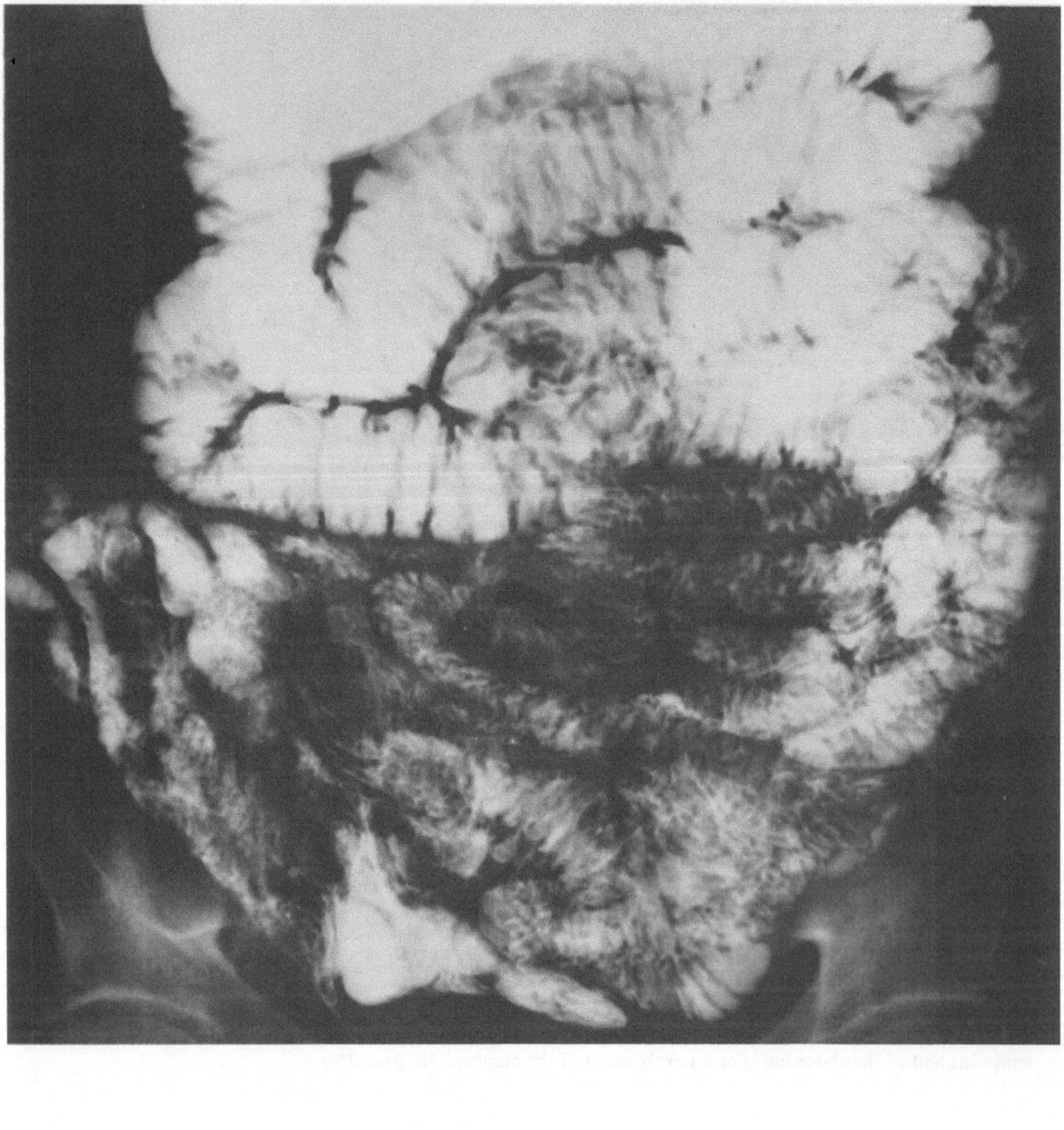

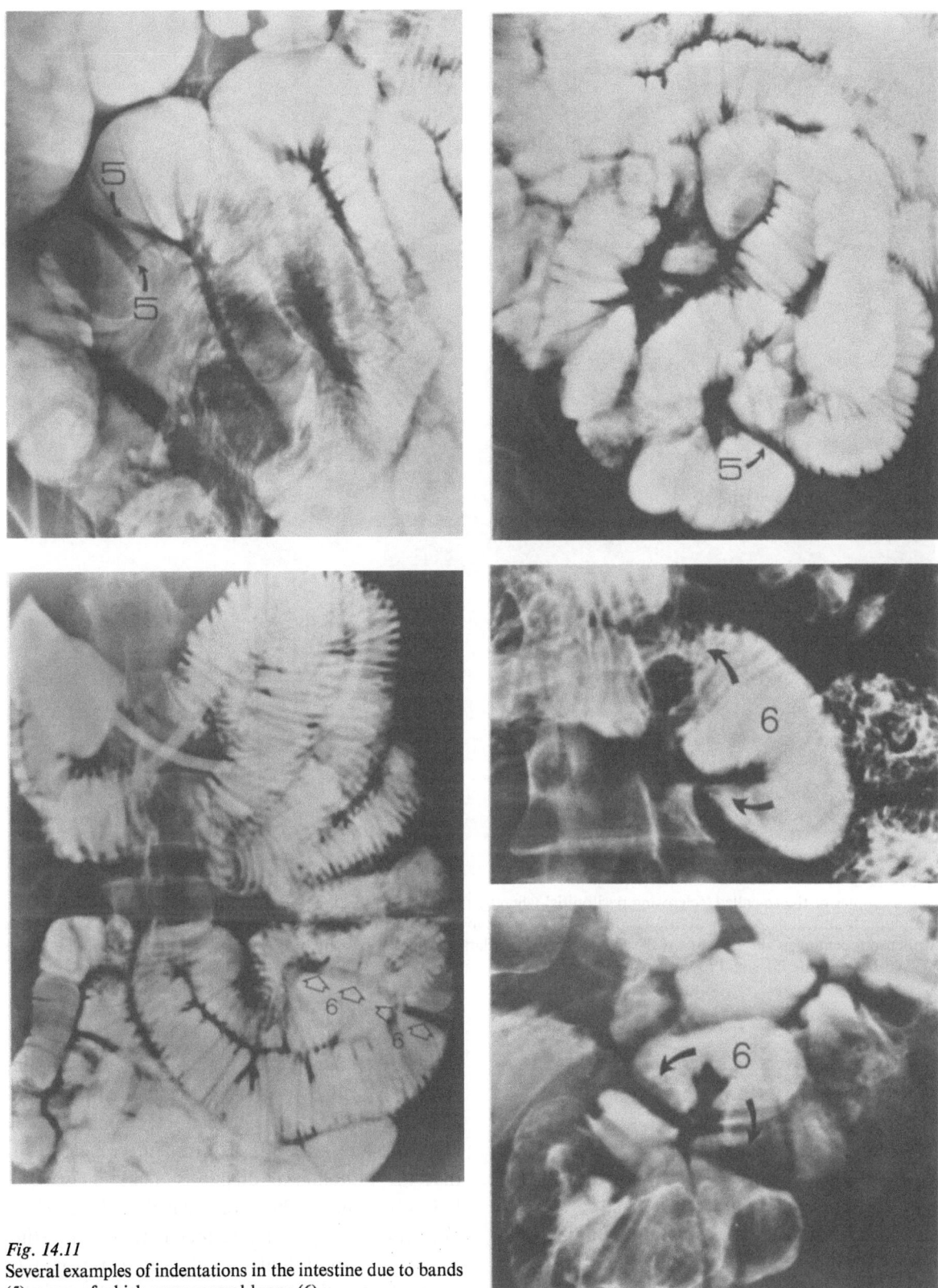

Fig. 14.11
Several examples of indentations in the intestine due to bands
(5), some of which cross several loops (6).

Fig. 14.10
Hypermotility of the intestine due to extensive adhesions. Jejunal loops are rather dilated because passage is somewhat impeded.

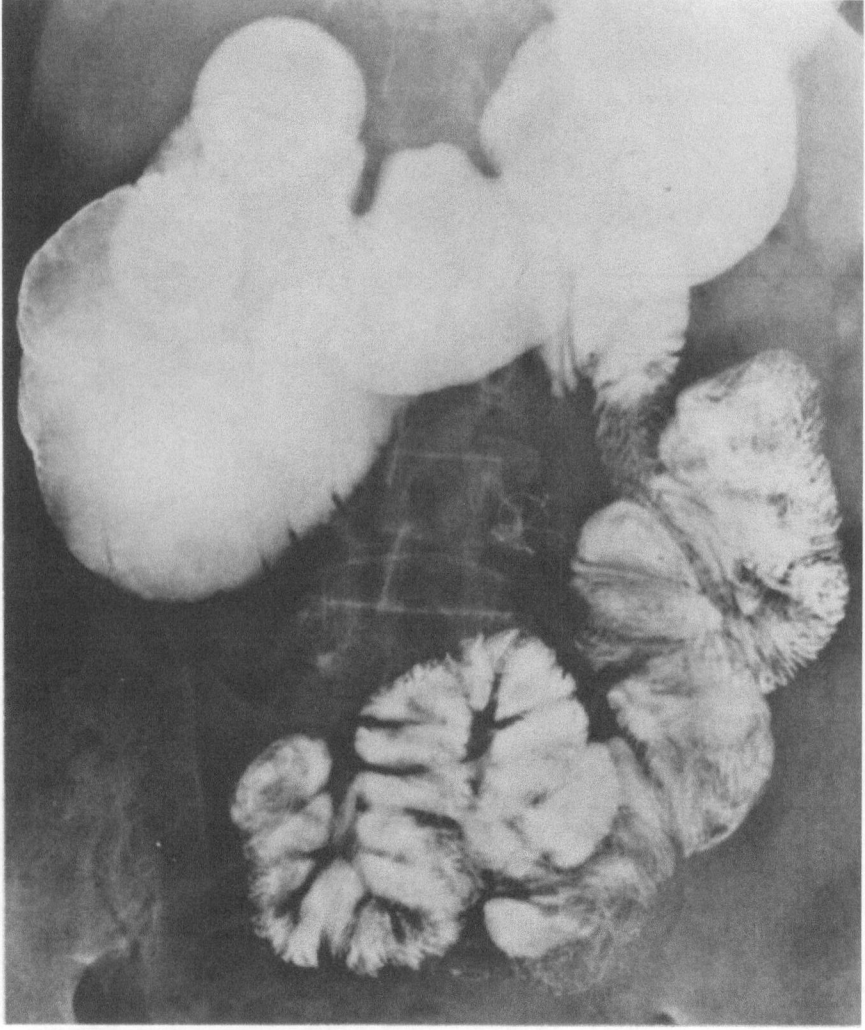

Fig. 14.12
Two examples of the so-called 'sclerosing peritonitis' whereby the mass of intestinal loops becomes more or less wedged in a continuously shriveling peritoneal sac. The intestineal loops show multiple indentations like those seen in fig. 14.11. Markedly swollen duodenum in the patient on the left; only slight dilatation in the patient to the right. The normal ileus pattern is masked because the intestinal loops are not able to dilate.

6. long band traversing several intestinal loops
7. hypermotility

A disorder, which possibly is due to occlusion of small vessels and can cause skin conditions which suggest psoriasis or lupus erythematodes, is the recently described sclerosing peritonitis which results from medication with the beta adrenergic blocking drug Practolol. Both the visceral and the parietal peritoneum show a gradually increasing fibrous shriveling such that the entire mass of loops of the small intestine is caught as it were in a strong net, thus being forced to assume an increasingly central position in the abdominal cavity. Although transit can be seriously impeded, the intestinal loops are not able to dilate which means that the radiological diagnosis 'ileus' is masked. It has been noted, however, that these loops show numerous widely scattered indentations suggesting bands or abrupt kinks so that it is possible to establish the diagnosis – if the possibility of this disorder is at least considered (fig. 14.12).

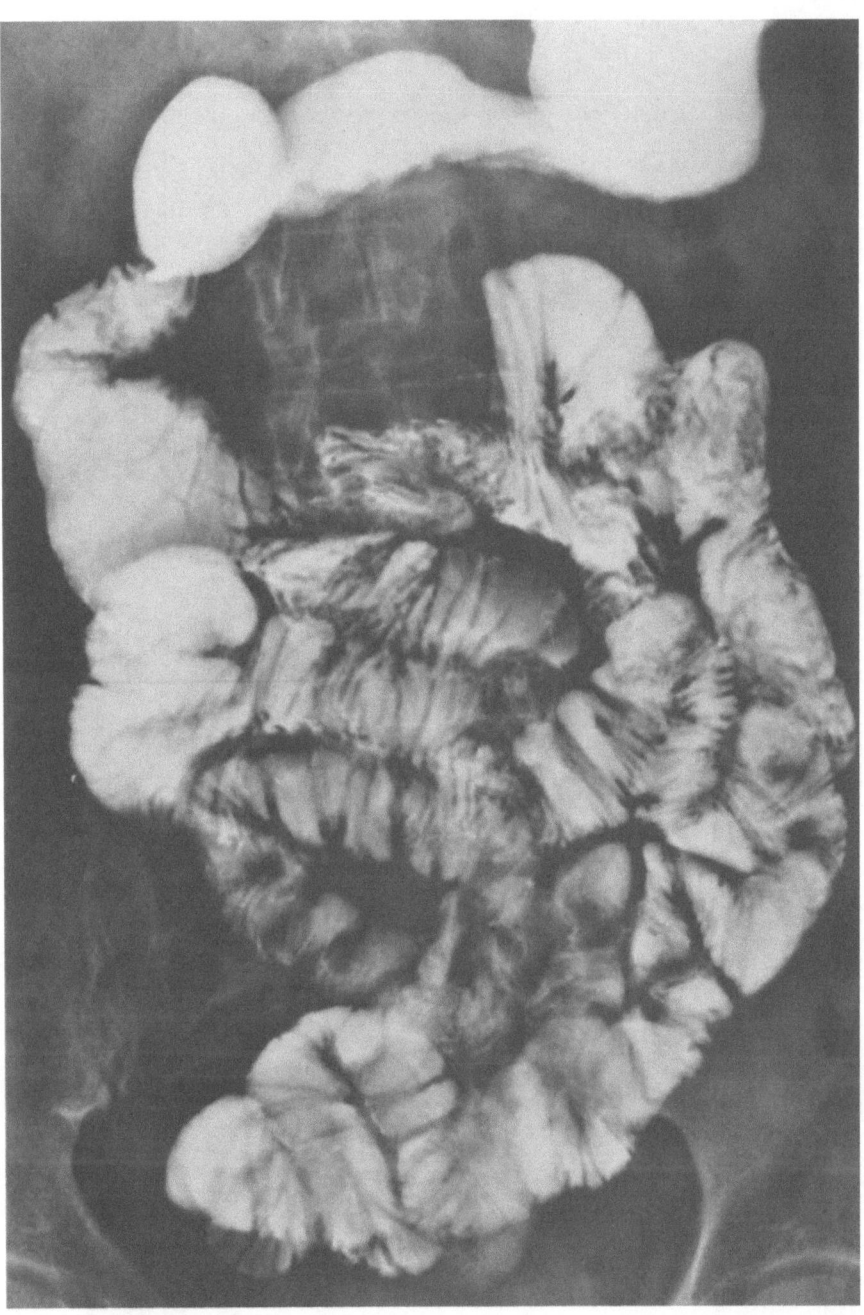

Fig. 14.12

3. Volvulus

Because of their constricting nature, bands sometimes cause a volvulus of the intestine. On the
roentgenogram the point of torsion of the volvulus
can often be identified by concentric rings of mucosal folds in the dilated intestinal loop which decrease
in size towards the center (fig. 14.13).

Volvulus of a mass of intestinal loops can be
caused by a particularly long mesentery or when
fixation of the mesentery to the posterior abdominal
wall is too short or inadequate. A good example
of the latter is shown in fig. 14.14; it can be seen
that the mass of intestinal loops changes position
very easily and as a result can cause intermittent
complaints. When, in a patient with unexplained

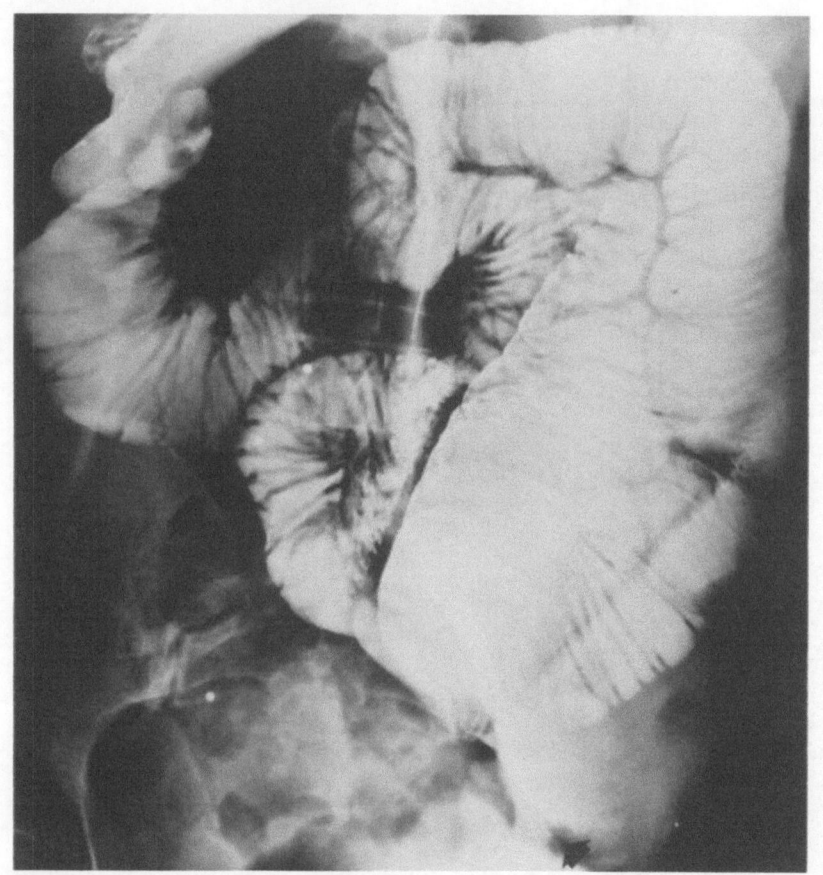

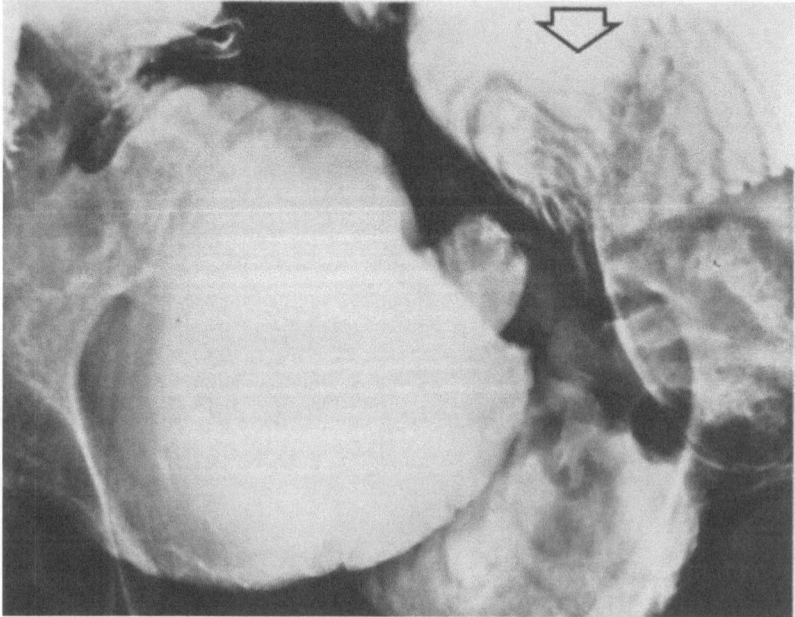

Fig. 14.13
Almost total obstruction of the small intestine because a band which runs from the upper right to the lower left quadrant (→ ←) in a patient with a 'short bowel' (Crohn's disease) contricted one loop completely and another quite markedly thus causing a volvulus. Survey film after administration of 1200 ml contrast fluid. Subsequently the site of obstruction was approached from the distal direction by filling of the colon. The point of torsion can be recognized on this roentgenogram by the mucosal folds which lie as concentric rings (→)

colic-like abdominal pain, a positional anomaly is demonstrated the possibility of a volvulus should always be considered (fig. 14.15). Often in volvulus the circulation is greatly disturbed in the involved intestinal segment; there can be signs of mucosal swelling due to elevated venous pressure as well as hyperperistalsis due to anoxia of the intestine (fig. 14.16).

4. Intussusceptions

Although it is known that small intestinal intussusceptions are not often recognized, it is interesting to note from the literature that this diagnosis is also often based on insufficient evidence. This also corroborates the statement sometimes made, but not really obvious, that intussusception in the small bowel can occur without causing symptoms and may be found accidentally.

An intussusception is seldom demonstrated, in spite of the more active peristalsis during an enteroclysis examination. A filling defect or clarification in the contrast column will be observed more readily with the enteroclysis examination than with conventional methods whereby generally less than 500 cc contrast medium is administered at a much lower rate of flow. In celiac disease in particular the intestinal loops are often dilated and the minute volume of the propulsive peristalsis may be greater than the stomach is able to pass on through the pylorus to the intestine; then large filling defects, sometimes due to air, may be seen in the contrast column which must be carefully differentiated from an intussusception. Because there are usually large quantities of fluid in the intestine in celiac

disease, the barium suspension very often flocculates during a conventional examination. Under these conditions, barium streamers may become visible in the center of the intestinal lumen where the rate of flow of the fluid is the greatest; these streamers may suggest an intussusception (fig. 14.17). As mentioned previously, x-rays should not be used for diagnosis if the intestinal loops are inadequately filled or if signs of flocculation are detected.

The roentgen pattern of an intussusception is complete if an otherwise well-filled intestinal loop shows a distalwards portio-like well-defined clarification with a barium streamer in the middle. In the intestinal loops containing the intussusception (the so-called intussuscipiens), the mucosal folds are pressed flat against the wall and are therefore not or barely visible (figs. 14.18 and 14.19 м). Understandably circulation in the intussuscipiens will be severely disturbed leading to marked mucosal edema, especially if the intussusception has existed for some time. The trio of phenomena which indicate the diagnosis of 'intussusception' (portio-like configuration; central barium streamers; visualization of a double intestinal wall) is, however, certainly not always (and in fact is usually not) complete so that unfortunately one must be satisfied with less. If the abnormality is but temporary and occurs only once so that the surgical indication is no longer present, confirmation of the radiolgical diagnosis, however probable it may be, is not always available (fig. 14.20).

In adults, an intussusception is almost always caused by a polyp or tumor of the intestinal mucosa; it is therefore found most frequently near the ileocecal junction where these abnormalities commonly occur (fig. 14.21).

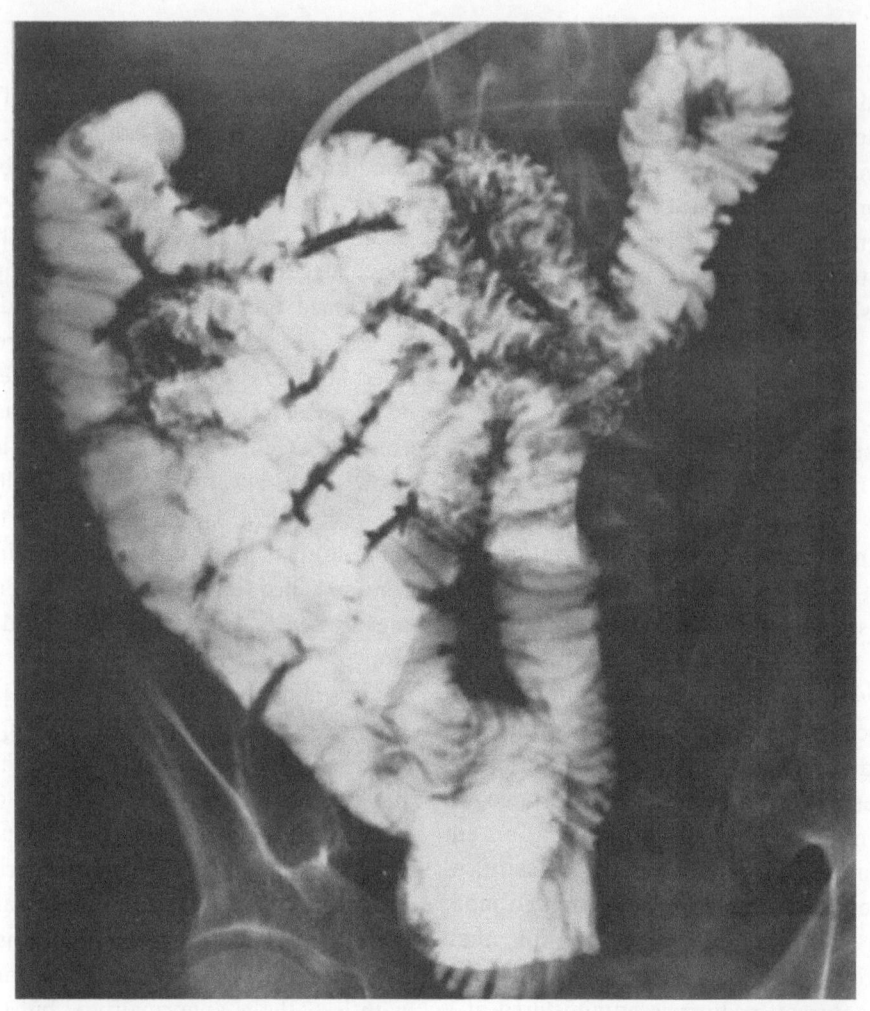

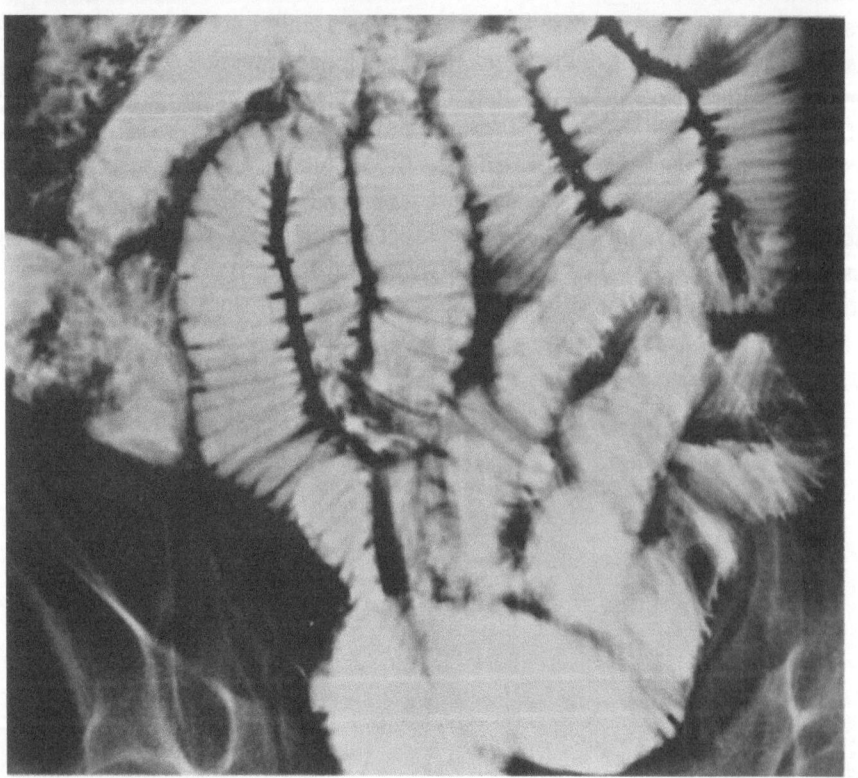

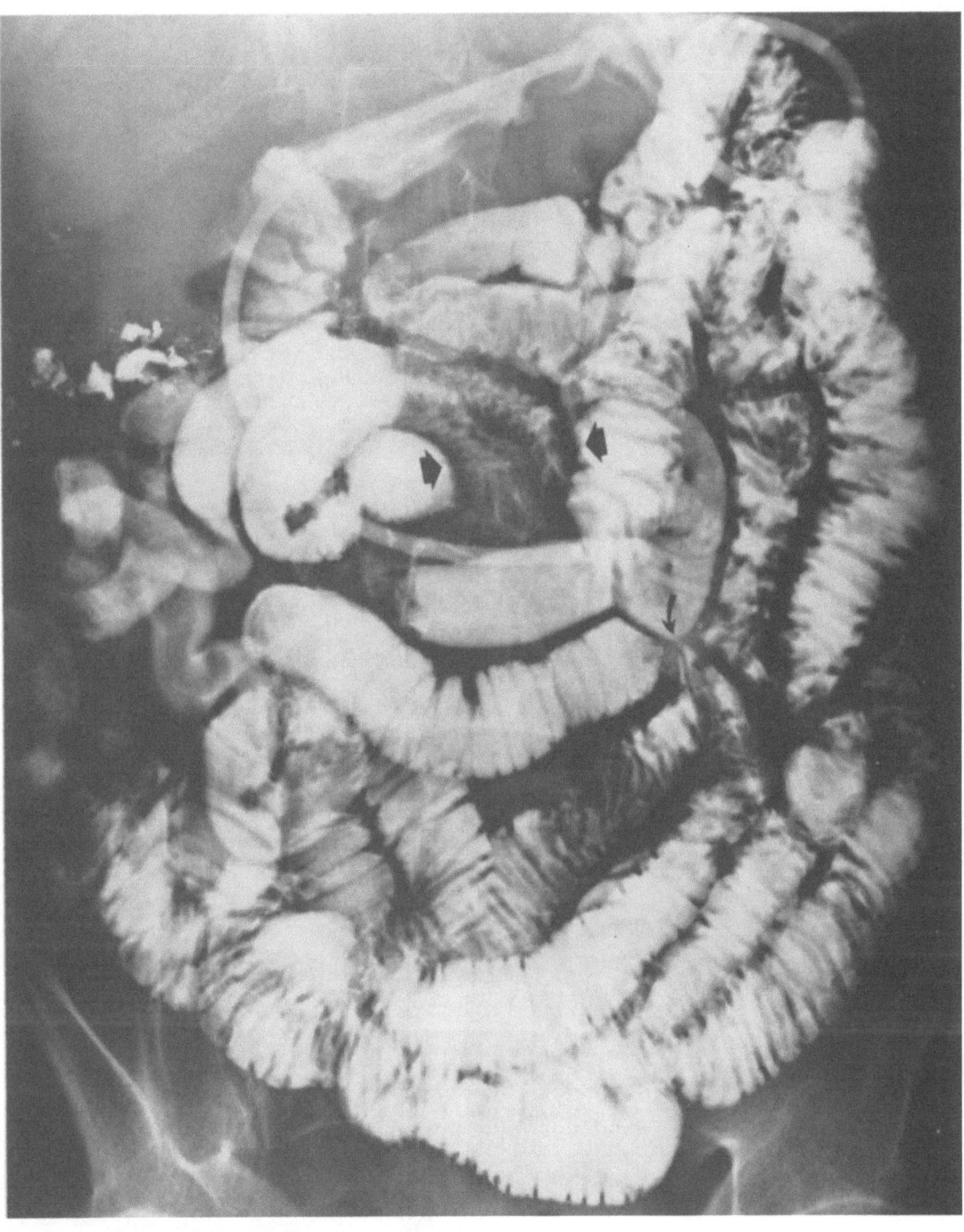

Fig. 14.14
Volvulus of the small intestine because the attachment of the mesentery was too short. The attack could be provoked by having the patient bend over as far as possible. The jejunum is in the upper right quadrant, the ileum in the lower left. The moderately dilated ileal loops show multiple indentations and the mucosal folds are stretched perpendicular to the axis of the intestine (left page). During periods without complaints the jejunum lies in the lower left quadrant and the ileum in the upper right. The mass of intestinal loops is therefore rotated through a 45° angle with respect to the normal position. To the left of the navel is an elongated intestinal loop with a pointed bulge (←) probably caused by a band. Local hypermotility with mucosal folds stretched in the perpendicular direction above the navel (→) (on right page).

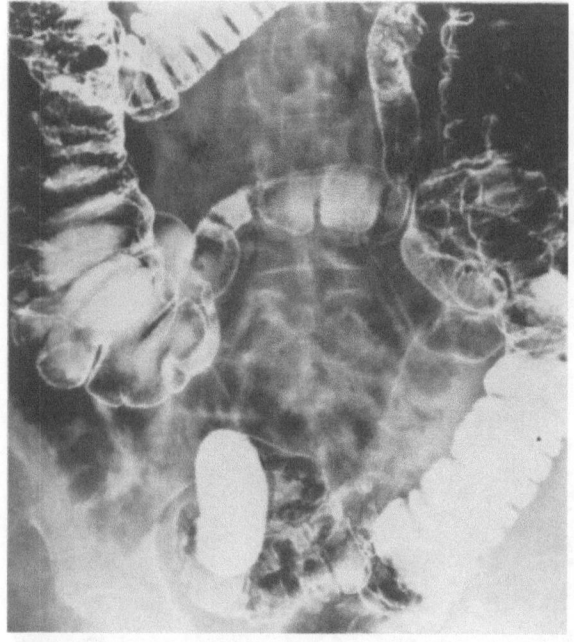

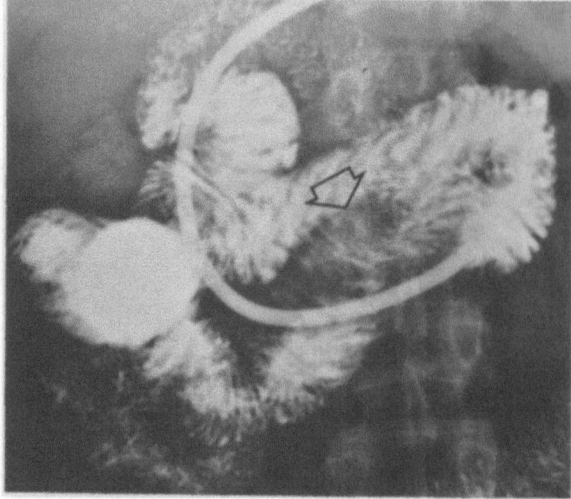

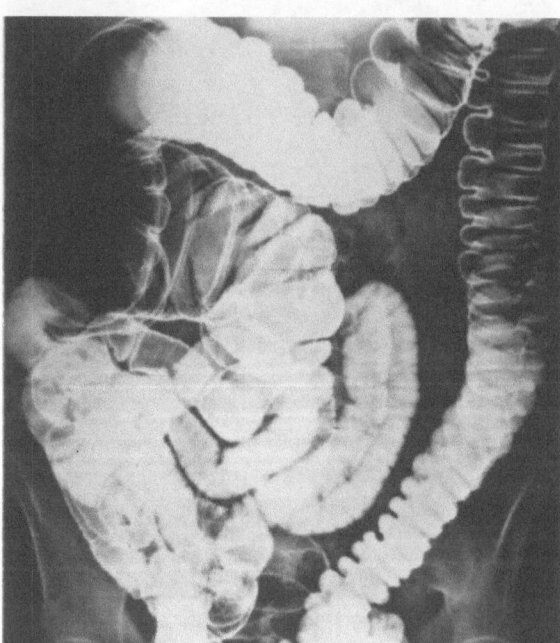

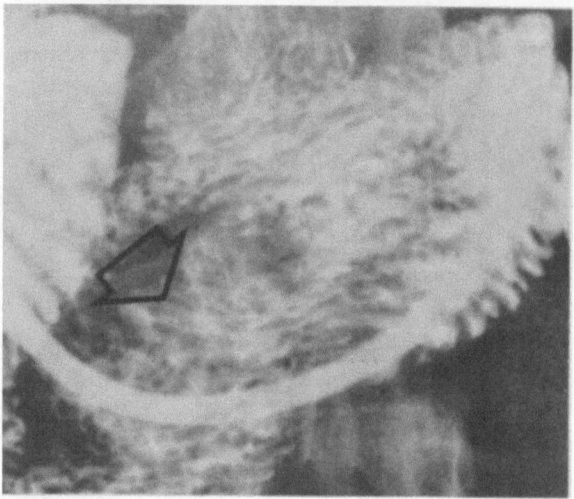

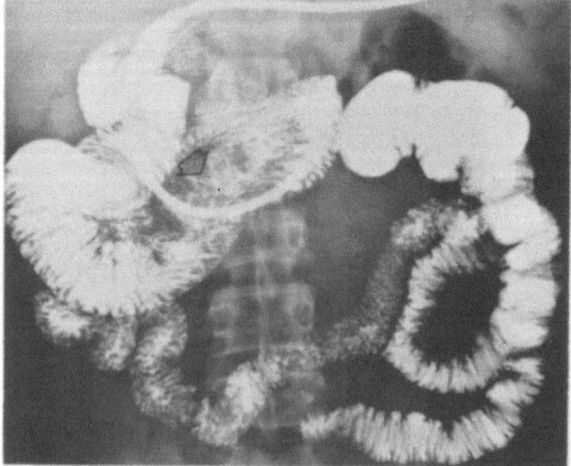

Fig. 14.15
Temporary moderately severe abdominal complaints connected with a change in the position of the distal half of the mass of ileal loops from the lover right (right) to the upper left (left) quadrant. Under all conditions the jejunum was to the left and in the center in the upper half of the abdomen and the proximal half of the ileum was in the middle in the lower abdomen. Probably this anomaly is due to the fact that part of the mesentery is too long.

Fig. 14.16
Intermittent moderately severe attacks of abdominal pain presumably connected with slight torsion of several proximal jejunal loops in the right upper quadrant. Locally there was quite strong hypermotility (→) so that it was not possible to visualize this segment of the intestine in a well-filled state.

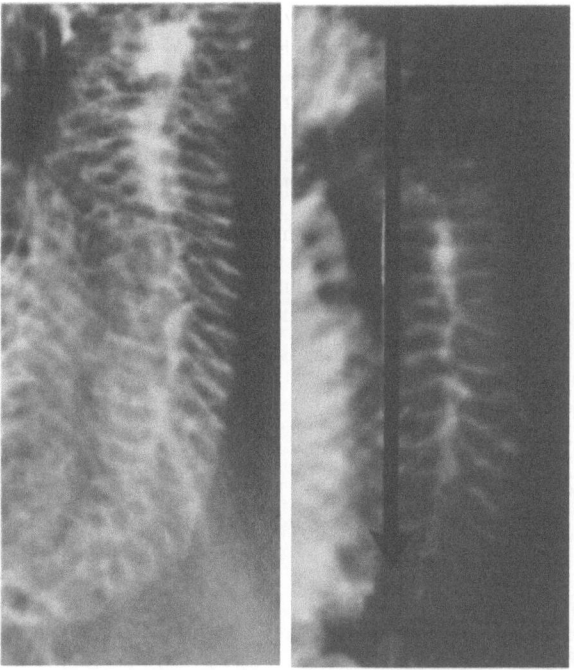

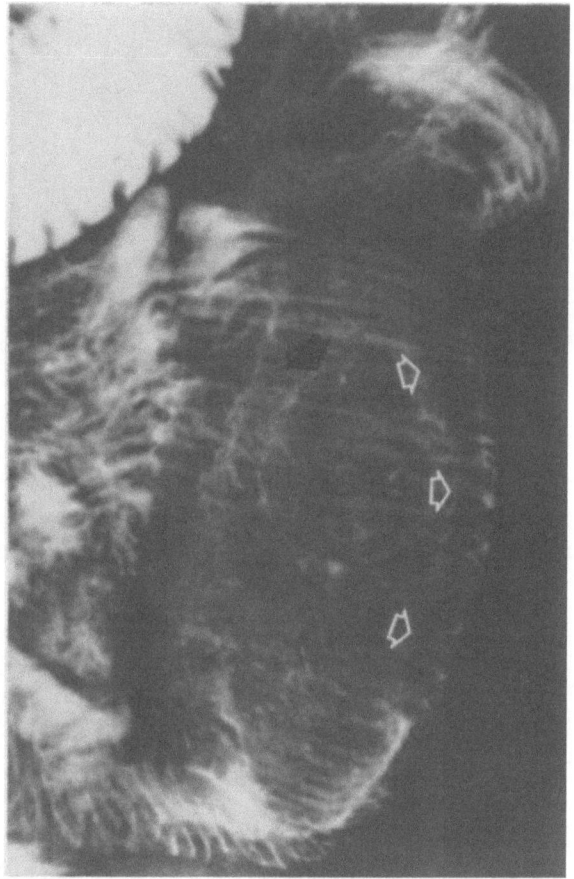

Fig. 14.17
Two barium streamers in the middle of an intestinal loop as
seen in cases of hypermotility. This misleading pattern suggesting an intussusception can develop in particular when
the lumen of the intestine is greatly dilated and disintegration
of the contrast fluid has occurred (as in some cases of celiac
disease).

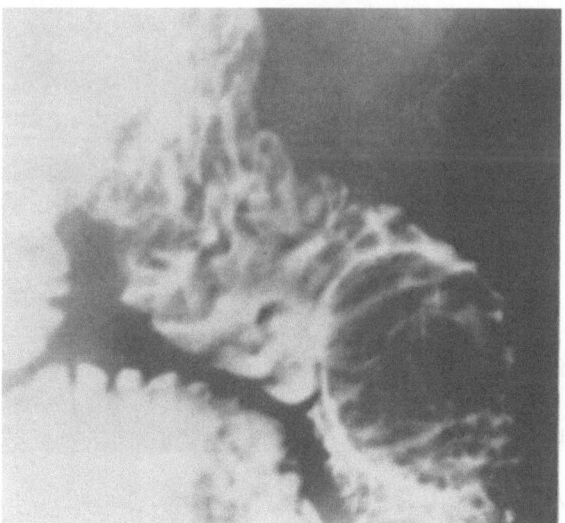

Fig. 14.18
Intussusception of jejunum into jejunum, caused by a lipoma
±2 cm in diameter (lower); the latter can be seen in the intussuscipiens ($\rightarrow \leftarrow$). The mucosal surface of the intussuscipiens is also just visible ($\uparrow\uparrow\uparrow$) about 0.5 cm inside the wall
of the enclosing intestinal loop.

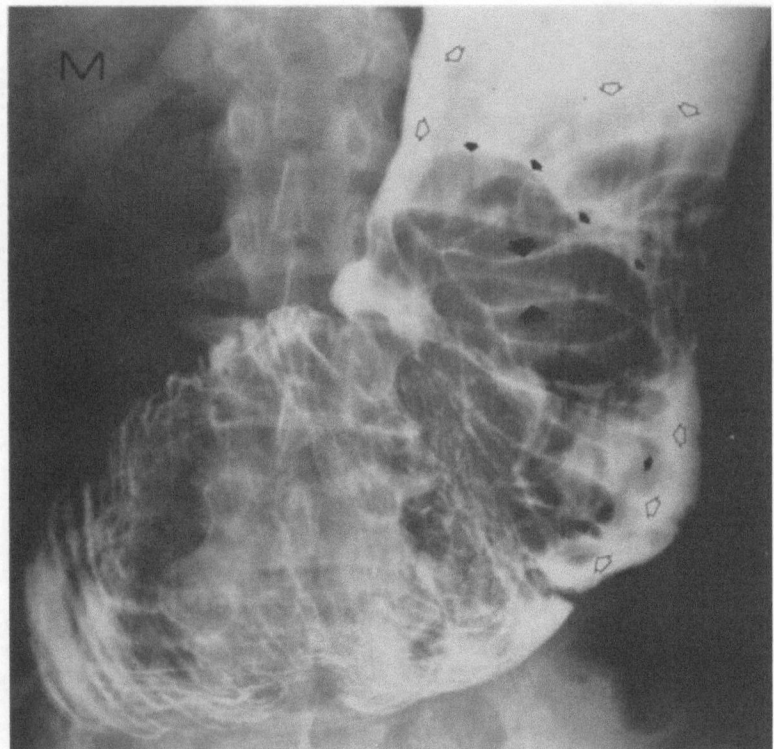

Fig. 14.19

M. Highly swollen mucosal folds
(→←) in a large intussuscipiens
after a BII gastrectomy. There was
a very complicated intussusception
consisting of that of the afferent
loop into the efferent loop and then
the retrograde intussusception of
both into the residual stomach. The
wall of the intussuscipiens is clearly
visible next to the inner wall of the
stomach.

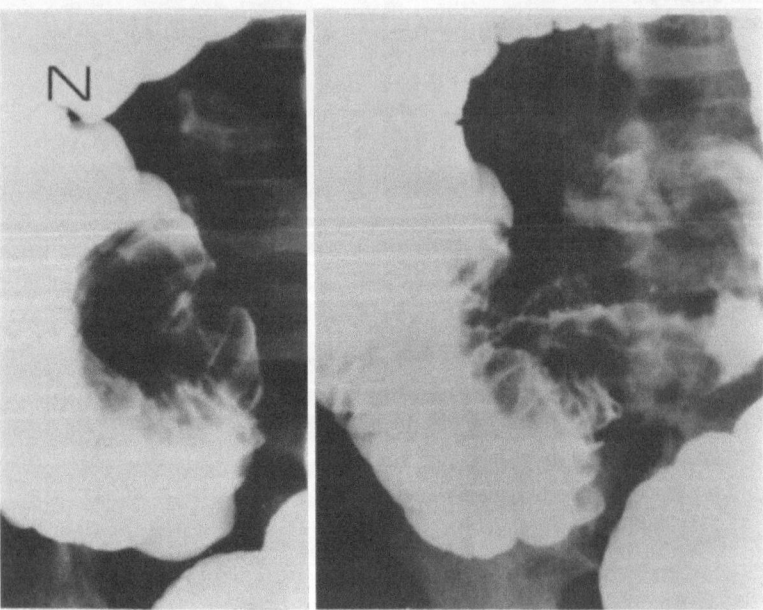

Fig. 14.19

N. Edematous swelling of the mucosa in the distal ileum and
Bauhin's valve immediately after reduction of an intussusception (of several days duration) which extended to the
left flexure of colon. Since the complaints were only
moderately severe, it was decided to try a conservative
reduction in spite of the prolonged duration of the
intussusception.

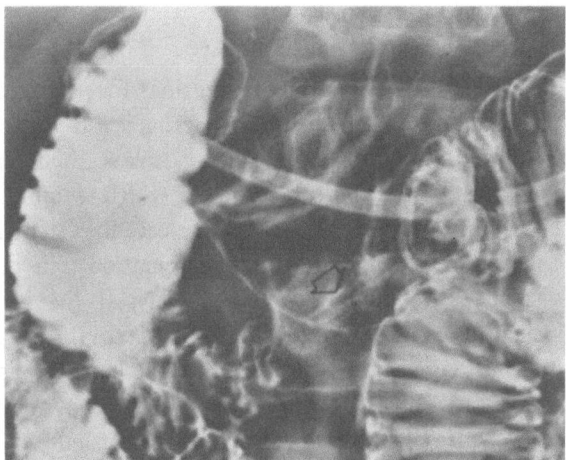

Fig. 14.20
Temporary subileus phenomenon. The examination taken after hypotonia was induced showed a streamer of contrast medium ±5 cm long in the distal duodenum which started abruptly and ended in a portio-like configuration. Since the complaints disappeared and abnormalities were no longer seen during a follow-up examination, surgical intervention was not required.

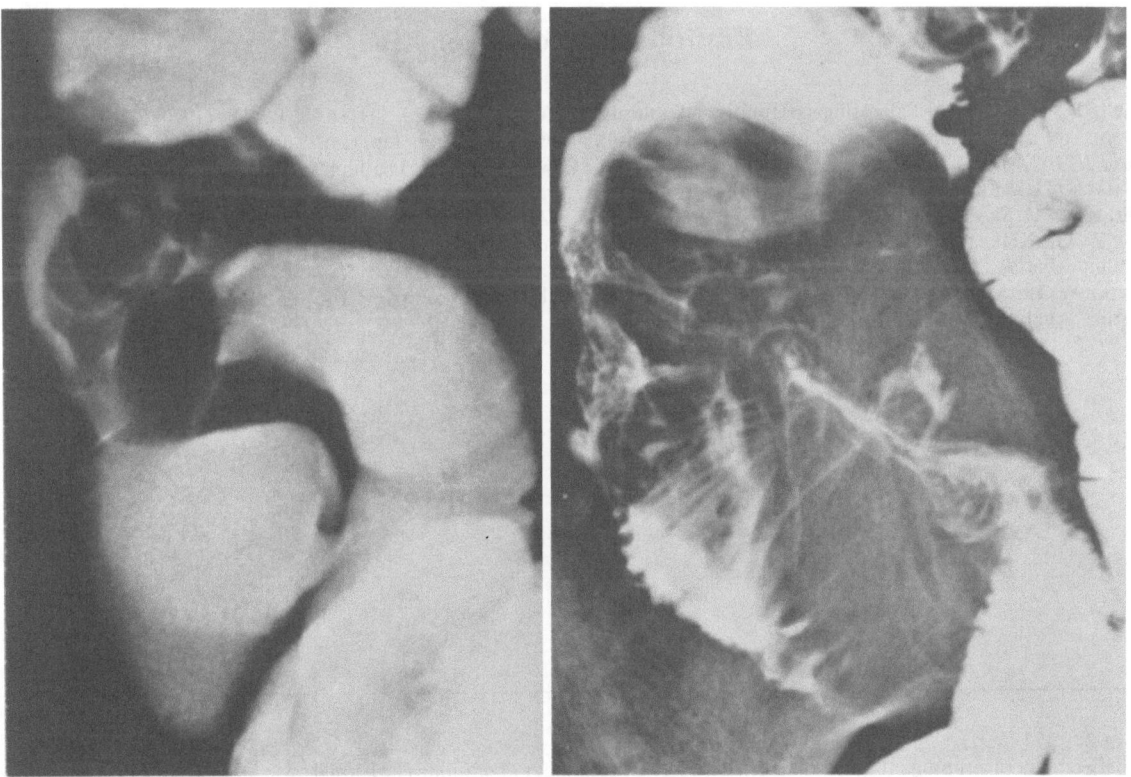

Fig. 14.21
Tumor in Bauhin's valve causing an intussusception in the cecum.

5. Incisional hernia

The presence of a mass of intestinal loops in an incisional or congenital inguinal hernia is a frequent finding. If the hernial opening is small, then an incarcerated hernia can develop which requires immediate surgery. It will be clear that when constriction occurs the venous circulation will be disturbed first and the most severely. If the obstruction of the venous flow is not total or is intermittent, then it is possible that the hematomas in the mucosa will not become so large that they cause acute obstruction. Moreover a transient and increasingly pronounced fibrosis during the recovery phase(s) can apparently prevent the development of necrosis. As discussed in Chapter X, after some time the results of a disturbance of the venous circulation can no longer be differentiated radio- logically from those of a disturbed arterial flow nor from Crohn's disease or a condition after radio- therapy.

A good example of an obstruction of the venous flow (in the rest phase) which proceeded so gradu- ally that the history was in fact 'clean' is seen in fig. 14.22. There is a large hernial sac which devel- oped in the incision of a previous kidney operation. The patient could in fact only report that the hernial sac was much smaller in the beginning and that it was not until later that he could force the intestinal loops in the sac back through the hernial opening into the abdominal cavity. It is interesting that the very rigid and stiff intestinal loops were easily palpable through the thin flabby wall of the hernial sac and that it could be established that the most lateral loops were fused with the wall of the hernial sac.

Bibliography chapter XIV

BROWN P.; et al. (1974) Sclerosing peritonitis, an unusual reaction to a beta-adrenergic-blocking drug (Practolol). *Lancet II*, 1477–1481.

DONHAUSER J. L.; KELLY R. C. (1950) Intussusception in the adult. *Amer. J. Surg. 79*, 673.

KERR W. G.; KIRKALDY-WILLIS W. H. (1946) Volvulus of the small intestine. *Br. med. J.* i, 799.

MORETZ W. H.; MORTON J. J. (1950) Acute volvulus of small intestine. Analysis of 36 cases. *Ann. Surg. 132*, 899.

RICCABONO X. J.; HASKINS R. M. (1970) Gastroduodenal intussusception: report of 2 cases. *Gastroenterology 38*, 995.

SAIDI F. (1969) The high incidence of intestinal volvulus in Iran. *Gut 10*, 838.

TALBOT C. H. (1960) Volvulus of the small intestine in adults. *Gut 1*, 76.

See also the nrs. 63–152–164–165–211–226 and 236 of the bibliography on pages 164 and following.

Fig. 14.22

A, B Lateral hernia through the abdominal wall after previous kidney operation. The hernial sac contains part of the ascending colon and a mass of jejunal loops which show the results of a disturbed venous flow. The abnormalities, consisting of multiple longitudinal ulcerations, asymmetric and circular shriveling, a markedly thickened intestinal wall and frequent spasms cannot be differentiated from those due to Crohn's disease or radiation enteritis.

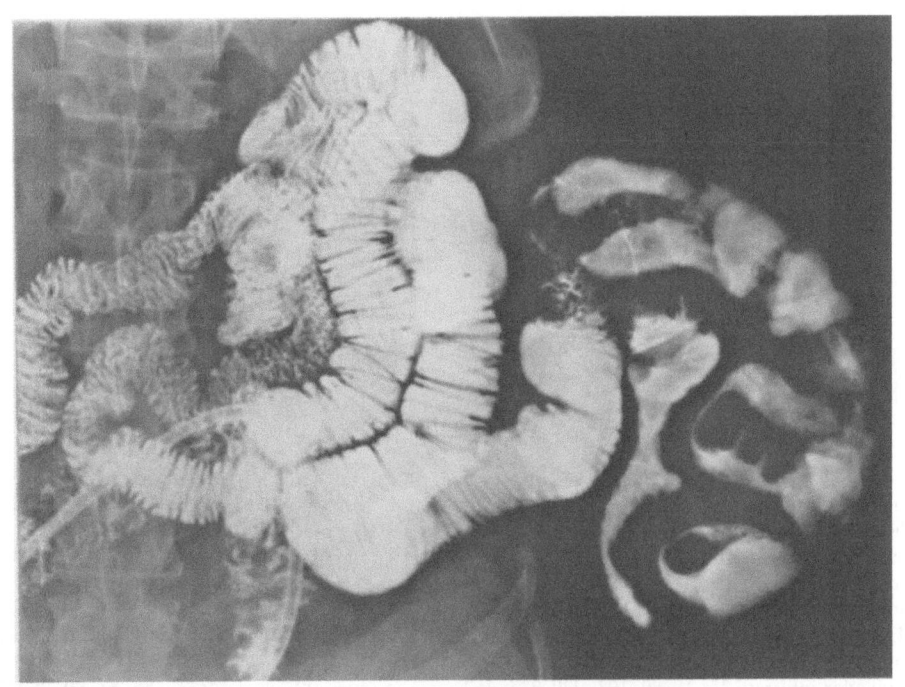

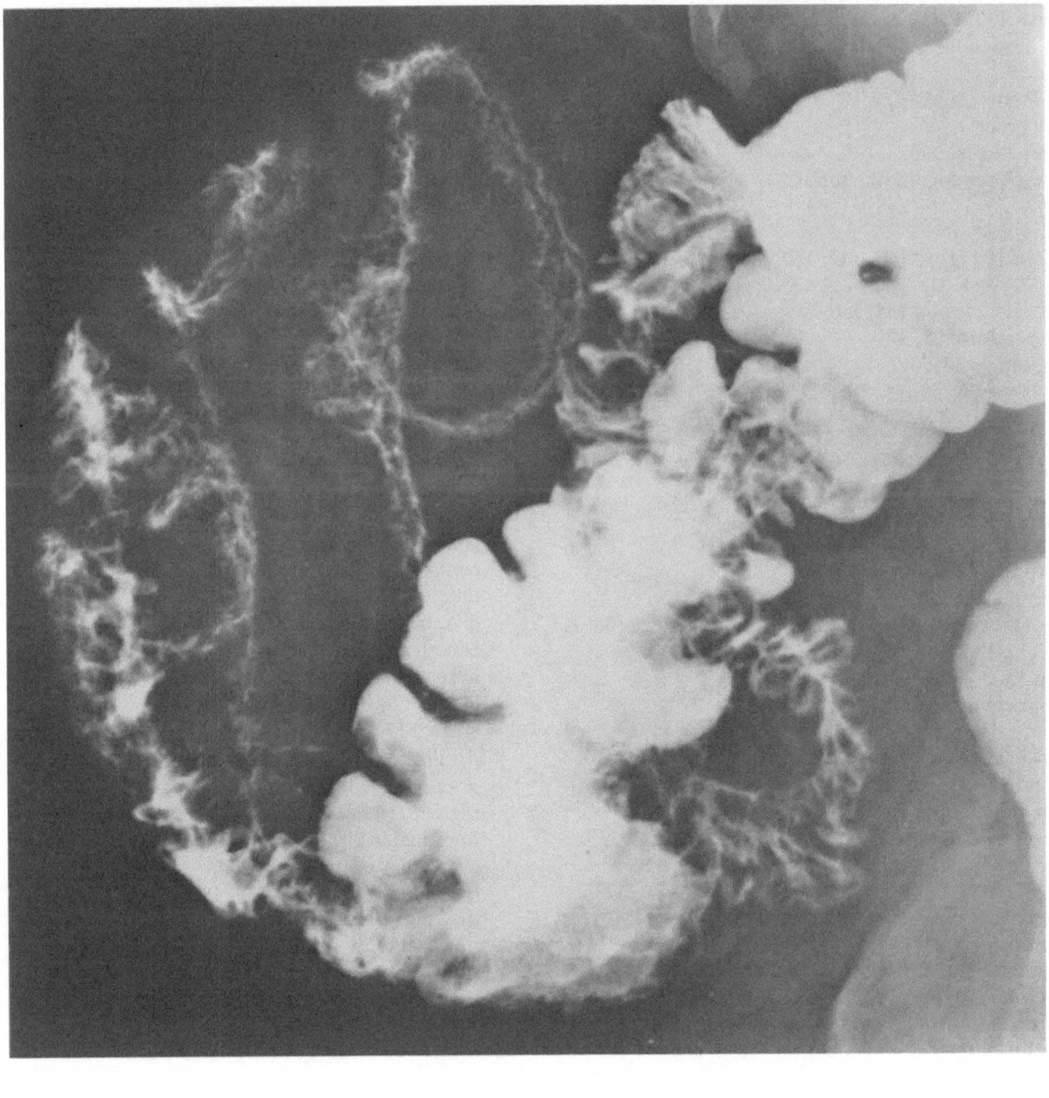

INDEX